Viruses, Cell Transformation and Cancer

PERSPECTIVES IN MEDICAL VIROLOGY

Volume 5

Series Editors

A.J. Zuckerman

Royal Free Hospital School of Medicine
University of London
London, UK

I.K. Mushahwar

Abbott Laboratories
Viral Discovery Group
North Chicago, IL, USA

Viruses, Cell Transformation and Cancer

Editor

R.J.A. Grand

CRC Institute for Cancer Studies
University of Birmingham
Edgbaston
Birmingham B15 2TT
UK

2001

ELSEVIER

Amsterdam – London – New York – Oxford – Paris – Shannon – Tokyo

ELSEVIER SCIENCE B.V.
Sara Burgerhartstraat 25
P.O. Box 211, 1000 AE Amsterdam, The Netherlands

First edition 2001

Library of Congress Cataloging in Publication Data
A catalog record from the Library of Congress has been applied for.

ISBN: 0-444-50496-6
ISSN: 0168-7069

⊖ The paper used in this publication meets the requirements of ANSI/NISO Z39.48-1992 (Permanence of Paper).
Printed in The Netherlands.

CONTENTS

INTRODUCTION...1
  Roger J.A. Grand

IMMORTALIZATION OF PRIMARY RODENT CELLS BY SV40 7
  Alison J. Darmon and Parmjit S. Jat

ADENOVIRUS EARLY REGION 1 PROTEINS: ACTION THROUGH INTERACTION.................43
  Roger J.A. Grand

POLYOMA VIRUS MIDDLE T-ANTIGEN: GROWTH FACTOR RECEPTOR MIMIC 85
  Philippa R. Nicholson and Stephen M. Dilworth

PATHOBIOLOGY OF HUMAN PAPILLOMAVIRUSES...129
  Margaret A. Stanley

THE FUNCTION OF THE HUMAN PAPILLOMAVIRUS ONCOGENES...................................145
  David Pim, Miranda Thomas and Lawrence Banks

HEPATITIS B VIRUS IN EXPERIMENTAL CARCINOGENESIS STUDIES 193
  Stephan Schaefer

EPSTEIN-BARR VIRUS AND ONCOGENESIS: FROM TUMORS TO TRANSFORMING GENES ...229
  Lawrence S.Young

HUMAN HERPESVIRUS-8 253
  Ruth F. Jarrett

HUMAN HERPESVIRUS-8: DYSREGULATION OF CELL GROWTH AND APOPTOSIS.............291
  Frank Neipel and Edgar Meinl

HUMAN T-CELL LEUKEMIA VIRUS TYPE I ONCOPROTEIN, TAX: CELL CYCLE
DYSREGULATION AND CELLULAR TRANSFORMATION 309
  Kenneth G. Low and Kuan-Teh Jeang

PROVIRAL TAGGING: A STRATEGY USING RETROVIRUSES TO IDENTIFY ONCOGENES......321
  Tarik Möröy, Martin Zörnig and Thorsten Schmidt

THE INDUCTION AND SUPPRESSION OF APOPTOSIS BY VIRUSES 351
  Ester M. Hammond and Roger J.A. Grand

EVASION OF THE IMMUNE SYSTEM BY TUMOR VIRUSES 413
  Nicola Philpott and Eric Blair

IMMUNITY TO HUMAN PAPILLOMAVIRUSES: IMPLICATIONS FOR VACCINE DESIGN 451
  Jane C. Steele

ADENOVIRUS CANCER GENE THERAPY 479
  Martin B. Powell and Gavin W. G. Wilkinson

LIST OF ADDRESSES 523

INTRODUCTION

Roger J.A. Grand

It is now firmly established that carcinogenesis is a multistage process that is the result of several causative events. Most commonly, many of these events result from genetic lesions attributable to environmental factors. The net result is a loss of growth control leading to the unregulated proliferation characteristic of the cancer cell. The identity of the majority of the environmental agents which cause the genetic mutations remains unknown although a few, such as tobacco smoke and ultra-violet radiation are now very familiar. Important cancer-causing environmental factors which do not induce mutation are tumor viruses. Their relevance to cancer in the context of this book is two-fold – firstly they induce tumors in the infected host and, secondly, they provide important models for studying neoplastic transformation as they transform cells in tissue culture and can also induce tumors in experimental animals.

Whilst viruses are not in general a major cause of cancer, it has recently been suggested that 10.3% of human cancers world-wide are attributable to viral infection. This was equivalent to about 835,000 cases in 1990 (Parkin et al., 1999). An additional 400,000 cancers are probably due to infection with non-viral agents such as *Helicobacter pylori*. Not surprisingly, a greater proportion of cancers arise from infection in developing countries (22.5% compared to 6.8% in developed countries [Parkin et al., 1999]). The viruses responsible for most of these cases are human papillomavirus (HPV), which is considered to be involved in about 90% of cervical cancers, Epstein-Barr virus (EBV) which has been linked to Burkitt's lymphoma, non-Hodgkin's lymphoma, Hodgkin's disease and nasopharyngeal carcinoma and Hepatitis B and C viruses (HBV and HCV) which are responsible for around half of the cases of liver cancer world-wide. In addition, HIV-infected individuals become susceptible to cancers due to further infection with other viruses such as human herpes virus 8 (HHV8) and EBV.

The realization that cancers can be linked to "infectious agents" is not recent. Leukemias and sarcomas in chickens were demonstrated to be transmissable in the first decade of this century (Ellerman and Bang, 1908; Rous, 1911). Similary, a predisposition to tumors of the breast in C3H mice was shown to be passed from mothers to offspring through milk (Bittner, 1936). A predisposition to lymphomas was also found to be due to viral infection (Gross, 1957). Since that time these cancers in mice have been attributed to infection with mouse mammary tumor virus (MMTV) and mouse leukemia virus (MLV) respectively. In the 1930s cancers were also shown to be caused by DNA viruses (although of course the difference was not realized at the time); for example, skin cancers were induced in cotton tail rabbits by infection by pox virus and papilloma virus (Shope, 1932; Shope and Hurst, 1933).

The study of DNA tumor viruses over the past fifty years has added greatly to our knowledge of how viruses cause tumors in mammals and, perhaps more significantly, has helped to identify some of the genes/proteins involved in non-virally induced tumorigenesis. It should be noted, however, that many of the most commonly studied

DNA tumor viruses such as Simian virus 40 (SV40), adenovirus, polyoma virus and BK and JC viruses are all considered to be non-oncogenic in humans although they can cause tumors in rodents. All of these, together with HPV, have small genomes, and this, taken in conjunction with the fact that the viral DNA can generally be used to transform cells in tissue culture has facilitated their study. Furthermore, it has become apparent that expression of only a small number of the viral genes is necessary for transformation or for oncogenesis. Studies using the small DNA tumor viruses have greatly enhanced our understanding of cell transformation and over the past twenty years it has become apparent that cellular proteins targeted by the DNA viruses are, in many cases, the products of genes mutated in human cancers. The most obvious examples of this are p53 and Rb. p53 was originally identified as a protein which formed a complex with SV40 T antigen (Lane and Crawford, 1979; Linzer and Levine, 1979) and was soon demonstrated to be a ubiquitous cellular component, which was often over-expressed and mutated in transformed cell lines and in tumor cells. It has now been confirmed as the most commonly mutated gene in human cancers (Levine et al., 1991) with about 60-65% of tumors expressing mutant p53 (Greenblatt et al., 1994). The retinoblastoma gene product pRb is also a target for the DNA tumor viruses and like p53 is mutated in an appreciable proportion of human cancers (Friend et al., 1986; Lee et al., 1988; Whyte et al., 1988; De Caprio et al., 1988).

Whilst our knowledge of how the small DNA viruses transform cells has increased greatly over the past two decades much less progress has been made with most of the viruses responsible for the majority of virally-induced human cancers. Thus, we understand reasonably well how the HPV E6 and E7 genes transform cells in culture and it is presumed that the same biochemical events play role in the early stages of cervical carcinoma. However, our understanding of the mechanism by which those viruses, other than HPV, initiate tumor development is rather more sketchy. Hepatitis B virus (HBV) is an important causative agent for an appreciable proportion of hepatocellular carcinomas (HCC) in Africa and Asia. Interestingly, infected individuals who are also exposed to aflatoxin have an appreciably increased incidence of the disease. This highlights a role for a particular virus as a co-carcinogen in conjunction with an environmental factor. Although the HBV genome is small (3kb) there is still considerable controversy over the mechanism by which the cancers arise. It has been suggested that chronic HBV infection can lead to inflammation and liver injury, followed by recurrent cellular regeneration. If genetic damage has been caused (for example, by chemical carcinogens) hepatocarcinomas could result. Perhaps more relevantly from the point of view of the theme of this book there is considerable evidence to suggest that the HBV HBx protein can play a role in hepatocarcinogenesis possibly by binding to p53, activating kinase pathways and increasing transcription. The activities of HBx are discussed in detail in Chapter 7 of this volume. In addition, it is possible that HBV surface antigens can act as oncogenic proteins and that integration of viral DNA into the host genome could play a role in transformation.

The situation with EBV is much more complex in that the viral genome is large (around 180kb) and encodes a number of proteins which may be involved in transformation and the production of tumors. In addition, EBV has been linked to several different cancers in both epithelial and lymphoid tissue – for example Burkitt's and other lymphomas, nasopharyngeal carcinoma (NPC), and Hodgkin's disease. Two viral proteins, EBV nuclear antigen 2 (EBNA2) and latent membrane protein 1 (LMP1) are essential for in vitro transformation of B cells but others also play a part. Furthermore, LMP1 is expressed in a number of EBV-associated tumors. The roles of the EBV proteins are considered in detail in Chapter 8 of this volume.

Human herpes virus 8 (HHV8) is a recent addition to the list of viruses which can cause tumors in humans and is now thought to be largely responsible for Karposi's sarcoma (KS) and primary effusion lymphoma (PEL). Of course, these are primarily a problem in immunosuppressed individuals but with increasing prevalence of HIV infection, particularly in Africa and Asia, the incidence of cancers attributable to HHV8 infection is likely to increase greatly in the near future. HHV8 (also known as Karposis's sarcoma-associated herpes virus [KSHV]) is a member of the γ-herpes virus subfamily and has a large genome (around 170kb) with in excess of 80 open reading frames. The fact that the virus was only identified a few years ago and the complexity of the genomic organisation has meant that our knowledge of its mode of action, both in transformation and tumorigenesis, is relatively limited. However, a detailed discussion of evidence linking HHV8 and KS and lymphoproliferative disease is presented in Chapter 9, together with a summary of the current knowledge of the properties of a number of virally-encoded proteins. The role of putative transforming proteins such as K1, K9, K12 and the K cyclin are presented in Chapters 9 and 10 as well as discussion of viral proteins (vFLIP and Bcl-2 homologues) which may inhibit apoptosis in the infected cell.

Retroviruses have been of immense assistance in helping us to understand the mechanisms of cellular transformation and the functions of a large number of important cellular proteins (the proto-oncogenes) such as Ras and Myc which function in the regulation of various aspects of cell growth. Whilst retroviruses can be tumorigenic in animals (for example, Rous sarcoma virus in chickens and Abelson leukaemia virus in mice) they appear to be directly responsible for few cancers in humans. However, human T-lymphotropic virus type I (HTLVI) is the causative agent of adult T cell leukaemia/lymphoma, whilst HTLVII probably causes hairy cell leukaemia. The number of cancers caused by HTLVI infection, worldwide, is relatively small (about 2600 in 1990) but as they are clustered in particular areas, giving a high prevalence in, for example, the southern tip of Japan, southern Gabon, northern Zaire and parts of the Caribbean they can pose a serious but geographically limited, health problem. The transforming protein of HTLVI is Tax which serves as a transcriptional activator. The activities of Tax with particular emphasis placed on its relationship to the cell cycle are described in Chapter 11.

Although few cancers in humans are directly caused by retroviruses it must be remembered that at the end of the twentieth century HIV is the infectious agent responsible for more deaths than any other. HIV does not appear to have a direct oncogenic capability but, by incapacitating the immune system, it is able to facilitate the development of cancers caused by other agents (e.g. KS and non-Hodgkin's lymphoma). Of course, many of the deaths due to AIDS are not a result of cancers but of opportunistic infections by non-cancer causing organisms. Despite the importance of HIV infection as a contributory cause of cancers it was considered that a detailed description of the properties of the virus was beyond the scope of this book. Similarly, the large number of animal retroviruses which have been so important in the elucidation of the mode of action of retroviral oncogenes have been ignored. This has been a somewhat arbitrary decision based more on limitation of space than lack of relevance. Whilst retroviruses such as avian erythroblastosis virus, avian myclecytomatosis virus-29 and Harvey sarcoma virus do not infect humans their study has highlighted the importance of cellular proto-oncogenes (in the case of those viruses *erbB, myc* and *H-ras* respectively). Furthermore, it is now well-known that either changes in protein expression due to chromosomal translocation (e.g. Myc and ErbB) or expression of an aberrant protein with an altered activity (e.g. H-ras) following mutation are of particular importance in the aetiology of some human cancers. In the examples mentioned it has been shown that *erbB* is amplified in tumors such as glioblastomas and squamous cell carcinomas, *myc* is amplified and over-expressed in, amongst others, tumors of the breast, lung and colon, as well as leukemias, whilst mutant *ras* is expressed in acute myeloid leukemias, colon and lung carcinomas. The subject of proto-oncogenes is so large and complex that if requires treatment in greater detail than could be justified in this book. Reluctantly, therefore discussion of proto-oncogenes has been omitted.

Within this volume the themes which I have very briefly touched upon here have been considered in detail. Although the DNA tumor viruses, with the notable exception of HPV, pose virtually no threat to humans, they have been discussed in considerable detail in Chapters 2, 3 and 4. I feel that this can be justified by their scientific importance in that results from the study of SV40, Ad and HPV have provided much of our basic knowledge of the mechanism of cell transformation. Those organisms which are the major causes the virally-induced cancers - HPV, HBV, EBV and the relatively recently discovered HHV8 - are dealt with in detail in the central portion of the book.

Retroviruses and their use in the search for novel oncogenes are discussed in Chapters 11 and 12 with emphasis placed on HTLV1 in the first of these. Towards the end of the volume more general themes are considered – in particular how viruses evade the host's immune system and how they either cause or limit an apoptotic response by the infected host. Finally, the possibilities of using viruses as therapeutic agents against human cancers have been discussed.

I believe that the broad-range of subjects covered will give a relatively up-to-date and fairly concise description of a very large body of scientific research. As the authors have concentrated on these aspects of the subject which they find of particular interest, it is hoped that their enthusiasm and knowledge will make this an illuminating and instructive account of a subject of relevance to scientists and clinicians, students and experienced researchers alike.

Finally, I should like to express my gratitude to all of the contributors and, in particular, to Nicola Waldron at the Institute for Cancer Studies, University of Birmingham for tireless endeavour in preparing this volume for publication.

References

Bittner, J.J. (1936) Some possible effects of nursing on the mammary gland tumor incidence in mice. Science 84, 162.

DeCaprio, J.A., Ludlow, J.W., Figge, J., Shew, J.Y., Huang, C.M., Lee, W.H., Marsilio, E., Paucha, E. and Livingston, D.M. (1988) SV40 large tumor antigen forms a specific complex with the product of the retinoblastoma susceptibility gene. Cell 54, 275-283.

Ellerman, V. and Bang, O. (1908) Experimentelle Leukemie bei Huhnern. Zentralbl Bakteriol Alet 46, 595-597.

Friend, S.H., Bernards, R., Rogelj, S., Weinberg, R.A., Rapaport, J.M., Albert, D.M. and Dryja, T.P. (1986). A human DNA segment with properties of the gene that predisposes to retinoblastoma and osteosarcoma. Nature 323, 643-646.

Greenblatt, M.S., Bennett, W.P., Holstein, M. and Harris, C.C. (1994) Mutations in the p53 tumor suppressor gene: clues to cancer etiology and molecular pathogenesis. Cancer Res. 54, 4855-4878.

Gross, L. (1957) Development and serial cell-free passage of a highly potent strain of mouse leukaemia virus. Proc. Soc. Exp. Biol. Med. 94, 767-771.

Lane, D.P. and Crawford, L.V. (1979) T antigen is bound to a host protein in SV40 transformed cells. Nature 278, 261-263.

Lee, E.Y., To, H., Shew, J.Y., Brookstein, R., Scully, P. and Lee, W.H. (1988) Inactivation of the retinoblastoma susceptibility gene in human breast cancers. Science 241, 218-221.

Levine, A.J., Momand, J. and Finlay, C.A. (1991) The p53 tumor suppressor gene. Nature 351, 453-456.

Linzer, D.I. and Levine, A.J. (1979) Characterization of a 54K dalton cellular antigen present in SV40-transformed cells and uninfected embryonal carcinoma cells. Cell 17, 43-52.

Parkin, D.M., Pisani, P., Munoz, N. and Ferlay, J. (1999) The global health burden of infection associated cancers. Cancer Surveys 33, 5-33.

Rous, P. (1911) A sarcoma of fowl transmissable by an agent separable from the tumor cells. J. Exp. Med. 13, 397-399.

Shope, R.E. (1932) A filtrable virus causing a tumor-like condition in rabbits and its relationship to virus myxomatosum. J. Exp. Med. 56, 803-822.

Shope, R.E. and Hurst, E.W. (1933) Infectious papillomatosis of rabbits. J. Exp. Med. 58, 607-623.

Whyte, P., Buchkovich, K.J., Horowitz, J.M., Friend, S.H., Raybuck, M., Weinberg, R.A. and Harlow, E. (1988) Association between an oncogene and an antioncogene: the adenovirus E1a proteins bind to the retinoblastoma gene product. Nature 334, 124-129.

IMMORTALIZATION OF PRIMARY RODENT CELLS BY SV40

Alison J. Darmon and Parmjit S. Jat

Ludwig Institute for Cancer Research, London

ABSTRACT

This review is predominantly concerned with the mechanisms by which simian virus 40 (SV40) induces immortalization of primary cells. Primary cells in culture have a finite mitotic life span, after which they undergo replicative senescence. Expression of SV40 in these cells, in particular the large tumor antigen (T antigen) of SV40, before they have senesced, allows them to overcome their finite mitotic life span and results in the establishment of immortal cell lines. The immortal state is dependent on the continued presence of T antigen, although whether all of the functions initially required to induce immortalization are required to maintain it is currently unclear. Here, we first discuss the growth restrictions of primary cells in culture, and define immortalization and transformation. We then briefly review cell cycle regulation and negative growth control in normal cells, with particular reference to the retinoblastoma family of proteins and p53, before discussing mechanisms used by SV40 to overcome these growth restrictions. Finally, we briefly mention *trans versus cis* complementation between T antigen mutants, initiation *versus* maintenance of immortalization, the putative role of the SV40 small t antigen, and the biological counting mechanism that measures the finite proliferative life span.

Immortalization *Versus* Transformation

When mammalian cells isolated from an embryo or an animal are cultured *in vitro*, they initially proliferate but stop dividing after a finite number of division (Hayflick and Moorhead, 1961). At this point the cultures undergo crisis and the cells senesce. Such senescent cells cannot be induced to enter mitosis, even if supplemented with fresh growth medium. However, the cells do not die but remain metabolically active (they continue to synthesize RNA and protein) and responsive to mitogens (some immediate early genes are expressed (Tavassoli and Shall, 1988). Analysis of senescent fibroblasts suggests that the cells arrest in the G_1, and possibly G_2, phases of the cell cycle. This is in contrast to the G_0 arrest for cells which enter quiescence in response to either serum deprivation or contact inhibition (Gelfant, 1977; Grove and Cristofalo, 1977).

It has been observed that cells from progressively older animals undergo progressively fewer divisions in culture before undergoing senescence, suggesting that there is an inverse correlation between the age of the animal and the *in vitro* life span of cells derived from that animal (Hayflick and Moorhead, 1961; Bierman, 1978; Rohme, 1981). Additionally, cells from the same animal species undergo a relatively constant number of divisions (approximately 30 population doublings for rodent embryo fibroblasts compared to 50-70 doublings for human fibroblasts), and the number of population doublings for a given cell type is highly reproducible. Thus, it has been suggested that cellular senescence may be a programmed event and that entry into senescence is a manifestation of aging at the cellular level (Kirkwood, 1996; Smith and Pereira-Smith, 1996).

The molecular basis for programmed entry into senescence is poorly-defined, although it has been suggested that it may be linked to the random accumulation of cellular damage (Orgel, 1973). This hypothesis suggests that as cells divide *in vitro* they accumulate mutations, karyotypic changes and other forms of DNA damage (such as loss of DNA methylation) and this leads to changes in the expression of positive and negative regulators of cell growth or to a predisposition to karyotypic instability, resulting in loss of proliferative potential (Sherwood et al., 1988).

Another hypothesis proposes that the progressive loss of telomeric DNA and other essential sequences from the ends of chromosomes determines the finite proliferative potential (Harley et al., 1990; Allsop et al., 1992). In this hypothesis, once the telomeres have shortened to a critical length, the cell stops dividing and becomes senescent. Although this mechanism probably operates in human cells, it is doubtful that it plays a role in regulating proliferative potential in murine cells (Zakian, 1995; Autexier and Greider, 1996; Lansdorp, 1997; Zakian, 1997; de Lange, 1998; Sedivy, 1998). Primary cells derived from telomerase-deficient mice enter senescence at the same time as primary cells from normal mice (Blasco et al., 1997) and are able to escape senescence at the same rate, suggesting no autonomous role for telomerase in regulating senescence in the murine system. In contrast, other workers (Bodnar et al., 1998; Vaziri and Benchimol, 1998) have found that ectopic expression of telomerase in normal human cells results in prolonged life spans in these cells.

Others have suggested that senescence is regulated via a genetic program (Pereira-Smith et al., 1989; Goldstein, 1990; Vojta and Barrett, 1995). A number of genes that may be involved in regulating senescence have been identified from senescent cells (Murano et al., 1991; Nuell et al., 1991; Noda et al., 1994).

When a cell overcomes senescence it is said to have become immortal, since it has acquired an infinite life span. A number of viral and cellular oncogenes can overcome senescence, including the large tumor antigen (T antigen) of simian virus 40 (SV40). Alternatively, serial cultivation of rodent embryo fibroblasts occasionally results in spontaneously immortal cell lines which have escaped senescence (Todaro and Green, 1963; Curatolo et al., 1984). The cellular lesions responsible for this escape from senescence are poorly-defined, however, mutations in the negative growth regulator p53 and increased expression of c-*myc* have been observed in some immortal cell lines (Tavassoli and Shall, 1988; Harvey and Levine, 1991; Rittling and Denhardt, 1992).

Immortalization has been suggested to be one of two steps required to bring about the complete malignant transformation of rodent cells *in vitro* (Weinberg, 1985). In contrast to fully transformed cells, immortal cells remain dependent on the presence of mitogens (although they have a reduced requirement for them), cannot overgrow a confluent monolayer and cannot form tumors in nude mice. The continued expression of the immortalizing oncogene is required to maintain the immortal state, however whether all the functions which were initially required to overcome the finite life span of the primary cells, or a subset of these functions, are required to maintain the immortal state has not been determined.

Immortal cells can be transformed into fully malignant cells by either the introduction of a second oncogene (Land et al., 1983; Ruley, 1983) or, at a low frequency, through the occurrence of spontaneous second events such as chromosomal mutations (Land et al., 1986).

Somatic cell fusions of normal diploid human fibroblasts with several immortal cell lines, including HeLa and SV40-transformed cells, have suggested that senescence is dominant over proliferation. The hybrids resulting from such fusions only proliferate for a limited period of time prior to undergoing senescence (Bunn and Tarrant, 1980; Pereira-Smith and Smith, 1981; *Ibid.*, 1988; Pereira-Smith et al., 1990). This is consistent with the idea that the inactivation of specific senescence-promoting genes may be important for cells to escape from senescence, and that activation of specific dominant oncogenes can overcome senescence.

Immortalization requires not only the ability to overcome the limited proliferation of primary cells but also requires the inhibition of programmed cell death by apoptosis. It is thought that apoptosis may be a cellular defense against deregulated growth in inappropriate conditions. Thus, in order to successfully immortalize a cell, an oncogene must not only deregulate cell growth but also overcome the apoptotic pathway(s) which may be activated in response to this deregulated cell growth (King and Cidlowski, 1998).

It is unknown whether immortalization has a role to play in tumorigenesis *in vivo*, or whether it is merely required for the *in vitro* establishment of transformed cell lines (Strauss and Griffin, 1990; Stamps et al., 1992). While it is hard to envisage a situation where a tumor could be derived without first overcoming the finite mitotic life span, it remains to be demonstrated whether this is a critical step in tumorigenesis.

Before focusing on the mechanisms used by SV40 to overcome senescence, we will first present a very brief review of cell cycle regulation in normal (that is, uninfected) cells.

Cell Cycle Control

In order to understand how SV40 can induce cellular proliferation and immortalization, it is first necessary to understand how cell cycling is regulated in the absence of SV40. This section presents an overview of cell cycle control (summarized in Figure 1) so that the affects of SV40 infection on cells can be more clearly understood. More in-depth reviews of cell cycle regulation are presented elsewhere.

Cyclins, Cdks, and Cdk Inhibitors

Progression of eukaryotic cells through the cell cycle is regulated by the sequential assembly and activation of key cyclin and cyclin-dependent kinase (cdk) complexes. The cyclins constitute the regulatory subunit of the complex, while the cdk is the

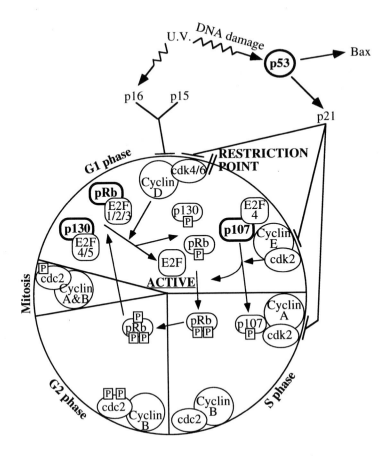

Fig. 1.   Summary of Cell Cycle Regulation. A simplified summary of eukaryotic cell cycle regulation is shown.   The proteins with which T antigen interacts are indicated in bold.   The cyclin-cdk complexes whose activities are associated with each phase of the cell cycle are shown. DNA damage results in p53-dependent transcriptional activation of p21 and Bax. The amount of damage incurred determines the cellular fate - irrepairable damage results in cell death by apoptosis, whereas lower levels of damage result in cell cycle arrest until the damage is repaired. See text for details.   Adapted from Hunter & Pines, 1994.

catalytic subunit. The levels of the various cyclins oscillate throughout the cell cycle and regulation is through modulation of transcription and degradation rates. In contrast, the levels of the cdks are relatively constant throughout the cell cycle and regulation of their activity is achieved by phosphorylation and association with specific inhibitors, as well as association with a cyclin subunit (Nigg, 1995; Sherr and Roberts, 1995; Lew and Kornbluth, 1996; Morgan, 1997). Different cyclin-cdk complexes are required at different stages of the cell cycle, thus, cdk4/6-cyclin D complexes form during early G_1, whereas cyclin E activates cdk2 during the G_1/S transition. Cyclin A binds cdk2 or cdc2 during S phase and at the G_2/M transition, and cyclin B-cdc2 functions during the G_2/M transition.

One method of inhibiting cyclin-cdk complexes is through the activity of a number of cdk inhibitors (Morgan, 1997). There are two families of cdk inhibitors: the Cip/Kip family, consisting of p21, p27 and p57; and the Ink4 family, consisting of p15, p16, and p18. The Cip/Kip family inhibits the cdk4/6- and cdk2-cyclin complexes involved in G_1 and G_1/S control, while the Ink4 family has a much narrower specificity for cdk4/6-cyclin D complexes (Morgan, 1997). The levels of both p21 (Tahara et al., 1995) and p16 (Serrano et al., 1996; Palmero et al., 1997; Zindy et al., 1997) increase as cells approach senescence suggesting a link between the cdk inhibitors and the induction of senescence (Noble et al., 1996; Brown et al., 1997; Uhrbom et al., 1997; McConnell et al., 1998; Vogt et al., 1998). Implications of these increased levels are discussed below.

pRb and Related Proteins

When a cell has finished mitosis it returns to G_1. At this stage, it must assess environmental conditions (for example, the presence of mitogens) and decide whether to divide again (i.e., continue through G_1 and the remaining stages of the cell cycle to M) or to become quiescent (i.e., enter G_0). This decision is made approximately two thirds of the way through G_1, at the "restriction (R) point" (Pardee, 1989). If the cell decides at R to continue cycling, the remainder of the cell cycle proceeds, unless an unforeseen event occurs (e.g., DNA damage). Once R is passed, growth is no longer dependent on the presence of mitogens.

Interestingly, transition through R appears to coincide with phosphorylation of the retinoblastoma susceptibility protein pRb (Weinberg, 1995; Bartek et al., 1996). That is, prior to R (in early G_1), pRb is present in an underphosphorylated form, but transition through R involves phosphorylation of pRb and results in hyperphosphorylated pRb (Buchkovich et al., 1989). Additionally, pRb is also phosphorylated during S, and again at G_2/M (DeCaprio et al., 1992) prior to dephosphorylation in M (Nelson et al., 1997), suggesting that pRb may play additional roles in cell cycle regulation besides its role at R.

How is it that once pRb is phosphorylated the cell proceeds through G_1? Underphosphorylated pRb is found in association with the transcription factor E2F (Chellappan et al., 1991; Chittenden et al., 1991; Hiebert et al., 1992; Flemington et al., 1993; Lees et al., 1993; Qin et al., 1995). Upon phosphorylation of pRb, E2F is released from this inhibitory complex and goes on to transactivate genes which contain an E2F site in their promoter (Suzuki-Takahashi et al., 1995; Sladek, 1997). These genes include c-*myc*, N-*myc*, c-*myb*, dihydrofolate reductase, thymidine kinase, DNA polymerase α, *cdc2*, EGF receptor, p107 and the *E2F-1* gene itself (Dalton, 1992; Neuman et al., 1994; Anderson et al., 1996; Sladek, 1997). Thus it seems that pRb regulates cell cycle progression by sequestering E2F. Once conditions are deemed to be suitable for cell division, pRb is phosphorylated and releases E2F, which goes on to induce transcription of important growth regulatory genes (Qin et al., 1994; Shan and Lee, 1994).

Although this model is fairly simple, the situation *in vivo* is actually more complicated. There exist two cellular proteins, p107 and p130, which have homology to pRb in the "pocket" domain (Ewen et al., 1991; Li et al., 1993; Mayol et al., 1993; Zhu et al., 1993). In addition, the E2F transcription factors consist of five family members. Underphosphorylated pRb associates with E2F-1, E2F-2, and E2F-3; while p107 associates with E2F-4 and p130 associates with E2F-4 and E2F-5 (Dyson et al., 1993; Beijersbergen et al., 1994; Ginsberg et al., 1994; Hijmans et al., 1995; Vairo et al., 1995). Thus, it seems that the pRb proteins associate with various E2F proteins to regulate transcriptional activity mediated by E2F. Each pRb protein may control a different cell cycle step: p130 is the predominant E2F-associated protein in G_0/early G_1 (following serum stimulation of quiescent cells); pRb associates with E2F during early-to mid-G_1, and p107 is the predominant E2F-associated protein near the G_1/S border (Figure 1). The pRb and p107/p130-associated E2F proteins regulate different sets of genes, allowing specificity throughout the cell cycle (Hurford et al., 1997).

Cyclin D-dependent kinases are most often implicated in the phosphorylation of pRb (Kato et al., 1993). The D-type cyclins (D1, D2 and D3) are unique in that they are the only cyclins able to bind pRb directly and it has been suggested that this binding targets pRb for phosphorylation by either cdk4 or cdk6 (Dowdy et al., 1993; Ewen et al., 1993). In fact, activity of cdk4/6-cyclin D can be regulated by the cdk inhibitors p21 (Harper et al., 1993; Xiong et al., 1993) and p16 (Serrano et al., 1993; Hall et al., 1995a). As mentioned above, the levels of both p21 and p16 are upregulated in senescent cells and senescent cells contain only the underphosphorylated (growth-inhibitory) form of pRb (Stein et al., 1990). Thus, it is tempting to speculate that the increased p21 and/or p16 levels promote senescence by regulating the phosphorylation of pRb.

Besides affecting transcriptional activity due to E2F, the pocket proteins (at least pRb and p107) can also directly repress or activate transcription from a number of promoters (Bremner et al., 1995; Dagnino et al., 1995). This activity is again regulated by phosphorylation. This transcriptional activity is mediated through interaction with tissue-specific transcription factors or the basal transcriptional machinery. Thus, in general, the pRb proteins regulate transcription in a cell cycle-dependent manner by interacting with cellular transcription factors.

p53

Once the cell has passed R, it has committed itself to completing the cell cycle. The next point of control is the G_1/S boundary. At this point, the cell checks that everything is in order before initiating DNA replication. While pRb is active at R, another protein, p53, plays a critical role at G_1/S (Levine, 1997; Wiman, 1997).

If a cell's DNA is damaged, by radiation for instance, this results in stabilization of the normally short-lived p53 protein (Maltzman and Czyzyk, 1984; Kastan et al., 1991; Kuerbitz et al., 1992). The outcome of this p53 activity is dependent on the extent of the damage (Figure 1). Minimal damage (i.e., repairable), results in p53-induced cell cycle arrest at G_1/S which allows the cell to repair the damaged DNA before proceeding through S, therefore ensuring that any mutations are not passed on to the daughter cells. It should be noted at this point that the cdk inhibitor p16 also participates in a G_1 arrest in response to DNA damage, and that this checkpoint operates in a p53-null background (Robles and Adami, 1998; Shapiro et al., 1998) suggesting that other mechanisms besides those mediated by p53 can induce growth arrest in response to damage. If the damage is extensive and cannot be repaired, p53 induces exit from the cell cycle and death by apoptosis. Besides acting at G_1/S, p53 can also halt DNA replication during S phase should damage be incurred. Again, minimal damage results in arrest until repairs are made, while extensive damage leads to apoptosis. Thus, p53 plays a critical role in determining cell fate.

The affects of p53 are mediated through transcriptional activation of genes containing a p53 responsive element. Examples of genes that are activated by p53 include the cdk inhibitor p21, the apoptotic protein Bax, and the p53 inhibitor mdm2 (Wu et al., 1993; El-Deiry et al., 1994; Miyashita et al., 1994). In addition, p53 can suppress transcription of other genes including those encoding Bcl-2, pRb, the transcription factors c-*fos*, c-*jun*, and c-*myc* and the proliferating cell nuclear antigen (PCNA) (Ginsberg et al., 1991; Mercer et al., 1991; Moberg et al., 1992; Shiio et al., 1992; Miyashita et al., 1994).

How do these various proteins carry out the functions attributed to p53? As outlined above, p21 can inhibit the cyclin D complexes responsible for phosphorylating pRb, thereby maintaining pRb in the underphosphorylated form which sequesters E2F. Since transcriptionally active E2F is not released, the cell does not express genes required for cell cycle progression and the cell cycle arrests. Additionally, p21 competes for binding to PCNA (Cox, 1997; Warbrick, 1998). PCNA is a component of the DNA replication machinery and is therefore required for both DNA replication and repair. When p21 is bound to PCNA, PCNA-dependent DNA replication is impaired, but PCNA-dependent nucleotide excision repair remains intact (Flores-Rozas et al., 1994; Li et al., 1994; Waga et al., 1994). Thus, by inducing p21 activity, p53 ensures repair of damaged DNA before the cell replicates the DNA in S phase.

Gadd45 also binds PCNA and stimulates DNA excision repair but inhibits entry into S phase (Smith et al., 1994; Hall et al., 1995b), which may also contribute to cell cycle arrest induced by p53.

In senescent cells p53 is active (Atadja et al., 1995; Kulju and Lehman, 1995; Bond et al., 1996) and the addition of wild-type p53 to p53-null cells can induce the senescence program (Sugrue et al., 1997). Gire and Wynford-Thomas (1998) have recently shown that p53 activity is critical for the maintenance of senescence, since microinjection of anti-p53 antibodies into senescent cells induces DNA synthesis and reversion to the "young" morphology. This is in contrast to the traditional view that senescence is irreversible and must be confirmed through future work. Nevertheless, it is clear that p53 plays a key role in the maintenance of the senescent phenotype.

In the presence of damage which cannot be repaired, p53 induces the expression of the apoptotic protein Bax and represses the transcription of a related protein, Bcl-2

(Miyashita et al., 1994). Bax heterodimerizes with other cellular Bcl-2 family members and induces apoptosis while Bcl-2 protects from apoptosis (Oltvai et al., 1993; Chao and Korsmeyer, 1998). Indeed, the relative levels of Bcl-2 and Bax are thought to determine a cell's propensity to undergo apoptosis (Hengartner, 1998). The actual mechanism used by the Bcl-2 proteins to induce apoptosis is unclear, but is thought to involve the release of cytochrome c from the mitochondria, which results in the activation of a family of cysteine proteases, the caspases, which are implicated as apoptotic mediators (Cryns and Yuan, 1998; Kidd, 1998). Clearly p53-dependent apoptosis is not this straightforward however, since DNA damage results in apoptosis in Bax-deficient thymocytes (Knudson et al., 1995). Other genes induced by p53 which may play a role in apoptosis include the Fas/APO-1 gene and the related gene for KILLER/DR5 which encode cell surface "death receptors" (Wu et al., 1997; Sheikh et al., 1998), the insulin-like growth factor binding protein 3 (Buckbinder et al., 1995) which could block an insulin-like growth factor survival signal and thereby promote death, and a zinc finger protein which promotes apoptosis (Israeli et al., 1997).

By using transcriptional activation of specific genes, p53 can determine whether a cell halts to repair damage or undergoes apoptosis. Indeed, the level of damage determines cellular fate: low levels of p53 (in response to low levels of damage) induce cell cycle arrest while higher levels induce apoptosis (Chen et al., 1996). In the absence of DNA damage, p53 is not stabilized and therefore doesn't induce transcription, and the cell proceeds into S phase.

SV40

As briefly outlined above the large tumor antigen (T antigen) protein of SV40 enables primary rodent cells to overcome senescence. Here, we review SV40 and the nature of the virus, before focusing on large T and the mechanisms it utilizes to overcome the finite proliferative potential of cells.

Simian virus 40 (SV40; 5243 bp) is a member of the papovavirus group of small icosahedral DNA viruses which contain double-stranded DNA genomes (Tooze, 1981). Sequence comparisons suggest that these viruses have co-evolved with their hosts (SV40 with monkey, polyoma virus with mouse, and the JC and BK viruses with human) from a common ancestor (Soeda et al., 1980). Lytic infection of cells permissive for viral infection results in full viral gene expression, synthesis of progeny particles and eventually cell death. In contrast, non-permissive cells survive viral infection and progeny particles are not produced, however, the early viral proteins are expressed.

The location of the coding sequences on the viral genome for the SV40 proteins is shown in Figure 2. Lytic infection by SV40 can be divided into two phases, early and late, defined by the onset of viral DNA replication. During the early phase of infection the viral genes from the "early" region (Figure 2) are expressed. These genes alter and/or recruit cellular proteins to participate in virus production, block any cellular antiviral systems, and participate directly in viral replication. They also drive the infected cell to enter the cell cycle in order to ensure that the cellular proteins required

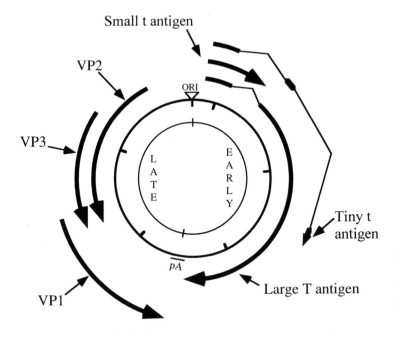

Fig. 2. Structure of the SV40 viral genome. The structure of the viral genome is shown, with the origin of replication (ORI) at the top. The early and late regions, and their associated proteins, are indicated. The polyadenylation signal sequence is shown as pA.

for viral replication, transcription and virion assembly are synthesized. Following viral and cellular DNA replication the "late" region genes are expressed (Figure 2) which encode the structural components of the virus particle. SV40 DNA has a single origin of replication which is located in the region that regulates transcription for both the early and late genes (Figure 2).

The SV40 early region encodes three early proteins, designated the large T, small t and tiny t antigens. These proteins are translated from differentially spliced mRNAs which have common translational start sites (Griffin, 1981). Thus, the tiny t, small t and large T antigens have homologous amino termini (amino acids 1-82, designated the T/t common region). The late region of SV40 encodes three proteins, VP1, VP2 and VP3, which are the structural components of the virion. VP3 corresponds to the carboxy-terminal portion of VP2 and this coding sequence partially overlaps the VP1 coding sequence (Figure 2). The late region mRNAs comprise a short 5'-untranslated leader segment attached to alternative body segments (Ziff, 1980) which contain the two large open reading frames from which the proteins are translated (Griffin, 1981). In contrast to the early region mRNAs, no splicing occurs within the late protein coding regions.

The different mRNAs are generated by juxtaposing the 5'-"leader" segment to alternative downstream initiation codons.

Since SV40 large T antigen is sufficient to immortalize primary rodent embryo fibroblasts in culture, we shall focus primarily on the role of this protein. However, small t antigen shall be mentioned briefly, later. Tiny t has only recently been identified and thus very little is know about its function (Zerrahn et al., 1993).

SV40 Large T Antigen

SV40 causes a lytic infection of monkey cells and an abortive infection of either rat or mouse cells. The replication of the viral genome in the lytic infection of monkey cells is entirely dependent on cellular chromosomal replication proteins and cellular metabolism, except for the SV40-encoded large T antigen which is required for the initiation of replication (Tegtmeyer, 1972; Tooze, 1981; Li and Kelly, 1984). This dependence on cellular replication proteins means that SV40 DNA replication can only occur in the S phase of the cell cycle. Thus, the SV40 early gene products have evolved the ability to stimulate cell growth and cellular DNA synthesis so that the cell can support viral replication. SV40 infection of monkey cells results in the production of thousands of daughter virions per cell and cell lysis after no more than a few days (Tooze, 1981). However, infection of rodent cells is abortive. If an early protein, the large T antigen, is expressed, following integration of the SV40 DNA into the genome, these cells display altered growth properties (i.e., they have become immortal; Risser and Pollack, 1974) and often they become fully transformed due to the occurrence of a second event. Thus immortalization by T antigen is thought to be due to T antigen stimulating cell growth despite the infection being abortive. It is interesting to note that some of the regions that are required for immortalization by the large T antigen are also required for inducing DNA synthesis, confirming a link between the immortalizing properties of large T antigen and its ability to drive a cell into the cell cycle (Fanning and Knippers, 1992).

SV40 large T antigen is a multifunctional phosphoprotein of 708 amino acids and is predominantly localized to the cell nucleus (Soule and Butel, 1979), although a small fraction is found in the plasma membrane (Santos and Butel, 1982). Several biochemical activities are associated with T antigen (reviewed in Fanning, 1992; Fanning and Knippers, 1992). It localizes to the nucleus by virtue of a nuclear localization signal between amino acids 126 to 132 (Kalderon et al., 1984; Lanford and Butel, 1984). T antigen has ATPase activity (Tjian and Robbins, 1979); DNA and RNA helicase activity (Scheffner et al., 1989; Stahl et al., 1986); topoisomerase activity (Marton et al., 1993); binds RNA covalently (Carroll et al., 1988); and is capable of both specific and non-specific binding of DNA (Carroll et al., 1974; Tjian et al., 1978; Prives et al., 1982; Damania and Alwine, 1996). While these activities are necessary for viral DNA replication, none of them are required for the immortalization or transformation of rodent cells (Stringer, 1982; Manos and Gluzman, 1984; 1985; Peden et al., 1990). T antigen is also capable of both activating and repressing transcription from a number of viral and cellular promoters (Alwine et al., 1977; Hansen et al., 1981; Mitchell et al., 1987; Saffer et al., 1990; Zhu et al., 1991a; Gilinger and Alwine, 1993; Gruda et al., 1993; Rice and Cole, 1993; Rushton et al., 1997). It binds a number of host cellular proteins such as p53 (Lane and Crawford, 1979; Linzer and Levine, 1979; Harlow et al., 1981); pRb (DeCaprio et al., 1988); p107 (Dyson et al., 1989); p130 (Hannon et al., 1993); p185 (Kohrman and Imperiale, 1992); DNA polymerase α (Smale and Tjian, 1986; Gannon and Lane, 1987; Dornreiter et al., 1990); the heat shock protein hsc70 (Sawai and Butel, 1989; Sawai et al., 1994) topoisomerase 1 (Simmons et al., 1996); a family of transcription factors related to CREB-binding protein (CBP; Avantaggiati et al., 1996; Eckner et al., 1996); and preliminary evidence suggests that it may also bind the SUG1 regulatory component of the proteasome (Grand et al., 1999). Finally, the amino terminal region of T antigen has homology to the J domain of the DnaJ family of molecular chaperones, and evidence suggests that T antigen is able to bind and activate the ATPase activity of DnaK proteins through this domain (Srinivasan et al., 1997). The specific regions of T antigen which are required for the interaction with some of these proteins and some of its biochemical activities have been identified and are shown in Figure 3.

SV40 Large T Antigen and Immortalization

Since we are only interested in the functions of T antigen required in immortalization, we shall focus on the domains of T antigen involved in this activity. Furthermore, we focus on immortalization of rodent cells, since in human cells SV40 causes an extension of life span but the cells still undergo crisis (reviewed by Sedivy, 1998). However, first, we shall briefly mention the nature of the assays used to measure immortalizing and transforming activity.

Introduction of large T antigen into primary rodent cells results in the cells acquiring an infinite proliferative potential but does not necessarily result in them becoming fully transformed (Petit et al., 1983; Jat and Sharp, 1986; Conzen and Cole, 1994). Only a small proportion of these immortal cells progress to the transformed state. Inactivation of the T antigen in these immortal cells results in a rapid and irreversible loss of proliferative potential in either the G_1 or G_2 phases of the cell cycle demonstrating that the T antigen protein is continuously required to maintain the proliferative state (Jat and Sharp, 1989; Radna et al., 1989; Tsuyama et al., 1991; Gonos et al., 1996). Introduction of large T antigen into established cell lines, however, can result in these cell lines acquiring a more fully transformed phenotype (Kriegler et al., 1984; Brown et al., 1986; Jat et al., 1986; Jat and Sharp, 1986; Chen and Paucha, 1990).

A large amount of research has been carried out to identify the functions of T antigen which are required for its ability to stimulate growth and induce immortalization. As a result a number of cellular assays have been used to investigate the growth stimulatory affects of SV40 large T antigen mutants. These assays have studied the ability of T antigen to induce DNA synthesis in quiescent cells; to immortalize primary cells from different species; to transform primary cells in co-operation with a second, cytoplasmic oncogene such as activated *ras* or polyoma virus

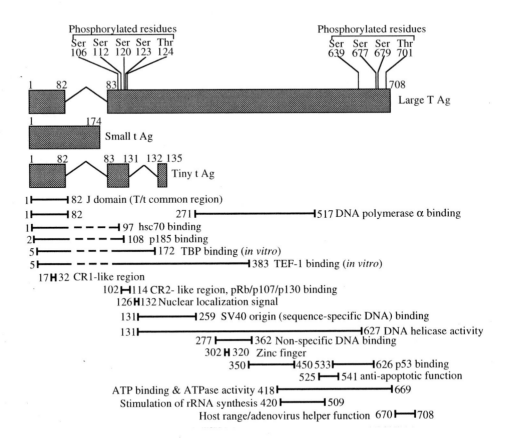

Fig. 3. *T antigen-associated functions and their locations. The various biochemical activities of the T antigens, and any regions required for binding cellular proteins are shown. References can be found within the text.*

middle T antigen; to allow anchorage-independent growth of established cells; to allow growth of established cells in low serum concentrations or at high saturation densities; and to induce tumors in experimental animals. Some of the regions identified by these various assays appear to be similar, however, other regions which have been identified as necessary in one assay are not required in others. It is clear therefore that the functions required by T antigen to stimulate growth are different depending on the cellular growth assay used.

Most of the studies that aim to identify activities of T antigen involved in immortalization have used the infection or transfection of various cell types by wild-type *versus* mutant T antigens in order to compare their activities. The cell type used for infection is critical in these assays. For example, REF52 and C3H10T1/2 cells are spontaneously immortalized rat and mouse fibroblast lines, respectively. When T antigen is introduced into these cells, they form dense colonies which can easily be identified under the microscope or by staining. Many conclusions have been drawn from studies using these cell lines, however, it is important to note that these assays measure transforming activity rather than immortalizing activity. Additionally, it should be remembered that any established cell line has already undergone the changes necessary for immortalization (i.e., these cells are already genetically abnormal), so these cells may have a reduced requirement for T antigen activities compared to normal primary cells.

Immortalization assays therefore should be performed on primary rat or mouse cells. Indeed, even these assays can cause confusion as different read-outs have been used by different groups and the requirements for immortalization seem to differ between mouse and rat cells. One read-out measures the number of colonies present in dishes of cultures transfected with the DNA of interest, at the time when non-transfected control cells are undergoing senescence. However, subsequent studies have revealed that the presence of colonies is not necessarily an indication of immortalization but could simply be an extension of life span (i.e., the cells eventually senesce; Conzen and Cole, 1995). A true measure of immortalization is the ability to expand colonies from the transfected cultures and continue their growth through a number of population doublings. For example, mouse embryo fibroblasts (MEFs) derived from the thorax of day 12-16 C57BL/6 embryos have an average *in vitro* life span of 16-17 days (that is, 6-8 population doublings). Thus, these cells can be considered immortal when they have undergone >60 population doublings and continue to grow exponentially. It should be noted that primary MEFs senesce at an earlier passage than primary rat embryo fibroblasts (REFs). This means that MEFs have less time to undergo somatic mutations *in vitro* that could contribute to immortalization. However, MEFs have a greater propensity for spontaneous immortalization than primary cells from other species (Macieira-Coelho and Azzarone, 1988). Thus, results in either system should be considered in view of the possibility of somatic mutations which may lead to spontaneous immortalization which is unrelated to the presence of T antigen. During these assays, the cells should be seeded at low density so that no monolayer is formed in order to avoid selective pressure which would enable the outgrowth of cells which have spontaneously acquired mutations allowing them to overcome contact inhibition.

Using assays such as those outlined above and a number of SV40 T antigen mutants, three regions of T antigen have been shown to be required for immortalization of rodent cells (Conzen and Cole, 1995). These regions are the amino terminal 82 amino acids (the T/t common region), amino acids 102-114 and amino acids 350-560. While all three regions are required for immortalization, C3H10T1/2 cells are still transformed by T antigen with mutations in the second or third regions but mutations in amino acids 1-82 results in non-transformation of C3H10T1/2. This illustrates the reduced requirement of T antigen functions for transformation of established lines *versus* immortalization of primary cells.

Below, we summarize some of the activities associated with these three regions and their relevance to immortalization.

AMINO ACIDS 1-82

The amino terminal 82 amino acids of T antigen are homologous to the amino terminal 82 amino acids of t antigen, thus, this region is known as the T/t common region.

One region in the amino terminal domain of T antigen is homologous to a region located towards the amino terminus of the adenovirus E1A oncogene. This region is designated conserved region 1 (CR1), since it is conserved between different adenovirus serotypes. In T antigen the CR1-like domain stretches from amino acids 17-32 of T antigen (Figge et al., 1988; Figure 3). In E1A, this region is required for interaction with the cellular protein p300, a protein with which T antigen also interacts (Yaciuk et al., 1991). Although it was originally thought that T antigen also interacts with p300 through its CR1, it is now known that interaction with p300 occurs through a different mechanism (see below).

For many years, the T/t common region of T antigen had an unknown function. Although mutations in this region could perturb many SV40 functions (e.g., immortalization and transformation, as well as viral DNA replication and morphogenesis), no biochemical function was ascribed to it.

Computer-assisted similarity searches suggested that the T/t common region was related to the J domain region of the DnaJ family of molecular chaperones (Kelley and Landry, 1994; reviewed in Brodsky and Pipas, 1998; Kelley, 1998; Figure 3). This region includes the conserved tripeptide HPD which is found in all DnaJ proteins. DnaJ proteins bind to and stimulate the ATPase activity of DnaK proteins, a function which requires the HPD sequence. DnaK proteins, in turn, interact with protein substrates in an ATP-dependent manner to prevent aggregation and promote protein folding. Thus, it is not surprising to learn that T antigen interacts with a human homologue of DnaK, hsc70 (Sawai and Butel, 1989; Sawai et al., 1994).

Recently, evidence has accumulated to suggest that the T antigen amino terminal domain actually functions as a J domain. Firstly, it was demonstrated that the SV40 T antigen J domain could functionally substitute for the J domain of E. coli DnaJ. Additionally, mutations in the histidine of the conserved tripeptide HPD could abolish this function (Kelley and Georgopoulos, 1997). Additional in vivo studies revealed that the T antigen J domain was necessary for efficient viral replication and that chimeric proteins generated from the J domain region of Hsj1 or DnaJ2 (human DnaJ proteins) fused to the central and carboxy terminal domains of T antigen could also promote efficient viral DNA replication (Campbell et al., 1997). Again, mutation of the histidine of the conserved HPD tripeptide in either intact T antigen or in the chimeric proteins could affect DNA replication. Furthermore, mutations in the HPD tripeptide or other conserved residues could prevent interactions between T antigen and a DnaK protein (hsc70).

Srinivasan et al. (1997) have recently demonstrated that the amino terminus of T antigen possesses two of the hallmarks of a DnaJ protein. Namely, this domain stimulates the ATPase activity of a DnaK protein, and promotes the ATP-dependent release of an unfolded polypeptide substrate from the DnaK protein. Thus, T antigen is thought to contain an active J domain. The consequences of this activity will be discussed below.

AMINO ACIDS 102-114

Amino acids 102-114 of T antigen have homology to the conserved region 2 (CR2) domain of adenovirus E1A and the human papilloma virus type 16 E7 protein (Figure 3). As with E1A and HPV 16 E7, it is the CR2 domain of T antigen which is responsible for its interactions with the pRb "pocket" proteins (pRb, p107, p130; DeCaprio et al., 1988; Moran, 1988; Munger et al., 1989). T antigen binds only the underphosphorylated (growth suppressing) form of pRb during G_1 (Ludlow et al., 1989; 1990). This binding of T antigen to a pRb-E2F complex disrupts the complex, resulting in release of E2F, allowing it to activate transcription and the cell to enter S phase. Similarly, T antigen targets p107 and p130, thereby disrupting their interactions with E2F proteins. Additionally, T antigen perturbs the phosphorylation status of p107 and p130 and increases degradation of these proteins (Stubdal et al., 1996).

Recent results from Srinivasan et al. (1997) suggest that pRb may not be the critical target of T antigen, but rather, the related proteins p107 and p130 may be more important for immortalization. These authors used two mutants of T antigen, 3213 and K1, which contain mutations within the CR2 domain (E107K, E108K for 3213, E107K for K1; Peden and Pipas, 1992), and studied their ability to transform the C3H10T1/2 cell line, both in the context of full-length T antigen and an amino terminal truncation mutant containing only amino acids 1 to 136 (TN136). Both the full-length T antigen and TN136 could transform C3H10T1/2 cells. In the context of full-length T antigen, both 3213 and K1 could transform C3H10T1/2, albeit with decreased efficiency compared to wild-type T antigen. However, in the context of TN136, neither 3213 nor K1 could transform these cells. Furthermore, the 3213 mutant in the context of full-length T antigen was found to interact with both p107 and p130, although at decreased levels compared to wild-type T antigen, whereas this interaction was eliminated when the mutations were in the context of TN136. In neither context did these mutants interact with pRb. The conclusions from these experiments are two-fold. Firstly, it would seem that p107 and p130 contact not only the CR2 domain of T antigen, but also sequences in the carboxy terminus of the protein. In contrast, pRb appears only to require the CR2 sequences for interaction with T antigen. Secondly, interaction with p107 and p130 appears to have some impact on transforming ability of T antigen. Thus, in full-length T antigen, although 3213 and K1 have reduced ability to interact with p107 and p130, the remaining interaction with the carboxy terminus may be sufficient for transformation to proceed. In the absence of a carboxy terminus and an intact CR2, p107 and p130 interaction is eliminated and the T antigen is transformation-defective. Thus, while interaction with pRb may be required for efficient transformation, it seems that interactions with p107 and p130 are sufficient for transformation of C3H10T1/2.

Through interacting with the pRb proteins, T antigen is able to interfere with the regulation of a range of other transcription factors besides E2F with which these pocket proteins interact. Each of these transcription factors may be involved, to a greater or lesser extent, in regulating the expression of genes involved in cell cycle progression. Thus the ability of T antigen to inactivate the pRb family may reflect its ability to deregulate cellular proliferation.

AMINO ACIDS 350-560

Towards the carboxy terminus of T antigen is the domain responsible for T antigen's interaction with p53 (Zhu et al., 1991b; Kierstead and Tevethia, 1993). The domain required for this interaction is actually bi-partite, consisting of amino acids 350-450 and 533-560 (Figure 3). It is generally accepted that the carboxy-terminus of T antigen beyond amino acid 627 can be removed without loss of immortalization, transformation or tumorigenic activity (Tevethia et al., 1988).

When T antigen binds to p53, the protein is stabilized. In non-transformed tissues the half-life of p53 is very short, approximately 10-20 minutes. However, in cells transformed by SV40 T antigen, the half-life of p53 is increased to as much as 20 hours (Oren et al., 1981). Thus, cells transformed by SV40 have much higher levels of p53 than normal cells. However, the p53 in these transformed cells is sequestered by T antigen, and is therefore unavailable for transcriptional activation or repression (Mietz et al., 1992). Thus, the G_1 checkpoint is unoperational, and cells proceed into S phase regardless of whether DNA damage is present. Indeed, it is thought that the increased occurrence of mutations in SV40-immortalized cells is due to the failure of p53 to monitor the genome and thus increased plasticity of the genome (Ray et al., 1990; Stewart and Bacchetti, 1991; Woods et al., 1994).

Additionally, sequestration of p53 may also abrogate p53-mediated apoptosis (McCarthy et al., 1994). While the inactivation of T antigen in cell lines conditionally immortalized by a temperature-sensitive mutant of T antigen (Jat and Sharp (1989) results in these cell lines growth-arresting without significant cell death, similar cell lines isolated by other investigators have been reported to undergo cell death by apoptosis when T antigen is inactivated (Yanai and Obinata, 1994). This is thought to be due to the sudden release of a large amount of stable p53.

In addition to p53 binding, this region may be responsible for the interaction between T antigen and the CBP/p300 proteins. The CBP/p300 proteins are a family of transcriptional co-activators implicated in a number of cellular processes including cell cycle control, transcriptional regulation and development (reviewed by Giles et al., 1998). Although it was originally thought that T antigen must bind the CBP/p300 proteins through the CR1 domain (by analogy to adenovirus; Yaciuk et al., 1991), Lill et al. (1997a) have found that T antigen still associates with p300 and p400 in the absence of amino acids 1-127 or 127-250. However, if the p53-binding region of T antigen was removed then p300 and p400 binding was also lost. Additionally, immunoprecipitated complexes were always found to contain p300, p400 and CBP, as well as p53 and T antigen. Thus, it seems likely that the CBP/p300 proteins are able to associate with T antigen by virtue of their interaction with p53 (Lill et al., 1997a). The CBP/p300 proteins may act as regulators of p53 (Avantaggiati et al., 1997; Gu et al., 1997; Gu and Roeder, 1997; Lill et al., 1997b) and this regulatory function may be disrupted by interaction with T antigen. Additional studies should help to clarify the affect on the CBP/p300 proteins of binding to T antigen.

In a similar manner, T antigen also interacts with the p53 inhibitor mdm2 through its interaction with p53 (Henning et al., 1997). Thus, in SV40-transformed cells, mdm2 is found either in a complex with p53 (which is an inhibitory complex), or a trimeric complex consisting of p53, T antigen, and mdm2. T antigen is not found in a complex with mdm2 alone. Indeed, p53 and T antigen bind an overlapping domain of mdm2 (Brown et al., 1993). One theory suggests that T antigen targets mdm2 in order to prevent mdm2-directed degradation of p53, thereby leading to stabilization of p53 in SV40-transformed cells (Henning et al., 1997).

In addition to p53 (and CBP/p300) binding, the carboxy terminus of T antigen also contains a novel anti-apoptotic function (recall from above that in addition to stimulating cell growth, the small DNA tumor viruses must also overcome apoptosis in response to deregulated cell growth). Conzen et al. (1997) found that if primary MEFs are transfected with a T antigen which is defective for p53 binding (and therefore can't abrogate p53-mediated apoptosis), the cells are neither immortal nor apoptotic, but rather they enter senescence. This is in contrast to transfection with only the amino terminus of T antigen, which results in apoptosis. Thus, the authors reasoned that T antigen must contain an anti-apoptotic function which is independent of p53 binding. They identified a region of T antigen which protects against apoptosis and contains a stretch of sixteen amino acids (amino acids 525-541; Figure 3) which has >60% homology with a domain found in adenovirus 5 E1B 19K protein, a protein previously shown to be essential for preventing E1A-induced apoptosis (White et al., 1991; Rao et al., 1992). This domain had previously been identified as homologous to the Bcl-2 family's BH1 domain, which is necessary but not sufficient for the interaction between E1B 19K and Bax (Yin et al., 1994; Han et al., 1996). Thus, it seems that in addition to inactivating p53 (and thereby overcoming p53-dependent apoptosis), T antigen may also be able to associate with Bcl-2 family members and inactivate apoptosis independently of p53.

The three regions discussed above are relatively well-defined as to their individual roles, however, there is evidence to suggest that some proteins can interact with both amino and carboxy termini of T antigen. Although pRb binds the CR2 it has been shown that the carboxy terminus of T antigen can compensate for mutations in both the J domain and CR2, suggesting that p107 and p130 may contact residues in the carboxy terminus of T antigen, as well as within CR2 (Srinivasan et al., 1997). Likewise, Yaciuk et al. (1991) have shown that amino acids 17-27 are critical for modulating the CBP/p300-associated functions of T antigen, but it is likely that these proteins bind to T antigen through the intermediacy of p53 (i.e., the carboxy terminus; Lill et al., 1997b). Additionally, a D44N mutant of T antigen (a mutation in the conserved aspartic acid residue of the J domain HPD motif, thus rendering the J domain non-functional) transforms established cell lines with nearly wild-type frequency, in the context of full length T antigen. On the other hand, in the context of an amino terminal deletion mutant, the D44N mutation is transformation-defective (Srinivasan et al., 1997). One possible explanation for this result is that hsc70, which interacts with the J domain, may also contact residues in the carboxy terminus of T antigen. Thus, in the full length protein, although the J domain is non-functional, the T antigen produced may be able to bind sufficient hsc70 through its carboxy terminus to function, however, in the absence of the carboxy terminus, hsc70 binding is completely defective.

PUTTING IT ALL TOGETHER

As briefly mentioned above, the sequences of T antigen implicated in immortalization depends upon the assay used. It is only recently that we are beginning to understand all of the data in terms of a single model, although, of course, there is still some confusion. For the sake of simplicity, we will attempt to avoid the specifics and stick to the generalities.

The region that one determines to be required for immortalization depends on the assay used to measure immortalizing ability. When REFs are transfected with T antigen mutants, it has been found that only the amino terminus (amino acids 1-147, 1-137 or 1-121) is necessary for immortalization (Asselin and Bastin, 1985; Sompayrac and Danna, 1985; 1988; 1991; 1992).

In contrast, when primary MEFs are transfected with T antigen mutants, it has been found that p53 binding (that is, the carboxy terminus of T antigen) is necessary for immortalization and the remainder of the molecule is dispensable (Tevethia et al., 1988; Thompson et al., 1990; Zhu et al., 1991b; Kierstead and Tevethia, 1993).

In transgenic mice, the generation of choroid plexus tumors is considered the hallmark of T antigen expression. In addition to choroid plexus tumors, wild-type T antigen also induces T and B cell lymphomas (Chen et al., 1992). The generation of transgenic mice represents another assay, albeit lengthy, for the regions of T antigen required for transformation. In this assay, *dl*1135 (lacking amino acids 17-27 and therefore a functional J domain), which fails to transform cells in culture, could specifically induce T cell lymphomas and occasionally choroid plexus tumors, but not B cell lymphomas (Symonds et al., 1993). The lack of transformation of B cells and the very low incidence of choroid plexus tumors in the presence of *dl*1135 could reflect the different requirements for transformation, depending on cell type, and that not all T antigen functions may be required for transformation of all cells.

Additionally, Chen et al. (1992) have shown that binding to p53 is not required for generating choroid plexus tumors but binding to pRb/p107, and probably p130, is. Mutant *dl*1137 (encoding only amino acids 1-121 and thus having an intact J domain and pRb binding domain but no p53 binding domain) could still induce choroid plexus tumors (but not T or B cell lymphomas) but these tumors developed much more slowly (8 months) than those induced by wild-type T antigen (1-2 months) (Robles et al., 1994). However, in a p53-null background, tumor progression occurred at a much higher rate with *dl*1137 (Symonds et al., 1994), suggesting that the extended latency period observed with *dl*1137 is directly attributable to failure to inactivate p53. Introducing the K1 mutation into *dl*1137, which disrupts binding to the pocket proteins, resulted in no brain abnormalities, implying a requirement for the pocket proteins for *in vivo* transforming activity.

The results with *dl*1137 suggest an explanation for the conflicting results between MEFs and REFs. As mentioned earlier, MEFs enter senescence after fewer divisions than REFs, and therefore have less time to undergo somatic mutation. Thus, although it appears that the amino terminus alone is sufficient to immortalize REFs, during the course of this assay somatic changes may have occurred which inactivate p53. These mutations could then co-operate with the amino terminus of T antigen to induce immortalization. Since immortalization of MEFs may not require the amino terminus of T antigen, it is possible that MEFs are more susceptible to inactivation of the pRb pathway.

In the *in vitro* experiments, the end-point of the assay used is also relevant to the conclusions drawn. When the number of colonies surviving at the time when normal MEFs are undergoing senescence is used as an end-point, only p53 binding (that is, the carboxy terminal region) appears to be required for immortalization. However, it is now known that this end-point does not necessarily indicate immortalization but only extension of life span (Conzen and Cole, 1995). We now know that either p53 binding alone or the activities of the amino terminus (J domain and pRb family binding) can independently extend the life span of primary MEFs. However, only when co-expressed will these activities promote immortalization (Tevethia et al., 1998). Thus, it now seems that all three domains are required for immortalization.

ROLE OF THE J DOMAIN

As outlined above, the amino terminus of T antigen contains a domain with activities similar to a J domain (reviewed in Brodsky and Pipas, 1998). Specifically, this domain stimulates the ATPase activity of a DnaK protein, and promotes the release of an unfolded polypeptide from a DnaK protein (Srinivasan et al., 1997).

Naturally, this leads one to ponder the role of the J domain in T antigen function. Recent work is starting to illuminate this role. Using polyoma virus large T antigen (which has homology to SV40 T antigen), Sheng et al. (1997) have shown that the J domain of T antigen is required for a productive interaction between T antigen and the pRb family of pocket proteins (pRb p107, p130), which bind a site adjacent to the J domain. Using transactivation of E2F-dependent promoters as a measure of pRb binding (i.e., in a productive interaction with pRb, E2F is released and promotes transcription), these workers showed that although T antigen could bind the pRb family members when its J domain was mutated, this interaction was unproductive (i.e., did not result in E2F-dependent transcription). Furthermore, the J domain activity could not be complemented in *trans* meaning that an intact J domain is required adjacent to the pocket protein binding domain.

The current model for J domain function postulates that the J domain directs the association of hsc70 (or another DnaK chaperone) to multiprotein complexes that are formed with T antigen. For example, during the T antigen-induced release of E2F from pRb family-containing complexes, the J domain may direct hsc70 to the T antigen-bound pRb/p107/p130-E2F complex, and hsc70 may mediate the disassembly of this complex (Sheng et al., 1997; Stubdal et al., 1997; Zalvide et al., 1998). Furthermore, Srinivasan et al. (1997) have demonstrated that the J domain also acts on an activity of T antigen localized to the carboxy terminus. As outlined above, p53 binds the carboxy terminus of T antigen, and it is thought that the CBP/p300 proteins and mdm2 interact with T antigen through p53. Thus, one possibility is that the J domain acts on a p53/CBP, p53/p300, p53/p400 or p53/mdm2 complex bound at the carboxy terminus (Lill et al., 1997b), thereby altering the complex. Transformation by adenovirus E1A is mediated in part through binding to the CBP/p300 proteins. Currently, any affect of T antigen on a p53/CBP or p53/mdm2 protein complex is unclear.

Thus, it is currently assumed that in the absence of a functional J domain, any interaction between T antigen and the pRb proteins is not productive. However, our recent results appear to contradict this (Powell et al., 1999). We have shown that *dl*1135, which lacks a functional J domain, can complement the temperature-sensitive growth phenotype of REF cell lines conditionally immortalized with a temperature-sensitive T antigen. Furthermore, we have found that *dl*1135 can productively interact with p130 to activate transcription from a p130 target gene. Thus, at least in this assay, the J domain does not seem to be required for productive interaction with pRb proteins. Obviously, more work is required to resolve these apparently conflicting results.

Cis versus *Trans Complementation*

Another contentious issue is whether functions of T antigen can be complemented in *trans* (i.e., by a separate T antigen molecule) or whether complementation can only occur in *cis* (i.e., on the same T antigen molecule).

Tevethia et al. (1998) have reported that co-expression of T antigen fragments containing amino acids 1-147 and 251-708 results in immortalization whereas neither fragment can immortalize alone, suggesting that complementation can occur in *trans*. Other groups have reported that the amino terminus of T antigen can be complemented by the homologous region in small t, again suggesting complementation in *trans* (Montano et al., 1990; Porrás et al., 1996). Furthermore, small t can activate the p53 binding domain of large T when the proteins are co-expressed (Zerrahn et al., 1996). However, other groups have found that the J domain and the pocket protein binding domain need to be present in *cis* for a productive interaction to occur (Sheng et al., 1997; Srinivasan et al., 1997).

Some of these results may be difficult to interpret. It is thought that mutations in the amino terminus can affect carboxy terminus activity and *vice versa*. For instance, *dl*1135 is a T antigen mutant which lacks amino acids 17-27. Thus, this protein lacks a functional J domain since this mutation removes a portion of the predicted α–1 helix of the J domain. Although the *dl*1135 protein is still able to bind pRb/p107/p130 and p53, this protein lacks ATPase activity (which is localized to the carboxy terminus of T antigen; Collins and Pipas, 1995; Figure 3), presumably due to a conformational change in T antigen. This makes it difficult to interpret *cis versus trans* complementation experiments, since complementation in some instances may be possible, but is prevented due to a change in conformation of T antigen. Ongoing experiments in our lab are designed to address the question of complementation between T antigen mutants.

Initiation versus *Maintenance of Immortalization*

It is currently unclear whether all of the functions initially required by T antigen to induce the immortal state are required to maintain it.

Our results suggest that initiation and maintenance of immortalization require different activities of T antigen (Powell et al., 1999). In these studies, we have used the *dl*1135 deletion mutant, which lacks amino acids 17-27 and therefore contains no functional J domain, and a conditionally immortal cell line to examine whether *dl*1135 can maintain immortalization. These cells contain a temperature-sensitive mutant of T antigen which is wild-type at the permissive temperature, but inactive at the non-permissive temperature (Jat and Sharp, 1989; Gonos et al., 1996). Thus, when cells are moved to the non-permissive temperature, they senesce within 72 hours. This defect can be complemented by wild-type T antigen, adenovirus E1A, or HPV type 16 E7 protein (Vousden and Jat, 1989; Riley et al., 1990).

When these cells were transfected with plasmids expressing *dl*1135, and then moved to the non-permissive temperature, the cells were found to continue proliferating. These data, combined with the failure of *dl*1135 to immortalize primary cells, suggests that *dl*1135 contains all the functions necessary for maintenance of immortalization, but lacks a function(s) required for initiation of immortalization. Consequently, it seems that not all of the functions required by T antigen to initiate the immortal state are required to maintain it.

The deletion in *dl*1135 results in the loss of the J domain, but also alters the conformation of the carboxy terminus of T antigen, as demonstrated by the loss of ATPase activity of *dl*1135. *dl*1135 is still able to interact with the pRb family and p53 proteins. The current hypothesis suggests that in the absence of an active J domain these interactions are non-productive. However, as outlined earlier, we have demonstrated that the interaction with p130 is still productive in the absence of a J domain. It is currently unclear what function (or lack thereof) causes *dl*1135 to fail to initiate immortalization. Perhaps a functional J domain is only required during initiation of immortalization, and its primary role may not be the disassembly of pRb family-E2F complexes, but rather a novel, poorly-defined role. Future work should help clarify this question.

Role of Small T Antigen

It has been shown that small t antigen is not required for immortalization, transformation or tumorigenicity of SV40. However, small t enhances the transformation activity of SV40 when levels of T antigen are limiting (Rubin et al., 1982; Bikel et al., 1987), especially in non-replicating cells, and is necessary for the low frequency of transformation of human cells by SV40. Small t antigen also activates the carboxy terminal p53-binding domain of T antigen (Zerrahn et al., 1996) and co-operates in the metabolic stabilization of p53 (Tiemann et al., 1995).

Adjacent to the T/t common region (which encodes a J domain, see above), small t contains two X-Cys-X-X-Cys clusters which co-ordinate the binding of two zinc ions per molecule of small t (Turk et al., 1993). This zinc-binding domain directs the interaction of the trimeric protein phosphatase 2A (PP2A) with small t. Following the binding of small t to the A and C subunits of PP2A, the B regulatory subunit is released from the phosphatase trimer, and phosphatase activity is inhibited (Yang et al., 1991; Mungre et al., 1994). Srinivasan et al. (1997) have postulated that the J domain may direct hsc70 to the t antigen-bound PP2A, and the chaperone protein promotes disassembly of PP2A and thus stimulates induction of the MAP kinase cascade (Sontag et al., 1993). However, Porrás et al. (1996) have reported that the HPD tripeptide of the J domain is unlikely to be involved in inhibition of PP2A and mutations here don't affect the ability of small t to activate MAPK and MEK (assays that reflect inhibition of PP2A). Thus, as for large T antigen, there are conflicts between the model and the data. Hopefully, future work will assist in resolving the role of the J domains of the T and t antigens, as well as shed some light on the role of small t antigen.

The Biological Counting Mechanism

Cells immortalized by a temperature-sensitive mutant of T antigen enter senescence upon inactivation of T antigen (Jat and Sharp, 1989; Radna et al., 1989; Tsuyama et al., 1991; Gonos et al., 1996). This suggests that the endogenous life span has elapsed in these cells and that the biological clock which counts cell divisions is still active in the presence of T antigen. This is indeed the case. We have shown that in the presence of T antigen, the biological clock still counts cell divisions, thus, all the proteins and signals necessary for senescence are present in SV40-infected cells but entry into the post-mitotic state of senescence has been over-ridden (Ikram et al., 1994).

Besides p16 and p21, which accumulate in cells approaching senescence (see above), other proteins implicated in the biological clock and hence senescence control include p27, p19^{ARF}, p24, and p33^{ING1}. p27 is a cdk inhibitor, related to p21, which accumulates in oligodendrocyte precursor cells and therefore may determine when proliferation stops and differentiation begins (Casaccia-Bonnefil et al., 1997; Durand et al., 1997; Ibid., 1998). (Senescence can be thought of as a type of terminal differentiation occurring once mitosis has stopped, thus, the mechanisms of counting prior to differentiation or senescence are expected to be similar; Groves et al., 1991). Indeed, p27-null mice are abnormally large and have increased numbers of cells in many organs, suggesting a role for p27 in limiting cell proliferation in many cell lineages (Fero et al., 1996; Kiyokawa et al., 1996; Nakayama et al., 1996).

p19^{ARF} is the alternatively spliced product of the p16 genomic sequence. Since it is translated from a different reading frame than p16, p19^{ARF} is not a cdk inhibitor (Quelle et al., 1995) but nevertheless can induce cell-cycle arrest in a p53-dependent manner (Kamijo et al., 1997). p19^{ARF} interacts directly with the p53 inhibitor mdm2, and thereby promotes degradation of mdm2 and stabilization of p53 (Pomerantz et al., 1998; Zhang et al., 1998), resulting in cell cycle arrest. Loss of p19^{ARF} in a transgenic mouse yields MEFs which fail to enter senescence suggesting a role for p19^{ARF} in the biological clock (Kamijo et al., 1997).

Two novel proteins have also been implicated in the biological counting mechanism and senescence. p24 is a protein that accumulates in primary cells as they approach senescence and also accumulates in the presence of T antigen (Mazars and Jat, 1997).

Garkavtsev and Riabowol (1997) have described another protein, p33^{ING1}, whose expression levels increase as cells approach senescence and whose growth inhibitory affects can be suppressed by T antigen, resulting in extension of life span. Thus, a number of proteins have been implicated in the biological counting mechanism. It is currently unclear whether any of these proteins play a direct role in regulating senescence.

Conclusions

As outlined above, T antigen can immortalize primary cells by overriding their senescence program. The activities that allow T antigen to perform this function include the J domain at the amino terminus, the CR2-like domain which is responsible for binding the pRb family of pocket proteins, and the carboxy terminal domain, which is responsible for binding p53, the CBP/p300 family of proteins, mdm2, and contains an anti-apoptotic function. The J domain is thought to mediate the changes in these complexes which are brought about by binding T antigen, by recruiting a DnaK chaperone, possibly hsc70, to the complex. The chaperone then disassembles the complex.

A number of questions regarding the activities of T antigen remain. Firstly, is the J domain required for a productive interaction with the pRb proteins? Some reports suggest that it is, while our own data suggest that it isn't. Possibly the J domain is only required under certain circumstances. Secondly, can the T antigen functions operate in *trans*, or only in *cis*? What is the role of small t antigen? What functions are required for the initiation of immortalization, and are these same functions, or only a sub-group of them, required for maintenance of immortalization? Finally, how do the many interactions of T antigen promote immortalization? Is this simply through inhibiting the growth-suppressive activities of the pRb proteins and p53, or are other mechanisms involved? How might these mechanisms be related to the biological counting mechanism that counts cell divisions, and how is this counting mechanism in turn related to immortalization and senescence?

Future work should further illuminate how T antigen induces immortalization, and should hopefully clarify how senescence is induced under normal circumstances.

References

Allsop, R.C., Vaziri, H., Patterson, C., Goldstein, S., Younglai, E.V., Futcher, A.B., Greider, C.W., and Harley, C.B. (1992). Telomere length predicts replicative capacity of human fibroblasts. Proc. Natl. Acad. Sci. USA 89, 10114-10118.

Alwine, J.C., Reed, S.I., and Stark, G.R. (1977). Characterisation of the autoregulation of simian virus 40 gene A. J. Virol. 62, 285-296.

Anderson, M.M., Chen, J., Cole, C.N., and Conrad, S.E. (1996). Activation of the human thymidine kinase (tk) promoter by simian virus 40 large T antigen requires both the T antigen pRb family-binding domain and tk promoter sequences resembling E2F-binding sites. J. Virol. 70, 6304-6313.

Asselin, C., and Bastin, M. (1985). Sequences from polyomavirus and simian virus 40 large T genes capable of immortalizing primary rat embryo fibroblasts. J. Virol. 56, 958-968.

Atadja, P., Wong, H., Garkavtsev, I., Veillette, C., and Riabowol, K. (1995). Increased activity of p53 in senescing fibroblasts. Proc. Natl. Acad. Sci. USA 92, 8348-8352.

Autexier, C., and Greider, C.W. (1996). Telomerase and cancer: Revisiting the telomere hypothesis. Trends Biochem. Sci. 21, 387-391.

Avantaggiati, M.L., Carbone, M., Graessmann, A., Nakatani, Y., Howard, B., and Levine, A.S. (1996). The SV40 large T antigen and adenovirus E1a oncoproteins interact with distinct isoforms of the transcriptional co-activator, p300. EMBO J. 15, 2236-2248.

Avantaggiati, M.L., Ogryzko, V., Gardner, K., Giordano, A., Levine, A.S., and Kelly, K. (1997). Recruitment of p300/CBP in p53-dependent signal pathways. Cell 89, 1175-1184.

Bartek, J., Bartkova, J., and Lukas, J. (1996). The retinoblastoma protein pathway and the restriction point. Curr. Opin. Cell Biol. 8, 805-814.

Beijersbergen, R.L., Kerkhoven, R.M., Zhu, L., Carlee, L., Voorhoeve, P.M., and Bernards, R. (1994). E2F-4, a new member of the E2F gene family, has oncogenic activity and associates with p107 *in vivo*. Genes Dev. 8, 2680-2690.

Bierman, E.L. (1978). The effect of donor age on the *in vitro* life span of cultured human arterial smooth muscle cells. In Vitro 14, 951-955.

Bikel, I., Montano, X., Agha, M.E., Brown, M., McCormack, M., Boltax, J., and Livingston, D.M. (1987). SV40 small t antigen enhances the transformation activity of limiting concentrations of SV40 large T antigen. Cell 48, 321-330.

Blasco, M.A., Lee, H.-W., Hande, M.P., Samper, E., Lansdorp, P.M., DePinho, R.A., and Greider, C.W. (1997). Telomere shortening and tumor formation by mouse cells lacking telomerase RNA. Cell 91, 25-34.

Bodnar, A.G., Ouellette, M., Frolkis, M., Holt, S.E., Chiu, C.-P., Morin, G.B., Harley, C.B., Shay, J.W., Lichtsteiner, S., and Wright, W.E. (1998). Extension of life-span by introduction of telomerase into normal human cells. Science 279, 349-352.

Bond, J.A., Haughton, M., Blaydes, J., Wynford-Thomas, D., and Wyllie, F.S. (1996). Evidence that transcriptional activation by p53 plays a direct role in the induction of cellular senescence. Oncogene 13, 2097-2104.

Bremner, R., Cohen, B.L., Sopta, M., Hamel, P.A., Ingles, C.J., Gallie, B.L., and Phillips, R.A. (1995). Direct transcriptional repression by pRB and its reversal by specific cyclins. Mol. Cell. Biol. 15, 3256-3265.

Brodsky, J.L., and Pipas, J.M. (1998). Polyomavirus T antigens: Molecular chaperones for multiprotein complexes. J. Virol. 72, 5329-5334.

Brown, M., McCormack, M., Zinn, K.G., Farrel, M.P., Bikel, I., and Livingston, D.M. (1986). A recombinant murine retrovirus for simian virus 40 large T cDNA transforms mouse fibroblasts to anchorage-independent growth. J. Virol. 60, 290-293.

Brown, D.R., Deb, S., Munoz, R.M., Subler, M.A., and Deb, S.P. (1993). The tumor suppressor p53 and the oncoprotein simian virus 40 T antigen bind to overlapping domains on the MDM2 protein. Mol. Cell. Biol. 13, 6849-6857.

Brown, J.P., Wei, W., and Sedivy, J.M. (1997). Bypass of senescence after disruption of p21[CIP1/WAF1] gene in normal diploid human fibroblasts. Science 177, 831-834.

Buchkovich, K., Duffy, L.A., and Harlow, E. (1989). The retinoblatoma protein is phosphorylated during specific phases of the cell cycle. Cell 58, 1097-1105.

Buckbinder, L., Talbott, R., Velasco-Miguel, S., Takenaka, I., Faha, B., Seizinger, B.R., and Kley, N. (1995). Induction of the growth inhibitor IGF-binding protein 3 by p53. Nature 377, 646-649.

Bunn, C.L., and Tarrant, G.M. (1980). Limited lifespan in somatic cell hybrids and cybrids. Exp. Cell Res. 127, 385-396.

Campbell, K.S., Mullane, K.P., Aksoy, I.A., Stubdal, H., Zalvide, J., Pipas, J.M., Silver, P.A., Roberts, T.M., Schaffhausen, B.S., and DeCaprio, J.A. (1997). DnaJ/hsp40 chaperone domain of SV40 large T antigen promotes efficient viral DNA replication. Genes Dev. 11, 1098-1110.

Carroll, R.B., Hager, L., and Dulbecco, R. (1974). Simian virus 40 T antigen binds to DNA. Proc. Natl. Acad. Sci. USA 71, 3754-3757.

Carroll, R.B., Samad, A., Mann, A., Harper, J., and Anderson, C.W. (1988). RNA is covalently linked to SV40 large T antigen. Oncogene 2, 437-444.

Casaccia-Bonnefil, P., Tikoo, R., Kiyokawa, H., Friedrich, V. Jr., Chao, M.V., and Koff, A. (1997). Oligodendrocyte precursor differentiation is perturbed in the absence of the cyclin-dependent kinase inhibitor p27^{Kip1}. Genes Dev. 11, 2335-2346.

Chao, D.T., and Korsmeyer, S.J. (1998). Bcl-2 family: Regulators of cell death. Annu. Rev. Immunol. 16, 395-419.

Chellappan, S.P., Hiebert, S., Mudryj, M., Horowitz, J.M., and Nevins, J.R. (1991). The E2F transcription factor is a cellular target for the RB protein. Cell 65, 1053-1061.

Chen, S., and Paucha, E. (1990). Identification of a region of simian virus 40 large T antigen required for cell transformation. J. Virol. 64, 3350-3357.

Chen, J., Tobin, G.J., Pipas, J.M., and Van Dyke, T. (1992). T-antigen mutant activities *in vivo*: Roles of p53 and pRB binding in tumorigenesis of the choroid plexus. Oncogene 7, 1167-1175.

Chen, X., Ko, L.J., Jayaraman, L., and Prives, C. (1996). p53 levels, functional domains, and DNA damage determine the extent of the apoptotic response of tumor cells. Genes Dev. 10, 2438-2451.

Chittenden, T., Livingston, D.M., and Kaelin, W.G. (1991). The T/E1a binding domain of the retinoblastoma product can interact specifically with a sequence specific DNA binding protein. Cell 65, 1073-1082.

Collins, B.S., and Pipas, J.M. (1995). T antigens encoded by replication-defective simian virus 40 mutant-*dl*1135 and mutant-5080. J. Biol. Chem. 270, 15377-15384.

Conzen, S.D., and Cole, C.N. (1994). The transforming proteins of simian virus 40. Sem. Virol. 5, 349-356.

Conzen, S.D., and Cole, C.N. (1995). The three transforming regions of SV40 T antigen are required for immortalization of primary mouse embryo fibroblasts. Oncogene 11, 2295-2302.

Conzen, S.D., Snay, C.A., and Cole, C.N. (1997). Identification of a novel antiapoptotic functional domain in simian virus 40 large T antigen. J. Virol. 71, 4536-4543.

Cox, L.S. (1997). Who binds wins: Competition for PCNA rings out cell-cycle changes. Trends Cell Biol. 7, 493-498.

Cryns, V., and Yuan, J. (1998). Proteases to die for. Genes Dev. 12, 1551-1570.

Curatolo, L., Erba, E., and Morasca, L. (1984). Culture conditions induce the appearance of immortalized C3H mouse cell lines. In Vitro 20, 597-601.

Dagnino, L., Zhu, L., Skorecki, K.L., and Moses, H.L. (1995). E2F-independent transcriptional repression by p107, a member of the retinoblastoma family of proteins. Cell Growth Differ. 6, 191-198.

Dalton, S. (1992). Cell cycle regulation of the human *cdc2* gene. EMBO J 11, 1797-1804.

Damania, B., and Alwine, J.C. (1996). TAF-like function of SV40 large T antigen. Genes Dev. 10, 1369-1381.

de Lange, T. (1998). Telomeres and senescence: Ending the debate. Science 279, 334-335.

DeCaprio, J.A., Ludlow, J.W., Figge, J., Shew, J.-Y., Huang, C.-M., Lee, W.-H., Marsilio, E., Paucha, E., and Livingston, D.M. (1988). SV40 large tumor antigen forms a specific complex with the product of the retinoblastoma susceptibility gene. Cell 54, 275-283.

DeCaprio, J.A., Furukawa, Y., Ajchenbaum, F., Griffin, J.D., and Livingston, D.M. (1992). The retinoblastoma susceptibility gene product becomes phosphorylated in multiple stages during cell cycle entry and progression. Proc. Natl. Acad. Sci. USA 89, 1795-1798.

Dornreiter, I., Hoss, A., Arthur, A.K., and Fanning, E. (1990). SV40 T antigen binds directly to the large subunit of purified DNA polymerase alpha. EMBO J. 9, 3329-3336.

Dowdy, S.F., Hinds, P.W., Louis, K., Reed, S.I., Arnold, A., and Weinberg, R.A. (1993). Physical interactions of the retinoblastoma protein with human cyclins. Cell 73, 499-511.

Durand, B., Gao, F.-B., and Raff, M. (1997). Accumulation of the cyclin-dependent kinase inhibitor p27/Kip1 and the timing of oligodendrocyte differentiation. EMBO J. 16, 306-317.

Durand, B., Fero, M.L., Roberts, J.M., and Raff, M.C. (1998). p27Kip1 alters the response of cells to mitogen and is part of a cell-intrinsic timer that arrests the cell cycle and initiates differentiation. Curr. Biol. 8, 431-440.

Dyson, N., Buchkovich, K., Whyte, P., and Harlow, E. (1989). The cellular 107K protein that binds to adenovirus E1A also associates with the large T antigens of SV40 and JC virus. Cell 58, 249-255.

Dyson, N., Dembski, M., Fattaey, A., Ngwu, C., Ewen, M., and Helin, K. (1993). Analysis of p107-associated proteins: p107 associates with a form of E2F that differs form pRB-associated E2F-1. J. Virol. 67, 7641-7647.

Eckner, R., Ludlow, J.W., Lill, N.L., Oldread, E., Arany, Z., Modjtahedi, N., DeCaprio, J.A., Livingston, D.M., and Morgan, J.A. (1996). Association of p300 and CBP with simian virus 40 large T antigen. Mol. Cell. Biol. 16, 3454-3464.

El-Deiry, W.S., Harper, J.W., O'Connor, P.M., Velculescu, V.E., Canman, C.E., Jackman, J., Pietenpol, J.A., Burrell, M., Hill, D.E., Wang, Y., Wiman, K.G., Mercer, W.E., Kastan, M.B., Kohn, K.W., Elledge, S.J., Kinzler, K.W., and Vogelstein, B. (1994). *WAF1/CIP1* is induced in *p53*-mediated G$_1$ arrest and apoptosis. Cancer Res. 54, 1169-1174.

Ewen, M.E., Xing, Y.G., Lawrence, J.B., and Livingston, D.M. (1991). Molecular cloning, chromosomal mapping, and expression of the cDNA for p107, a retinoblastoma gene product-related protein. Cell 66, 1155-1164.

Ewen, M.E., Sluss, H.K., Sherr, C.J., Matsushime, H., Kato, J., and Livingston, D.M. (1993). Functional interactions of the retinoblastoma protein with mammalian D-type cyclins. Cell 73, 487-497.

Fanning, E. (1992). Simian virus 40 large T antigen: The puzzle, the pieces and the emerging picture. J. Virol. 66, 1289-1293.

Fanning, E., and Knippers, R. (1992). Structure and function of simian virus 40 large tumor antigen. Annu. Rev. Biochem. 61, 55-85.

Fero, M.L., Rivkin, M., Tasch, M., Porter, P., Carow, C.E., Firpo, E., Polyak, K., Tsai, L.H., Broudy, V., Perlmutter, R.M., Kaushansky, K., and Roberts, J.M. (1996). A syndrome of multiorgan hyperplasia with features of gigantism, tumorigenesis, and female sterility in p27(Kip1)-deficient mice. Cell 85, 733-744.

Figge, J., Webster, T., Smith, T.H., and Paucha, E. (1988). Prediction of similar transformating regions in SV40 large T, adenovirus E1A and myc oncogenes. J. Virol. 62, 1814-1818.

Flemington, E.K., Speck, S.H., and Kaelin, W.G., Jr. (1993). E2F-1-mediated transactivation is inhibited by complex formation with the retinoblastoma susceptibility gene product. Proc. Natl. Acad. Sci. USA 90, 6914-6918.

Flores-Rozas, H., Kelman, Z., Dean, F.B., Pan, Z.-Q., Harper, W.J., Elledge, S.J., O'Donnell, M., and Hurwitz, J. (1994). Cdk-interacting protein 1 directly binds with proliferating cell nuclear antigen and inhibits DNA replication catalyzed by the DNA polymerase δ holoenzyme. Proc. Natl. Acad. Sci. USA 91, 8655-8659.

Gannon, J.V., and Lane, D.P. (1987). p53 and DNA polymerase α compete for binding to SV40 T antigen. Nature 329, 456-458.

Garkavtsev, I., and Riabowol, K. (1997). Extension of the replicative life span of human diploid fibroblasts by inhibition of the p33^{ING1} candidate tumor suppressor. Mol. Cell. Biol. 17, 2014-2019.

Gelfant, S. (1977). A new concept of tissue and tumour cell proliferation. Cancer Res. 37, 3845-3862.

Giles, R.H., Peters, D.J.M., and Breuning, M.H. (1998). Conjunction dysfunction: CBP/p300 in human disease. Trends Genet. 14, 178-183.

Gilinger, G., and Alwine, J.C. (1993). Transcriptional activation by simian virus 40 large T antigen: Requirements for simple promoter structures containing either TATA or initiator elements with variable upstream factor binding sites. J. Virol. 67, 6682-6688.

Ginsberg, D., Mechta, F., Yaniv, M., and Oren, M. (1991). Wild type p53 can down-modulate the activity of various promoters. Proc. Natl. Acad. Sci. USA 88, 9979-9983.

Ginsberg, D., Vairo, G., Chittenden, T., Xiao, Z.X., Xu, G., Wydner, K.L., DeCaprio, J.A., Lawrence, J.B., and Livingston, D.M. (1994). E2F-4, a new member of the E2F transcription factor family, interacts with p107. Genes Dev. 8, 2665-2679.

Gire, V., and Wynford-Thomas, D. (1998). Reinitiation of DNA synthesis and cell division in senescent human fibroblasts by microinjection of anti-p53 antibodies. Mol. Cell. Biol. 18, 1611-1621.

Goldstein, S. (1990). Replicative senesncence: The human fibroblast comes of age. Science 249, 1129-1132.

Gonos, E.S., Burns, J.S., Mazars, G.R., Kobrna, A., Riley, T.E.W., Barnett, S.C., Zafarana, G., Ludwig, R.L., Ikram, Z., Powell, A.J., and Jat, P.S. (1996). Rat embryo fibroblasts immortalized with simian virus 40 large T antigen undergo senescence upon its inactivation. Mol. Cell. Biol. 16, 5127-5138.

Grand, R.J.A., Turnell, A.S., Mason, G.G.F., Wang, W., Milner, A.E., Mymryk, J.S., Rookes, S.M., Rivett, A.J., and Gallimore, P.H. (1999). Adenovirus early region 1A protein binds to mammlian SUG1 - a regulatory component of the proteasome. Oncogene.......

Griffin, B.E. (1981). Structure and genomic organisation of SV40 and polyoma virus. *In* "Molecular Biology of tumor viruses: DNA tumor viruses", 2 ed. (J. Tooze, Ed.). NY: Cold Spring Harbor Laboratory.

Grove, G.L., and Cristofalo, V.J. (1977). Characterisation of the cell cycle of cultured human diploid cells: Effects of ageing and hydrocortisone. J. Cell Physiol. 90, 415-422.

Groves, A.K., Bögler, O., Jat, P.S., and Noble, M. (1991). The cellular measurement of time. Curr. Opin. Cell Biol. 3, 224-229.

Gruda, M.C., Zabolotny, J.M., Xiao, J.H., Davidson, I., and Alwine, J.C. (1993). Transcriptional activation by simian virus 40 large T antigen: Interactions with multiple components of the transcription complex. Mol. Cell. Biol. 13, 961-969.

Gu, W., and Roeder, R.G. (1997). Activation of p53 sequence-specific DNA binding by acetylation of the p53 C-terminal domain. Cell 90, 595-606.

Gu, W., Shi, X.-L., and Roeder, R.G. (1997). Synergistic activation of transcription by CBP and p53. Nature 387, 819-823.

Hall, M., Bates, S., and Peters, G. (1995a). Evidence for different modes of action of cyclin-dependent kinase inhibitors: p15 and p16 bind to kinases, p21 and p27 bind to cyclins. Oncogene 11, 1581-1588.

Hall, P.A., Kearsey, J.M., Coates, P.J., Norman, D.G., Warbrick, E., and Cox, L.S. (1995b). Characterisation of the interaction between PCNA and Gadd45. Oncogene 10, 2427-2433.

Han, J., Sabbatini, P., Perez, L., Rao, D., Modha, D., and White, E. (1996). E1B 19K protein blocks apoptosis by interacting with and inhibiting the p53-inducible and death-promoting Bax protein. Genes Dev. 10, 461-477.

Hannon, G.J., Demetrick, D., and Beach, D. (1993). Isolation of the Rb-related p130 through its interaction with CDK2 and cyclins. Genes Dev. 7, 2378-2391.

Hansen, U., Tenen, D.G., Livingston, D.M., and Sharp, P. (1981). T antigen repression of SV40 early transcription from two promoters. Cell 27, 603-612.

Harley, C.B., Futcher, A.B., and Greider, C.W. (1990). Telomeres shorten during ageing of human fibroblasts. Nature 345, 458-460.

Harlow, E., Pim, D.C., and Crawford, L.V. (1981). Complex of simian virus 40 large-T antigen and host 53,000-molecular-weight protein in monkey cells. J. Virol. 37, 564-573.

Harper, J.W., Adami, G.R., Wei, N., Keyomarsi, K., and Elledge, S.J. (1993). The p21 cdk-interacting protein Cip1 is a potent inhibitor of G1 cyclin-dependent kinases. Cell 75, 805-816.

Harvey, D.M., and Levine, A.J. (1991). p53 alteration is a common event in the spontaneous immortalization of primary BALB/c murine embryo fibroblasts. Genes Dev. 5, 2375-2385.

Hayflick, L., and Moorhead, P.S. (1961). The serial cultivation of human diploid cell strains. Exp. Cell Res. 25, 585-621.

Hengartner, M.O. (1998). Death cycle and Swiss army knives. Nature 391, 441-442.

Henning, W., Rohaly, G., Kolzau, T., Knippschild, U., Maacke, H., and Deppert, W. (1997). MDM2 is a target of simian virus 40 in cellular transformation and during lytic infection. J. Virol. 71, 7609-7618.

Hiebert, S.W., Chellappan, S.P., Horowitz, J.M., and Nevins, J.R. (1992). The interaction of RB with E2F coincides with an inhibition of the transcriptional activity of E2F. Genes Dev. 6, 177-185.

Hijmans, E.M., Voorhoeve, P.M., Beijersbergen, R.L., van 't Veer, L., and Bernards, R. (1995). E2F-5, a new E2F family member that interacts with p130 *in vivo*. Mol. Cell. Biol. 15, 3082-3089.

Hunter, T., and Pines, J. (1994). Cyclins and cancer II: Cyclin D and CDK inhibitors come of age. Cell 79, 573-582.

Hurford, R.K. J., Cobrinik, D., Lee, M.-H., and Dyson, N. (1997). pRB and p107/p130 are required for regulated expression of different sets of E2F responsive genes. Genes Dev. 11, 1447-1463.

Ikram, Z., Norton, T., and Jat, P.S. (1994). The biological clock that measures the mitotic life-span of mouse embryo fibroblasts continues to function in the presence of simian virus 40 large tumor antigen. Proc. Natl. Acad. Sci. USA 91, 6448-6452.

Israeli, D., Tessler, E., Haupt, Y., Elkeles, A., Wilder, S., Amson, R., Telerman, A., and Oren, M. (1997). A novel p53-inducible gene, PAG680, encodes a nuclear zinc finger protein whose over-expression promotes apoptosis. EMBO J. 16, 4384-4392.

Jat, P.S., Cepko, C.L., Mulligan, R.C., and Sharp, P.A. (1986). Recombinant retroviruses encoding SV40 large T antigen and polyomavirus large and middle T antigens. Mol. Cell. Biol. 6, 1204-1217.

Jat, P.S., and Sharp, P.A. (1986). Large T antigens of simian virus 40 and polyomavirus efficiently establish primary fibroblasts. J. Virol. 59, 746-750.

Jat, P.S., and Sharp, P.A. (1989). Cell lines established by a temperature-sensitive simian virus 40 large-T-antigen gene are growth restricted at the non permissive temperature. Mol. Cell. Biol. 9, 1672-1681.

Kalderon, D., Richardson, W.D., Markham, A.F., and Smith, A.E. (1984). Sequence requirements for nuclear location of simian virus 40 large-T antigen. Nature 311, 33-38.

Kamijo, T., Zindy, F., Roussel, M.F., Quelle, D.E., Downing, J.R., Ashmun, R.A., Grosveld, G., and Sherr, C.J. (1997). Tumor suppression at the mouse INK4a locus mediated by the alternative reading frame product p19^{ARF}. Cell 91, 649-659.

Kastan, M.B., Onyekwere, O., Sidransky, D., Vogelstein, B., and Craig, R.W. (1991). Participation of p53 protein in the cellular response to DNA damage. Cancer Res. 51, 6304-6311.

Kato, J.-Y., Matsuoka, M., Hiebert, S.W., Ewen, M.E., and Sherr, C.J. (1993). Direct binding of cyclin D to the retinoblastoma gene product (pRb) and pRb phosphorylation by the cyclin D-dependent kinase CDK4. Genes Dev. 7, 331-342.

Kelley, W.L. (1998). The J-domain family and the recruitment of chaperone power. Trends Biochem. Sci. 23, 222-227.

Kelley, W.L., and Landry, S.J. (1994). Chaperone power in a virus? Trends Biochem. Sci. 19, 277-278.

Kelley, W.L., and Georgopoulos, C. (1997). The T/t common exon of simian virus 40, JC and BK polyomavirus T antigens can functionally replace the J-domain of the Escherichia coli DnaJ molecular chaperone. Proc. Natl. Acad. Sci. USA 94, 3674-3684.

Kidd, V.J. (1998). Proteolytic activities that mediate apoptosis. Annu. Rev. Physiol. 60, 533-573.

Kierstead, T.D., and Tevethia, M.J. (1993). Association of p53 binding and immortalization of primary C57BL/6 mouse embryo fibroblasts by using simian virus 40 T-antigen mutants bearing internal overlapping deletion mutations. J. Virol. 67, 1817-1829.

King, K.L., and Cidlowski, J.A. (1998). Cell cycle regulation and apoptosis. Annu. Rev. Physiol. 60, 601-617.

Kirkwood, T.B.L. (1996). Human senescence. BioEssays 18, 1009-1016.

Kiyokawa, H., Kineman, R.D., Manova-Todorova, K.O., Soares, V.C., Hoffman, E.S., Ono, M., Khanam, D., Hayday, A.C., Frohman, L.A., and Koff, A. (1996). Enhanced growth of mice lacking the cyclin-dependent kinase inhibitor function of p27(Kip1). Cell 85, 721-732.

Knudson, C.M., Tung, K.S.K., Tourtellotte, W.G., Brown, G.A.J., and Korsmeyer, S.J. (1995). Bax-deficient mice with lymphoid hyperplasia and male germ cell death. Science 270, 96-99.

Kohrman, D.C., and Imperiale, M.J. (1992). Simian virus 40 large T antigen complexes with a 185-kilodalton host protein. J. Virol. 66, 1752-1760.

Kriegler, M., Perez, C.F., Hardy, C., and Botchan, M. (1984). Transformation mediated by the SV40 T antigens: Separation of the overlapping SV40 early genes with a retroviral vector. Cell 38, 483-491.

Kuerbitz, S.J., Plunkett, B.S., Walsh, W.V., and Kastan, M.B. (1992). Wild type p53 is a cell cycle checkpoint determinant following irradiation. Proc. Natl. Acad. Sci. USA 89, 7491-7495.

Kulju, K.S., and Lehman, J.M. (1995). Increased p53 protein associated with aging in human diploid fibroblasts. Exp. Cell Res. 217, 336-345.

Land, H., Parada, L.F., and Weinberg, R.A. (1983). Tumourigenic conversion of primary embryo fibroblasts requires at least two cooperative oncogenes. Nature 314, 596-602.

Land, H., Chen, A.C., Morgensten, J.P., Parada, L.F., and Weinberg, R.A. (1986). Behaviour of myc and ras oncogenes in transformation of of rat embryo fibroblasts. Mol. Cell. Biol. 6, 1917-1925.

Lane, D.P., and Crawford, L.V. (1979). T antigen is bound to a host protein in SV40-transformed cells. Nature 278, 261-263.

Lanford, R.E., and Butel, J.S. (1984). Construction and characterization of an SV40 mutant defective in nuclear transport of T antigen. Cell 37, 801-813.

Lansdorp, P.M. (1997). Lessons from mice without telomerase. J. Cell Biol. 139, 309-312.

Lees, J.A., Saito, M., Vidal, M., Valentine, M., Look, T., Harlow, E., Dyson, N., and Helin, K. (1993). The retinoblastoma protein binds to a family of E2F transcription factors. Mol. Cell. Biol. 13, 7813-7825.

Levine, A.J. (1997). p53, the cellular gatekeeper for growth and division. Cell 88, 323-331.

Lew, D.J., and Kornbluth, S. (1996). Regulatory roles of cyclin-dependent kinase phosphorylation in cell cycle control. Curr. Opin. Cell Biol. 8, 795-804.

Li, J.J., and Kelly, T.J. (1984). Simian virus 40 DNA replication in vitro. Proc. Natl. Acad. Sci. USA 81, 6973-6977.

Li, Y., Graham, C., Lacey, S., Duncan, A.M.V., and Whyte, P. (1993). The adenovirus E1A-associated 130-kD protein is encoded by a member of the retinoblastoma gene family and physically interacts with cyclins A and E. Genes Dev. 7, 2366-2377.

Li, R., Waga, S., Hannon, G.J., Beach, D., and Stillman, B. (1994). Differential effects by the p21 CDK inhibitor on PCNA-dependent DNA replication and repair. Nature 371, 534-537.

Lill, N.L., Tevethia, M.J., Eckner, R., Livingston, D.M., and Modjtahedi, N. (1997a). p300 family members associate with the carboxyl terminus of simian virus 40 large tumor antigen. J. Virol. 71, 129-137.

Lill, N.L., Grossman, S.R., Ginsberg, D., DeCaprio, J., and Livingston, D.M. (1997b). Binding and modulation of p53 by p300/CBP coactivators. Nature 387, 823-827.

Linzer, D.I.H., and Levine, A.J. (1979). Characterization of a 54K dalton cellular SV40 tumor antigen present in SV40-transformed cells and uninfected embryonal carcinoma cells. Cell 17, 43-52.

Ludlow, J.W., DeCaprio, J.A., Huang, C.M., Lee, W.H., Paucha, E., and Livingston, D.M. (1989). SV40 large T antigen binds preferentially to an underphosphorylated member of the retinoblastoma susceptibility gene product family. Cell 56, 57-65.

Ludlow, J.W., Shon, J., Pipas, J.M., Livingston, D.M., and DeCaprio, J.A. (1990). The retinoblastoma susceptibility gene product undergoes cell cycle-dependent dephosphorylation and binding to and release from SV40 large T. Cell 60, 387-396.

Macieira-Coelho, A., and Azzarone, B. (1988). The transition from primary culture to spontaneous immortalization in mouse fibroblast populations. Anticancer Res. 8, 669-676.

Maltzman, W., and Czyzyk, L. (1984). UV irradiation stimulates levels of p53 cellular tumor antigen in nontransformed mouse cells. Mol. Cell. Biol. 4, 1689-1694.

Manos, M.M., and Gluzman, Y. (1984). Simian virus 40 large T-antigen point mutants that are defective in viral DNA replication but competent in oncogenic transformation. Mol. Cell. Biol. 4, 1125-1133.

Manos, M.M., and Gluzman, Y. (1985). Genetic and biochemical analysis of transformation-competent, replication-defective simian virus 40 large T antigen mutants. J. Virol. 53, 120-127.

Marton, A., Jean, D., Delbecchi, L., Simmons, D.T., and Bourgaux, P. (1993). Topoisomerase activity associated with SV40 large tumor antigen. Nucl. Acids Res. 21, 1689-1695.

Mayol, X., Grana, X., Baldi, A., Sang, N., Hu, Q., and Giordano, A. (1993). Cloning of a new member of the retinoblastoma gene family (pRb2) which binds to the E1A transforming domain. Oncogene 8, 2561-2566.

Mazars, G.R., and Jat, P.S. (1997). Expression of p24, a novel p21$^{WAF1/Cip1/Sdi1}$-related protein, correlates with measurement of the finite proliferative potential or rodent embryo fibroblasts. Proc. Natl. Acad. Sci. USA 94, 151-156.

McCarthy, S.A., Symonds, H.S., and Van Dyke, T. (1994). Regulation of apoptosis in transgenic mice by simian virus 40 T antigen-mediated inactivation of p53. Proc. Natl. Acad. Sci. USA 91, 3979-3983.

McConnell, B.B., Starborg, M., Brookes, S., and Peters, G. (1998). Inhibitors of cyclin-dependent kinases induce features of replicative senescence in early passage human diploid fibroblasts. Curr. Biol. 8, 351-354.

Mercer, W.E., Shields, M.T., Lin, D., Appella, E., and Ullrich, S.J. (1991). Growth suppression induced by wild-type p53 protein is accompanied by selective down-regulation of proliferating-cell nuclear antigen expression. Proc. Natl. Acad. Sci. USA 88, 1958-1962.

Mietz, J.A., Unger, T., Huibregtse, J.M., and Howley, P.M. (1992). The transcriptional transactivation function of wild-type p53 is inhibited by SV40 large T-antigen and by HPV-16 E6 oncoprotein. EMBO J. 11, 5013-5020.

Mitchell, P.J., Wang, C., and Tjian, R. (1987). Positive and negative regulation of transcription *in vitro*: Enhancer-binding protein AP-2 is inhibited by SV40 T antigen. Cell 50, 847-861.

Miyashita, T., Krajewski, S., Krajewska, M., Wang, H.G., Lin, H.K., Liebermann, D.A., Hoffman, B., and Reed, J.C. (1994). Tumor suppressor p53 is a regulator of bcl-2 and bax gene expression in vitro and in vivo. Oncogene 9, 1799-1805.

Moberg, K.H., Tyndall, W.A., and Hall, D.J. (1992). Wild-type murine p53 represses transcription from the murine c-myc promoter in a human glial cell line. J. Cell Biochem. 49, 208-215.

Montano, X., Millikan, R., Milhaven, J.M., Newsom, D.A., Ludlow, J.W., Arthur, A.K., Fanning, E., Bikel, I., and Livingston, D.M. (1990). Simian virus 40 small tumor antigen and an amino-terminal domain of large tumor antigen share a common transforming function. Proc. Natl. Acad. Sci. USA 87, 7448-7452.

Moran, E. (1988). A region of SV40 large T antigen can substitute for a transforming domain of the adenovirus E1A products. Nature 334, 168-170.

Morgan, D.O. (1997). Cyclin-dependent kinases: Engines, clocks and microprocessors. Annu. Rev. Cell Dev. Biol. 13, 261-291.

Munger, K., Werness, B.A., Dyson, N., Phelps, W.C., Harlow, E., and Howley, P.M. (1989). Complex formation of human papillomavirus E7 proteins with the retinoblastoma tumor suppressor gene product. EMBO J. 8, 4099-4105.

Mungre, S., Enderle, B., Turk, B., Porrás, A., Wu, Y.-Q., Mumby, M.C., and Rundell, K. (1994). Mutations which affect the inhibition of protein phosphatase 2A by simian virus 40 small-t antigen in vitro decrease viral transformation. J. Virol. 68, 1675-1681.

Murano, S., Thweatt, R., Reis, R.J.S., Jones, R.A., Moerman, E.J., and Goldstein, S. (1991). Diverse gene sequences are overexpressed in Werner syndrome fibroblasts undergoing premature replicative senescence. Mol. Cell. Biol. 11, 3905-3914.

Nakayama, K., Ishida, N., Shirane, M., Inomata, A., Inoue, T., Shishido, N., Horii, I., Loh, D.Y., and Nakayama, K. (1996). Mice lacking p27(Kip1) display increased body size, multiple organ hyperplasia, retinal dysplasia, and pituitary tumors. Cell 85, 707-720.

Nelson, D.A., Krucher, N.A., and Ludlow, J.W. (1997). High molecular weight protein phosphatase type 1 dephosphorylates the retinoblastoma protein. J. Biol. Chem. 272, 4528-4535.

Neuman, E., Flemington, E.K., Sellers, W.R., and Kaelin, W.G., Jr. (1994). Transcription of the E2F-1 gene is rendered cell-cycle dependent by E2F DNA-binding sites within its promoter. Mol. Cell. Biol. 14, 6607-6615.

Nigg, E.A. (1995). Cyclin-dependent protein kinases: Key regulators of the eukaryotic cell cycle. BioEssays 17, 471-480.

Noble, J.R., Rogan, E.M., Neumann, A.A., Bryan, T.M., and Reddel, R.R. (1996). Association of extended in vitro proliferative potential with loss of p16INK4 expression. Oncogene 13, 1259-1268.

Noda, A., Ning, Y., Venable, S.F., Pereira-Smith, O.M., and Smith, J.R. (1994). Cloning of senescent cell-derived inhibitors of DNA synthesis using an expression screen. Exp. Cell Res. 211, 90-98.

Nuell, M.J., Stewart, D.A., Walker, L., Friedman, V., Wood, C.M., Owens, G.A., Smith, J.R., Schneider, E.L., Dell'Orco, R., Lumpkin, C.K., Danner, D.B., and McClung, J.K. (1991). Prohibitin, an evolutionarily conserved intracellular protein that blocks DNA synthesis in normal fibroblasts and HeLa cells. Mol. Cell. Biol. 11, 1372-1381.

Oltvai, Z.N., Milliman, C.L., and Korsmeyer, S.J. (1993). Bcl-2 heterodimerises in vivo with a conserved homolog, Bax, that accelerates programmed cell death. Cell 74, 609-619.

Oren, M., Maltzman, W., and Levine, A.J. (1981). Post-translational regulation of the 54K cellular tumor antigen in normal and transformed cells. Mol. Cell. Biol. 1, 101-110.

Orgel, L.E. (1973). Aging of clones of mammalian cells. Nature 243, 441-445.

Palmero, I., McConnell, B., Parry, D., Brookes, S., Hara, E., Bates, S., Jat, P., and Peters, G. (1997). Accumulation of p16INK4a in mouse fibroblasts as a function of replicative senescence and not of retinoblastoma gene status. Oncogene 15, 495-503.

Pardee, A.B. (1989). G1 events and regulation of cell proliferation. Science 246, 603-608.

Peden, K.W., Spence, S.L., Tack, L.C., Cartwright, C.A., Srinivasan, A., and Pipas, J.M. (1990). A DNA replication-positive mutant of simian virus 40 that is defective for transformation and the production of infectious virions. J. Virol. 64, 2912-2921.

Peden, K.W., and Pipas, J.M. (1992). Simian virus 40 mutants with amino-acid substitutions near the amino terminus of large T antigen. Virus Genes 6, 107-118

Pereira-Smith, O.M., and Smith, J.R. (1981). Expression of SV40 large T antigen in finite life-span hybrids of normal and SV40-transformed fibroblasts. Somat. Cell Genet. 7, 411-421.

Pereira-Smith, O.M., and Smith, J.R. (1988). Genetic analysis of indefinite division in human cells: Identification of four complementation groups. Proc. Natl. Acad. Sci. USA 85, 6042-6046.

Pereira-Smith, O.M., Spiering, A.L., and Smith, J.R. (1989). Cellular senescence: The result of a genetic program. In "Growth control during cell aging" (E. Wang, and H. R. Warner, Eds.) Boca Raton: CRC Press Inc.

Pereira-Smith, O.M., Robetorye, S., Ning, Y., and Orson, F.M. (1990). Hybrids from fusion of normal human T lymphocytes with immortal human cells exhibit limited life span. J. Cell Physiol. 144, 546-549.

Petit, C.A., Gardes, M., and Feunteun, J. (1983). Immortalisation of rat embryo fibroblasts by SV40 is maintained by the A gene. Virology 127, 74-82.

Pomerantz, J., Schreiber-Agus, N., Liegeois, N.J., Silverman, A., Alland, L., Chin, L., Potes, J., Chen, K., Orlow, I., Lee, H.W., Cordon-Cardo, C., and DePinho, R.A. (1998). The Ink4a tumor suppressor gene product, p19Arf, interacts with MDM2 and neutralizes MDM2's inhibition of p53. Cell 92, 713-723.

Porrás, A., Bennett, J., Howe, A., Tokos, K., Bouck, N., Henglein, B., Sathyamangalam, S., Thimmapaya, B., and Rundell, K. (1996). A novel simian virus 40 early-region domain mediates transactivation of the cyclin A promoter by small-t antigen and is required for transformation in small-t antigen-dependent assays. J. Virol. 70, 6902-6908.

Powell, A.J., Gonos, E.S., Peden, K.W.C., Pipas, J.M., and Jat, P.S. (1999). Oncogene 18, 7343-7350.

Prives, C. (1990). The replication functions of SV40 T antigen are regulated by phosphorylation. Cell 61, 735-738.

Prives, C., Barnet, B., Scheller, A., Khoury, G., and Gilbert, J. (1982). Discrete regions of simian virus 40 large T antigen are required for nonspecific and viral origin-specific DNA binding. J. Virol. 43, 73-82.

Qin, X.-Q., Livingston, D.M., Kaelin, W.G., Jr., and Adams, P.D. (1994). Deregulated E2F-1 transcription factor expression leads to S-phase entry and p53-mediated apoptosis. Proc. Natl. Acad. Sci. USA 91, 10918-10922.

Qin, X.-Q., Livingston, D.M., Ewen, M., Sellers, W.R., Arany, Z., and Kaelin, W.G., Jr. (1995). The transcription factor E2F-1 is a downstream target of RB action. Mol. Cell. Biol. 15, 742-755.

Quelle, D.E., Zindy, F., Ashmun, R.A., and Sherr, C.J. (1995). Alternative reading frames of the INK4a tumor suppressor gene encode two unrelated proteins capable of inducing cell cycle arrest. Cell 83, 993-1000.

Radna, L.R., Caton, Y., Jha, K.K., Kaplan, P., Li, G., Traganos, F., and Ozer, H.L. (1989). Growth of immortal SV40 tsA-tansformed human fibroblasts is temperature dependent. Mol. Cell. Biol. 9, 3093-3096.

Rao, L.M., Debbas, M., Sabbatini, P., Hockenbery, D., Korsmeyer, S., and White, E. (1992). The adenovirus E1A proteins induce apoptosis which is inhibited by the E1B 19K and Bcl-2 proteins. Proc. Natl. Acad. Sci. USA 89, 7742-7746.

Ray, F.A., Peabody, D.S., Cooper, J.L., Cram, L.S., and Kraemer, P.M. (1990). SV40 T antigen alone drives karyotype instability that precedes neoplastic transformation of human diploid fibroblasts. J. Cell. Biochem. 42, 13-31.

Rice, P.W., and Cole, C.N. (1993). Efficient transcriptional activation of many simple modular promoters by simian virus 40 large T antigen. J. Virol. 67, 6689-6697.

Riley, T.E.W., Follin, A., Jones, N.C., and Jat, P.S. (1990). Maintenance of cellular proliferation by adenovirus early region 1A in fibroblasts conditionally immortalized by using simian virus 40 large T antigen requires conserved region 1. Mol. Cell. Biol. 10, 6664-6673.

Risser, R., and Pollack, R. (1974). A nonselective analysis of SV40 transformation of mouse 3T3 cells. Virology 59, 477-489.

Rittling, S.R., and Denhardt, D.T. (1992). p53 mutations in spontaneously immortalized 3T12 but not 3T3 mouse embryo cells. Oncogene 7, 935-942.

Robles, M.T.S., Symonds, H., Chen, J., and Van Dyke, T. (1994). Induction versus progression of brain tumor development: Differential functions for the pRb-targeting and p53-targeting domains of simian virus 40 T antigen. Mol. Cell. Biol. 14, 2686-2698.

Robles, S.J., and Adami, G.R. (1998). Agents that cause DNA double strand breaks lead to p16INK4a enrichment and the premature senescence of normal fibroblasts. Oncogene 16, 1113-1123.

Rohme, D. (1981). Evidence for a relationship between longevity of mammalian species and life spans of normal fibroblasts *in vitro* and erythrocytes *in vivo*. Proc. Natl. Acad. Sci. USA 78, 5009-5013.

Rubin, H., Figge, J., Bladon, M.T., Chen, L.B., Ellman, M., Bikel, I., Farell, M., and Livingston, D.M. (1982). Role of small t antigen in the acute transforming activity of SV40. Cell 30, 469-480.

Ruley, H.E. (1983). Adenovirus E1a enables cellular and viral genes to transform primary cells in culture. Nature 304, 602-606.

Rushton, J.J., Jiang, D., Srinivasan, A., Pipas, J.M., and Robbins, P.D. (1997). Simian virus 40 T antigen can regulate p53-mediated transcription independent of binding p53. J. Virol. 71, 5620-5623.

Saffer, J.D., Jackson, S.P., and Thurston, S.J. (1990). SV40 stimulates expression of the *trans*-acting factor Sp1 at the mRNA level. Genes Dev. 4, 659-666.

Santos, M., and Butel, J.S. (1982). Association of SV40 large tumor antigen and cellular proteins on the surface of SV40-transformed mouse cells. Virology 120, 1-17.

Sawai, E.T., and Butel, J.S. (1989). Association of a cellular heat shock protein with simian virus 40 large T antigen in transformed cells. J. Virol. 63, 3961-3973.

Sawai, E.T., Rasmussen, G., and Butel, J.S. (1994). Construction of SV40 deletion mutants and delimitation of the binding domain for heat shock protein to the amino terminus of large T-antigen. Virus Res. 31, 367-378.

Scheffner, M., Knippers, R., and Stahl, H. (1989). RNA unwinding activity of SV40 large T antigen. Cell 57, 955-963.

Sedivy, J.M. (1998). Can ends justify the means?: Telomeres and the mechanisms of replicative senescence and immortalization in mammalian cells. Proc. Natl. Acad. Sci. USA 95, 9078-9081.

Serrano, M., Hannon, G.J., and Beach, D, (1993). A new regulatory motif in cell-cycle control causing specific inhibition of cyclin D/CDK4. Nature 366, 704-707.

Serrano, M., Lee, H.-W., Chin, L., Cordon-Cardo, C., Beach, D., and DePinho, R.A. (1996). Role of the *INK4a* locus in tumor suppression and cell mortality. Cell 85, 27-37.

Shan, B., and Lee, W.-H. (1994). Deregulated expression of E2F-1 induces S-phase entry and leads to apoptosis. Mol. Cell. Biol. 14, 8166-8173.

Shapiro, G.I., Edwards, C.D., Ewen, M.E., and Rollins, B.J. (1998). p16^{INK4A} participates in a G_1 arrest checkpoint in response to DNA damage. Mol. Cell. Biol. 18, 378-387.

Sheikh, M.S., Burns, T.F., Huang, Y., Wu, G.S., Amundson, S., Brooks, K. S., Fornace, A.J. J., and El-Deiry, W.S. (1998). p53-dependent and -independent regulation of the death receptor KILLER/DR5 gene expression in response to genotoxic stress and tumor necrosis factor alpha. Cancer Res. 58, 1593-1598.

Sheng, Q., Denis, D., Ratnofsky, M., Roberts, T.M., DeCaprio, J.A., and Schaffhausen, B. (1997). The DnaJ domain of polyomavirus large T antigen is required to regulate Rb family tumor suppressor function. J. Virol. 71, 9410-9416.

Sherr, C.J., and Roberts, J.M. (1995). Inhibitors of mammalian G1 cyclin-dependent kinases. Genes Dev. 9, 1149-1163.

Sherwood, S.W., Rush, D., Ellsworth, J.L., and Schimke, R.T. (1988). Defining cellular senescence in IMR-90 cells: A flow cytometric analysis. Proc. Natl. Acad. Sci. USA 85, 9086-9090.

Shiio, Y., Yamamoto, T., and Yamaguchi, N. (1992). Negative regulation of Rb expression by the p53 gene product. Proc. Natl. Acad. Sci. USA 89, 5206-5210.

Simmons, D.T., Melendy, T., Usher, D., and Stillman, B. (1996). Simian virus 40 large T antigen binds topoisomerase 1. J. Virol. 222, 365-374.

Sladek, T.L. (1997). E2F transcription factor action, regulation and possible role in human cancer. Cell Prolif. 30, 97-105.

Smale, S.T., and Tjian, R. (1986). T-antigen-DNA polymerase α complex implicated in simian virus 40 DNA replication. Mol. Cell. Biol. 6, 4077-4087.

Smith, M.L., Chen, I.T., Zhan, Q., Bae, I., Chen, C.Y., Gilmer, T.M., Kastan, M.B., O'Connor, P.M., and Fornace, A.J., Jr. (1994). Interaction of the p53-regulated protein Gadd45 with proliferating cell nuclear antigen. Science 266, 1376-1380.

Smith, J.R., and Pereira-Smith, O.M. (1996). Replicative senescence: Implications for in vivo aging and tumor suppression. Science 273, 63-67.

Soeda, E., Maruyama, T., Arrand, J.R., and Griffin, B.E. (1980). Host-dependent evolution of three papova viruses. Nature 285, 165-167.

Sompayrac, L., and Danna, K.J. (1985). The simian virus 40 sequences between 0.169 and 0.423 units are not essential to immortalise early-passage rat embryo cells. Mol. Cell. Biol. 5, 1191-1194.

Sompayrac, L., and Danna, K.J. (1988). A new SV40 mutant that encodes a small fragment of T antigen transforms established rat and mouse cells. Virology 163, 391-396.

Sompayrac, L., and Danna, K. J. (1991). The amino-terminal 147 amino acids of SV40 large T antigen transform secondary rat embryo fibroblasts. Virology 181, 412-415.

Sompayrac, L., and Danna, K.J. (1992). An amino-terminal fragment of SV40 T antigen transforms REF52 cells. Virology 191, 439-442.

Sontag, E., Fedorov, S., Kamibayashi, C., Robbins, D., Cobb, M., and Mumby, M. (1993). The interaction of SV40 small t antigen with protein phosphatase 2A stimulates the Map kinase pathway and induces cell proliferation. Cell 75, 887-897.

Soule, H.R., and Butel, J.S. (1979). Subcellular localisation of simian virus 40 large tumor antigen. J. Virol. 30, 523-532.

Srinivasan, A., McClellan, A.J., Vartikar, J., Marks, I., Cantalupo, P., Lin, Y., Whyte, P., Rundell, K., Brodsky, J.L., and Pipas, J.M. (1997). The amino-terminal transforming region of simian virus 40 large T and small t antigens functions as a J domain. Mol. Cell. Biol. 17, 4761-4773.

Stahl, H., Droge, P., and Knippers, R. (1986). DNA helicase activity of SV40 large tumor antigen. EMBO J. 5, 1939-1944.

Stamps, A.C., Gusterson, B.A., and O'Hare, M.J. (1992). Are tumours immortal? Eur. J. Cancer 28A, 1495-1500.

Stein, G.H., Beeson, M., and Gordon, L. (1990). Failure to phosphorylate the retinoblastoma gene product in senescent human fibroblasts. Science 249, 666-669.

Stewart, N., and Bacchetti, S. (1991). Expression of SV40 large T antigen, but not small t antigen, is required for the induction of chromosomal aberrations in transformed human cells. Virology 180, 49-57.

Strauss, M., and Griffin, B.E. (1990). Cellular immortalization- An essential step or merely a risk factor in DNA virus-induced transformation? Cancer Cells 2, 360-365.

Stringer, J.R. (1982). Mutant of simian virus 40 large T-antigen that is defective for viral DNA synthesis, but competent for transformation of cultured rat cells. J. Virol. 42, 854-864.

Stubdal, H., Zalvide, J., and DeCaprio, J.A. (1996). Simian virus 40 large T antigen alters the phosphorylation state of the RB-related proteins p130 and p107. J. Virol. 70, 2781-2788.

Stubdal, H., Zalvide, J., Campbell, K.S., Schweitzer, C., Roberts, T.M., and DeCaprio, J.A. (1997). Inactivation of pRB-related proteins p130 and p107 mediated by the J domain of simian virus 40 large T antigen. Mol. Cell. Biol. 17, 4979-4990.

Sugrue, M.M., Shin, D.Y., Lee, S.W., and Aaronson, S.A. (1997). Wild-type p53 triggers a rapid senescence program in human tumor cells lacking functional p53. Proc. Natl. Acad. Sci. USA 94, 9648-9653.

Suzuki-Takahashi, I., Kitagawa, M., Saijo, M., Higashi, H., Ogino, H., Matsumoto, H., Taya, Y., Nishimura, S., and Okuyama, A. (1995). The interactions of E2F with pRB and with p107 are regulated via the phosphorylation of pRB and p107 by a cyclin-dependent kinase. Oncogene 10, 1691-1698.

Symonds, H.S., McCarthy, S.A., Chen, J., Pipas, J.M., and Van Dyke, T. (1993). Use of transgenic mice reveals cell-specific transformation by a simian virus 40 T-antigen amino-terminal mutant. Mol. Cell. Biol. 13, 3255-3265.

Symonds, H., Krall, L., Remington, L., Saenz-Robles, M., Lowe, S., Jacks, T., and Van Dyke, T. (1994). p53-dependent apoptosis suppresses tumor growth and progression in vivo. Cell 78, 703-711.

Tahara, H., Sato, E., Noda, A., and Ide, T. (1995). Increase in expression level of $p21^{sdi1/cip1/waf1}$ with increasing division age in both normal and SV40-transformed human fibroblasts. Oncogene 10, 835-840.

Tavassoli, M., and Shall, S. (1988). Transcription of the c-*myc* oncogene is altered in spontaneously immortalised rodent fibroblasts. Oncogene 2, 337-345.

Tegtmeyer, P. (1972). SV40 DNA synthesis: The viral replicon. J. Virol. 10, 591-598.

Tevethia, M.J., Pipas, J.M., Kierstead, T., and Cole, C. (1988). Requirements for immortalization of primary mouse embryo fibroblasts probed with mutants bearing deletions in the 3' end of SV40 gene A. Virology 162, 79-89.

Tevethia, M.J., Lacko, H.A., and Conn, A. (1998). Two regions of simian virus 40 large T-antigen independently extend the life span of primary C57BL/6 mouse embryo fibroblasts and cooperate in immortalization. Virology 243, 303-312.

Thompson, D.L., Kalderon, D., Smith, A.E., and Tevethia, M.J. (1990). Dissociation of Rb-binding and anchorage-independent growth from immortalization and tumorigenicity using SV40 mutants producing N-terminally truncated large T antigens. Virology 178, 15-34.

Tiemann, F., Zerrahn, J., and Deppert, W. (1995). Cooperation of simian virus 40 large T and small t antigens in metabolic stabilization of tumor suppressor p53 during cellular transformation. J. Virol. 69, 6115-6121.

Tjian, R., Fey, G., and Graessmann, A. (1978). Biological activity of purified simian virus 40 T antigen proteins. Proc. Natl. Acad. Sci. USA 75, 1279-1283.

Tjian, R., and Robbins, R. (1979). Enzymatic activities associated with purified simian virus 40 T antigen-related protein. Proc. Natl. Acad. Sci. USA 76, 610-615.

Todaro, G.J., and Green, H. (1963). Quantitative studies of the growth of mouse embryo cells in culture and their development into established cell lines. J. Cell Biol. 17, 299-313.

Tooze, J., Ed. (1981). "Molecular biology of tumor viruses: DNA tumor viruses", 2 ed. NY: Cold Spring Harbor Laboratory.

Tsuyama, N., Miura, M., Kitahira, M., Ishibashi, S., and Ide, T. (1991). SV40 T-antigen is required for maintenance of immortal growth in SV40-transformed human fibroblasts. Cell Struct. Funct. 16, 55-62.

Turk, B., Porrás, A., Mumby, M.C., and Rundell, K. (1993). Simian virus 40 small-t antigen binds two zinc ions. J. Virol. 67, 3671-3673.

Uhrbom, L., Nister, M., and Westermark, B. (1997). Induction of senescence in human malignant glioma cells by p16INK4A. Oncogene 15, 505-514.

Vairo, G., Livingston, D.M., and Ginsberg, D. (1995). Functional interaction between E2F-4 and p130: Evidence for distinct mechanisms underlying growth suppression by different retinoblastoma protein family members. Genes Dev. 9, 869-881.

Vaziri, H., and Benchimol, S. (1998). Reconstitution of telomerase activity in normal human cells leads to elongation of telomeres and extended replicative life span. Curr. Biol. 8, 279-282.

Vogt, M., Haggblom, C., Yeargin, J., Christiansen-Weber, T., and Haas, M. (1998). Independent induction of senescence by p16^{INK4a} and p21^{CIP1} in spontaneously immortalized human fibroblasts. Cell Growth Differ. 9, 139-146.

Vojta, P.J., and Barrett, J.C. (1995). Genetic analysis of cellular senescence. Biochim. Biophys. Acta 1242, 29-41.

Vousden, K.H., and Jat, P.S. (1989). Functional similarity between HPV16E7, SV40 large T and adenovirus E1a proteins. Oncogene 4, 153-158.

Waga, S., Hannon, G.J., Beach, D., and Stillman, B. (1994). The p21 inhibitor of cyclin-dependent kinases controls DNA replication by interaction with PCNA. Nature 369, 574-578.

Warbrick, E. (1998). PCNA binding through a conserved motif. BioEssays 20, 195-199.

Weinberg, R.A. (1985). The action of oncogenes in the cytoplasm and the nucleus. Science 230, 770-776.

Weinberg, R.A. (1995). The retinoblastoma protein and cell cycle control. Cell 81, 323-330.

White, E., Cipriani, P., Sabbatini, P., and Denton, A. (1991). Adenovirus E1B 19-kilodalton protein overcomes the cytotoxicity of E1A proteins. J. Virol. 65, 2968-2978.

Wiman, K.G. (1997). p53: Emergency brake and target for cancer therapy. Exp. Cell Res. 237, 14-18.

Woods, C., LeFeuvre, C., Stewart, N., and Bacchetti, S. (1994). Induction of genomic instability in SV40 transformed human cells: Sufficiency of the N-terminal 147 amino acids of large T antigen and role of pRB and p53. Oncogene 9, 2943-2950.

Wu, X., Bayle, J.H., Olson, D., and Levine, A.J. (1993). The p53-mdm2 autoregulatory feedback loop. Genes Dev. 7, 1126-1132.

Wu, G.S., Burns, T.F., McDonald, E.R., 3rd, Jiang, W., Meng, R., Krantz, I.D., Kao, G., Gan, D.D., Zhou, J.Y., Muschel, R., Hamilton, S.R., Spinner, N.B., Markowitz, S., Wu, G., and El-Deiry, W.S. (1997). KILLER/DR5 is a DNA damage-inducible p53-regulated death receptor gene. Nature Genet. 17, 141-143.

Xiong, Y., Hannon, G.J., Zhang, H., Casso, D., Kobayashi, R., and Beach, D. (1993). p21 is a universal inhibitor of cyclin kinases. Nature 366, 701-704.

Yaciuk, P., Carter, M.C., Pipas, J.M., and Moran, E. (1991). Simian virus 40 large-T antigen expresses a biological activity complementary to the p300-associated transforming function of the adenovirus E1A gene products. Mol. Cell. Biol. 11, 2116-2124.

Yanai, N., and Obinata, M. (1994). Apoptosis is induced at nonpermissive temperature by a transient increase in p53 in cell lines immortalized with temperature-sensitive SV40 large T-antigen gene. Exp. Cell Res. 211, 296-300.

Yang, S.-I., Lickteig, R.L., Estes, R., Rundell, K., Walter, G., and Mumby, M.C. (1991). Control of protein phosphatase 2A by simian virus 40 small-t antigen. Mol. Cell. Biol. 11, 1988-1995.

Yin, X.-M., Oltvai, Z.N., and Korsmeyer, S.J. (1994). BH1 and BH2 domains of Bcl-2 are required for inhibition of apoptosis and heterodimerization with Bax. Nature 369, 321-323.

Zakian, V.A. (1995). Telomeres: Beginning to understand the end. Science 270, 1601-1607.

Zakian, V.A. (1997). Life and cancer without telomerase. Cell 91, 1-3.

Zalvide, J., Stubdal, H., and DeCaprio, J.A. (1998). The J domain of simian virus 40 large T antigen is required to functionally inactivate RB family proteins. Mol. Cell. Biol. 18, 1408-1415.

Zerrahn, J., Knippschild, U., Winkler, T., and Deppert, W. (1993). Independent expression of the transforming amino-terminal domain of SV40 large T antigen from an alternatively spliced third SV40 early mRNA. EMBO J. 12, 4739-4746.

Zerrahn, J., Tiemann, F., and Deppert, W. (1996). Simian virus 40 small t antigen activates the carboxyl-terminal transforming p53-binding domain of large T antigen. J. Virol. 70, 6781-6789.

Zhang, Y., Xiong, Y., and Yarbrough, W.G. (1998). ARF promotes MDM2 degradation and stabilizes p53: ARF-INK4a locus deletion impairs both the Rb and p53 tumor suppression pathways. Cell 92, 725-734.

Zhu, J.Y., Rice, P.W., Chamberlain, M., and Cole, C.N. (1991a). Mapping the transcriptional transactivation function of simian virus 40 large T antigen. J. Virol. 65, 2778-2790.

Zhu, J., Abate, M., Rice, P.W., and Cole, C.N. (1991b). The ability of simian virus 40 large T antigen to immortalize primary mouse embryo fibroblasts cosegregates with its ability to bind to p53. J. Virol. 65, 6872-6880.

Zhu, L., van den Heuvel, S., Helin, K., Fattaey, A., Ewen, M., Livingston, D., Dyson, N., and Harlow, E. (1993). Inhibition of cell proliferation by p107, a relative of the retinoblastoma protein. Genes Dev. 7, 1111-1125.

Ziff, E.B. (1980). Transcription and RNA processing by the DNA tumour viruses. Nature 287, 491-499.

Zindy, F., Quelle, D.E., Roussel, M.F., and Sherr, C.J. (1997). Expression of the p16[INK4a] tumor suppressor versus other INK4 family members during mouse development and aging. Oncogene 15, 203-211.

ADENOVIRUS EARLY REGION 1 PROTEINS: ACTION THROUGH INTERACTION.

Roger J.A. Grand

CRC Institute for Cancer Studies, University of Birmingham, UK

1. Introduction

The significance of adenoviruses in the context of this book rests on two seminal sets of observations. Firstly, in the early 1960s it was demonstrated that group A adenoviruses (Ad12, Ad18 and Ad31) could induce tumors after injection into newborn rodents (Trentin et al., 1962; Yabe et al., 1962; 1964; Green and Pina, 1964). Secondly, it was shown, about ten years later, that a region located towards the left-hand end of the Ad genome, which encoded the early region 1 (E1) proteins, could transform rodent cells in culture (Gallimore et al., 1974; Graham et al., 1974). Since that time adenoviruses have become a much-studied model for virus-induced cell transformation with the early region 1A (E1A) protein being considered a paradigm for viral transforming proteins.

Adenovirus early region 1 encodes four major proteins – two from E1A and two from E1B. The two homologous E1A components, which only differ by the inclusion of a 30-40 amino acid polypeptide located towards the C-terminus of the larger molecule, are essential for Ad-mediated transformation and, to all intents and purposes, for viral infection. Two quite distinct proteins are transcribed from E1B and these greatly increase the frequency of Ad E1A-mediated transformation by acting as anti-apoptosis factors and play major roles in viral infection. It now appears that none of the adenovirus E1 proteins possesses enzymic activity – therefore, it seems that they exert their influence, both during viral infection and during cellular transformation, through a complex series of protein-protein interactions with important cellular components. It is this ability to form complexes which is the subject of this chapter. Adenovirus virology and biochemistry has recently been considered at great length in a three volume monograph (Doerfler and Bohm, 1995) as well as in a series of review articles (see for example, Boulanger and Blair, 1991; Moran, 1994; Bayley and Mymryk, 1994; Shenk, 1996; Flint and Shenk, 1997). In addition, the role of Ad E1 proteins in the induction and suppression of apoptosis has been described at some length in this book (see Chapter 13) and elsewhere (White, 1996; 1998; Chinnadurai, 1998; Teodoro and Branton, 1997a). Therefore this review will concentrate on a discussion of recent advances in our understanding of the relationship between the adenovirus E1 proteins and the cellular components with which they interact. Hopefully this will shed new light on the means by which adenoviral E1 proteins affect target cells both during transformation and infection. In addition, it may provide pointers to general mechanisms of cell transformation and oncogenesis.

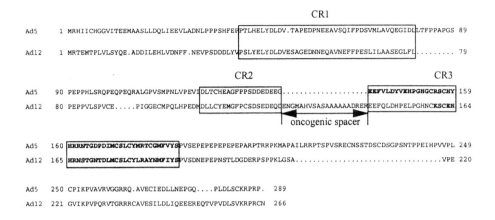

Fig. 1. Comparison of the amino acid sequences of Ad5 and Ad12 early region 1A proteins. The sequences are arranged to give maximum homology. The dimensions of conserved regions (CR) 1, 2 and 3 are shown, as is the 'oncogenic spacer' or 'unique' region present only in the Ad12 protein. The amino acid sequences present only in the proteins translated from 13S mRNAs are indicated in bold type.

2. Adenovirus Early Region 1A

a. *Strucure of Ad E1A*

Ad E1A is the first protein to be expressed during viral infection and is essential for Ad-mediated transformation. It is encoded within the first 1500bp of the Ad genome. Whilst there are a number of E1A proteins expressed during infection (see for example Boulanger and Blair, 1991) two major polypeptides are translated from 13S and 12S mRNAs following infection or transfection of Ad E1A DNA. In all virus serotypes the proteins translated from these mRNAs are identical except from the presence of a unique region located towards the C-terminus of the larger molecule (Figure 1).

Comparison of the amino acid sequences of Ad E1As from different virus serotypes has allowed the definition of three regions of marked homology – conserved regions (CR) 1, 2 and 3 (Figure 1). These sequences are the sites for interaction with a large number of E1A-binding proteins and are responsible for many of the properties of E1A. In addition, there are less well-conserved regions, such as the N-terminus, which are also sites of interaction and are important for the biological activity of E1A. Overall, about half of the amino acids are identical in Ad2/5 and Ad12 E1As but the conservation is appreciably greater in the conserved regions (Figure 1). E1A also has limited areas of homology to other viral oncoproteins such as SV40 Tag and HPV E7 and, more interestingly, to cellular proteins such as cyclin D (Dowdy et al., 1993; Kato et al., 1993), C-terminal binding protein (CtBP) interacting protein (CtIP) (Schaeper et al., 1998), E2F (Trouche and Kouzarides, 1996) and the recently characterised cellular repressor of E1A stimulated genes (CREG) (Veal et al., 1998). These regions of homology to non-viral proteins are generally in sites of interaction with cellular components. Thus, for example, the binding sites for pRb on E1A and cyclin D, for CtBP on E1A and CtIP and for CBP and pRb on E1A and E2F1 all have marked similarity. This point is considered in more detail below.

It can be seen from Figure 1 that there is a region present in Ad12 E1A to which there is no homologous Ad5 sequence (amino acids 125-144). This is known as the "unique", or "spacer" region. Using chimaeric Ad5/Ad12 E1A proteins and mutational analysis this region has been shown to be, at least partly, responsible for the ability of Ad12 transformed cells to induce tumors in the syngeneic host (Telling and Williams, 1994; Jelinek et al., 1994; Williams et al., 1995). Whilst other regions of E1A probably play a role in determining tumorigenicity (in particular by down-regulation of MHC1 expression or regulating NK susceptibility of transformants [Jelinek et al., 1994; Pereira et al., 1995]), there is now little doubt that the spacer region has a profound influence on the oncogenicity of the virus perhaps by binding to an, as yet unidentified, cellular protein. This is discussed in more detail in chapter 14 of this volume and in Williams et al. (1995).

E1As are of 25 to 30K molecular weight and contain a preponderance of acidic amino acids giving the protein a PI of 4-5 depending on serotype. E1A is phosphorylated at a number of residues, although the significance of some of these phosphorylation events is not clear. In most cases serine residues are the target for the kinase activity, although occasionally threonine residues are phosphorylated – no reports of tyrosine phosphorylation have been made. In the Ad2/5 protein S^{89} and S^{219} appear to be primary sites for phosphorylation by a cdk-like kinase – probably cdc2 or cdk2 (Tsukamoto et al., 1986; Tremblay et al., 1988; 1989; Dumont and Branton, 1992; Mal et al., 1996). To date, no marked biological effects have been observed from phosphorylation at these sites. Slightly more recently it has been noted that phosphorylation of S^{132} reduced the apoptosis-inducing ability of the Ad5 289a.a. protein thus increasing its transforming potential (Whalen et al., 1996). Due to the proximity of S^{132} to the pRb binding motif (LTCHE) in CR2 (see below) it is quite possible that phosphorylation causes a conformational change facilitating binding. Additional MAPK phosphorylation sites are present in CR3 at S^{185} and S^{188} and these amino acids are dephosphorylated in response to cAMP (Whalen et al., 1997). Phosphorylation at these residues affects the ability of E1A to regulate transactivation of the E4 promoter (Whalen et al., 1997).

Overall, the effects of phosphorylation on E1A activity appear to be subtle but it is possible that examination in a variety of assay systems may allow the linking of particular phosphorylation sites to changes in certain protein binding properties. The observation that phosphorylation can cause marked changes in the conformation of E1A, apparent in large variations in mobility following SDS PAGE (Dumont et al., 1989), would tend to support this suggestion.

Within conserved region 3, which is only present in E1A proteins translated from the 13S mRNA, is a highly conserved motif which binds 1 atom of Zn^{2+} (Culp et al., 1988). Integrity of this C4-type zinc finger is necessary for the transactivation properties of the CR3 region (Culp et al., 1988; Webster and Ricciardi, 1991) — mutation of any of the cysteine residues leads to loss of metal ion binding and transactivation properties. It is not clear whether the zinc finger motif is directly involved in protein binding (in this case with TATA binding protein [TBP] — see below) or is necessary for the maintenance of the correct three-dimensional structure of the region.

Although Ad E1A can be considered as the paradigm for DNA viral oncogenes and has been the object of exhaustive study for well over two decades, we have very little knowledge of its secondary or tertiary structure. Presumably, a number of workers have embarked on cystalographic or nuclear magnetic resonance (NMR) studies without success. It has been suggested that Ad E1A adopts a relatively extended conformation such that it is able to interact with the multitude of binding proteins so far characterised (see for example Bayley and Mymryk, 1994). This idea is based largely on the observation that mutations in the binding site on E1A for one protein have virtually no effect on other sites but is, as yet, unsupported by direct observation.

NMR studies carried out using synthetic peptides identical to the binding sites on E1A for TBP and C-terminal binding protein (CtBP) have, however, shown that these regions adopt stable three-dimensional structures in solution (Molloy et al., 1998; 1999). Thus, the N-terminal portion of CR3 which is a TBP binding site forms an α helix, whilst the CtBP binding site comprises a series of β turns. Significantly, mutations in the CtBP binding site which interfere with CtBP binding also cause disruption of the peptide structure (Molloy et al., 1998). The problem with studies of this sort is to know to what extent the structures of synthetic peptides reflect those present in the intact protein. It is interesting to note, however, that on binding to CtBP a conformational change is observed in synthetic peptides which suggests that the CtBP binding site becomes α helical (D. Molloy and R. Grand, unpublished data). Additionally, it has been observed, using CD spectroscopy, that there is a marked increase in helical content of an exon 2 polypeptide on CtBP binding. Whilst these observations do not, in themselves, add significantly to our knowledge of E1A function they do confirm that the protein is not simply an elongated polypeptide chain waiting to have structure imposed on it by the binding proteins.

b. *Biological significance of Ad E1A expression*

Ad E1A is the first protein to be expressed after the onset of adenovirus infection. From a viral viewpoint the primary role of E1A is to regulate transcription of other viral genes and to stimulate the host-cell DNA synthetic machinery. (The larger Ad E1B protein ensures that it is primarily viral proteins which are ultimately produced). To achieve this Ad E1A induces progression into S phase of the cell cycle. The effects of Ad E1A following transfection of DNA into mammalian cells, either alone, or more usually, in conjunction with Ad E1B or mutant *ras*, are largely attributable to the same properties which are important during viral infection. However, in the somewhat altered circumstances, specifically the absence of expression of other viral genes, this leads to immortalization and transformation. Ad E1A also produces various other effects when introduced alone into mammalian cells. It induces quiescent cells into cycle, inhibits differentiation or causes apoptosis. In view of the observations that Ad E1A has no enzymic activity and is unable to bind to DNA directly it is apparent that it exerts its effects through protein:protein interactions. The cellular targets for E1A are involved, directly or indirectly, in transcriptional regulation and it now appears that disruption of the normal cellular transcription, either by repression or activation, ultimately leads to effects as diverse as apoptosis, cell cycle progression, proliferation, the inhibition of differentiation, and cell transformation. The biological effects of Ad E1A are now well-established and have previously been described in considerable detail (see, for example, Boulanger and Blair, 1991; various contributions to Doerfler and Bohm, 1995 but most usefully the seminal review by Bayley and Mymryk, 1994). There is no necessity to repeat these descriptions here. The important question now is not what Ad E1A does but how it does it – in the first half of this chapter I will attempt to summarize some of the more interesting recent observations which provide answers to this question.

c. Interaction of the N-terminal domain of E1A

The N-terminal region of E1A is taken, for convenience, as the amino acid sequence from the N-terminus to the beginning of CR1. It is not highly conserved but in both Ad2/5 and Ad12 it is responsible, in conjunction with CR1, for interaction with p300/CBP and with TBP. In addition, in Ad5 it has been shown to bind SUG1, and p400, TBP, Id proteins as well as a number of other cellular components. Proteins interacting with Ad E1A are summarized in Table 1.

p300 was originally identified as an Ad E1A binding protein (Howe et al., 1990; Stein et al., 1990; Eckner et al., 1994) but is now recognised as a member of the highly conserved CBP (CREB [cyclic AMP response element binding protein] binding protein) / p300 family of transcriptional co-activators (reviewed in Shikama et al., 1997; Giles et al., 1998; Snowden and Perkins, 1998). Other homologues include p270 (Dallas et al., 1998) and p400 (Barbeau et al., 1994) which has also been identified as an E1A binding protein. CBP and p300 have been studied in most detail – they share 63% overall identity with appreciably greater homology in the various regions identified as binding sites for other proteins (see Figure 2). p300/CBP serve as bridges between a large number of sequence specific DNA binding general transcription factors and basal transcription machinery playing an important role in transcriptional transactivation. The interacting transcription factors include c-Fos, E2F, cJun, c-Myb, CREB, NF-κB and p53 amongst others (see Shikama et al., 1997 for a comprehensive discussion). With regard to the basal transcription machinery p300/CBP binds directly to RNA helicase A facilitating interaction with RNA polymerase II (Nakajima et al., 1997; Kee et al., 1996), TFIIB and TBP (Yuan et al., 1996; Kwok et al., 1994). The binding of Ad E1A to p300/CBP will result in disruption of many of these complex interactions giving rise to aberrant gene expression.

TABLE 1

Cellular proteins binding to Adenovirus E1A.

Site of interaction	Binding protein	Reference
1. N terminal region	p400	Barbeau *et al.*, 1994.
	Myogenin and E12	Taylor *et al.*, 1993.
	SUG1	Grand *et al.*, 1999a.
	Id-1H and Id-2H	Nakajima *et al.*, 1998.
	Stat 1	Look *et al.*, 1998.
	TBP	Song *et al.*, 1995; 1997.
N terminal region + CR1	p300/CBP	Howe *et al.*, 1990; Stein *et al.*, 1990; Eckner *et al.*, 1994.
2. CR1	p/CAF	Reid *et al.*, 1998.
3. CR1 + CR2	pRb, p107, p130	Whyte *et al.*, 1988; Ewen *et al.*, 1991; Li *et al.*, 1993; Hannon *et al.*, 1993.
4. CR3	TBP	Lee *et al.*, 1991; Horikoshi *et al.*, 1991.
	ATF2	Liu and Green, 1990; Chatton *et al.*, 1993.
	YY1	Lewis *et al.*, 1995.
	BS69	Hateboer *et al.*, 1995
5. C terminal region	CtBP	Boyd *et al.*, 1993.
		Schaeper *et al.*, 1995.

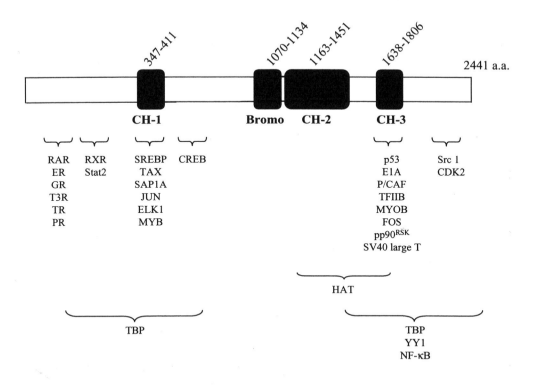

Fig. 2. Domain structures of p300. Diagrammatic representation of the domains of p300 is shown together with the suggested binding sites for various interacting cellular and viral proteins (modified from figures in Shikama et al., 1997, Giles et al., 1998 and Snowden and Perkins, 1998). CH domains: cysteine, histidine rich domains; bromo: bromodomain; HAT domain, region required for histone acetyl transferase activity.

A second crucially important property of p300/CBP proteins is their histone acetyl transferase (HAT) activity. Acetylation of the lysine residues in the N-terminal tail of histones results in reduction in positive charge on the protein, reducing its affinity for DNA thereby increasing the accessibility of target gene promoters (Bannister and Kouzarides, 1996; Yang et al., 1996; Ogryzko et al., 1996) and stimulating transcription (Martinez-Balbas et al., 1998). Uniquely amongst HATs so far characterised, p300/CBP can acetylate all of the four core histones. In addition, further HATs can form complexes with p300/CBP. One of these, the p300/CBP associated factor (P/CAF) also binds directly to E1A (see below).

The interaction of Ad E1A with p300/CBP usually results in inactivation of the HAT activity and is required for correct E1A functioning (Chakravarti et al., 1999). In addition, binding of E1A to CBP/p300 or P/CAF causes the disruption of the p300/CBP : P/CAF complex (Yang et al., 1996) with direct binding to P/CAF reducing its own HAT activity (Reid et al., 1998; Chakravarti et al., 1999). Depending on the system used, however, it has been suggested that Ad E1A can cause an increase in CBP HAT activity similar to that seen following phosphorylation, perhaps by CDK2 (Ait-Si-Ali et al., 1998).

As well as acetylating histones p300/CBP can also modify a number of other proteins such as p53 (Gu and Roeder, 1997) and members of the basal transcription machinery TFII E β and TFII F (Imhof et al., 1997). Acetylation of p53 modifies its ability to bind DNA but whether this activity is affected by E1A has yet to be demonstrated.

There are two binding sites on Ad E1A for p300, one located in the N-terminal domain and the other towards the centre of CR1 (Barbeau et al., 1994; Bannister and Kouzarides, 1995). The binding site for p400 also appears to be in the N-terminal region and perhaps in CR1 although definitive information is, so far, unavailable (Barbeau et al., 1994). Mutations in E1A CR1 or CR2 which impair interaction with the Rb family of proteins do not affect binding to p300/CBP. The observation that there are essentially two separate binding sites on E1A for p300/CBP might suggest that there are two recognition sites on p300. However, in studies using Ad2/5 E1A it has been shown that the C/H3 domain encompasses the region required for interaction with E1A (Arany et al., 1995). This site is also involved in binding to a variety of other proteins such as SV40 T ag, P/CAF, and specific transcription factors like Fos, p53, Myo D, E2F and Stat 1 as well as the general transcription factors TFII B and TBP (Shikama et al., 1997 and references therein). Interestingly, a second site within p300 (a.a. 1999-2200) appears to bind to Ad12 E1A but not the Ad5 homologue (Lipinski et al., 1999), the significance of this will have to await further investigation.

The biological implications of the binding of Ad E1A to p300/CBP are considerable. Of particular importance is the observation that p300 binding is responsible for the transcription repression activity of E1A (Rochette-Egly et al., 1990; Stein et al., 1990; Wang et al., 1993; Arany et al., 1995; Smits et al., 1996). Thus, it is supposed that complex formation prevents p300 interaction with transcription factors (Jones, 1995). Whilst definitive evidence for the effect of E1A on the full gamut of p300/CBP-binding transcription factors is not yet available it has been shown, for example, that CBP-induced stimulation of cFos, cJun and p53 activity is counteracted by binding of E1A (Bannister and Kouzarides, 1995; Lee et al., 1996; Lill et al., 1997; Avantaggiati et al., 1997; Somasundaram and El-Deiry, 1997). This repression activity mediated through p300/CBP can then affect a number of important biological processes such as development and differentiation, cell cycle regulation and apoptosis. Whilst it is beyond the scope of this review to consider the role of p300/CBP in detail it is appropriate to draw the reader's attention to a few important observations (see Shikama et al., 1997; Giles et al., 1998). p300/CBP are negative regulators of the cell cycle and mutant Ad E1A, which fails to bind pRb but can interact with p300, causes entry into S phase (Howe et al., 1990; Wang et al., 1993). In addition, p300 has a role in Ad E1A-induced p53-mediated apoptosis. Thus, whilst it now appears that the induction of p53 by E1A is attributable to up-regulation of p19[ARF] which, in turn requires the integrity of the pRb binding sites (de Stanchina et al., 1998; see this volume chapter 13) p300 also plays a role. Ad E1A proteins which do not interact with p300 also fail to induce p53 in rodent cells and some but not all human cells (Querido et al., 1997a; Chiou and White, 1997; Somasundaram and El-Deiry, 1997). In this context p300 is able to bind to p53 and MDM2 through the C/H1 domain. Both interactions are required for the normal proteasome-mediated degradation of p53, with over-production of p300/CBP C/H1 leading to p53 stabilization (Grossman et al., 1998). Additionally, it has been suggested that p300/CBP is required for transactivation of the *mdm2* gene by p53 (Thomas and White, 1998). Quite how all of these observerations fit together to form a coherent picture is not clear at the moment.

It has long been established that Ad E1A suppresses muscle-specific transcription and differentiation (Webster et al., 1988) and that this is attributable to its ability to interact with p300/CBP (Mymryk et al., 1992; Eckner et al., 1996). In myotubes p300/CBP, P/CAF and MyoD form a multimeric complex which can be disrupted by E1A (Puri et al., 1997). The HAT activity of P/CAF is essential for up-regulation of p21 expression and terminal cell cycle arrest. Thus, it appears that it is the recruitment of this activity to MyoD through p300/CBP which Ad E1A abrogates (Puri et al., 1997). Whether the ability to increase expression of p21 is the sole function of P/CAF that is required for muscle differentiation is not yet clear. Ad E1A also directly interacts, through its N terminal region, with the bHLH domains of myogenin and E12 which are involved in myocyte differentiation (Taylor et al., 1993). It has been suggested that this may contribute to the inhibition of differentiation.

When interferon α (IFNα) binds to its receptor it causes the formation of the ISGF3 complex which activates transcription of cellular "antiviral genes" (Darnell et al., 1994; Qureshi et al., 1996). Stat 1, Stat 2 and the DNA binding component p48 are all components of ISGF3. p300/CBP interacts with Stat2 through its CH1 domain, Ad E1A being able to repress Stat 2 transactivation by its binding to p300/CBP (Bhattacharya et al., 1996). This will have the effect of, at least partly, inhibiting the cellular response by relieving IFNα-mediated blockade of viral replication. Significantly, recent evidence suggests that Ad E1A will also interact directly with Stat 1 (Look et al., 1998). Again, the binding site on Ad E1A is in the region between amino acids 2 and 36. Thus, interaction is partly responsible for inhibition of IFN-γ dependent expression. (Look et al., 1998). Stat 1 is involved in the regulation of transcription of a number of genes involved in the host cell antiviral response such that Stat 1 regulatory sites have been identified in ICAM-1, IRF-1 and TAP1 genes. IRF-1, in turn, plays a part in the induction of IFN-β and MHC class I (discussed in more detail in Look et al., 1998).

A basic helix loop helix protein, Twist, expressed during embryogenesis in neural crest cells is able to bind p300 and P/CAF and directly inhibit their HAT activities (Hamamori et al., 1999). Through this activity it is considered that Twist can inhibit differentiation in a number of different cell types such as neuronal (Lee et al., 1995a) and muscle cells (Hebrok et al., 1994). The obvious similarity between the effects of Ad E1A and Twist on cellular differentiation and acetyl transferase activity of p300 and P/CAF has allowed Hamamori et al. (1999) to suggest that the biological activities of

E1A might reflect some of the physiological functions regulated by Twist (Hamamori et al., 1999).

Up to now there have been no reports of the p300 homologue p270 interacting with Ad E1A. Interestingly, however, p270 has been shown to be a component of the mammalian SW1/SNF complex (Dallas et al., 1998) which is involved in chromatin remodelling (reviewed Peterson and Tamkun, 1995). When E1A is expressed in yeast it produces a "slow-growth" phenotype which has been attributed to targeting of the SW1/SNF complex, specifically through interaction of E1A with SNF12 (Miller et al., 1996). The N-terminal region of Ad E1A, including CR1 (residues 1-82) is responsible for the growth inhibitory effects and for disruption of SW1/SNF-dependent transcription (Miller et al., 1996). It is tempting to speculate that Ad E1A could directly affect SW1/SNF complex in mammals through binding either to p270 or perhaps to other components homologous to yeast proteins such as SNF12 (this possibility is considered by Mymryk and Smith, 1997). Perhaps of some relevance is the observation that Rb family members can bind to BRG1 and hBRM – two components of the mammalian SW1/SNF complex (Danaief et al., 1994; Strober et al., 1996). Sites of interaction on hBRG1 and hBRM have been mapped to LXCXE motifs (Dunaief et al., 1994; Strober et al., 1996). Ad E1A can compete for the pocket domain on Rb disrupting the complexes and inhibiting the growth inhibitory effects of the interaction of Rb with hBRG1 and hBRM (Dunaief et al., 1994; Strober et al., 1996).

In addition, to Ad E1A-mediated transcriptional repression through binding to p300/CBP it has also been suggested that there is an additional repression domain located towards the N-terminus of E1A which binds to TBP (Song et al., 1995; 1997; Lipinski et al., 1998). The interaction of E1A with TBP has the effect of dissociating the latter protein from the TATA box promoter complex. This disruptive effect of Ad E1A can be blocked in vitro by the addition of TFIIB (Song et al., 1997). In the context of transcriptional repression the major site of interaction for TBP on E1A is between amino acids 4 and 25, although other residues within the N-terminal 80 amino acids may play a role (Song et al., 1997). It should be borne in mind that TBP binds to p300/CBP (Yuan et al., 1996) and therefore it might be suggested that Ad E1A could inhibit transcriptional activation by TBP by interfering with its interaction with p300. However, the in vitro studies presented by Song et al. (1995; 1997) would argue strongly in favour of a direct effect. The TBP binding transcriptional repression domain at the N-terminus of E1A is quite distinct from the activation sequences located in CR3 (see below).

It has recently been shown that Id (inhibitors of differentiation) proteins Id-1H and Id-2H bind to the N-terminal region of Ad E1A (Nakajima et al., 1998). The binding site for the Id proteins has been mapped to residues 1-16 and/or 24-36 on E1A (Nakajima et al., 1998). Both Id proteins and Ad E1A are positive regulators of S phase entry; indeed it has been shown that after expression of either of these proteins in the rat cell line 3Y1 cells accumulate in S phase, then undergo apoptosis. The significance of the interaction between E1A and Id proteins for this effect is not clear at present.

A further cellular protein which binds to the N-terminus of Ad E1A is SUG1, a multi-functional 45K phosphoprotein (Grand et al., 1999a). SUG1 is a regulatory component of the 26S proteasome (reviewed Coux et al., 1996), a DNA helicase (Fraser et al., 1997), and an intermediary between nuclear receptors and the basal transcriptional machinery (vom Baur et al., 1995; Lee et al., 1995b). The binding site on Ad5 E1A for this protein has been mapped to the region between amino acids 4 and 25 (Turnell and Grand, unpublished results). The interaction appears to be direct, not requiring the presence of any of the other known E1A N-terminal binding proteins (Grand et al., 1999a; Turnell and Grand, unpublished data). The biological significance of this interaction is not clear but, to date, it has been shown that Ad12 E1A is able to inhibit the ability of 26S proteasomes to degrade p53 in *in vitro* assays (Grand et al., 1999a, Turnell et al., unpublished observations). Ad E1A cannot, however, SUG1 helicase activity, intrinsic ATPase activity or thyroid hormone receptor activity (Turnell, Zhang and Grand, unpublished data). The binding of SUG1 to cFos suggests that it may play a role in transcriptional regulation (Wang et al., 1996) – activation or inhibition of this by E1A would be consistent with its other well-characerised activities.

d. *Interaction of Rb family of proteins with E1A conserved regions 1 and 2*

Conserved regions 1 and 2, together with the N-terminal domain (see above), have long been known to be essential for E1A-mediated regulation of gene expression, induction of cell cycle progression, DNA synthesis and mitosis and cell transformation (see Bayley and Mymryk, 1994 for a comprehensive review of the literature up to that time). CR1 forms part of the binding site for p300 (which has been discussed in the previous section), probably the whole binding site for p/CAF and, together with CR2, the site for interaction with the Rb family of proteins.

pRb was originally identified as the protein encoded by a gene mutated in retinoblastoma cells. Inactivation of the *Rb* gene has since been shown to be a common event in many human cancers. In normal cells Rb exerts a growth inhibitory effect in mid to late G1 stage of the cell cycle, controlling the cell's commitment to DNA replication (i.e. the G1 to S phase transition). The activity of Rb is regulated by phosphorylation by cyclin-dependent kinases with the hypophosphorylated (relatively dephosphorylated) form binding to, and inhibiting the transactivation properties of, the E2F family of transcription factors. In addition, bound hypophosphorylated Rb also causes E2F to become an active repressor at certain promoters. Phosphorylation of Rb by cyclin A/cdk2, cyclin E/cdk2 and cdk4/6 and D type cyclins causes dissociation from E2F which is then free to activate transcription of a number of genes, many of which are involved in DNA synthesis. Thus during G1 Rb is predominantly dephosphorylated – the hyperphosphorylated form appears as cells enter S phase and continues during G2 and M.

The interaction of Ad E1A with Rb causes dissociation of the Rb/E2F complex; simplistically this can be seen as a duplication of the effect of phosphorylation. The major binding site on E1A for Rb is the LXCXE motif present in the N-terminal half of CR2. This sequence is conserved amongst the oncoproteins of small DNA tumor viruses – e.g. T ag in SV40 and E7 in HPV (Whyte et al., 1988; Dyson et al., 1989; 1990; 1992; Munger et al., 1989; Chellappan et al., 1992). These viral proteins interact with a site on

Rb known as the A/B pocket which comprises two amino acid sequences (379-572 and 646-772) which are separated by an 'insert' or 'spacer' domain which is not involved in complex formation. (Kaelin et al., 1990; Hu et al., 1990; Huang et al., 1990). Crystalographic studies have shown that LXCXE binds to a groove region in the B box component of the A/B pocket. This amino acid sequence is highly conserved amongst Rb proteins from many species and the p130 and p107 homologues (see below). The A box is considered to be involved in the stable folding of B (Lee et al., 1998). A second protein binding site, the 'large A/B pocket', comprises amino acids 379-870 and is involved in interaction with E2F and has growth suppression properties.

As already mentioned, phosphorylation regulates the interaction of Rb with E2F but it also has a significant effect on binding of the viral oncoproteins. For example, phosphorylation of T821/826 of Rb inhibits binding to Tag. Similarly, Ad E1A binds to the hypophosphorylated form of Rb (Mittnacht et al., 1994). On the other hand, the phosphorylation of E1A enhances Rb binding and its ability to disrupt Rb/E2F complexes (Mal et al., 1996). It is not clear which sites on E1A are of particular importance in modulating its binding activity but it serves as a substrate for cdk2, cdk4 and cdc2 in vitro, with similar sites being phosphorylated in vivo (Mal et al., 1996). Cdk2/cyclin A and cdk2/cyclin E complexes are associated with Ad E1A in vivo (probably in complexes with p107) and these could play an important role in regulation of its ability to disrupt the cell cycle in normal cells (Faha et al., 1993).

Both Rb and E2F are, in fact, members of families of homologous proteins. p107 and p130 were first identified as viral oncoprotein-binding proteins with appreciable homology to Rb (Ewen et al., 1991; Cobrinik et al., 1993; Hannon et al., 1993; Li et al., 1993). The topography of the interaction of E1A with p107 and p130 is similar to that seen for Rb in that interaction is through both CR1 and CR2 with the LXCXE motif being of particular significance. The basic domain structure of p107 and p130 is also similar to that seen for Rb. Some differences have been noted, however, in that the two larger proteins can form complexes with cdk2 and cyclins A and E (Pines and Hunter, 1990; Ewen et al., 1992; Faha et al., 1992; Hannon et al., 1993; Li et al., 1993) whilst Rb does not. p107 and p130 do not interact with c-Abl, whilst Rb possesses a C-terminal C pocket (amino acids 768-928) binding site (Welch and Wang, 1993; Knudsen and Wang, 1998).

E2F is a heterodimeric transcription factor, comprising two subunits each encoded by a member of two related families: E2F and DP. Up to now, five E2F components and three DP components have been isolated (see Dyson 1998 for a comprehensive review of E2F). Various combinations of E2F, DP and Rb family of proteins have been identified. Both p107 and p130 preferentially interact with E2F-4 and E2F-5, whereas Rb binds predominantly to E2F-1, E2F-2 and E2F-3. Differences have been observed in the appearances of the different E2F/Rb family proteins complexes during the cell cycle. For example, E2F-1, 2 and 3 bound to hypophosphorylated Rb are found predominantly in G1 and to a lesser extent in S phase when most Rb becomes phosphorylated (Chellappan et al., 1991; Cao et al., 1992; Lees et al., 1993). E2F/p130 complexes predominate in G0 and in G1 and bind to cyclin E-cdk2 (Cobrinik et al., 1993). E2F/p107 predominates in G1 and S, becoming associated with cyclin A-cdk2 in

S phase (Devoto et al., 1992; Shirodkar et al.,1 992; Lees et al., 1992; Schwarz et al., 1993). Thus, the binding of E1A to different members of the Rb family and disruption of the complex with E2F may exert an effect at different points in the cell cycle.

A number of novel properties of Rb have recently been demonstrated which suggest an additional level of sophistication in regulation of the cell cycle. Although phosphorylation of Rb is essential for the well-characterized G1/S transition it is also important for continued progress through S phase and completion of DNA replication. Obviously, binding of E1A to Rb will ensure that E2F is "free" throughout the cycle (Knudsen et al., 1998).

As well as repressing E2F activity by masking the E2F activation domain it now appears that the pocket proteins can repress transcription by recruiting the histone deacetylase HDAC1. Deacetylation of histones favours the binding of histones to DNA, reducing accessibility of transcription factors (Magnaghi-Jaulin et al., 1998; Brehm et al., 1998; Luo et al., 1998). Binding to HDAC1 has been demonstrated for p107 and p130 as well as Rb (Ferreira et al., 1998). Interaction with the Rb family appears to be through an LXCXE-like motif located towards the C-terminus of HDAC1 (the actual sequence is IACEE). It seems reasonable to suppose that this interaction between the pocket protein family and HDAC1 is a further target for Ad E1A and other viral oncoproteins and this has been confirmed for the HPV oncoprotein E7 (Brehm et al., 1998).

The relative contributions of CR1 and CR2 to the interaction with the pocket proteins are still a matter of some debate. Whilst the major binding motif LXCXE occurs in CR2 deletions point mutations in CR1 reduce the binding of E1A to Rb, p107 and p130 (Whyte et al., 1989; Howe et al.,1990; Howe and Bayley, 1992; Giordano et al., 1991; Wang et al., 1993). Whether this means that there are two distinct sites of interaction in Rb, p107 and p130 for E1A has not been confirmed but it is certainly possible.

Recently, direct binding of the histone acetyltransferase P/CAF to the CR1 of Ad E1A has been demonstrated (Reid et al., 1998). P/CAF is a transcriptional activator which is able to function independently of its ability to bind p300/CBP (Yang et al., 1996). The histone acetyltransferase activity is essential for the ability of P/CAF to regulate transcription, with binding to E1A resulting in inactivation (Reid et al., 1998). The binding site for P/CAF on E1A has been mapped to the central segment of CR1 (residues 55-60 in Ad5), quite distinct from the region required for interaction with CBP/p300 and Rb (Reid et al., 1998). Interestingly, deletion of a similar region in E1A abrogated its ability to block myogenesis (Sandmoller et al., 1996).

e. Interaction of Ad E1A conserved region 3 with cellular transcriptional activators

As discussed above, conserved region 3 in unique to the larger 289 amino acid component of Ad2/5 E1A, although in Ad12 the N-terminal third of it is present in both the 13S and 12S products (Figure 1). The integrity of CR3 is essential for the activation of all adenoviral genes. In addition, this region of E1A is also involved in transcriptional activation of a number of cellular genes. CR3-mediated regulation by E1A has been shown to be attributable to binding of this short 48 amino acid sequence to a number of different cellular transcription factors, which possess different specificities and modes of action. Amongst the targets for CR3 are components of transcription factor IID (TFIID) a multisubunit protein complex required for transcription by promoters targeted by RNA polymerase II, specifc DNA-binding proteins such as ATF and the activator/repressor YY1 and the repressor BS69. Detailed analysis of transcriptional regulation by CR3 is beyond the scope of this chapter and readers in need of more information are referred to excellent reviews by Jones (1995) and Flint and Shenk (1997).

CR3 contains a C4 type zinc finger, the integrity of which is essential for the full transcriptional activation by E1A (Culp et al., 1988; Webster and Ricciardi, 1991). Mutational analysis has shown that the zinc finger domain and the adjacent amino acids N-terminal to it form a binding site for TBP, the DNA binding subunit of TFIID (Horikoshi et al., 1991; Lee et al., 1991; Geisberg et al., 1994). The N-terminal portion of CR3 forms an α helix (Molloy et al., 1999) which could interact with helices in the basic region between residues 221 and 271 of TBP. p53 also binds to TBP in this area and it is probable that interaction with Ad E1A displaces p53 from TBP, relieving p53-mediated repression (Horikoshi et al., 1995).

Ad E1A also interacts with other subunits of TFIID – the TBP-associated factors (TAFs). CR3 has been shown to be important for binding of E1A to human TAFII 250, TAFII 55 and TAFII 135 as well as the *Drosophila* homologue of TAF II 135-TAFII 110 (Mazzarelli et al., 1995; 1997; Chiang and Roeder, 1995; Geisberg et al., 1995; Tanese et al., 1996). The binding sites for human TAFII 250 and *Drosophila* TAFII 110 have been mapped to the C-terminus of CR3 (amino acids 180-188 in Ad5) (Geisberg et al., 1995). Deletions elsewhere in CR3 have relatively little effect on the interaction. Interestingly, deletions at either end of CR3 (amino acids 140-146 and 180-188) cause marked reduction in binding to TAFII 135 (Mazzarelli et al., 1997). As with TAFII 250 elimination of sequences encompassing the zinc finger domain have little effect (Mazzarelli et al., 1997). It is possible therefore that different sites on CR3 may be involved in this interaction with different TAFs, although this has yet to be confirmed. TAFII 135 binds to TFIIA, which in turn stabilizes the interaction of TFIID with the promoter. It has been suggested that complex formation between E1A and TAFII 135 might favour binding of TFIIA to TFIID, thus activating transcription (Mazzarelli et al., 1997).

In addition to interaction with TFIID the CR3 region can also bind to activating transcription factors (ATFs). The major targets for E1A are ATF2 and ATFa (Liu and Green, 1990; Flint and Jones, 1991; Chatton et al., 1993) and it is largely through this binding that E1A is able to activate transcription from the early adenovirus promoters. ATFs have basic region leucine zipper (bZIP) domains which are required for dimerization and binding to other members of the ATF and Jun/Fos families. The bZIP motifs are necessary for protein binding to cAMP response element (CRE) sites on DNA. E1A interacts with the leucine zipper of ATF2 (Liu and Green, 1994; Livingstone et al., 1995) – this is considered to cause a conformational change in the protein exposing the N-terminal transcriptional activation domain (Flint and Jones, 1991; Abdel-Hafiz et al., 1993). Phosphorylation of two amino acids (T69 and T71) in the N-terminal domain of ATF2 by stress activated protein kinases (SAPK) is necessary for transcriptional activation by the N-terminal domain and for intact ATF-2 to respond to E1A (Livingstone et al., 1995; see also Jones, 1995).

A further interaction of CR3 is with the multi-functional transcription factor yin yang 1 (YY1) (Lewis et al., 1995). YY1 is a zinc finger transcriptional factor which has been implicated in the control of a variety of different promoters (reviewed Shi et al., 1997). It is capable of activating or repressing transcription depending on the context of its binding to other proteins and to DNA. Interaction with CR3 has been shown to relieve YY1-mediated repression (Lewis et al., 1995). Furthermore, YY1 can also bind to the N-terminal region of E1A although this is probably through interaction with p300/CBP. A novel protein, BS69, has been shown to inhibit transactivation activity of the 289a.a. Ad5 E1A component, perhaps by competing with TBP for the binding site in CR3 (Hateboer et al., 1995). BS69 appears to be expressed highly in kidney and brain but its normal cellular function is not yet clear.

Interaction of transcriptional regulators with the CR3 domain of E1A results in changes in expression of a number of cellular proteins. Thus, for example, there is a large panel of cellular genes transcribed by RNA polymerase II that are induced by E1A; examples include c-fos, c-jun, cyclin A and heat shock proteins 70 and 90 (see Bayley and Mymryk, 1994 for a full listing). The importance of an increase in expression of these proteins for E1A-mediated cell transformation has not been firmly established, most attention having been paid to the regulation by the Rb family of proteins and p300 (as described above). However, it is obvious that increases in levels of the AP1 family of transcription factors (e.g. Jun and Fos), cyclins and cdks amongst many other proteins cannot help but have profound effects on the growth properties of cells expressing E1A. Whether there is any selectivity in the action of CR3 on cellular gene expression has not been established. It seems reasonable to suppose that there is not a profound increase in expression of all genes transcribed, by, for example, RNA polymerase II but how this selectivity by E1A might work in practice remains to be established.

f. Binding of E1A to C-terminal binding protein CtBP

Exon 2 of Ad E1A, which stretches from CR3 to the C-terminus is much less well-characterised than exon 1. It has been shown to be essential for immortalization of primary BRK cells (Quinlan et al., 1988; Subramanian et al., 1989; Gopalakrishnan et al., 1997) but not for DNA mediated transformation in co-operation with activated *ras* genes (Zerler et al., 1986; Quinlan et al., 1988; Schneider et al., 1987; Subramanian et al., 1989). Indeed, it has been demonstrated that deletions in exon 2 of E1A enhance the transformation efficiency in conjunction with *ras* with the resulting transformants being more tumorigenic in syngeneic animals (Subramanian et al., 1989; Douglas et al., 1991; Linder et al., 1992; Boyd et al., 1993). To date the only protein demonstrated to bind to the C-terminal region of E1A (i.e. encoded by exon 2) is a 48K nuclear phosphoprotein which has been termed C-terminal binding protein (Boyd et al., 1993). CtBP interacts with E1A through a highly conserved motif (PXDLSXK/R) which is located very close to the C-terminus (amino acids 233-239 in Ad2 E1A 243a.a. component) (Schaeper et al., 1995; Molloy et al., 1998). In addition, it has been shown that deletion of the CtBP binding site gives rise to an E1A mutant with increased transformation potential in conjunction with activated *ras* (Boyd et al., 1993). A homologue, CtBP2, has also been identified (Katsanis and Fisher, 1998) and this can homodimerize and heterodimerize with CtBP1 (the originally identified CtBP protein) (Sewalt et al., 1999).

It is likely that in normal cells CtBP interacts with several more proteins which have the conserved PXDLSXK/R sequence in the binding site. The gene encoding one such protein has been isolated from human cells (Schaeper et al., 1998). The protein, termed C-terminal interacting protein (CtIP), is of 125K and appears also to bind to the BRCA1 tumor suppressor gene product (Yu et al., 1998). BRCA1 regulates gene expression at the level of RNA transcription. This is probably attributable to the tandemly repeated BRCT domains, located at the C-terminus, which are also binding sites for CtIP (Yu et al., 1998). BRCT domains can activate RNA transcription *in vitro* (Chapman and Verma, 1996; Monteiro et al., 1996) whilst the intact protein co-purifies with RNA polymerase II (Scully et al., 1997). Interestingly, mutations in BRCA1 associated with tumor production occur in the C-terminal BRCT domains – thus it has been suggested that the BRCA1-CtIP interaction might be required for tumor suppression (Yu et al., 1998). CtBP also binds to the human homologue of a *Xenopus* polycomb protein (HPC2), again through a sequence similar to Ad E1A (in this case PIDLRS) (Sewalt et al., 1999). CtBP does not bind to a second polycomb protein (M33) which lacks the PXDLS motif. HPC2, like the *Xenopus* protein (XPc) is a repressor of gene activity and it has been suggested that CtBP acts as a co-repressor in conjunction with it (Sewalt et al., 1999).

A *Drosophila* homologue of mammalian CtBP has been cloned and a number of interacting polypeptides isolated (Nibu et al., 1998; Poortinga et al., 1998). All of these binding proteins possess the conserved motif PXDLSXK/R. This amino acid sequence appears to be quite widespread in *Drosophila* but it is not clear, at present, whether its possession always generates interaction with CtBP. The three most closely characterised dCtBP binding proteins (Hairy, Knirps and Snail) are transcriptional repressors (Poortinga et al., 1998; Nibu et al., 1998). Hairy is a promoter-bound repressor, binding to particular sites on DNA where it recruits the Groucho co-repressor of basal and activated transcription (Jimenez et al., 1996; Fisher et al., 1996). Knirps and Snail are also short-range repressors which control segmentation of the abdomen and establishment of a boundary between the mesoderm and neurogenic ectoderm respectively.

The role of CtBP in mammalian cells has yet to be unequivocally established but, by analogy with the *Drosophila* system and based on *in vitro* studies, it is involved in transcriptional repression, for example being able to inhibit E1A CR1-dependent transactivation *in vitro* (Sollerbrant et al., 1996). In addition, CtBP is able to bind to HDAC1 *in* vitro (Sundqvist et al., 1998).

3. Adenovirus Early Region 1b

The Ad E1B gene encodes two major proteins – of 19K and 58K/54K. During viral infection and during DNA-mediated transformation the smaller of these acts as an anti-apoptosis factor. The larger E1B protein (54K in Ad12 and 58K in Ad2/5) also suppresses Ad E1A-induced apoptosis during transformation but during viral infection is primarily, although not exclusively, involved in the regulation of transport of viral and cellular mRNAs. All of these processes appear to be mediated through protein-protein interactions.

a. *Adenovirus early region 1B 19K protein*

The Ad E1B 19K protein is a functional and amino acid sequence homologue of Bcl-2, playing an anti-apoptotic role during both viral infection and during DNA-mediated transformation. *In vivo*, this normally means that E1B 19K protects cells from E1A-induced p53-mediated apoptosis but *in vitro* introduction of the viral gene into cells protects from other apoptotic stimuli such as TNFα and Fas. The role of Ad E1B in protecting cells from apoptosis is considered in detail in chapter 13 of this book, attention being given here only to a discussion of the 19K binding proteins. In addition, reviews of the roles of Ad E1 proteins in apoptosis have recently been written by the two workers responsible for the most important advances in understanding the biochemistry of Ad E1B 19K (Chinnadurai, 1998; White, 1998). Readers in need of more information are referred to these reports.

Structure of Ad E1B 19K protein. Adenovirus E1B 19K protein has limited amino acid sequence homology to the Bcl-2 family of protein (for review see for example Brown, 1997; Adams and Cory, 1998; Reed, 1997). At least four well-conserved regions in Bcl-2 can be distinguished by comparison of amino acid sequences in the proteins from various species and other members of the family. These are termed Bcl-2 homology (BH) domains with BH1 and BH3 being most highly conserved in Ad E1B 19K protein (Figure 3). The Bcl-2 family of proteins regulate apoptosis in normal cells through a series of homo- and hetero-dimerisation protein-protein interactions, such that certain interactions favour apoptosis whilst others favour viability. Thus, for example, it has been considered that Bcl-2 homodimerisation and formation of the Bcl-2-Bax heterodimer gives a powerful anti apoptotic signal. Similarly, other members of the Bcl-2 family can exert their influence on the cell through comparable interactions. Obviously, the expression of the Ad E1B 19K protein against this background will have a profound effect on the balance of Bcl-2 family protein binding activities.

Appreciable effort has been put into the isolation of Ad E1B 19K binding proteins. To date seven interacting polypeptides have been demonstrated (Boyd et al., 1994; 1995; Farrow et al., 1995; Han et al., 1996a; 1996b; Chen et al., 1996; Rao et al., 1997), Bak, Bax and Bik are Bcl-2 homologues but appear to have pro-apoptotic functions. These three proteins bind to E1B 19K (Farrow et al., 1995; Chen et al., 1996; Boyd et al., 1995). Thus, simplistically it may be that interaction of these with the viral protein supresses their activity, favouring cell viability. Bax and Bak have extensive homology

Pro-survival

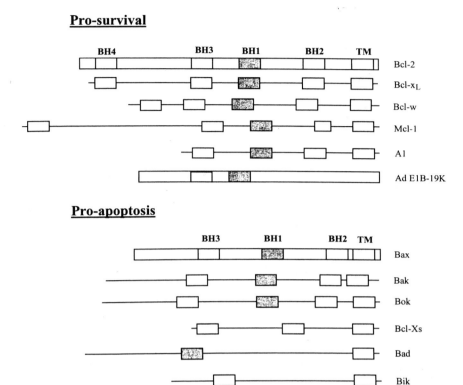

Pro-apoptosis

Fig. 3. Domain structures of members of the Bcl-2 family of apoptotic regulators. Bcl-2 homology (BH) domains are shown as are the hydrophobic transmembrane TM domains. Domain assignments are based on amino acid sequence homology.

to Bcl-2 – containing BH1, 2 and 3 domains as well as the C-terminal transmembrane TM domain. Bik, however, is considerably less similar with only BH3 and TM domains. The BH3 domain in these and other pro-apoptosis proteins is important for homodimerization, heterodimerization and induction of cell death (see for example Chittenden et al., 1995; Zha et al., 1996). The BH3 domain of Bax (aminoacids 50-78) is the binding site for the Ad E1B 19K protein (and Bcl-2) (Han et al., 1996a; 1998a) and it seems reasonable to suppose that the homologous domains in Bik and Bak are also targets for the adenovirus protein (Han et al., 1998a). Some difficulties have been experienced in closely mapping the binding site for Bax on E1B 19K. Deletion of N- and C-terminal fragments of Ad E1B 19K gives rise to truncated proteins with BH1, 2 and 3 intact, which will bind exon 3 of Bax but not the full length molecule (Han et al., 1996a). Point mutations at F51 and S87 (in BH3 and BH1 respectively) also disrupt complex formation and the ability to inhibit apoptosis (Han et al., 1996a). Han et al.,

(1996a) concluded that BH3 is required but not sufficient for the interaction between E1B 19K and Bax. This proposition is consistent with the observed inability of E1B 19K to interact with Bad, which does not contain a BH3 domain (Chen et al., 1996). Bik, which contains a BH3 domain but no BH1, 2 or 4, binds to E1B 19K – presumably through BH3. The binding determinants on E1B 19K for Bik are comparable to those required for interaction with Bax (Han et al., 1996b). Thus, only a small deletion at the C-terminus left the binding capability intact, whilst other deletions had a profound effect. Point mutations at residues 51 and 87 also abolished the interaction (Han et al., 1996b).

In the original yeast two-hybrid screen for Ad E1B 19K binding proteins Boyd et al. (1994) isolated cDNAs encoding three interacting proteins which they termed NIP1, 2 and 3 (nineteen K-interacting protein). These polypeptides also bound to Bcl-2 and homologous regions in E1B 19K and Bcl-2 were necessary for the interaction (Boyd et al., 1994). As with Bax and Bik point mutations in amino acids 50 and 51 of the E1B 19K protein interferred with binding; similarly a small deletion (amino acids 90-96) in the putative BH1 domain impaired the interaction (Boyd et al., 1994). In the original study limited homology between NIP1, 2 and 3 and diverse cellular proteins was noted. However, it now seems likely that NIPs are probably rather distant members of the Bcl-2 family. NIP3 (also now called BNIP3) can homodimerize, induce apoptosis-inducing signals and locates to the mitochondrion (Chen et al., 1997a; Yasuda et al., 1998). In addition, it contains transmembrane and BH3 domains which are required for activity (Chen et al., 1997a; Yasuda et al., 1998). NIP1 also contains a TM domain capable of localizing it to mitochondrial and nuclear membranes (Yasuda et al., 1998).

Mode of action of the Ad E1B 19K protein. It has long been known that mutations in the gene encoding E1B 19K protein give rise to adenoviruses which cause cytopathic effect and DNA degradation in infected cells (see Chapter 13). The full significance of these early observations was recognised when it was shown that Ad E1B 19K and Bcl-2 were essentially interchangeable and would protect infected and transformed cells from Ad E1A-induced p53-dependent and independent apoptosis (White et al., 1991; Rao et al, 1992; Debbas and White, 1993; Chiou et al., 1994a; b; Shen and Shenk, 1994; Teodoro et al., 1995). Recent close analysis has demonstrated that E1B 19K, Bcl-2 and Bcl-X_L have a very similar ability to protect different cell types from apoptosis induced by, for example, growth factor deprivation, cytotoxic drugs, γ-irradiation and glucocorticoids (Huang et al., 1997; see also Boulakia et al., 1996). It therefore seems reasonable to assume that Ad E1B 19K protein functions in a very similar manner to Bcl-2 (and presumably Bcl-X_L) and differences between them, particularly in primary stucture, may be, at least partly, attributable to different mechanisms of targeting to their site of action (see below).

Whilst there is still some doubt about the precise mode of action of the Bcl-2 family of proteins there is now sufficient evidence to allow a possible model to be proposed (see for example, Adams and Cory, 1998). In *C. elegans* it has been shown that the Bcl-2 homologue CED-9 interacts with the CED-4 protein which, in turn, binds to the caspase CED-3. A CED-4 homologue, Apaf-1, has been identified in the mammalian system (Zou et al., 1997) and this is able to interact with both Bcl-X_L (via its CED-4 homology domain) and with procaspase-9 at the N-terminus. It has been suggested that the association of pro-survival proteins such as Bcl-X$_L$ or Bcl-2 with Apaf-1 may prevent it from binding and activating the procaspase. The association of pro-apoptotic proteins such as Bax or Bik with Bcl-2 would prevent its association with Apaf-1 which would be free to trigger the caspase cascade. It is proposed that Ad E1B 19K could play an identical role to Bcl-2 and Bcl-X$_L$ in this scheme. Indeed, it has recently been shown that the viral protein interacts with CED-4 both in a yeast two-hybrid assay and in cell lysates (Han et al., 1998b). Furthermore Ad E1B 19K is able to inhibit CED-4-mediated FLICE-induced apoptosis but not apoptosis caused by FLICE in the absence of CED-4 (Perez and White, 1998; Han et al., 1998b). Mutational analysis has demonstrated that Bcl-2 and Bcl-X$_L$ bind to CED-4 through their N-terminal BH4 domains (Huang et al., 1998). However, it is suggested that this is not the site of interaction on Ad E1B 19K since deletion of the N-terminus ablated binding to Bax but not to CED-4 (Han et al., 1998b). As a result of the study by Han et al. (1998b) it was proposed that interaction was through BH3 and the central conserved region on Ad E1B 19K. Obviously further study is required to resolve this point.

Bcl-2 also helps to maintain organelle integrity. For example it inhibits release of cytochrome c from mitochondria (Yang et al., 1997; Kluck et al., 1997) and apoptosis. Cytochrome c is required for correct functioning of Apaf 1 and subsequent activation of caspase 9 (Li et al., 1997; Zou et al., 1997). Whether Ad E1B 19K will also duplicate this and other functions of Bcl-2 remains to be seen. It should be noted, however, that Ad E1B 19K does not localize to the mitochondria (White and Cipriani, 1989; 1990) although it can maintain the integrity of the organelle after over-expression of pro-apoptotic proteins such as Bax (Han et al., 1998a).

Sub-cellular localization of the Ad E1B 19K protein. In both infected and trans-formed cells Ad E1B 19K is primarily located in nuclear membranes and in the membranes of the endoplasmic reticulum (Persson et al., 1982; White et al., 1984; White and Cipriani, 1989; 1990). In addition, the protein has been shown to associate with intermediate filaments causing disruption of the normally observed pattern (White and Cipriani, 1989, 1990). The distribution of E1B 19K protein in the nucleus and ER is similar to that observed for Bcl-2. However, uniquely, E1B 19K binds directly to nuclear lamin A/C. Because of the insolubility of the proteins the interaction has been most convincingly demonstrated using the yeast two-hybrid system (Farrow et al., 1995; Rao et al., 1997). The interaction probably targets E1B 19K to its site of action in the nuclear envelope and it is interesting to note that incorrect localization (due to mutation of lamin) results in reduced ability to inhibit apoptosis (Rao et al., 1997).

It is possible that in the nuclear lamina E1B 19K is in an appropriate position to bind its target proteins such as Bak, Bax and Bik. Bcl-2 which plays a role largely comparable to 19K is similarly located but this is mainly due to the presence of a C-terminal membrane-spanning domain, missing from the viral protein (Hockenbery et al., 1990; Chen-Leavy and Cleary, 1990; Tanaka et al., 1993).

Expression of E1B 19K results in inhibition of capase-mediated lamin degradation and subsequent nuclear events, such as chromatin condensation, characteristic of apoptosis (Rao et al., 1996). However, it is probable that the stability of the lamins is not due to direct protein-protein interaction with E1B 19K but to a general inhibitory effect of the viral protein on caspase activity and apoptosis in general (Rao et al., 1992; 1997). Attempts to map a binding site for lamin on Ad E1B 19K protein have been largely unsuccessful with the N-terminal 146 amino acid fragment being required for interactions (Rao et al., 1997). Deletional mutation studies established amino acids 252-390 as the region on lamin A (and the homologue lamin C) as the binding site for the viral protein.

Apart from its ability to block apoptosis Ad E1B 19K also has transcriptional regulatory properties. It blocks p53-mediated transcriptional repression, probably contributing to its ability to block p53 induced apoptosis (Shen and Shenk, 1994; Sabbatini et al., 1995). It can also stimulate expression from early Ad promoters, as well as from enhancer-linked cellular promoters (Hermann et al., 1987; Yoshida et al., 1987). Recently, a mechanism for this transcriptional activation has been suggested (See and Shi, 1998). Ad E1B 19K activates c-Jun dependent transcription. It is considered that transcripitonal activation of c-Jun by Ad E1B 19K is mediated through the MEKK1 and MKK4 signalling pathways (See and Shi, 1998).

b. *Adenovirus early region 1B 54K/58K protein*

The larger Ad E1B proteins have distinct roles during infection and transformation. In the former case this is mainly, although not entirely, concerned with the regulation of mRNA metabolism and in the latter with the neutralization of p53 activity. During infection the Ad 5 E1B 58K protein interacts with the 34K E4 orf6 protein (Sarnow et al., 1984). This complex acts on late viral mRNAs after transcription but before translocation from the nucleus. It has been suggested that the viral complex binds to a cellular factor required for mRNA export and transports it to the site of viral replication and transcription – this has the effect of favouring late viral mRNA processing and reducing host cell mRNA metabolism (Ornelles and Shenk, 1991). Alternatively, the E4 orf6 : E1B 58K proteins could block nuclear retention of late viral mRNAs by interacting with, and neutralizing the activity of, cellular RNA binding proteins which carry nuclear retention signals (Dix and Leppard, 1993). It should be noted that the effects of the E4 orf6 : E1B 58K complex on viral mRNA metabolism are largely limited to some but not all late RNAs; early mRNAs are largely unaffected.

The Ad5 E1B 58K protein, has no nuclear localization signal (NLS) and in isolation is cytoplasmic. However, when bound to E4 orf6 the complex is nuclear, presumably due to an arginine-rich nuclear retention signal on E4 orf6 (Goodrum et al., 1996; Dobbelstein et al., 1997). The E4 orf6 : E1B 58K complex can act as a nucleocyto-plasmic transporter for viral mRNAs shuttling between the nucleus and cytoplasm. This is regulated by E4 orf6 which contains a nuclear export signal similar to that found in the rev and rex retroviral proteins (Dobelstein et al., 1997). It is possible that the E1B 58K protein acts as the RNA binding component of the complex as it has recently been demonstrated that in vitro it will bind to a variety of RNA probes (Horridge and Leppard, 1998). Whether such an interaction occurs in vivo has yet to be established.

Table 2. Comparison of the properties of Ad2/5 E1B 58K and Ad12 E1B 54K proteins

Property	Ad2/5 E1B 58K	Ad12 E1B 54K	Reference
A. Infected Cells			
Binding to E4orf6	Yes	Not known	Sarnow et al., 1984
Regulates mRNA metabolism	Yes	Not known	Babiss and Ginsberg, 1984; Babiss et al., 1985; Ornelles and Shenk, 1991
Binding to Ad E1B-AP5	Yes	Weakly	Gaber et al., 1998; Grand and Dobner, unpublished data
B. Ad E1-transformed cells			
Binding to p53	Strong	Weak	Sarnow et al., 1982; Grand et al., 1994
Repressor of p53 transcriptional activity	Yes	Yes	Yew and Berk, 1992; Yew et al., 1994
Effect on p53 expression	Increases	Increases	Zantema et al., 1985a,b; Grand et al., 1996
Subcellular localization	Cytoplasmic flecks	Predominantly nuclear but some homogeneous cytoplasmic distribution	Zantema et al., 1985a,b; Blair-Zajdel and Blair, 1998; Mak et al., 1998
p53 binding site	Amino acids 216-235	Amino acids 202-221	Grand et al., 1999b
Nuclear localization signal	None	Probably between amino acids 228 and 239	Grand et al., 1999b
Binding to E1B-AP5	Yes	Weakly	Gabler et al, 1998; Grand and Tobner, unpublished data
Quaternary structure	Dimer	Tetramer	Grand et al., 1995; Martin and Berk, 1998
Phosphorylation	Phosphorylated at serine 490 and 491 and threonine 495	No	Teodoro et al., 1994; Teodoro and Branton, 1997b; Grand, unpublished data
Binding to RNA	Yes	Not known	Horridge and Leppard, 1998

Interestingly, Ad5 E1A 58K protein forms a stable complex with a novel protein (termed E1B-AP5) in both infected and transformed cells (Gabler et al., 1998). E1B-AP5 is an RNA binding protein of the heterogeneous nuclear ribonucleoprotein (hnRNP) family related to hnRNP-U/SAF-A. The interaction is modulated by E4 orf6 with less E1B-AP5 bound to E1B 58K in the presence of the E4 component (Gabler et al., 1998). These data might suggest that there is no requirement for direct interaction for the Ad E1B 58K protein to play a role in the regulation of RNA metabolism – however, this remains to be established.

It is not clear whether the Ad12 E1B 54K protein acts in the same way as the Ad5 homologue during viral infection. A number of clues suggest that it might not but as yet no firm evidence is available. The Ad12 protein has a NLS located between amino 228 and 239 and therefore is present in the nucleus even in the absence of the Ad12 E4 orf6 (Grand et al., 1999b). It is quite possible that the Ad12 E1B 54K : Ad12 E4 orf6 may have different properties to the Ad5 proteins, particularly as there is somewhat limited homology, at the amino acid level, between Ad5 and Ad12 E4 components. The observation that the Ad5 and Ad12 E1B proteins behave very differently in Ad E1 transformed cells would lend credence to the suggestion that differences might be apparent during infection.

As well as the modulation of RNA metabolism it has long been established that the larger Ad E1B proteins are intimately concerned in the regulation of p53 activity. This is primarily evident in Ad E1 transformed cells (see below) but it appears that p53 is also a specific target during viral infection. It had been thought that p53 is lost during infection due to shut-down of host cell RNA metabolism, as described above, and proteasome-mediated degradation of the existing protein (Grand et al., 1994). However, recent evidence suggests that p53 is a specific target for Ad5 E1B 58K-E4orf6 resulting in very rapid degradation (Querido et al., 1997b; Steegenga et al., 1998).

Shortly after its identification as a binding protein for SV40 T antigen it was shown that p53 also interacts with Ad5 E1B 58K protein in transformed cells (Sarnow et al., 1982). Complex formation results in the over-expression of p53 and re-localization of the p53 from the nucleus to cytoplasmic dense bodies (Zantema et al., 1985a; b). In Ad12 E1 transformants interaction between p53 and the 54K E1B protein was thought to occur much less frequently and/or was appreciably weaker (Grand et al., 1994). In the latter case no redistribution of p53 was observed and the E1B protein was located predominantly in the nucleus but also to a limited extent in the cytoplasm. It appears likely that in the case of Ad12 E1 transformed cells complex formation takes place but is difficult to demonstrate by co-immunprecipitation techniques since in both Ad2/5 and Ad12 E1B-expressing cells transcriptional activation properties of p53 are neutralized (Yew and Berk, 1992).

Interestingly, both Ad5 and Ad12 E1B proteins can repress transcription, in vitro, when directed to DNA even in the absence of p53 (Yew et al., 1994). However, in vivo both viral proteins are targeted to p53-responsive genes, presumably though direct interaction, specifically repressing transcription possibly through interaction with RNA polymerase II transcription machinery (Yew et al., 1994; Martin and Berk, 1998). The transcriptional repression properties of Ad5 E1B 58K protein appear to be regulated by phosphorylation at sites close to the C-terminus. Thus mutation of S490, S491 and T495 to A results in a protein which has lost its ability to repress transcription as well as its ability to neutralize the p53-dependent apoptosis induced by Ad E1A (Teodoro et al., 1994; Teodoro and Branton, 1997b). Serines at residue 490 and 491 are possible substrates for casein kinase II, although the precise kinase responsible for phosphorylation has yet to be identified (Teodoro et al., 1994). It is worth bearing in mind, however, that Ad12 E1B 54K is not phosphorylated either in virally infected – or Ad E1 – transformed cells (RJAG, unpublished data). Thus, it is not likely that protein phosphorylation is a generalised regulatory mechanism for the control of Ad E1B activity.

In vitro and in vivo studies have suggested that the larger Ad E1B protein exists as a dimer or tetramer (Grand et al.,1995; Martin and Berk, 1998) as well as a member of a very high molecular weight complex (Grand et al., 1995). The polymerization appears to occur in the absence of a strong binding to p53 (i.e. in Ad12 E1 transformants) and may reflect interaction with a novel cellular protein such as AP5. Alternatively, the high molecular weight complex could represent an E1B/nucleic acid interaction.

In Ad E1-transformed cells the level of p53 is dramatically increased as a result of protein stabilization (increased half-life [van den Heuval et al., 1990; Grand et al., 1993]). Whilst this is partially attributable to Ad E1A expression (Lowe and Ruley, 1993) there is also a direct, more pronounced, effect of the larger Ad E1B protein (Grand et al., 1996). It is likely that stabilization of p53 by Ad E1B is caused by interference by the viral protein with binding to MDM2 which is considered to be responsible for targeting it to the proteasome (Haupt et al., 1997; Kubbutat et al., 1997). The binding sites on p53 for both MDM2 and Ad5 E1B 58K protein have been mapped to the N-terminal domain with amino acids 23-27 being of particular significance (Lin et al., 1994). The binding sites for p53 on the larger Ad2 and Ad12 E1B proteins have been mapped to homologous regions close to the centre of the molecule – between amino acids 216 and 235 on Ad2 E1B 58K and between 202 and 221 on Ad12 E1B 54K proteins (Grand et al.,1999b; Kao et al., 1990). In the case of the Ad12 protein this is close to the NLS at amino acids 228-239.

In Ad E1-transformed cells it appears that localization of p53 is governed by the E1B proteins. Thus the NLS on p53 is overridden in Ad2/5 E1 transformants, with the p53: Ad2/5 E1B 58K complex being apparent in large cytoplasmic dense bodies – the origin and structure of which are not clear (Zantema et al., 1985a, b). The NLS on Ad12 E1B 54K ensures its presence in the nucleus, together with p53, in Ad12 E1 transformed cells.

Interestingly, it has recently been shown that Ad E1B 58K does not interact with the p53 homologue, p73 (Higashino et al., 1998; Marin et al., 1998; Roth et al., 1998), nor does it affect the transcriptional regulatory activity of p73. The inability of p73 to interact with Ad2/5 E1B 58K protein is due to differences in amino acid sequence between it and p53 at the N-terminus. Thus, when [24]KLLPE[28] from p53 replaces [20]SSLEP[24] on p73 the latter protein is converted to a "strong" Ad E1B binder (Roth et al., 1998). These data suggest that inactivation of p73 is not necessary for Ad E1-induced transformation and mediation of p73 activity is not as important during viral infection. It should be noted, however, that the activity of p73 can be modulated by Ad E4 orf6 (Higashino et al., 1998).

As previously mentioned, during viral infection, the larger E1B protein functions in concert with E4 orf6 to regulate RNA metabolism. Over the past three years the ability of this protein to affect transformation has been examined. E4 orf6 binds strongly to p53, quite distinctly from any interaction via the E1B protein and is also able to block transcriptional activation (Dobner et al., 1996) and p53-mediated apoptosis (Moore et al., 1996). Binding sites for the two viral protein are in different domains of p53 with E1B interacting at the N-terminus and E4 orf6 between amino acids 318-360 (Dobner et al., 1996). More recent analysis has suggested that E4 orf6 may have an oncogenic potential. Thus, it can co-operate with Ad E1A to increase the transformation frequency of baby rat kidney cells (Moore et al., 1996; Nevels et al., 1997), can increase the growth rate of cells already expressing Ad E1 (Nevels et al., 1999a) and increases the tumorigenicity and malignancy of Ad transformants (Moore et al., 1996; Nevels et al., 1999a). It appears that this effect is primarily due to the interaction with p53 reducing its transcriptional activation properties and perhaps modulating its tumor suppressor functions. However, it is also important to note that E4 orf 6 reduces the steady state levels of p53 in Ad E1 transformed cells (Nevels et al., 1997; 1999a) as well as altering its location from the cytoplasmic dense bodies to the nucleus in human cells (Moore et al., 1996).

Ad5 E4 orf3 has also recently been shown to bind to the larger E1B protein in transformed cells (Nevels et al., 1999b), with both proteins co-localizing to PML oncogenic domains (POD) which are considered to be centres of DNA processing (Doucas et al., 1996; Nevels et al., 1999b; Konig et al., 1999). Like E4 orf6 E4 orf3 co-operates with Ad E1A to transform baby rat kidney cells and increases the growth rate and tumorigenicity of Ad E1 transformants (Nevels et al., 1999b). These activities are considered not to result from modulation of p53 transcriptional activation properties.

c. E1B-defective mutant adenovirus as an anti-tumor agent

Over the past two years there has been considerable controversy triggered by reports that mutant adenoviruses which fail to express the larger E1B protein can be used to kill preferentially human cells which lack functional p53. It has been further suggested that this offers a therapeutic tool for the treatment and perhaps eradication of certain human tumors (Bischoff et al.,1996; Heise et al., 1997; Kirn et al., 1998). However, in response to these claims there have been a number of studies which conclude that E1B 58K⁻ virus is no more efficacious in killing cells with mutant p53 than normal cells. Similarly, the mutant virus has comparable properties to wt in this situation.

In the original study by Bischoff et al. (1996) it was proposed that an adenovirus mutant virus (Ad5 dl1520) which did not express the larger E1B protein would have very limited replicative capacity in "normal" cells (i.e. expressing wt p53) but would be able to replicate (and therefore lyse/kill) in cells lacking functional p53. This was indeed the case using the cervical carcinoma cell line C33A (mutant p53) and the osteosarcoma cell line U20S(wt p53). In an expanded investigation using a number of other cell lines similar results were obtained (Heise et al., 1997). In addition, it was shown that tumors, induced in nude mice by injection of the cells (C33A) expressing mutant p53, were highly susceptible to virus with tumor regression occuring in more than half the cases. Administration of Ad5 *dl*1520 in combination with chemo-therapeutic agents resulted in considerably more pronounced tumor regression than with either agent alone (Hiese et al., 1997). So encouraging were these results that the virus has been used in clinical trials on patients with head and neck cancers. Preliminary results showed that there was appreciable regression of tumors (reduction of tumor mass by 40-100%) expressing mutant p53 after injection of virus (Kirn et al., 1998).

Unfortunately, these studies have not been received with universal enthusiasm (see for examples original comments in Pennisi [1996] as well as Goodrun and Ornelles, 1998; Rothmann et al., 1998; Hall et al., 1998; Turnell et al., 1999). Detailed studies of the cytopathic effects of the virus in a number of cell lines have suggested that the conclusions drawn by the "Onyx group" were an oversimplification. It appears that *dl*1520 is able to replicate in tumor cell lines wholly independently of p53 status (Rothmann et al., 1998; Hall et al., 1998; Goodrum and Ornelles, 1998; Turnell et al., 1999). Contrary to original suggestions, replication of the virus in normal primary human cells has also been observed (Rothmann et al., 1998; Turnell et al., 1999). In addition, the ability of Ad5 *dl*1520 to replicate seems to be dependent upon as yet unknown factors since – for example, C33A (mutant p53), A549 (wt p53) and U87 (wt p53) cells are highly permissive whilst U205 (wt p53) and U373 (mutant p53) are not (Rothmann et al., 1998). Similarly, some variations in the replicative capacity of wt Ad5 and Ad12 viruses with different cell lines has been observed, although this again appears to be independent of p53 status (Rothmann et al., 1998; Turnell et al., 1999).

The ability of *dl*1520 to kill the infected cell is of central importance to any consideration of its use as a therapeutic tool. The consensus amongst later reports is that cell killing is largely dependent on replicative capacity of the virus rather than p53 status (Goodrum and Ornelles, 1998; Rothmann, et al., 1998; Turnell et al., 1999). It has also been suggested that virus replication may be governed by the ability of the mutant virus to inhibit host cell apoptosis and therefore varies with level of expression of the E1B 19K protein (Turnell et al., 1999).

Despite arguments over how Ad5 *dl*1520 causes tumor regression preliminary results from clinical trials are encouraging as noted above. It may be that others factors which have been shown to be important in determining the activity of the virus in vitro, such as multiplicity of infection and cell cycle status of the target cell might combine fortuitously to promote infectivity, premature adenovirus-induced apoptosis and consequent death of tumor cells (Kirn et al., 1998; Goodrum and Ornelles, 1998; Turnell et al., 1999).

4. Concluding Remarks

Adenovirus E1A is a small protein of around 250 amino acids. Considering the many millions of hours (and dollars) which have been devoted to its study it might be expected that we should be close to understanding how it functions. Unfortunately, this is not the case. Whilst progress has been considerable in particular areas and we now understand, reasonably well, the way in which Ad E1A affects the interaction of the Rb family with E2F and perhaps how transcription is controlled through CR3 our grasp of its overall mode of action is still tentative. For example, it is still not clear what proportion of E1A interacts with each cellular component, whether E1A can bind more than one protein at the same time, how binding to one might affect interaction with a second or third and whether there remain other important unidentified targets. Recent reports of novel binding proteins would seem to support the idea that there are yet more partners to find (Reid et al., 1998; Grand et al., 1999a). Indeed, a number of novel proteins interacting with the N terminal region have been observed (Sang and Giordano, 1997). Whether any of these are identical to P/CAF (Reid et al., 1998) and SUG1 (Grand et al., 1999a) will have to await further investigation.

Even in the case of relatively well-characterized interacting proteins there is still a great deal to learn. We are only just coming to terms with the full implications of binding to p300/CBP and CtBP. It is becoming apparent that histone acetyl transferases are a major target for E1A with both p300/CBP and P/CAF forming complexes. HAT activity is obviously important in the regulation of gene expression and so it is not surprising that it is affected by E1A. Whether other HATs will be shown to be targets for E1A remains to be seen but it would perhaps be surprising if this were not the case. The observation that the unique or spacer region of Ad12 E1A is at least partially responsible for the oncogenicity of the Ad12 E1A protein (see Williams et al., 1995 and Chapter 14 of this volume) would suggest it plays a role in down-regulation of MHCI expression. This may be attributable to specific binding to novel cellular proteins. These are so far unidentified.

Concluding their review of the properties of the Ad E1 proteins in 1991, Boulanger and Blair considered that the approach most likely to elucidate their mode of action was to undertake studies using purified proteins after expression in bacteria or eukaryotic cells. Surprisingly, investigations of this kind have provided almost none of the significant advances over the last ten years. Most of the major recent discoveries in this field (like those in the past) have been made on the basis of "*in vivo*" studies using cells in culture. In fact, there has proved to be very little requirement for purified proteins in biochemical characterization of the Ad E1 components. However, to understand more fully the mode of action of Ad E1 proteins, and in particular Ad E1A, a structural analysis of proteins in their free and bound forms will have to be undertaken using either X-ray crystallography or nuclear magnetic resonance. Studies of this sort will provide the information necessary for understanding the effect of interaction with one partner protein on binding to a second or perhaps third cellular component. As already mentioned, investigation of the structure of Ad E1A has proved particularly difficult for a number of reasons. Ad E1A is expressed at high levels only in an insoluble form requiring denaturation for solublization, Ad E1A is difficult to crystallize (in our hands at least) and the limited evidence available suggests that the structure of the protein may be appreciably dependent on binding partners. However, there can be little doubt that results of biophysical/structural investigations would greatly increase our knowledge of

Ad E1A activity. Results of recent studies of HPV E7 and pRb support this contention (Lee et al., 1998).

The situation with the E1B proteins is rather different. Because of the marked similarity (in function if not in amino acid sequence) between Ad E1B 19K and Bcl-2, it seems likely that when we understand the mode of action of the latter protein then we will know fairly precisely how the viral protein protects both infected and transformed cells from apoptosis. The role of the larger E1B protein is far less clear. Considering the multiplicity of partners for E1A, it is difficult to believe that p53 and E4orf6 represent its only interacting components. Indeed, a further cellular protein (E1B-AP5 [Gabler et al., 1998]) has recently been described. It is surely not particularly perceptive to suggest that this is likely to be only the first of many Ad E1B binding proteins. Whether E1B-AP5 is involved in the Ad E1B-mediated regulation of mRNA metabolism (Babiss et al., 1985; Ornelles and Shenk, 1991) is not clear, but it is possible that other proteins intimately concerned with cellular mRNA metabolism will be isolated as E1B 58K/54K binding proteins in the near future.

Differences in the properties of the Ad2/5 E1B 58K and Ad12 E1B 54K proteins have been described in some detail (Table 2). Of particular interest is the fact that the Ad12 protein will inhibit p53 transcriptional activation, even though a complex between the two proteins can only be demonstrated with difficulty. This may, of course, be an artificial difference attributable to our experimental procedures but might be rather more significant, perhaps indicating the involvement of additional cellular components. The observation that Ad12 E1B 54K possesses a NLS (Grand et al., 1999b) suggests that Ad12 E4orf6 is less important in targeting it to the nucleus during viral infection (unlike the Ad2/5 situation). It is quite possible therefore that the Ad12 protein has a distinct function. Whether it possesses the p53 binding oncogenic properties of Ad2/5 E4orf6 is currently under investigation.

Whilst Ad E1B proteins have long been considered to have no transforming ability of their own and largely to function as "anti-apoptosis" factors, it has been demonstrated that Ad12 E1B 54K will extend appreciably the lifespan of mammalian cells in culture (Gallimore et al., 1997). How this is accomplished is not clear at present but it might suggest additional, as yet unknown, properties of the protein, or perhaps gives some indication of the specific contribution of the larger E1B protein to the Ad E1-transformed phenotype.

Recently, adenoviruses have assumed a new significance as therapeutic tools. Whilst many of the organisms used for gene delivery have deletions in the E1 region and are beyond the scope of this review (they are considered in detail in chapter 16) two other mutant adenoviruses appear to have considerable potential in the search for anti-tumor agents. The first of these is the ONYX-015 virus which, whilst the subject of criticism, seems to be proving effective in clinical trials. A second, more experimental, approach could be the use of mutant adenoviruses expressing "mini E1A". It has been shown that viruses expressing the N terminal third of E1A can suppress *neu*-mediated transformation without inducing transformation in their own right due to the lack of CR2 (Chen et al., 1997b). Obviously, such a virus is a very long way from a serious therapeutic agent at present but it is indicative of the potential of mutant adenoviruses in the treatment of human cancers.

It seems fitting that a virus which has taught us so much about the mechanism of transformation and has been responsible for the identification of important cellular components such as p300, p107, p130, CtBP and Bak, may provide novel weapons in the fight against human cancers in the near future.

Acknowledgements

I am must grateful to Andrew Turnell for invaluable discussion, Ester Hammond for the illustrations and Nicola Waldron for secretarial help. I also thank the Cancer Research Campaign for many years of financial support.

References

Abdel-Hafiz, H.A.M., Chen, C.-Y., Marcell, T., Kroll, D.J. and Hoeffler, J.P. (1993) Structural determinants outside of the leucine zipper influence the interactions of CREB and ATF2-interaction of CREB with ATF2 blocks E1a-ATF2 complex formation. Oncogene 8, 1161-1174.

Adams, J.M. and Cory, S. (1998) The Bcl-2 protein family : arbiters of cell survival. Science 281-1322-1326.

Ait-Si-Ali, S., Ramirez, S., Barre, F.-X., Dkhissi, F., Magnaghi-Jaulin, L., Girault, J.A., Robin, P., Knibiehler, M., Pritchard, L.L., Ducommun, B., Trouche, D. and Harel-Bellan, A. (1998) Histone acetyltransferase activity of CBP is controlled by cycle-dependent kinases and oncoprotein E1A. Nature 396, 184-186.

Arany, Z., Newsome, D., Oldread, E., Livingston, D.M. and Eckner, R. (1995) A family of transcriptional adaptor proteins targeted by the E1A oncoprotein. Nature 374, 81-84.

Avantaggiati, M.L., Ogryzko, V., Gardner, K., Giordano, A., Levine, A.S. and Kelly, K. (1997) Recruitment of p300/CBP in p53-dependent signal pathways. Cell 89, 1175-1184.

Babiss, L.E. and Ginsberg, H.S. (1984) Adenovirus type 5 early region 1B gene product is required for efficient shut off of host protein synthesis. J. Virol. 50, 202-212.

Babiss, L.E., Ginsberg, H.S. and Darnell, J.E. (1985) Adenovirus E1B proteins are required for accumulation of late viral mRNA and for effects on cellular mRNA translation and transport. Mol. Cell. Biol. 5, 2552-2558.

Bannister, A.J. and Kouzarides, T. (1995) CBP-induced stimulation of c-Fos activity is abrogated by E1A. EMBO J. 14, 4758-4762.

Bannister, A.J. and Kouzarides, T. (1996) The CBP co-activator is a histone acetyltransferase. Nature 384, 641-643.

Barbeau, D., Charbonneau, R., Whalen, S.G., Bayley, S.T. and Branton, P.E. (1994) Functional interactions within adenovirus E1A protein complexes. Oncogene 9, 359-373.

Bayley, S.T. and Mymryk, J.S. (1994) Adenovirus E1a proteins and transformation. Int. J. Onc. 5, 425-444.

Bhattacharya, S., Eckner, R., Grossman, S., Oldread, E., Arany, Z., D'Andrea, A. and Livingston, D.M. (1996) Cooperation of Stat2 and p300/CBP in signalling induced by interferon-α. Nature 383, 344-347.

Bischoff, J.R., Kirn, D.H., Williams, A., Heise, C., Horn, S., Muna, M., Ng, L., Nye, J.A., Sampson-Johannes, A., Fattaey, A., and McCormick, F. (1996) An adenovirus mutant that replicates selectively in p53-deficient human tumor cells. Science 274, 373-376.

Blair-Zajdel, M.E. and Blair, G.E. (1988) The intracellular distribution of the transformation-associated p53 in adenovirus transformed rodent cells. Oncogene 2, 579-584.

Boulakia, C.A., Chen, G., Ng, F.W.H., Teodoro, J.G., Branton, P.E., Nicholson, D.W., Poirier, G.G. and Shore, G.C. (1996) Bcl-2 and adenovirus E1B 19 kDa proteins prevent E1A-induced processing of CPP32 and cleavage of poly (ADP-ribose) polymerase. Oncogene 12, 529-535.

Boulanger, P.A. and Blair, G.E. (1991) Expression and interactions of human adenovirus oncoproteins. Biochem. J. 275, 281-299.

Boyd, J.M., Gallo, G.J., Elangovan, B., Houghton, A.B., Malstrom, S., Avery, B.J., Ebb, R.G., Subramanian, T., Chittenden, T., Lutz, R.J. and Chinnadurai, G. (1995) BIK, a novel death inducing protein shares a distinct sequence motif with bcl-2 family proteins and interacts with viral and cellular survival-promoting proteins. Oncogene 11, 1921-1928.

Boyd, J.M., Subramanian, T., Schaeper, U., La Regina, M., Bayley, S. and Chinnadurai, G. (1993) A region in the C-terminus of adenovirus 2/5 E1a protein is required for association with a cellular phosphoprotein and important for the negative modulation of T24-ras mediated transformation, tumourigenesis and metastasis. EMBO J. 12, 469-478.

Boyd, J.M., Malstrom, S., Subramanian, T., Venkatesh, L.K., Schaeper, U., Elangovan, B., D'Sa-Eipper, C. and Chinnadurai, G. (1994) Adenovirus E1B kDa and Bcl-2 proteins interact with a common set of cellular proteins. Cell 79, 341-351.

Brehm, A., Miska, E.A., McCance, D.J., Reid, J.L., Bannister, A.J. and Kouzarides, T. (1998) Retinoblastoma protein recruits histone deacetylase to repress transactivation. Nature 391, 597-601.

Brown, R. (1997) The bcl-2 family of proteins. Brit. Med. Bull. 53, 466-477.

Cao, L., Faha, B., Dembski, M., Tsai, L.H., Harlow, E. and Dyson, N. (1992) Independent binding of the retinoblastoma protein and p107 to the transcription factor E2F. Nature 355, 176-179.

Chakravarti, D., Ogryzko, V., Kao, H.-Y., Nash, A., Chen, H., Nakatani, Y. and Evans, R.M. (1999) A viral mechanism for inhibition of p300 and PCAF acetyltransferase activity. Cell 96, 393-403.

Chapman, M.S. and Verma, I.M. (1996) Transcriptional activation of BRCA1. Nature 382, 678-679.

Chatton, B., Bocco, J.L., Gaire, M., Hauss, C., Reimund, B., Goetz, J. and Kedinger, C. (1993) Transcriptional activation by the adenovirus larger E1a product is mediated by members of the cellular transcription factor ATF family which can directly associate with E1a. Mol. Cell. Biol. 13, 561-570.

Chellappan, S. Hiebert, S., Mudryj, M., Horowitz, J.M. and Nevins, J.R. (1991) The E2F transcription factor is a cellular target for the Rb protein. Cell 65, 1053-1061.

Chellappan, S., Kraus, V.B., Kroger, B., Munger, K., Howley, P.M., Phelps, W.C. and Nevins, J.R. (1992) Adenovirus-E1A, Simian virus-40 tumor-antigen and human papillomavirus –E7 protein share the capacity to disrupt the interaction between transcription factor-E2F and the retinoblastoma gene product. Proc. Natl. Acad. Sci. USA 89, 4549-4553.

Chen, G., Branton, P.E., Yang, E., Korsmeyer, S.J. and Shore, G.C. (1996) Adenovirus E1B 19-kDa death suppressor protein interacts with Bax but not with Bad. J. Biol. Chem. 271, 24221-24225.

Chen, G., Ray, R., Dubik, D., Shi, L., Cizeau, J., Bleackley, C., Saxena, S., Gietz, R.D., and Greenberg, A.H. (1997a) The E1B 19K/Bcl-2-binding protein Nip3 is a dimeric mitochondrial protein that activates apoptosis. J. Exp. Med. 186, 1975-1983.

Chen, H., Yu, D., Chinnadurai, G., Karungaran, D. and Hung, M.-C. (1997b) Mapping of adenovirus 5 E1A domains responsible for suppression of neu-mediated transformation via transcriptional repression of neu. Oncogene 14, 1965-1971.

Chen-Leavy, Z. and Cleary, M.L. (1990) Membrane topology of the Bcl-2 proto-oncogenic protein demonstrated in vitro. J. Biol. Chem. 265, 4929-4933.

Chiang, C.-M. and Roeder, R.G. (1995) Cloning of an intrinsic human TFIID subunit that interacts with multiple transcriptional activators. Science 267, 531-536.

Chinnadurai, G. (1998) Control of apoptosis by human adenovirus genes. Sems Virol. 8, 399-408.

Chiou, S.K., Rao, L. and White, E. (1994a) Bcl-2 blocks p53-dependent apoptosis. Mol. Cell. Biol. 14, 2556-2563.

Chiou, S.K., Tseng, C.C., Rao, L. and White, E. (1994b) Functional complementation of the adenovirus E1b 19-Kilodalton protein with Bcl-2 in the inhibition of apoptosis in infected cells. J. Virol. 68, 6553-6566.

Chiou, S.-K. and White, E. (1997) p300 binding by E1A cosegregates with p53 induction but is dispensable for apoptosis. J. Virol. 71, 3515-3525.

Chittenden, T., Flemington, C., Houghton, A.B., Ebb, R.G., Gallo, G.J., Elangovan, B., Chinnadurai, G. and Lutz, R.J. (1995) A conserved domain in Bak, distinct from BH1 and BH2, mediates cell death and protein binding functions. EMBO J. 14, 5589-5596.

Cobrinik, D., Whyte, P., Peeper, D.S., Jacks, T. and Weinberg, R.A. (1993) Cell cycle-specific association of E2F with the p130 E1A-binding protein. Genes. Dev. 7, 2392-2404.

Coux, O., Tanaka, K. and Goldberg, A.L. (1996) Structure and functions of the 20S and 26S proteasomes. Annu. Rev. Biochem. 65, 801-847.

Culp, J.S., Webster, L.C., Friedman, D.J., Smith, C.L., Huang, W.J., Hu, F. Y.-H., Rosenberg, M. and Riccardi, R.P. (1988) The 289-amino acid E1a protein of adenovirus binds zinc in a region that is important for transactivation. Proc. Natl. Acad. Sci. USA 85, 6450-6454.

Dallas, P.B., Cheney, I.W., Liao, D.-W., Bowrin, V., Byam, W., Pacchione, S., Kobayashi, R., Yaciuk, P. and Moran, E. (1998) p300/CREB binding protein-related protein p270 is a component of mammalian SWI/SNF complexes. Mol. Cell. Biol. 18, 3596-3603.

Darnell Jr., J.E., Kerr, I.M. and Stark, G.R. (1994) Jak-STAT pathways and transcriptional activation in responses to IFNs and other extracellular signaling proteins. Science 264, 1415-1421.

Debbas, M. and White, E. (1993) Wild-type p53 mediates apoptosis by E1a, which is inhibited by E1b. Genes Dev. 7, 546-554.

de Stanchina, E., McCurrach, M.E., Zindy, F., Shieh, S.-Y., Ferbeyre, G., Samuelson, A.V., Prives, C., Roussel, M.F., Sherr, C.J. and Lowe, S.W. (1998) E1A signaling to p53 involves the p19^{ARF} tumor suppressor. Genes Dev. 12, 2434-2442.

Devoto, S.H., Mudryj, M., Pines, J., Hunter, T. and Nevins, J.R. (1992) A cyclin A-protein kinase complex possesses sequence-specific DNA binding activity: p33^{cdk2} is a component of the E2F cyclin A complex. Cell 68, 167-176.

Dix, I. and Leppard, K.N. (1993) Regulated splicing of adenovirus type 5 E4 transcripts and regulated cytoplasmic accumulation of E4 mRNA. J. Virol. 67, 3226-3231.

Dobbelstein, M., Roth, J., Kimberly, W.T., Levine, A.J. and Shenk, T. (1997) Nuclear export of the E1B 55-kDa and E4 34-kDa adenoviral oncoproteins mediated by a rev-like signal sequence. EMBO J. 16, 4276-4284.

Dobner, T., Horikoshi, N., Rubenwolf, S. and Shenk, T. (1996) Blockage by adenovirus E4orf6 of transcriptional activation by the p53 tumor suppressor. Science 272, 1470-1473.

Doerfler, W. and Bohm, P. (editors) (1995) The molecular repertoire of adenovirus Volumes I, II and III Springer, Berlin.

Doucas, V., Ishov, A.M., Romo, A., Juguilon, H., Weitzman, M.D., Evans, R.G. and Maul, G.G. (1996) Adenovirus replication is coupled with the dynamic properties of the PML nuclear structure. Genes Dev. 10, 196-207.

Douglas, J.L., Gopalakrishnan, S. and Quinlan, M.P. (1991) Modulation of transformation of primary epithelial cells by the second exon of the Ad5 E1A 12S gene. Oncogene 6, 2093-2103.

Dowdy, S.F., Hinds, P.W., Louie, K., Reed, S.I., Arnold, A. and Weinberg, R.A. (1993) Physical interaction of the retinoblastoma protein with human D-cyclins. Cell 73, 499-511.

Dumont, D.J., Tremblay, M.L. and Branton, P.E. (1989) Phosphorylation at serine 89 induces a shift in gel mobility but has little effect on the function of adenovirus type 5 E1A proteins. J. Virol. 63, 987-991.

Dumont, D.J. and Branton, P.E. (1992) Phosphorylation of adenovirus E1A proteins by the p34^{cdc2} protein kinase. Virology 189, 111-120.

Dunaief, J.L., Strober, B.E., Guha, S., Khavari, P.A., Alin, K., Luban, J., Begemann, M., Crabtree, G.R. and Goff, S.P. (1994) The retinoblastoma protein and BRG1 form a complex and cooperate to induce cell cycle arrest. Cell 79, 119-130.

Dyson, N., Bernards, R., Friend, S.H., Gooding, L.R., Hassell, J.A., Major, E.O., Pipas, J.M., Vandyke, T. and Harlow, E. (1990) Large T antigens of many polyoma viruses are able to form complexes with the retinoblastoma protein. J. Virol. 64, 1353-1356.

Dyson, N., Howley, P.M., Munger, K. and Harlow, E. (1989) The human papilloma virus-16 E7 oncoprotein is able to bind to the retinoblastoma gene product. Science 243, 934-937.

Dyson, N., Guida, P., Munger, K. and Harlow, E. (1992) Homologous sequences in adenovirus E1a and human papilloma virus E7 proteins mediate interaction with the same set of cellular proteins. J. Virol. 66, 6893-6902.

Dyson, N. (1998) The regulation of E2F by pRB-family proteins. Genes Dev. 12, 2245-2262.

Eckner, R., Ewen, M.E., Newsome, D., Gerdes, M., DeCaprio, J., Lawrence, J.B. and Livingston, D.M. (1994) Molecular cloning and functional analysis of the adenovirus E1a-associated 300-kD protein (p300) reveals a protein with properties of a transcriptional adaptor. Genes Dev. 8, 869-884.

Eckner, R., Yao, T.P., Oldread, E. and Livingston, D.M. (1996) Interaction and functional collaboration of p300/CBP and bHLH factors in muscle and B-cell differentiation. Genes Dev. 10, 2478-2490.

Ewen, M.E., Xing, Y., Lawrence, J.B. and Livingston, D.M. (1991) Molecular cloning, chromosomal mapping and expression of the cDNA for p107, a retinoblastoma gene product related protein. Cell 66, 1155-1164.

Ewen, M.E., Faha, B., Harlow, E. and Livingston, D.M. (1992) Interaction of p107 with cyclin A independent of complex formation with viral oncoproteins. Science 255, 85-87.

Faha, B., Ewen, M.E., Tsai, L.H., Livingston, D.M. and Harlow, E. (1992) Interaction between human cyclin-A and adenovirus E1A-associated p107 protein. Science 255, 87-90.

Faha, B., Harlow, E. and Lees, E. (1993) The adenovirus E1a-associated kinase consists of cyclin E-p33cdk2 and cyclin A-p33cdk2. J. Virol. 67, 2456-2465.

Farrow, S.N., White, J.H.M., Martinou, I., Raven, T., Pun, K.-T., Grinham, C.J., Martinou, J.-C. and Brown, R. (1995) Cloning of a bcl-2 homologue by interaction with adenovirus E1B 19K. Nature 374, 731-733.

Ferreira, R., Magnaghi-Jaulin, L., Robin, P., Harel-Bellan, A. and Trouche, D. (1998) The three members of the pocket proteins family share the ability to repress E2F activity through recruitment of a histone deacetylase. Proc. Natl. Acad. Sci. USA 95, 10493-10498.

Fisher, A.L., Ohsako, S. and Caudy, M. (1996) The WRPW motif of the hairy-related basic helix-loop-helix repressor protein acts as a 4-amino-acid transcription repression and protein-protein interaction domain. Mol. Cell. Biol. 16, 2670-2677.

Flint, J. and Shenk, T. (1997) Viral transactivating proteins. Annu. Rev. Genet. 31, 177-212.

Flint, K.J. and Jones, N.C. (1991) Differential regulation of three members of the ATC/CREB family of DNA binding proteins. Oncogene 6, 2019-2026.

Fraser, R.A., Resignol, M., Heard, D.J., Egly, J.M. and Chambon, P. (1997) SUG1, a putative transcriptional mediator and subunit of the PA700 proteasome complex, is a DNA helicase. J. Biol. Chem. 272, 7122-7126.

Gabler, S., Schutt, H., Groitl, P., Wolf, H., Shenk, T. and Dobner, T. (1998) E1B 55-kilodalton-associated protein: a cellular protein with RNA-binding activity implicated in nucleocytoplasmic transport of adenovirus and cellular mRNAs. J. Virol. 72, 7960-7971.

Gallimore, P.H., Sharp, P.A. and Sambrook, J. (1974) Viral DNA in transformed cells. J. Mol. Biol. 89, 49-72.

Gallimore, P.H., Lecane, P.S., Roberts, S., Rookes, S.M. , Grand, R.J.A. and Parkhill, J. (1997) Adenovirus 12 early region 1B 54K protein significantly extends the life span of normal mammalian cells in culture. J. Virol. 6629-6640.

Geisberg, J.V., Lee, W.S., Berk, A.J. and Riccardi, R.P. (1994) The zinc finger region of the adenovirus E1a transactivating domain complexes with the TATA box binding protein. Proc. Natl. Acad. Sci. USA, 91, 2488-2492.

Geisberg, J.V., Chen, J.-L. and Ricciardi, R.P. (1995) Subregions of the adenovirus E1A transactivation domain target multiple components of the TFIID complex. Mol. Cell. Biol. 15, 6283-6290.

Giles, R.H., Peters, D.J.M. and Breuning, M.H. (1998) Conjunction dysfunction: CBP/p300 in human disease. Trends Genet. 14, 178-183.

Giordano, A., McCall, C., Whyte, P. and Franza Jr., B.R. (1991) Human cyclin A and the retinoblastoma protein interact with similar but distinguishable sequences in the adenovirus E1a gene product. Oncogene 6, 481-485.

Goodrum, F.D. and Ornelles, D.A. (1998) p53 status does not determine outcome of E1B 55-kilodalton mutant adenovirus lytic infection. J. Virol. 72, 9479-9490.

Goodrum, F.D., Shenk, T. and Ornelles, D.A. (1996) Adenovirus early region 4 34-kilodalton protein directs the nuclear localization of the early region 1B 55-kilodalton protein in primate cells. J. Virol. 70, 6323-6335.

Gopalakrishnan, S., Douglas, J.L. and Quinlan, M.P. (1997) Immortalization of primary epithelial cells by E1A 12S requires late, second exon-encoded functions in addition to complex formation with pRB and p300. Cell Growth and Diff. 8, 541-551.

Graham, F.L., van der Eb, A.J. and Heijneker, H.L. (1974) Size and location of the transforming region in human adenovirus type 5 DNA. Nature 251, 687-691.

Grand, R.J.A., Lecane, P.S., Roberts, S., Grant, M.L., Lane, D.P., Young, L.S., Dawson, C.W. and Gallimore, P.H. (1993) Overexpression of wild type p53 and c-Myc in human fetal cells transformed with adenovirus early region 1. Virology 193, 579-591.

Grand, R.J.A., Grant, M.L. and Gallimore, P.H. (1994) Ehanced expression of p53 in human cells infected with mutant adenoviruses. Virology 203, 229-240.

Grand, R.J.A., Mustoe, T., Roberts, S. and Gallimore, P.H. (1995) The quaternary structure of the adenovirus 12 early region 1B 54K protein. Virology 207, 255-259.

Grand, R.J.A., Owen, D., Rookes, S.M. and Gallimore, P.H. (1996) Control of p53 expression by adenovirus 12 early region 1A and early region 1B 54K proteins. Virology 218, 23-34.

Grand, R.J.A., Turnell, A.S., Mason, G.G.F., Wang, W., Milner, A.E., Mymryk, J.S., Rookes, S.M., Rivett, A.J. and Gallimore, P.H. (1999a) Adenovirus early region 1A protein binds to mammalian SUG1-a regulatory component of the proteasome. Oncogene 18, 449-458.

Grand, R.J.A., Parkhill, J., Szestak, T., Rookes, S.M., Roberts, S. and Gallimore, P.H. (1999b) Definition of a major p53 binding site on Ad2 E1B 58K protein and a possible nuclear localization signal on the Ad12 E1B 54K protein. Oncogene 18, 955-965.

Green, M. and Pina, M. (1964) Biochemical studies on adenovirus multiplication, VI. Properties of highly purified tumourigenic human adenoviruses and their DNAs. Proc. Natl. Acad. Sci. USA 51, 1251-1259.

Grossman, S.R., Perez, M., Kung, A.L., Joseph, M., Mansur, C., Xiao, Z.-X., Kumar, S., Howley, P.M. and Livingston, D.M. (1998) p300/MDM2 complexes participate in MDM2-mediated p53 degradation. Molec. Cell 2, 405-415.

Gu, W. and Roeder, R.G. (1997) Activation of p53 sequence-specific DNA binding by acetylation of the p53 C-terminal domain. Cell 90, 595-606.

Hall, A.R., Dix, B.R., O'Carroll, S.J. and Braithwaite, A.W. (1998) p53-dependent cell death/apoptosis is required for a productive adenovirus infection. Nature Medicine 4, 1068-1013.

Hamamori, Y., Sartorelli, V., Ogryzko, V., Puri, L.P., Wu, H.-Y., Wang, J.Y.J., Nakatani, Y. and Kedes, L. (1999) Regulation of histone acetyltransferases p300 and PCAF by the bHLH protein twist and adenoviral oncoprotein E1A. Cell 96, 405-413.

Han, J., Sabbatini, P., Perez, D., Rao, Lakshmi, Modha, D. and White, E. (1996a) The E1B 19K protein blocks apoptosis by interacting with and inhibiting the p53-inducible and death-promoting Bax protein. Genes and Dev. 10, 461-477.

Han, J., Sabbatini, P. and White, E. (1996b) Induction of apoptosis by human Nbk/Bik, a BH3-containing protein that interacts with E1B 19K. Mol. Cell. Biol. 16, 5857-5864.

Han, J., Modha, D. and White, E. (1998a) Interaction of E1B 19K with Bax is required to block Bax-induced loss of mitochondrial membrane potential and apoptosis. Oncogene 17, 2993-3005.

Han, J., Wallen, H.D., Nunez, G. and White, E. (1998b) E1B 19,000-molecular weight protein interacts with and inhibits CED-4-dependent, FLICE-mediated apoptosis. Mol Cell. Biol. 18, 6052-6062.

Hannon, G.J., Demetrick, D. and Beach, D. (1993) Isolation of the Rb related p130 through its interaction with cdk2 and cyclins. Genes and Dev. 7, 2378-2391.

Hateboer, G., Gennissen, A., Ramos, Y.F.M., Kerkhoven, R.M., Sonntag-Buck, V., Stunnenberg, H.G. and Bernards, R. (1995) BS69, a novel adenovirus E1A-associated protein that inhibits E1A transactivation. EMBO J. 14, 3159-3169.

Haupt, Y., Maya, R., Kazaz, A. and Oren, M. (1997) Mdm2 promotes the rapid degradation of p53. Nature 387, 296-299.

Hebrok, A., Wertz, K. and Fuchtbauer, E.M. (1994) M-twist is an inhibitor of muscle differentiation. Dev. Biol. 165, 537-544.

Heise, C., Sampson-Johannes, A., Williams, A., McCormick, F., Von Hoff, D.D. and Kirn, D.H. (1997) ONYX-015, an E1B gene-attenuated adenovirus, causes tumor-specific cytolysis and antitumoral efficacy that can be augmented by standard chemotherapeutic agents. Nature Med. 3, 639-645.

Hermann, C.H., Dery, C.V. and Mathews, M.B. (1987) Transactivation of host and viral genes by the adenovirus E1B 19K tumor antigen. Oncogene 2, 25-35.

Higashino, F., Pipas, J.M. and Shenk, T. (1998) Adenovirus E4orf6 oncoprotein modulates the function of the p53-related protein, p73. Proc. Natl. Acad. Sci. USA 95, 15683-15687.

Hockenbery, D., Nunez, G., Milliman, R.D., Schreiber, R.D. and Korsmeyer, S.J. (1990) Bcl-2 is an inner mitochondrial membrane protein that blocks programmed cell death. Nature 348, 334-336.

Horikoshi, N., Maguire, K., Kralli, A., Maldonado, E., Reinberg, D. and Weinmann, R. (1991) Direct interaction between adenovirus E1a protein and the TATA box binding transcription factor IID. Proc. Natl. Acad. Sci. USA 88, 5124-5128.

Horikoshi, N., Usheva, A., Chen, J., Levine, A., Weinmann, R. and Shenk, T. (1995) Two domains on p53 interact with the TATA binding protein and the adenovirus 13S E1A protein disrupts the association relieving p53-mediated transcriptional repression. Mol. Cell. Biol. 15, 227-234.

Horridge, J.J. and Leppard, K.N. (1998) RNA-binding activity of the E1B 55-kilodalton protein from human adenovirus type 5. J. Virol. 72, 9374-9379.

Howe, J.A. and Bayley, S.T. (1992) Effects of Ad5 E1a mutant viruses on the cell cycle in relation to the binding of cellular proteins including the retinoblastoma protein and cyclin A. Virology 186, 15-24.

Howe, J.A., Mymryk, J.S., Egan, C., Branton, P.E. and Bayley, S.T. (1990) Retinoblastoma growth suppressor and a 300-kDa protein appear to regulate cellular DNA synthesis. Proc. Acad. Sci. USA 87, 5883-5887.

Hu, Q., Dyson, N. and Harlow, E. (1990) The regions of the retinoblastoma protein needed for binding to adenovirus E1A or SV40 large T antigen are common sites for mutations. EMBO J. 9, 1147-1155.

Huang, S., Wang, N.P., Tseng, B.Y., Lee, W.H. and Lee, E.H. (1990) Two distinct and frequently mutated regions of retinoblastoma protein are required for binding SV40 antigen. EMBO J. 9, 1815-1822.

Huang, D.C.S., Cory, S. and Strasser, A. (1997) Bcl-2, Bcl-X_L and adenovirus protein E1B 19kD are functionally equivalent in their ability to inhibit cell death. Oncogene 14, 405-414.

Huang, D.C.S., Adams, J.M. and Cory, S. (1998) The conserved N-terminal BH4 domain of Bcl-2 homologues is essential for inhibition of apoptosis and interaction with CED-4. EMBO J. 17, 1029-1039.

Imhof, A., Yang, X.-J., Ogryzko, V.V., Nakatani, Y., Wolffe, A.P. and Ge, H. (1997) Acetylation of general transcription factors by histone acetyltransferases. Curr. Biol. 7, 689-692.

Jelinek, T., Pereira, D.S. and Graham, F.L. (1994) Tumorigenicity of adenovirus transformed rodent cells is influenced by at least two regions of adenovirus type 12 early region 1A. J. Virol. 68, 888-896.

Jimenez, G., Pinchin, S.M. and Ish-Horowicz, D. (1996) In vivo interactions of the Drosophila Hairy and Runt transcriptional repressors with target promoters. EMBO J. 15, 7088-7098.

Jones, N. (1995) Transcriptional modulation by the adenovirus E1A gene. Curr. Top. Microbiol. Immunol. 199/III, 59-80.

Kaelin, W.G., Ewen, M.E. and Livingston, D.M. (1990) Definition of the minimal simian virus 40 large T antigen and adenovirus E1A-binding domain in the retinoblastoma gene product. Mol. Cell. Biol. 10, 3761-3769.

Kao, C.C., Yew, P.R. and Berk, A.J. (1990) Domains required for in vitro association between cellular p53 and the adenovirus 2 E1B 55K proteins. Virology 179, 806-814.

Kato, J., Matsushime, H., Hiebert, S.W., Ewen, M.E. and Sherr, C.J. (1993) Direct binding of cyclin D to retinoblastoma gene product (pRb) and Rb phosphorylation by cyclin D-dependent kinase CDK4. Genes Dev. 7, 331-342.

Katsanis, N. and Fisher, E.M.C. (1998) A novel C-terminal binding protein (CtBP2) is closely related to CtBP1 an adenovirus E1A-binding protein and maps to human chromosome 21q21.3. Genomics 47, 294-299.

Kee, B., Arias, J. and Montminy, M. (1996) Adaptor mediated recruitment of RNA polymerase II to a signal dependent activator. J. Biol. Chem. 271, 2373-2375.

Kirn, D., Hermiston, T. and McCormick, F. (1998) ONYX-015 : Clinical data are encouraging. Nature Med. 4, 1341-1342.

Kluck, R.M., Bossy-Wetzel, E., Green, D.R. and Newmeyer, D.D. (1997) The release of cytochrome C from mitochondria: a primary site for Bcl-2 regulation of apoptosis. Science 275, 1132-1136.

Knudsen, E.S., Buckmaster, C., Chen, T.-T., Feramisco, J.R. and Wang, J.Y.J. (1998) Inhibition of DNA synthesis by RB: effects on G_1/S transition and S-phase progression. Genes Dev. 12, 2278-2292.

Knudsen, E.S. and Wang, J.Y.J. (1998) Hyperphosphorylated p107 and p130 bind to T-antigen: identification of a critical regulatory sequence present in RB but not in p107/p130. Oncogene 16, 1655-1663.

Konig, C., Roth, J. and Dobbelstein, M. (1999) Adenovirus type 5 E4orf3 protein relieves p53 inhibition by E1B-55-kilodalton protein. J. Virol. 73, 2253-2262.

Kubbutat, M.H.G., Jones, S.N. and Vousden, K.H. (1997) Regulation of p53 stability by Mdm2. Nature 387, 299-303.

Kwok, P.R.S., Lundblad, J., Chrivia, J., Richards, J., Bachinger, H., Brennan, R., Roberts, S., Green, M. and Goodman, R. (1994) Nuclear protein CBP is a coactivator for the transcription factor CREB. Nature 370, 223-226.

Lee, W.S., Kao, C.C., Bryant, G.O., Liu, X. and Berk, A.J. (1991) Adenovirus E1A activation domain binds the basic repeat in the TATA box transcription factor. Cell 67, 365-376.

Lee, J.E., Hollenberg, S.M., Snider, L., Turner, D.L., Lipnick, N. and Weintraub, H. (1995a) Conversion of Xenopus ectoderm into neurons by Neuro D, a basic helix loop helix protein. Science 268, 836-844.

Lee, J.W., Ryan, F., Swaffield, J.C., Johnston, S.A. and Moore, D.D. (1995b) Interaction of thyroid hormone receptor with a conserved transcription mediator. Nature 374, 91-94.

Lee, J.-S., See, R.H., Deng, T. and Shi, Y. (1996) Adenovirus E1A downregulates cJun- and JunB-mediated transcription by targeting their coactivator p300. Mol. Cell. Biol. 16, 4312-4326.

Lee, J.O., Russo, A.A. and Pavletich, N.P. (1998) Structure of the retinoblastoma tumour-suppressor pocket domain bound to a peptide from HPV E7. Nature 391, 859-865.

Lees, E., Faha, B., Dulic, V., Reed, S.I. and Harlow, E. (1992) Cyclin-E CDK2 and cyclin-A CDK2 kinases associate with p107 and E2F in a temporally distinct manner. Genes. Dev. 6, 1874-1885.

Lees, J.A., Saito, M., Vidal, M., Valentine, M., Look, T., Harlow, E., Dyson, N. and Helin, K. (1993) The retinoblastoma protein binds to a family of E2F transcripton factors. Mol. Cell. Biol. 13, 7813-7825.

Lewis, B.A., Tullis, G., Seto, E., Horikoshi, N., Weinmann, R. and Shenk, T. (1995) Adenovirus E1A proteins interact with the cellular YY1 transcription factor. J. Virol. 69, 1628-1636.

Li, P., Nijihawan, D., Budihardjo, L., Srinivasula, S.M., Ahmad, M., Alnemri, E.S. and Wang, X. (1997) Cytochrome c and dATP-dependent formation of Apaf1/caspase 9 complex initiates an apoptotic protease cascade. Cell 91, 479-489.

Li, Y., Graham, C., Lacy, S., Duncan, A.M.V. and Whyte, P. (1993) The adenovirus E1A associated 130-Kd protein is encoded by a member of the retinoblastoma gene family and physically interacts with cyclins A and E. Genes Dev. 7, 2366-2377.

Lill, N.L., Grossman, S.R., Ginsberg, D., DeCaprio, J. and Livingston, D.M. (1997) Binding and modulation of p53 by p300/CBP coactivators. Nature 387, 823-827.

Lin, J., Chen, J., Elenbaas, B. and Levine, A.J. (1994) Several hydrophobic amino acids in the p53 amino-terminal domain are required for transcriptional activation, binding to mdm-2 and the adenovirus 5 E1B 55-kD protein. Genes Dev. 8, 1235-1246.

Linder, S., Popowicz, P., Svensson, C., Marshall, H., Bondesson, M. and Akusjarvi, G. (1992) Enhanced invasive properties of rat embryo fibroblasts transformed by adenovirus E1a mutants with deletions in the carboxy-terminal exon. Oncogene 7, 439-443.

Lipinski, K.S., Esche, H. and Brockmann, D. (1998) Amino acids 1-29 of the adenovirus serotypes 12 and 2 E1A proteins interact with rap30 (TF$_{II}$F) and TBP in vitro. Virus Res. 54, 99-106.

Lipinski, K.S., Fax, P., Wilker, B., Hennemann, H., Brockmann, D. and Esche, H. (1999) Differences in the interactions of oncogenic adenovirus 12 early region 1A and nononcogenic adenovirus 2 early region 1A with the cellular coactivators p300 and CBP. Virology 255, 94-105.

Liu, F. and Green, M.R. (1994) Promoter targeting by adenovirus E1a through interaction with different cellular DNA-binding domains. Nature 368, 520-525.

Liu, F. and Green, M.R. (1990) A specific member of the ATF transcription factor family can mediate transcription activation by the adenovirus E1a protein. Cell 61, 1271-1224.

Livingstone, C., Patel, G. and Jones, N. (1995) ATF-2 contains a phosphorylation-dependent transcriptional activation domain. EMBO J. 14, 1785-1797.

Look, D.C., Roswit, W.T., Frick, A.G., Gris-Alvey, Y., Dickhaus, D.M., Walter, M.J. and Holtzman, M.J. (1998) Direct suppression of Stat1 function during adenoviral infection. Immunity 9, 871-880.

Lowe, S.W. and Ruley, H.E. (1993) Stabilisation of the p53 tumor suppressor is induced by adenovirus 5 E1a and accompanies apoptosis. Genes Dev. 7, 535-545.

Lundbad, J.R., Kwok, R.P.S., Laurance, M.E., Harter, M.L. and Goodman, R.H. (1995) Adenoviral E1A-associated protein p300 as a functional homologue of the transcriptional co-activator CBP. Nature 374, 85-88.

Luo, R.X., Postigo, A.A. and Douglas, C.D. (1998) Rb interacts with histone deacetylase to repress transcription. Cell 92, 463-473.

Magnaghi-Jaulin, L., Groisman, R., Naguibneva, I., Robin, P., Lorain, S., LeVillain, J.P., Troalen, F., Trouche, D. and Harel-Bellan, A. (1998) Retinoblastoma protein represses transcription by recruiting a histone deacetylase. Nature 391, 601-605.

Mak, I., Mak, S. and Benchimol, S. (1988) Expression of the cellular p53 protein in cells transformed by adenovirus 12 and viral DNA fragments. Virology 163, 201-204.

Mal, A., Piotrkowski, A. and Harter, M.L. (1996) Cyclin-dependent kinases phosphorylate the adenovirus E1A protein, enhancing its ability to bind pRb and disrupt pRb-E2F complexes. J. Virol. 70, 2911-2921.

Marin, M.C., Jost, C.A., Irwin, M.S., DeCaprio, J.A., Caput, D. and Kaelin, Jr. W.G. (1998) Viral oncoproteins discriminate between p53 and the p53 homology p73. Mol. Cell. Biol. 18, 6316-6324.

Martin, M.E.D. and Berk, A.J. (1998) Adenovirus E1B 55K represses p53 activation in vitro. J. Virol. 72, 3146-3154.

Martinez-Balbas, M.A., Bannister, A.J., Martin, K., Haus-Seuffert, P., Meisterernst, M. and Kouzarides, T. (1998) The acetyltransferase activity of CBP stimulates transcription. EMBO J. 17, 2886-2893.

Mazzarelli, J.M., Atkins, G.B., Geisberg, J.V. and Ricciardi, R.P. (1995) The viral oncoproteins Ad5 E1A, HPV E7 and SV40 Tag bind a common region of the TBP-associated factor-110. Oncogene 11, 1859-1864.

Mazzarelli, J.M., Mengus, G., Davidson, I. and Ricciardi, R.P. (1997) The transactivation domain of adenovirus E1A interacts with the C terminus of human TAF$_{II}$135. J. Virol. 71, 7978-7983.

Miller, M.E., Cairns, B.R., Levinson, R.S., Yamamoto, K.R., Engel, D.A. and Smith, M.M. (1996) Adenovirus E1A specifically blocks SWI/SNF-dependent transcriptional activation. Mol. Cell. Biol. 16, 5737-5743.

Mittnacht, S., Lees, J.A., Desai, D., Harlow, E., Morgan, D.O. and Weinberg, R.A. (1994) Distinct subpopulations of the retinoblastoma protein show a distinct pattern of phosphorylation. EMBO J. 13, 118-127.

Molloy, D.P., Milner, A.E., Yakub, I.K., Chinnadurai, G., Gallimore, P.H. and Grand, R.J.A. (1998) Structural determinants present in the C-terminal binding protein binding site of adenovirus early region 1A proteins. J. Biol. chem. 273, 20867-20876.

Molloy, D.P., Smith, K.J., Milner, A.E., Gallimore, P.H. and Grand, R.J.A. (1999) The structure of the site on adenovirus E1A responsible for binding to TATA box binding protein determined by NMR spectroscopy. J. Biol. Chem. 274, 3503-3512.

Monteiro, A.N.A., August, A. and Hanafusa, H. (1996) Evidence for a transcriptional activation function of BRCA1 C-terminal region. Proc. Nat. Acad. Sci. USA, 93, 13595-13599.

Moore, M., Horikoshi, N. and Shenk, T. (1996) Oncogenic potential of the adenovirus E4orf6 protein. Proc. Acad. Natl. Sci. USA 93, 11295-11301.

Moran, E. (1994) Mammalian cell growth controls reflected through protein interactions with the adenovirus E1a gene products. Sems. Virol. 5, 327-340.

Munger, K., Werness, B.A., Dyson, N., Phelps, W.C., Harlow, E. and Howley, P.M. (1989) Complex formation of human papillomavirus E7 proteins with the retinoblastoma tumor suppressor gene product. EMBO J. 8, 4099-4105.

Mymryk, J.S., Lee, R.W.H. and Bayley, S.T. (1992) Ability of adenovirus 5 E1A proteins to suppress differentiation of BC$_3$H1 myoblasts correlates with their binding to a 300Kda cellular protein. Mol. Biol Cell 3, 1107-1115.

Mymryk, J.S. and Smith, M.M. (1997) Influence of the adenovirus 5 E1A oncogene on chromatin remodelling. Biochem. Cell Biol. 75, 95-102.

Nakajima, T., Uchida, C., Anderson, S.F., Lee, C.-G., Hurwitz, J., Parvin, J.D. and Montminy, M. (1997) RNA helicase A mediates association of CBP with RNA polymerase II. Cell 90, 1107-1112.

Nakajima, T., Yageta, M., Shiotsu, K., Morita, K., Suzuki, M., Tomooka, Y. and Oda, K. (1998) Suppression of adenovirus E1A-induced apoptosis by mutated p53 is overcome by coexpression with Id proteins. Proc. Natl. Acad. Sci. USA 95, 10590-10595.

Nevels, M., Rubenwolf, S., Spruss, T., Wolf, H. and Dobner, T. (1997) The adenovirus E4orf6 protein can promote E1A/E1B-induced focus formation by interfering with p53 tumor suppression function. Proc. Natl. Acad. Sci. USA 94, 1206-1211.

Nevels, M., Spruss, T., Wolf, H. and Dobner, T. (1999a) The adenovirus E4orf6 protein contributes to malignant transformation by antagonizing E1A-induced accumulation of the tumor suppressor protein p53. Oncogene 18, 9-17.

Nevels, M., Tauber, B., Kremmer, E., Spruss, T., Wolf, H. and Dobner, T. (1999b) Transforming potential of the adenovirus type 5 E4orf3 protein. J. Virol. 73, 1591-1600.

Nibu, Y., Zhang, H. and Levine, M. (1998) Interaction of sort-range repressors with *Drosophila* CtBP in the embryo. Science 280, 101-104.

Ogryzko, V.V., Schiltz, R.L., Russanova, V., Howard, B.H. and Nakatani, Y. (1996) The transcriptional coactivators p300 and CBP are histone acetyltransferases. Cell 87, 953-959.

Ornelles, D.A. and Shenk, T. (1991) Localisation of the adenovirus early region 1B 55 kilodalton protein during lytic infection : association with nuclear viral inclusions requires the early region 4 34 kilodalton protein. J. Virol. 65, 434-429.

Pennisi, E. (1996) Will a twist of viral fate lead to a new cancer treatment? Science 274, 342-343.

Pereira, D.S., Rosenthal, K.L. and Graham, F.L. (1995) Identification of adenovirus E1A regions which affect MHC class I expression and susceptibility to cytotoxic T lymphocytes. Virology 211, 268-277.

Perez, D. and White, E. (1998) E1B 19K inhibits Fas-mediated apoptosis through FADD-dependent sequestration of FLICE. J. Cell. Biol. 141, 1255-1266.

Persson, H., Katze, M.G. and Philipson, L. (1982) Purification of a native membrane-associated adenovirus tumor antigen. J. Virol. 42, 905-917.

Peterson, C.L. and Tamkun, J.W. (1995) The SW1-SNF complex : a chromatin remodelling machine. Trends Biochem. Sci. 20, 143-146.

Pines, J. and Hunter, T. (1990) Human cyclin A is adenovirus E1a-associated protein p60 and behaves differently from cyclin B. Nature 346, 760-763.

Poortinga, G., Watanabe, M. and Parkhurst, S.M. (1998) Drosophila CtBP: a Hairy-interacting protein required for embryonic segmentation and Hairy-mediated transcriptional repression. EMBO J. 17, 2067-2078.

Puri, P.L., Sartorelli, V., Yang, X.-J. , Hamamori, Y., Ogryzko, V.V., Howard, B.H., Kedes, L., Wang, J.Y.J., Graessmann, A., Nakatani, Y. and Levrero, M. (1997) Differential roles of p300 and PCAF acetyltransferases in muscle differentiation. Mol. Cell 1, 35-45.

Querido, E., Teodoro, J.G. and Branton, P.E. (1997a) Accumulation of p53 induced by the adenovirus E1A protein requires regions involved in the stimulation of DNA synthesis. J. Virol. 71, 3526-3533.

Querido, E., Marcellus, R.C., Lai, A., Charbonneau, R., Teodoro, J.G., Ketner, G. and Branton, P.E. (1997b) Regulation of p53 levels by the E1B 55-kilodalton protein and E4orf6 in adenovirus-infected cells. J. Virol. 71, 3788-3798.

Quinlan, M.P., Whyte, P. and Grodzicker, T. (1988) Growth factor induction by the adenovirus type 5 E1a 12S protein is required for immortalisation of primary epithelial cells. Mol. Cell. Biol. 8, 3191-3203.

Qureshi, S.A., Leung, S., Kerr, I.M., Stark, G.R. and Darnell, Jr. J.E. (1996) Function of Stat2 protein in transcriptional activation by alpha interferon. Mol. Cell. Biol. 16, 288-293.

Rao, L., Debbas, M., Sabbatini, P., Hockenbery, D., Korsmeyer, S. and White, E. (1992) The adenovirus E1a proteins induce apoptosis, which is inhibited by the E1b 19-Kda and Bcl-2 proteins. Proc. Natl. Acad. Sci. USA 89, 7742-7746.

Rao, L., Perez, D. and White, E. (1996) Lamin proteolysis facilitates nuclear events during apoptosis. J. Cell Biol. 135, 1441-1455.

Rao, L., Modha, D. and White, E. (1997) The E1B 19K protein associates with lamins *in vivo* and its proper localization is required for inhibition of apoptosis. Oncogene 15, 1587-1597.

Reed, J.C. (1997) Double identity for proteins of the Bcl-2 family. Nature 387, 773-776.

Reid, J.L., Bannister, A.J., Zegerman, P., Martinez-Balbas, M.A. and Kouzarides, T. (1998) E1A directly binds and regulates the P/CAF acetyltransferase. EMBO J. 17, 4469-4477.

Rochette-Egly, C., Fromental, C. and Chambon, C. (1990) General repression of enhanson activity by adenovirus-2 E1A proteins. Genes Dev. 4, 137-150.

Roth, J., Konig, C., Weinzek, S., Weigel, S., Ristea, S. and Dobbelstein, M. (1998) Inactivtion of p53 but not p73 by adenovirus type 5 E1B 55-kilodalton and E4 34-kilodalton oncoproteins. J. Virol. 72, 8510-8516.

Rothmann, T., Hengstermann, A., Whitaker, N.J., Scheffner, M. zur Hausen, H. (1998) Replication of ONYX-015, a potential anticancer adenovirus, is independent of p53 status in tumor cells. J. Virol. 72, 9470-9478.

Sabbatini, P., Chiou, S.-K., Rao, L. and White, E. (1995) Modulation of p53-mediated transcriptional repression and apoptosis by the adenovirus E1B 19K protein. Mol. Cell. Biol. 15, 1060-1070.

Sandmoller, A., Meents, H. and Arnold, H.H. (1996) A novel E1A domain mediates skeletal-muscle-specific enhancer repression independently of pRb and p300 binding. Mol. Cell. Biol. 16, 5846-5856.

Sang, N. and Giordano, A. (1997) Extreme N terminus of E1A oncoprotein specifically associates with a new set of cellular proteins. J. Cell. Physiol. 170, 182-191.

Sarnow, P., Ho, Y.S., Williams, J. and Levine, A. (1982) Adenovirus E1b-58kd tumour antigen and SV40 large tumour antigen are physically associated with the same 54kd cellular protein in transformed cells. Cell 28, 387-394.

Sarnow, P., Hearing, P., Anderson, C.W., Halbert, D.N., Shenk, T. and Levine, A.J. (1984) Adenovirus early region 1b 58,000-Dalton tumour antigen is physically associated with an early region 4 25,000-Dalton protein in productively infected cells. J. Virol. 49, 692-700.

Schaeper, U., Boyd, J.M., Verma, S., Uhlmann, E., Subramanian, T. and Chinnadurai, G. (1995) Molecular cloning and characterization of a cellular phosphoprotein that interacts with a conserved C-terminal domain of adenovirus E1A involved in a negative modulation of oncogenic transformation. Proc. Natl. Acad. Sci. USA 92, 10467-10471.

Schaeper, U., Subramanian, T., Lim, L., Boyd, J.M. and Chinnadurai, G. (1998) Interaction between a cellular protein that binds to the C-terminal region of adenovirus E1A (CtBP) and a novel cellular protein is disrupted by E1A through a conserved PLDLS motif. J. Biol. Chem. 273, 8549-8552.

Schneider, J.F., Fisher, F., Goding, C.R. and Jones, N.C. (1987) Mutational analysis of the adenovirus E1a gene: the role of transcriptional regulation in transformation. EMBO J. 6, 2053-2060.

Scully, R., Anderson, S.F., Chao, D.M., Wei, W., Ye, L., Young, R.A., Livingston, D.M. and Parvin, J.D. (1997) BRCA1 is a component of RNA polymerase II holoenzyme. Proc. Natl. Acad. Sci. USA 94, 5605-5610.

Schwarz, J.K., Devoto, S.H., Smith, E.J., Chellappan, S.P., Jakoi, L. Nevins, J.R. (1993) Interactions of the p107 and Rb proteins with E2F during the cell proliferation response. EMBO J. 12, 1013-1020.

See, R.H. and Shi, Y. (1998) Adenovirus E1B 19,000-molecular weight protein activates c-Jun N-terminal kinase and c-Jun mediated transcription. Mol. Cell. Biol. 18, 4012-4022.

Sewalt, R.G.A.B., Gunster, M.J., van der Vlag, J., Satijn, D.P.E. and Otte, A.P. (1999) C-terminal binding protein is a transcriptional repressor that interacts with a specific class of vertebrate polycomb proteins. Mol. Cell. Biol. 19, 777-787.

Shen, V. and Shenk, T. (1994) Relief of p53 mediated transcriptional repression by the adenovirus E1B 19-kDa protein or the cellular Bcl-2 protein. Proc. Natl. Acad. Sci. USA 91, 8940-8944.

Shenk, T. (1996) Adenoviridae : the viruses and their replication in Fields Virology 3rd edition (edited by Fields, B.N., Knipe, D.M. and Howley, P.M.) pp2111-2148. Lippincott-Raven, Philadelphia New York.

Shi, Y. Lee, J.-S., Galvin, K.M. (1997) Everything you have ever wanted to know about Yin Yang 1..... Biochim. Biophys. Acta. 1332, F49-F66.

Shikama, N., Lyon, J. and La Thangue, N.B. (1997) The p300/CBP family: integrating signals with transcription factors and chromatin. Trends. Cell Biol. 7, 230-236.

Shirodkar, S., Ewen, M., DeCaprio, J.A., Morgan, J., Livingston, D.M. and Chittenden, T. (1992) The transcription factor E2F interacts with the retinoblastoma product and a p107-cyclin A complex in a cell-cycle-regulated manner. Cell 68, 157-166.

Smits, P.H., de Wit, L., van der Eb, A.J. and Zantema, A. (1996) The adenovirus E1A-associated 300 kDa adaptor protein counteracts the inhibition of the collagenase promoter by E1A and represses transformation. Oncogene 12, 1529-1535.

Snowden, A.W. and Perkins, N.D. (1998) Cell cycle regulation of the transcriptional coactivators p300 and CREB binding protein. Biochem. Pharmacol. 55, 1947-1954.

Sollerbrant, K., Chinnadurai, G. and Svensson, C. (1996) The CtBP binding domain in the adenovirus E1A protein controls CR1-dependent transactivation. Nucl. Acids. Res. 24, 2578-2584.

Somasundaram, K. and El-Deiry, W.S. (1997) Inhibition of p53-mediated transactivation and cell cycle arrest by E1A through its p300/CBP-interacting region. Oncogene 14, 1047-1057.

Song, C.Z., Loewenstein, P.M., Toth, A. and Green, M. (1995) TFIID is a direct functional target of the adenovirus E1A transcription-repression domain. Proc. Natl. Acad. Sci. USA 92, 10330-10333.

Song, C.Z., Loewenstein, P.M., Toth, K, Tang, Q., Nishikawa, A. and Green, M. (1997) The adenovirus E1A repression domain disrupts the interaction between the TATA binding protein and the TATA box in a manner reversible by TFIIB. Mol. Cell. Biol. 17, 2186-2193.

Steegenga, W.T., Riteco, N., Jochemsen, A.G., Fallaux, F.J. and Bos, J.L. (1998) The large E1B protein together with the E4orf6 protein target p53 for active degradation in adenovirus infected cells. Oncogene 16, 349-357.

Stein, R.W., Corrigan, M., Yaciuk, P., Whelan, J. and Moran, E. (1990) Analysis of E1A-mediated growth regulation functions : binding of the 300-kilodalton cellular product correlates with E1A enhancer repression function and DNA synthesis-inducing activity. J. Virol. 64, 4421-4427.

Strober, B.E., Dunaief, J.L., Guha, S. and Goff, S.P. (1996) Functional interactions between the hBRM/hBRG1 transcriptional activators and the pRb family of proteins. Mol. Cell. Biol. 16, 1576-1583.

Subramanian, T., La Regina, M. and Chinnadurai, G. (1989) Enhanced ras oncogene mediated cell transformation and tumorigenesis by adenovirus 2 mutants lacking the C terminal region of E1a protein. Oncogene 4, 415-420.

Sundqvist, A., Sollerbrant, K. and Svensson, C. (1998) The carboxy-terminal region of adenovirus E1A activates transcription through targeting of a C-terminal binding protein-histone deacetylase complex. FEBS Letts. 429, 183-188.

Tanaka, S., Saito, K. and Reed, J. (1993) Structure function analysis of Bcl-2 oncoprotein. J. Biol. Chem. 268, 10920-10926.

Tanase, N., Saluja, D., Vassallo, M.F., Chen, J.-L. and Admon, A. (1996) Molecular cloning and analysis of two subunits of the human TFIID complex hTAF II 130 and hTAF II 100. Proc. Natl. Acad. Sci. USA 93, 13611-13616.

Tao, Y., Kassatly, R.F., Cress, W.D. and Horowitz, J.M. (1997) Subunit composition determines E2F DNA-binding site specificity. Mol. Cell. Biol. 17, 6994-7007.

Taylor, D.A., Kraus, V.B., Schwarz, J.J., Olson, E.N. and Kraus, W.E. (1993) E1A-mediated inhibition of myogenesis correlates with a direct physical interaction of E1A$_{12S}$ and basic helix-loop-helix proteins. Mol. Cell. Biol. 13, 4714-4727.

Telling, G.C. and Williams, J. (1994) Constructing chimeric type 12/type 5 adenovirus E1A genes and using them to identify an oncogenic determinant of adenovirus type 12. J. Virol. 68, 877-887.

Teodoro, J.G., Halliday, T., Whalen, S.G., Takayesu, D., Graham, F.L. and Branton, P.E. (1994) Phosphorylation at the carboxy terminus of the 55-kilodalton adenovirus type 5 E1b protein regulates transforming activity. J. Virol. 68, 776-786.

Teodoro, J.G., Shore, G.C. and Branton, P.E. (1995) Adenovirus E1A proteins induce apoptosis by both p53-dependent and p53-independent mechanisms. Oncogene 11, 467-474.

Teodoro, J.G. and Branton, P.E. (1997a) Regulation of apoptosis by viral gene products. J. Virol. 71, 1739-1746.

Teodoro, J.G. and Branton, P.E. (1997b) Regulation of p53-dependent apoptosis, transcriptional repression, and cell transformation by phosphorylation of the 55-kilodalton E1B protein of human adenovirus type 5. J. Virol. 71, 3620-3627.

Thomas, A. and White, E. (1998) Suppression of the p300-dependent mdm2 negative-feedback loop induces the p53 apoptotic function. Genes Dev. 12, 1975-1985.

Tremblay, M.L., McGlade, C.J., Gerber, G.E. and Branton, P.E. (1988) Idenification of the phosphorylation sites in early region 1A proteins of adenovirus type 5 by amino acid sequencing of peptide fragments. J. Biol. Chem. 263, 6375-6383.

Tremblay, M.L., Dumont, D.J. and Branton, P.E. (1989) Analysis of phosphorylation sites in the exon 1 region of E1A proteins of human adenovirus type 5. Virology 169, 397-407.

Trentin, J., Yabe, Y. and Taylor, G. (1962) The quest for human cancer viruses. Science 137, 835-841.

Trouche, D. and Kouzarides, T. (1996) E2F1 and E1A 12S have a homologous activation domain regulated by RB and CBP. Proc. Natl. Acad. Sci. USA 93, 1439-1442.

Tsukamoto, A.S., Ponticelli, A., Berk, A.J. and Gaynor, R.B. (1986) Genetic mapping of a major site of phosphorylation in adenovirus type 2 E1A proteins. J. Virol. 59, 14-22.

Turnell, A.S., Grand, R.J.A. and Gallimore, P.H. (1999) The replicative capacities of large E1B-null group A and group C adenoviruses are independent of host cell p53 status. J. Virol. 73, 2074-2083.

Van den Heuval, S.J.L., van Laar, T., Kast, W.M., Melief, C.J.M., Zantema, A. and van der Eb, A.J. (1990) Association between the cellular p53 and the adenovirus 5 E1B 55Kd proteins reduces the oncogenicity of Ad transformed cells. EMBO J. 9, 2621-2629.

Veal, E., Eisenstein, M., Tseng, Z.H. and Gill, G. (1998) A cellular repressor of E1A-stimulated genes that inhibits activation of E2F. Mol. Cell. Biol. 18, 5032-5041.

Vom Bauer, E., Zechel, C., Heery, D., Heine, M.J.S., Garnier, J.M., Vivat, V., Le Douarin, B., Gronemeyer, H., Chambon, P. and Losson, R. (1995) Differential ligand-dependent interactions between the AF-2 activating domain of nuclear receptors and theputative transcriptional intermediary factors mSUG1 and TIFI. EMBO J. 15, 110-124.

Wang, H.G.H., Yakiuk, P., Riccardi, R.P., Green, M., Yokoyama, K. and Moran, E. (1993) The E1a products of onogenic adenovirus serotype 12 include amino-terminally modified forms able to bind the retinoblastoma protein but not p300. J. Virol. 67, 4804-4813.

Wang, W., Chevray, P.M. and Nathans, D. (1996) Mammalian Sug1 and c-Fos in the nuclear 26S proteasome. Proc. Natl. Acad. Sci. USA 93, 8236-8240.

Wang, H.-G.H., Rikitake, Y., Carter, M.C., Yaciuk, P., Abraham, S.E., Zerler, B. and Moran, E. (1993) Identification of specific adenovirus E1A N-terminal residues critical to the binding of cellular proteins and to the control of cell growth. J. Virol. 67, 476-488.

Webster, K.A., Muscat, G.E.O. and Kedes, L. (1988) Adenovirus E1A products suppress myogenic differentiation and inhibit transcripton from muscle-specific promoters. Nature 332, 553-557.

Webster, L.C. and Ricciardi, R.P. (1991) Trans-dominant mutants of E1a provide genetic evidence that the zinc finger of the transactivating domain binds a transcription factor. Mol. Cell. Biol. 11, 4287-4296.

Welch, P.J. and Wang, J.Y. (1993) A C-terminal protein binding domain in the retinoblastoma protein regulates nuclear C-Abl tyrosine kinase in the cell cycle. Cell 75, 779-790.

Whalen, S.G., Marcellus, R.C., Barbeau, D. and Branton, P.E. (1996) Importance of the Ser-132 phosphorylation site in cell transformation and apoptosis induced the adenovirus type 5 E1A protein. J. Virol. 70, 5373-5383.

Whalen, S.G., Marcellus, R.C., Whalen, A., Ahn, N.G., Ricciardi, R.P. and Branton, P.E. (1997) Phosphorylation within the transactivation domain of adenovirus E1A protein by mitogen-activated protein kinase regulates expression of early region 4. J. Virol. 71, 3545-3553.

White, E. (1996) Life death and the pursuit of apoptosis. Genes Dev. 10, 1-15.

White, E. (1998) Regulation of apoptosis by adenovirus E1A and E1B oncogenes. Sem. Virol. 8, 505-513.

White, E., Blose, S.H. and Stillman, B. (1984) Nuclear envelope localisation of an adenovirus tumor antigen maintains the integrity of cellular DNA. Mol. Cell. Biol. 4, 2865-2875.

White, E. and Cipriani, R. (1989) Specific disruption of intermediate filaments and the nuclear lamina by the 19-kDa product of the adenovirus E1B oncogene. Proc. Natl. Acad. Sci. USA 86, 9886-9890.

White, E. and Cipriani, R. (1990) Role of adenovirus E1B proteins in transformation: altered organization of intermediate filaments in transformed cells that express the 19-kilodalton protein. Mol. Cell. Biol. 10, 120-130.

White, E., Cipriani, R., Sabbatini, P. and Denton, A. (1991) The adenovirus E1B 19 kilodalton protein overcomes the cytotoxicity of E1A proteins. J. Virol. 65, 2968-2978.

Whyte, P., Buchkovich, K.J., Horowitz, J.M., Friend, S.H., Raybuck, M., Weinberg, R.A. and Harlow, E. (1988) Association between an oncogene and an anti-oncogene: the adenovirus E1A proteins bind to the retinoblastoma gene product. Nature 334, 124-129.

Whyte, P., Williamson, N.M. and Harlow, E. (1989) Cellular targets for transformation by the adenovirus E1A proteins. Cell 56, 67-75.

Williams, J., Williams, M., Liu, C. and Telling, G. (1995) Assessing the role of E1A in the differential oncogenicity of group A and group C human adenoviruses. Curr. Top. Microbiol. Immunol. 199/III 149-175.

Yabe, Y., Samper, L., Byran, E., Taylor, G. and Trentin, J.J. (1964) Oncogenic effect of human adenovirus type 12, in mice. Science 143, 46-47.

Yabe, Y., Trentin, J.J. and Taylor, G. (1962) Cancer induction in hamsters by human type 12 adenovirus. Effect of age and virus dose. Procs. Soc. Exp. Biol. 111, 343-344.

Yang, X.-J., Ogryzko, V.V., Nishikawa, J.-I., Howard, B.H. and Nakatani, Y. (1996) A p300/CBP-associated factor that competes with the adenovirus oncoprotein E1A. Nature 382, 319-324.

Yang, J., Liu, X.S., Bhalla, K., Kim, C.N., Ibrado, A.M., Cai, J.Y., Peng, T.I., Jones, D.P. and Wang, X.D. (1997) Prevention of apoptosis by Bcl2 : release of cytochrome C from mitochondria blocked. Science 275, 1129-1132.

Yasuda, M, Theodorakis, P., Subramanian, T. and Chinnadurai, G. (1998) Adenovirus E1B-19K/BCL-2 interacting protein BNIP3 contains a BH3 domain and a mitochondrial targeting sequence. J. Biol. Chem. 273, 12415-12421.

Yew, P.R., and Berk, A.J. (1992) Inhibition of p53 transactivation required for transformation by adenovirus E1B 55K protein. Nature 357, 82-85.

Yew, P.R., Liu, X. and Berk, A.J. (1994) Adenovirus E1B oncoprotein tethers a transcriptional repression domain to p53. Genes Dev. 8, 190-202.

Yoshida, K., Venkatesh, L., Kuppuswamy, M. and Chinnadurai, G. (1987) Adenovirus transforming 19-kD T antigen has an enhancer dependent transactivation function and relieves enhancer repression mediated by viral and cellular genes. Genes Dev. 1, 645-658.

Yu, X., Wu, L.C., Bowcock, A.M., Aronheim, A. and Baer, R. (1998) The C-terminal (BRCT) domains of BRCA1 interact in vivo with CtIP, a protein implicated in the CtBP pathway of transcriptional repression. J. Biol. Chem. 273, 25388-25392.

Yuan, W., Condorelli, G., Caruso, M., Felsani, A. and Giordano, A. (1996) Human p300 is a co-activator for the transcription factor MyoD. J. Biol. Chem. 271, 9009-9013.

Zantema, A., Fransen, J.A.M., Davis-Olivier, A., Ramaekers, F.C.S., Vooijs, G.P., de Leys, B. and van der Eb A.J. (1985a) Localisation of the E1b proteins of adenovirus 5 in transformed cells as revealed by interaction with monoclonal antibodies. Virology 142, 44-58.

Zantema, A., Schrier, P.I., Davis-Olivier, A., van Laar, T., Vaessen, R.T.M.J. and van der Eb, A.J. (1985b) Adenovirus serotype determines association and localisation of the large E1b tumour antigen with cellular tumour antigen p53 in transformed cells. Mol. Cell. Biol. 5, 3084-3091.

Zerler, B., Moran, B., Maruyama, K., Moomaw, J., Grodzicker, T. and Ruley, H.E. (1986) Adenovirus E1a coding sequences that enable ras and pmt oncogenes to transform cultured primary cells. Mol. Cell. Biol. 6, 887-899.

Zha, H., Aime-Sempe, C., Sato, T. and Reed, J.C. (1996) Pro-apoptotic protein Bax heterodimerises with Bcl-2 and homodimerizes with Bax via a novel domain (BH3) distinct from BH1 and BH2. J. Biol. Chem. 271, 7440-7444.

Zou, H., Henzel, W.J., Liu, X., Lutschg, A. and Wang, X. (1997) Apaf1, a human protein homologous to C.elegans CED-4 participates in cytochrome c-dependent activation of caspase-3. Cell 90, 405-414.

POLYOMA VIRUS MIDDLE T-ANTIGEN:
GROWTH FACTOR RECEPTOR MIMIC

Philippa R. Nicholson and Stephen M. Dilworth

Department of Metabolic Medicine, Imperial College School of Medicine, London

ABSTRACT

Polyoma is a small, double stranded DNA, mouse virus that normally propagates by a lytic infectious cycle. Under some circumstances, however, polyoma virus can induce the formation of a wide variety of tumors. The early proteins, or T-antigens, exert this oncogenic effect, which is paralleled by an ability to transform cells in culture. The three T-antigens co-operate to induce tumorigenesis, but the main transforming role is contained within one polypeptide, the middle T-antigen (MT). MT interacts with, and alters the regulation of, a number of host proteins that control cell proliferation. MT binds the A and C subunits of protein phosphatase 2A, and this complex then associates with a member of the *src*-family of non-receptor tyrosine protein kinases. As a consequence, the kinase is activated, and MT itself becomes tyrosine phosphorylated on at least three residues. These act as binding sites for the SH2 domains of phosphatidylinositol (3') kinase and phospholipase Cγ-1, and the phosphotyrosine-binding domain of Shc. Each of these polypeptides is in turn phosphorylated on tyrosine residues, which initiates a series of intracellular events culminating in transformation. These pathways are the same as those stimulated by tyrosine kinase associated growth factor receptors, leading to the conclusion that MT acts as a functional homologue of such a receptor. MT, therefore, not only supplies us with information about the mechanisms behind tumor induction *in vivo* and transformation in cell culture, but can also be used to examine the molecular details of signal transduction induced by growth factor receptors. MT also interacts with the constitutively synthesised heat shock protein 70, and some members of the 14-3-3 family of polypeptides, but the role of these interactions is less clear.

Introduction

In order to devise effective measures to counter tumor growth, the alterations responsible for the cell's aberrant proliferation need to be understood at the molecular level. Within the animal, these changes are difficult to investigate, but the development of tissue culture transformation assays that mimic some of the alterations occurring *in vivo* held out the hope that the molecular basis of transformation could be defined as a first step. Initially, viruses were the only model transformation systems that could be easily manipulated, so were extensively studied. This work provided the foundations on which most of our current knowledge of cell transformation is based. With the advent of molecular biology, and the ability to study cellular genes directly, viruses became less popular models for a time. However, the realisation that a number of viruses are

85

involved in human tumorigenesis has now reversed this trend, and viral models are proving a useful approach when investigating the processes underlying carcinogenesis.

Generally, DNA tumor viruses have probably not evolved to be oncogenic, as tumor formation yields little advantage to the virus itself in most cases. So why do a number of viruses encode potent oncogenes? Most cells in higher, multi-cellular, organisms are quiescent, clearly not an ideal environment when the host cell machinery is required to synthesise viral DNA. Therefore, it is likely that DNA viruses encode a protein with a mitogenic activity in order to provide the conditions for duplication of their own genome. Normally, the cell dies when viral progeny are produced, so this activity has little effect on the organism. If the cell survives and continues to synthesise this mitogenic protein, however, it could potentially be oncogenic. Tumorigenesis, then, probably occurs when expression of the encoded replication promoting polypeptide is uncoupled from a lytic cycle. Viruses have constraints when evolving such a protein, notably the limitations on genome size imposed by the viral capsid. Therefore, it is not unexpected that a remarkable level of refinement in the function of DNA viral oncogenes has been found, each protein often having multiple actions. As they precisely target cell growth control mechanisms, viruses can be used to identify the proteins involved in regulating cell proliferation. As confirmation of this, studies of viral oncogenes first discovered such important proteins as p53, p107Rb, p130Rb, p300, and PI3K, and the existence of tyrosine phosphorylations, to list just a few. It would be naive to assume that we currently understand completely how the components involved in controlling cell growth function, so DNA viral oncogenes are still valuable models for studying the molecular changes that result in cell transformation and growth.

In 1953, Gross first reported that an infectious agent in cell free filtrates from mouse leukaemias caused parotid gland tumors when inoculated back into mice (Gross 1953). The virus was then shown to cause a variety of tumors, which led to it being named polyoma (Eddy et al. 1958). Since then, polyoma virus (PyV) has been widely studied as a model of viral lytic infection, and tumorigenesis. Polyoma virus is a small, double stranded DNA virus found endemically in wild mouse populations that causes few overt deleterious effects. When injected into new-born animals, however, it induces with high efficiency, and a short latency period, a wide variety of tumors (reviewed in Gross 1983). It has a number of close relatives in other species, including a hamster variant, SV40 from rhesus monkeys, and the human viruses JC and BK (for review see Pipas, 1992).

The Lytic Cycle

The PyV genome consists of 5297 base pairs of closed circular DNA (latest GenBank submission; Figure 1). It is organised into two transcription units, separated by a non-coding region which contains the origin of DNA replication and transcriptional promoters and enhancers. On infection of permissive cells (i.e., those that can support a full lytic infection) the virion penetrates the plasma membrane, and probably migrates to the nucleus, where the capsid proteins are removed and the viral chromatin transcribed. Initially, RNA is produced from only the "early" region, and is spliced

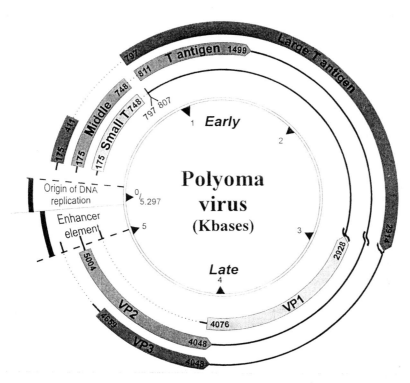

*Fig. 1. Physical Map of the Polyoma Virus Genome. The closed circular DNA of PyV is repre-
sented schematically, together with the mRNA (solid line) and coding regions (shaded boxes)
indicated around the outside. The base pair numbering of the start and finish points of each
coding region are shown, together with the identification of the polypeptide synthesised by each
mRNA. Regions of RNA removed by splice reactions are indicated by dotted lines. The non-
coding regions required for DNA replication initiation and transcription enhancer activity are
also marked. Base pair numbering are taken from the latest GenBank entry.*

using two donor and two acceptor sites to form four mRNAs. These encode three
known proteins, or T-antigens (see later). The largest of these, large T (LT), is
translocated to the nucleus where it interacts with the viral genome at the origin of DNA
replication, located between the two gene cistrons. Through the intrinsic helicase
activity of LT (Wang and Prives, 1991), and its ability to bind the host cell DNA
polymerase α (Murakami et al. 1986), DNA replication is initiated at this point, and
proceeds bi-directionally to produce new viral genomes. As DNA replication starts, the
other transcription promoter is activated to produce "late" RNA. This is again spliced to
produce a number of mRNAs, which synthesise the three capsid proteins, VP1, 2 and 3.
These actively accumulate in the nucleus where new virions are assembled. When the
cell contains many thousands of virions, it lyses to release mature viral particles
(reviewed in Tooze 1980).

Abortive Transformation

Not all rodent cells can support a full lytic infection cycle. Those that do are termed permissive, and consist mainly of mouse fibroblast and epithelial cells. Other mouse cells are non or semi-permissive, often due to the absence of transcriptional control factors such as enhancer binding proteins. Cells from other rodent species support variable levels of viral replication. Hamster cells are semi-permissive, producing small numbers of infectious particles, whereas rat cells are non-permissive. In these cases, DNA replication does not occur, probably due to the inability of PyV LT to interact with DNA polymerase α from different species (Murakami et al. 1986). The episomal viral genome is then lost as the cell divides. The phenotype of these infected cells alters dramatically whilst they are synthesising the early proteins. They lose their actin cable network, enter the cell cycle, and show increased membrane fluidity and activity. As the viral genome is lost, these properties also disappear, leading to the process being called "abortive transformation" (Stoker 1968). In a small proportion of infected cells, however, possibly as a result of LT action, the viral genome becomes integrated into the host cell genome, and the early proteins are continuously expressed. In this case the cell permanently acquires these altered properties and becomes "transformed". Integration appears not to be site specific, and does not influence transformation, which remains dependent upon continued expression of the viral proteins. PyV-transformed cells exhibit a large number of altered properties including a loss of contact inhibition of growth and movement, resulting in an ability to overgrow one another to form foci, and the capacity to grow without anchorage, and so divide in semi-solid media. Together with these phenotypic changes, PyV transformed cells can form tumors when inoculated back into syngeneic animals. It is this ability to transform cells in culture as well as in the animal that has made PyV such an attractive model for studying the mechanisms underlying transformation and tumorigenesis.

The T-Antigens

Sera from animals carrying PyV-induced tumors contain antibodies that recognize the non-cellular, viral proteins present in transformed cells. These antibodies enabled the proteins responsible for inducing transformation to be first identified and studied. As they are recognized by sera from tumor bearing animals, these proteins were named the tumor (T) antigens. Three T-antigens are found in PyV-transformed cells, the large T-antigen (LT), middle T-antigen (MT), and small T-antigen (ST), and these are encoded by the early region. The DNA sequence of PyV, together with genetic, protein, and RNA studies, allowed the amino acid sequence of each protein to be predicted (reviewed in Griffin and Dilworth 1983; Tooze 1980). Isolation of cDNAs then enabled each T-antigen to be expressed independently (Zhu et al. 1984), so the precise role of each T-antigen could be examined. LT was found to be vital for viral replication, but it also has an ability to immortalise cells in culture, and lower the serum requirement for cell growth (Rassoulzadegan et al. 1982; Rassoulzadegan et al. 1983). MT expression is sufficient to transform established cells in culture (Treisman et al. 1981), making it the principle oncogene in PyV. A definite role for ST is still being sought, although a number of studies have suggested it can potentiate the activity of MT (see later), and is required for efficient viral replication. As ST contains mainly a subset of the MT sequences, it is sensible to consider ST first when discussing their properties.

Small T-Antigen

ST is a 22kDa protein found both in the nucleus and the cytoplasm (Noda et al. 1986; Silver et al. 1978; Zhu et al. 1984). It has the same N-terminal 79 amino acids as LT and MT, then shares residues 79 to 192 with MT, and finally, has 4 unique amino acids at the C-terminus (see Figure 1). As with many DNA virus-encoded oncogenes, ST does not appear to have any enzymatic activity of its own. Instead, it exerts an effect on cells by interacting with host polypeptides, and altering the way their function is regulated. As the majority of ST sequences are also present in MT, we will assume that binding to proteins within the common region is similar, and that results derived from one T-antigen are also applicable to the other, although this may not always have been demonstrated.

The major polypeptides found co-precipitated with ST are the regulatory A and catalytic C subunits of protein phosphatase 2A (PP2A) (Pallas et al., 1990). By analogy with MT (Pallas et al. 1989; Walter et al. 1987), ST also binds the constitutively expressed heat shock 70 protein (Hsc70) when a mutation is made to the PP2A binding site. The closely related SV40 ST has been more extensively studied than that of PyV, so it is tempting to draw comparisons between the two. However, there are suggestions that PyV ST and SV40 ST do not bind to PP2A in the same manner. For instance, where SV40 ST binds to repeats 3 to 6 of PP2A.A, polyoma MT and ST interact with repeats 2 to 8 (Ruediger et al., 1992). It is not yet clear whether this means they have different effects on the activity of the phosphatase. Consequently, we will concentrate mainly on the polyoma results here, but draw from the SV40 ST information when it is relevant.

Homologies Between ST Species

The amino acid sequences of the ST polypeptides encoded by a number of polyoma viruses share extensive homology. This suggests they may have similar functions, and that the important residues involved in protein interaction may be identified as the amino acids highly conserved between species (Figures 2 and 3). Some notable areas of homology are readily apparent from these comparisons. The N-terminal region of ST, up to amino acid 30, shows extensive homology between species, especially in the disposition of hydrophobic residues such as leucines (Figure 2). Mutations in the extreme N-terminal region of MT disrupt PP2A binding (Glenn and Eckhart, 1995), although this has yet to be repeated with ST. Amino acids 9 to 19 show similarity to the conserved region (CR) 1 region of adenovirus E1A (Wang et al., 1993). This area of E1A is involved in binding p300, a member of a family of transcriptional activators including the CREB binding protein, CBP (Arany et al., 1994; Eckner et al., 1994). E1A

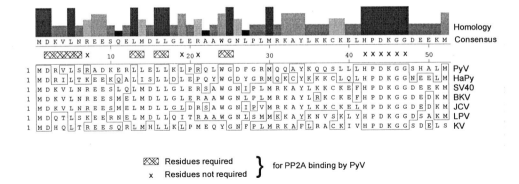

Fig. 2. *Sequence Homology Between the N-terminal Regions of ST Species. The N-terminal sequences of a number of ST species from related polyoma viruses are shown aligned to maximise homology. The virus encoding the ST is indicated on the right, mouse polyoma virus (PyV), hamster polyoma virus (HaPy), Rhesus monkey SV40 (SV40), human BK and JC viruses (BKV and JCV), African green monkey lymphotropic virus (LPV), and the mouse K virus (KV) are shown. A consensus sequence derived from this homology is shown above the main sequences, together with a bar graph showing the level of homology. Residues that have been shown to be required for PyV ST (or MT) binding to PP2A are indicated by hatched boxes, and those that have been demonstrated not to be required by an x. Not all residues within a region are necessarily involved, merely the overall area has been shown to be required. Sequences are taken from the latest SwissProt database, and the sequences of Bovine polyoma virus (BPyV) and Budgerigar Fledgling Disease Virus (BFDV) have been omitted as they have lower homology and so may function differently.*

binding to p300 probably results in cells exiting from G0, an inhibition of differentiation, and alterations in gene transcription. As SV40 LT binds p300 through the LT unique region (Lill et al., 1997), it is unlikely that this region in ST binds p300 alone. However, the SV40 ST sequence can functionally replace the CR1 of E1A (Yaciuk et al., 1991), so this region may have a supplementary role in p300 interaction. In PyV, mutations to this sequence disrupt PP2A binding and transformation by MT (Glenn and Eckhart, 1995). However, this does not apply to SV40 ST, as the homologous region here is not required for interaction with PP2A (Sontag et al., 1993). Therefore, the exact role of this region in either PyV or SV40 is still not clear.

The next ST region with strong homology between species is a HPDKGG sequence at residues 42 to 47 (Figure 2). This sequence is found in all ST species, and is similar to a motif present in the DnaJ family of proteins in bacteria, which interact with the ATPase domain of the heat shock 70 group of polypeptides. Through this association, DnaJ acts as a molecular chaperone involved in assembling multi-subunit complexes, so it is feasible that this region is similarly involved in forming the complexes centred on ST and MT (see below). The HPDKGG sequence is required for ST binding to Hsc70 (Campbell et al., 1997), and the N-terminus of SV40 can act as a functional J domain

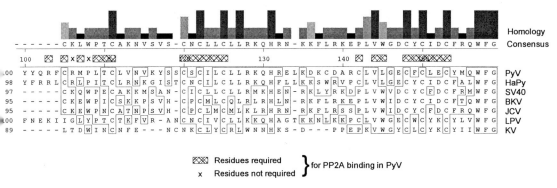

Fig. 3. *Sequence homology between the C-terminal Region of ST Species. The homologies between ST sequences near the C-terminal end are shown. Representation are as in Figure 2.*

(Kelley and Georgopoulos, 1997; Srinivasan et al., 1997). Deletion of this sequence decreases PyV ST binding to PP2A *in vitro*, but has little effect on MT binding *in vivo* (Campbell et al., 1995; Glenn and Eckhart, 1995). SV40 ST mutants defective in this DnaJ domain do not fully activate the E6/E7 promoter of human papilloma virus (Smits et al., 1992), or transactivate the adenovirus E2 promoter (Mungre et al., 1994) and the cyclin A promoter (Porras et al., 1996).

Two CXCXXC motifs at amino acids 120-125 and 148-153, and sequences surrounding them, are also highly conserved between all ST species (Figure 3). Disruption of either site in PyV ST probably prevents PP2A binding (Campbell et al., 1995; Markland and Smith 1987), although the second repeat may not be required for SV40 ST PP2A binding (Sontag et al., 1993). Cys and His are frequently involved in co-ordinating Zn^{2+} ions, and SV40 ST (Turk et al., 1993) and PyV MT (Rose and Schaffhausen, 1995) have both been shown to bind zinc. Therefore this region, probably interacts with zinc ions, and may maintain the structural integrity of the region.

Finally, a region surrounding residue 180 in polyoma ST is also conserved amongst other species (not shown). An Ile insertion between residues 178 and 179 is responsible for the defect in the hr-t mutant, NG59 (Markland and Smith 1987), which inhibits PP2A binding to MT (Grussenmeyer et al. 1987; Pallas et al. 1988). Deletion of residues 180 to 189 in MT, which includes two highly conserved leucines, also disrupts association with PP2A (Brewster et al., 1997).

Effects of ST on PP2A Activity

ST binds mainly to the A subunit of PP2A (Ruediger et al., 1992), although the C subunit potentiates binding. The regulatory B subunits of PP2A interact with similar regions of the A polypeptide, suggesting ST may act as a virally-encoded B subunit.

Whether ST binds to a free AC complex, or displaces the B subunit from PP2A, possibly through the action of Hsc70, is not yet clear, though the identification of a large pool of the PP2A.AC core enzyme in cells suggests the former may be correct (Kremmer et al., 1997). The effect that binding to polyoma ST (or MT) has on PP2A enzymatic activity has not been investigated to the same extent as SV40 ST (reviewed in Mumby, 1995). *In vitro*, SV40 ST lowers the catalytic activity of the PP2A.AC complex 50 to 75%, though this depends greatly on the substrate used. This effect is similar to the inhibition observed on addition of the B' subunit (Scheidtmann et al., 1991; Yang et al., 1991). Binding to MT and ST seems to modulate the phosphatase activity of PP2A, rather than inhibiting it non-specifically, and it is feasible that activity towards a particular substrate could be stimulated by interaction, as well as inhibited. In addition, the action of PP2A in cells could be altered by the T-antigen sequestering PP2A to a sub-cellular site where it can no longer access its substrates. All of these factors make it difficult to determine exactly how the ST-PP2A interaction influences other events within the cell merely by examining the effects *in vitro*.

In vivo *Actions of ST*

PyV ST can potentiate the transforming action of MT (Asselin et al. 1984; Noda et al. 1987), and is required with MT to stimulate the growth of epithelial cells in semi-solid media. In isolation, PyV ST expression promotes cell growth, to the extent that the cells can form small colonies in soft agar (Cherington et al. 1986; Noda et al. 1986), but do not develop into tumors when injected into animals. In addition, the actin microfilament arrangement is unaltered by PyV ST expression, unlike the effect of SV40 ST (Bikel et al. 1983; Graessmann et al. 1980). PyV ST can also potentiate the mitogenic activities of LT (Ogris et al., 1992). During the viral lytic cycle, LT alone is sufficient for viral DNA replication in cultured fibroblasts, but with low yields. Co-expression of ST, but not full length MT, can increase this efficiency dramatically (Berger and Wintersberger 1986; Templeton et al. 1986). Interestingly, truncated MT lacking the hydrophobic membrane binding domain can stimulate replication, indicating it is the sub-cellular location of the T-antigen, rather than any intrinsic defect, that causes this effect (Templeton et al. 1986). The ability to promote MT transformation, stimulate viral DNA synthesis, and influence the maturation of infectious particles, have been shown by mutational analysis to be separable (Martens et al. 1989). The defect in stimulating viral DNA synthesis correlates with PP2A binding, whereas the other two effects do not (Campbell et al., 1995). The molecular basis for these other properties remains to be determined

SV40 ST inhibits the dephosphorylation of phosphorylated active ERK and MEK by PP2A in cells, so preventing inactivation of the MAP Kinase cascade (Sontag et al., 1993). This is not the only effect of ST, though, as dominant negative mutants of ERK cannot completely inhibit the growth promoting properties of SV40 ST. *In vitro* experiments suggest that the phosphatase activity towards ERK1 is reduced by ST binding to the AC core enzyme (Sontag et al., 1993), though whether this fully accounts for the effects on ERK activity *in vivo* is not known. Dephosphorylation and inactivation of the transcription factors AP-1 (Frost et al., 1994) and CREB (Wheat et al., 1994), has also been shown to be inhibited by SV40 ST. SV40 ST binding to PP2A also activates the atypical protein kinase Cζ (PKCζ) (Sontag et al., 1997). This leads to activation of MEK and probably through a separate route, degradation of I-κB α and activation of NF-κB-dependent gene transcription. Both activation of MEK and NF-κB, and the stimulation of cell growth by SV40 ST, are dependent upon PI3K activity, in an interesting possible link to MT action (see later). PyV ST has not yet been investigated for these activities, but it is likely that they provide a plausible explanation for the growth-promoting and MT-complementing actions of ST.

Middle T-Antigen

MT is a virally encoded, 55kDa protein present in the membranes of cells lytically infected, or transformed, by PyV (Ito et al. 1977a; Silver et al. 1978). The first 192 amino acids of MT are also present in ST, then a further 229 MT unique residues are encoded by mRNA following the splice site (Figure 1). The 421 amino acids in MT predict a molecular weight of around 49kDa, though the size measured by SDS-PAGE is in the region of 55kDa. It seems that sequences in the 300 to 330 region of MT are responsible for most of this anomalous gel migration, rather than any modification (Ito et al. 1980). In the polyoma family of viruses, only the mouse and hamster species encode a MT polypeptide, and there is limited homology between the unique areas of these two polypeptides.

MT alone can fully transform established fibroblasts in culture (Treisman et al. 1981). Inducible promoters have been used to show that MT transformation depends upon continued expression of the protein (Azarnia and Loewenstein 1987; Heiser and Eckhart 1985; Raptis et al. 1985; Strauss et al., 1990), and is reversible when MT synthesis is inhibited. MT is also required for both viral replication and tumorigenesis in the mouse (Freund et al., 1992b). In tissue culture cells, PyV mutants with a defective MT replicate poorly in some cell types that support a normal wild type infection. This seems to be related to a MT-induced phosphorylation of VP1, which is required for efficient assembly of the capsid (Garcea et al. 1985; Garcea and Benjamin 1983). The kinase responsible for this phosphorylation is active in some cell types, but MT is required to stimulate it in others, so accounting for the host range defect. Interestingly, this ability does not seem to be related to MT-induced transformation (Garcea et al. 1989).

Two properties of MT are required for its oncogenic action, the capacity to bind to cellular membranes, and its association with a series of host proteins.

A. *Membrane Association*

MT from PyV-infected cells purifies with a cell fraction that consists mainly of plasma membrane (Ito et al. 1977a; Silver et al. 1978). MT contains a stretch of 22 hydrophobic amino acids near its C-terminus that acts as a membrane-binding domain. MT lacking this sequence no longer associates with membranes, and does not transform (Carmichael et al. 1982). There are only six amino acids C-terminal to this hydrophobic region, and these seem to have little influence on MT function (Dahl et al., 1992), although drastic changes in this area can lower transforming efficiency (Novak and Griffin 1981). Consequently, the majority, or even all, of MT is likely to be on one side of the membrane. No signal sequence to direct co-translational membrane insertion is found anywhere within the MT coding region, and there is evidence that MT is synthesised on free polysomes. Attempts to label MT on the outside of cells have failed (Ito and Spurr 1980), and MT is sensitive to trypsin digestion only in inside-out membrane preparations (Schaffhausen et al. 1982). It is likely, therefore, that MT is synthesised as a soluble form in the cytoplasm, then associates with the cytoplasmic face of membranes through the hydrophobic region.

Replacement of the hydrophobic sequence at the C-terminus of MT with a membrane binding sequence from vesicular stomatitis virus glycoprotein G (VSV-G) generates a species that retains membrane association, but not the ability to transform (Templeton et al. 1984). In addition, point mutations within the hydrophobic region of MT can inhibit transformation without affecting association with membranes (Markland et al. 1986a). It is possible, then, that the MT hydrophobic domain has some specific action, either interacting with factors, such as proteins or lipids, within the membrane environment, or targeting MT to particular membranes. The amino acid sequence of this region also shows homology with a similar area in the hamster polyoma virus, again suggesting it may have a specific role (Markland and Smith 1987).

The "CAAX" sequence present in the *ras* family of membrane-associated polypeptides is modified with a lipid moiety in cells, and is responsible for locating these proteins to a membrane site. A MT species with the hydrophobic domain replaced with a "CAAX" sequence can still transform (Elliott et al., 1998), unlike the situation with VSV G-derived amino acids. Interestingly, a region of predominately basic residues adjacent to the hydrophobic domain in MT co-operates with the "CAAX" motif to provide the membrane specificity required of a fully functional MT. This basic sequence may target MT to a cytoskeleton attached internal membrane site, rather than the plasma membrane, and has been shown to be important for MT transformation (Dahl et al., 1992; Templeton and Eckhart 1984).

Immunofluorescence and electron microscopy studies indicate that a large proportion of MT in infected cells is associated with the cytoplasmic face of most internal cell membranes (Dilworth et al. 1986). Using new monoclonal antibodies and transformed cells, we can also detect a significant amount of MT at the cell periphery (Brewster et al., 1997). This location is not uniform, but seems to be concentrated in discrete spots. Using a number of MT mutants that are defective in binding various polypeptides we have shown that the association with the *src*-family of protein kinases (see later) has no observable effect on the distribution of MT, but disruption of PP2A binding makes a dramatic difference. MT that fails to bind PP2A is no longer found at the cell periphery, but instead concentrates at internal membrane sites close to the nucleus. This work has been extended to include a number of other PP2A binding defective MT mutants (Figure 4C), and all show the same effect, whereas MT lacking

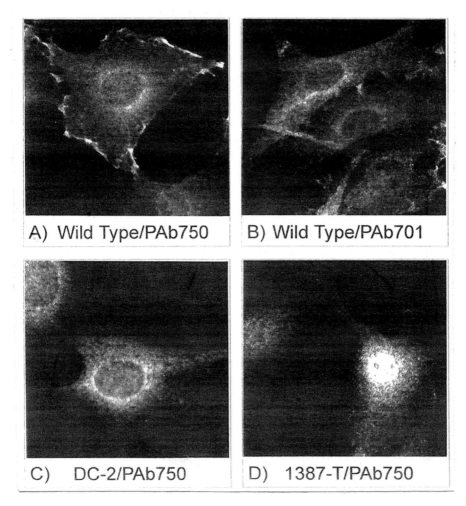

A) Wild Type/PAb750   B) Wild Type/PAb701

C)   DC-2/PAb750   D)   1387-T/PAb750

Fig. 4. Sub-cellular Distribution of MT With and Without Associated PP2A. Immunofluorescence analysis of Rat2 fibroblasts expressing various MT mutants is shown. The MT species expressed, and the monoclonal antibody used, are indicated beneath each panel. PAb750 recognizes all MT forms, whereas PAb701 recognizes only MT that is not associated with PP2A. Mutant DC-2 removes the second CXCXXC motif from MT, and does not interact with PP2A. Note that only MT bound to PP2A is found at the cell periphery.

the hydrophobic domain is found throughout the cytoplasm (Figure 4D). In addition, a specific monoclonal antibody that detects wild type MT only when it is not associated with PP2A (PAb701 Dilworth and Griffin 1982) also does not react with MT at the plasma membrane (Figure 4B). How PP2A binding results in MT re-distribution to the plasma membrane remains to be uncovered, although two different hypotheses can be suggested. Firstly, PP2A could expose a cryptic localising site in MT, possibly by dephosphorylating a MT sequence that acts as a specific membrane protein-binding region. Secondly, PP2A itself might relocate the MT with which it associates to peripheral membranes. This latter theory would only be viable if PP2A was found at the plasma membrane. Although for many years PP2A was considered a ubiquitous cytoplasmic phosphatase, many reports have now demonstrated that a fraction of PP2A is found at membrane sites (for example see Hansra et al., 1996; Pitcher et al., 1995; Ulug et al., 1992). This membrane-bound PP2A is thought to be involved in the de-sensitisation of some signal transduction proteins (Hansra et al., 1996), and may be targeted by MT. It would be an unexpected aspect of MT function if in addition to stimulating many signalling pathways (see next section), it had also evolved a means of preventing this activation being reversed by the normal actions of membrane-bound PP2A.

B. *Protein Binding*

Once again, MT has no overt enzymatic activity of its own. Instead, it transforms by interacting with the host cell proteins that control proliferation. Consequently, defining the polypeptides bound to MT, and the effect interaction has on the activity of each polypeptide, is vital to understanding MT-induced transformation. Most non-transforming MT mutants have a defect in a region required for protein binding, so identifying the polypeptides associated with MT frequently involves examining the polypeptides found co-immunoprecipitated with mutant MT species. The results of a number of such experiments are summarised in Figure 5, where the MT sites required for association with cellular proteins are shown, together with the location of some of the significant MT mutants that helped in identifying these binding species. At least 13 different polypeptides are so far known to associate with MT. Many of these are linked in a sequence of binding interactions that progress along the molecule, so we will consider them in the order the sites are found in the MT polypeptide.

PROTEIN PHOSPHATASE 2A
Immunoprecipitates formed with sera from animals bearing polyoma-induced tumors contain prominent polypeptides with molecular weights of around 35-37 and 60-63kDa in addition to the known T-antigens (Hutchinson et al. 1978; Ito et al. 1977b; Schaffhausen et al. 1978; Silver et al. 1978). These two species associate with PyV MT (Grussenmeyer et al. 1987; Grussenmeyer et al. 1985; Pallas et al. 1988) and ST, and are homologous to the polypeptides bound to SV40 ST (Walter et al. 1988). Partial amino acid sequencing identified these as the catalytic, C (35kDa), and regulatory, A (60kDa) subunits of protein phosphatase 2A (PP2A) (Pallas et al., 1990; Walter et al. 1989; Walter et al., 1990).

Site recognized in MT. It is likely that the PP2A binding site in MT is within the N-terminal region that is incommon with ST, as both interact with the phosphatase. Not all the known mutations in this area have been examined for an effect on PP2A association, as many were isolated before the identity of the 60 and 35kDa proteins had been established. However, where binding has been investigated, all of the mutations in the

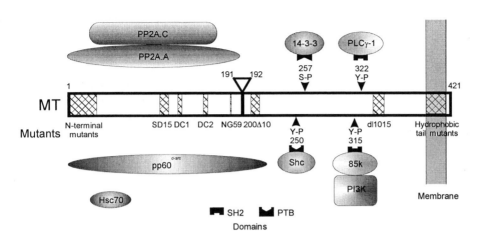

Fig. 5. *Schematic representation of the Binding Sites on MT for Associated Proteins. MT is represented schematically, together with the regions required for association with host proteins to occur. The membrane binding hydrophobic region is also indicated, together with the method of association involved (SH2/PTB domain, etc.) where known. Also indicated within MT (hatched boxes) are a number of significant mutants that were involved in identifying these binding sites.*

MT/ST common region that affect transformation also disrupt PP2A binding, and every mutant with a lesion outside the MT/ST common sequence associates with PP2A as well as wild type MT. No mutant has been isolated that does not bind PP2A but does transform, suggesting that the interaction is required for MT transformation. As with ST, a number of sequences in MT are required for PP2A association, including the N-terminal 30 amino acids, the two conserved CXCXXC motifs, and a region either side of amino acid 180 (Brewster et al., 1997; Markland and Smith, 1987) (see Figures 2 and 3). Interestingly, the region with the highest homology between various ST species (see above), the sequence HPDKGG, is not required for PP2A binding (Campbell et al., 1995; Glenn and Eckhart, 1995), or transformation.

Site recognized in PP2A. PP2A.A consists of 15 non-identical repeat units (Walter et al. 1989), arranged in a rod-like structure (Ruediger et al., 1994). MT binds to repeats 2 to 8 in the A subunit, though addition of PP2A.C promotes the interaction (Ruediger et al., 1992), and the C subunit interacts with repeats 11 to 15. The PP2A.B subunits also bind the central repeating units in A, so, like ST, MT resembles a virally encoded B polypeptide. No homology between the sequences of various B species and MT has been observed, with the exception of the sequence DKGG present in the B'α subunit (Pallas et al., 1992). However, this sequence in MT is not required for PP2A binding.

Effects of the interaction. As with ST, it is still not clear what effect association with MT has on PP2A action. Phosphatase activity can easily be detected in MT immunoprecipitates (Pallas et al., 1990; Ulug et al., 1992), so an overall inhibition of the enzyme does not occur. Another possible effect of association with MT could be an alteration in the substrate specificity of the phosphatase. In support of this, an increase in the activity towards phosphorylated tyrosine residues has been reported (Cayla et al., 1993). As interaction with MT brings PP2A into contact with a number of other polypeptides bound to MT, such as $pp60^{c-src}$ or Shc (see below), it is also feasible that complex formation results in the phosphatase acting on these molecules. There is no evidence for this as yet, however. Much of the work on T-antigen binding to PP2A has been performed using SV40 ST (see above), and it is tempting to extrapolate from these results to MT. However, a number of reports suggest MT cannot perform all the roles of ST in cells (Asselin et al. 1984; Berger and Wintersberger 1986; Noda et al. 1987; Templeton et al. 1986), probably as a result of their different sub-cellular distributions. The location of MT in cellular membranes originally suggested that MT might re-direct PP2A activity to membrane proteins not normally accessible to the phosphatase. However, the report that MT does not change the overall level of PP2A activity in membranes (Ulug et al., 1992), and the demonstration that PP2A binding influences the location of MT (Brewster et al., 1997), suggest that MT targets a sub-population of PP2A already present in the membrane. Therefore, the MT/PP2A complex may have quite separate roles to ST/PP2A. MT mutants have been isolated that bind PP2A but not $pp60^{c-src}$, and still associate with cellular membranes (Brewster et al., 1997). These mutant MT species do not induce any overt changes in the phenotype of cells, but may help determine how MT association with PP2A influences phosphatase, and cell, behaviour.

Whether association with MT influences PP2A activity, then, remains unclear. However, the methodologies to examine the consequences of MT binding to PP2A are now available. PP2A interaction with MT, however, does appear to be required for the subsequent association with $pp60^{c-src}$ (see below).

SRC-FAMILY MEMBERS

$pp60^{c-src}$ was the first protein associated with MT to be identified (Courtneidge and Smith 1983; Courtneidge and Smith 1984). The src-family of tyrosine kinases share extensive sequence homology, and $pp62^{c-yes}$ (Kornbluth et al. 1987) and $pp59^{c-fyn}$ (Cheng et al. 1988a; Horak et al. 1989; Kypta et al. 1988), the other src-family kinases present in fibroblast cells, also bind to MT. Although the interaction between MT and $pp60^{c-src}$ has been the most extensively studied, analogous results with $pp62^{c-yes}$ and $pp59^{c-fyn}$ have been found when they were examined, so it is assumed that all three associations occur through similar mechanisms. The demonstration that MT can transform $pp60^{c-src}$ null cells (Kiefer et al., 1994a; Thomas et al., 1993), presumably through an interaction with $pp62^{c-yes}$ and $pp59^{c-fyn}$, indicates that the effects induced are similar, at least. However, one notable difference has been reported; whereas MT binding to $pp60^{c-src}$ (Bolen et al. 1984; Courtneidge 1985), and $pp62^{c-yes}$ (Kornbluth et al. 1987) activates their kinase activity, MT binding to $pp59^{c-fyn}$ does not (Cheng et al. 1988a; Horak et al. 1989; Kypta et al. 1988). The basis for this difference, and the effect it may have in cells, remains unclear.

Site recognized in MT. All of the MT mutants that disrupt PP2A binding also inhibit association with pp60^{c-src}, suggesting these two interactions are closely related (Campbell et al., 1995; Glenn and Eckhart, 1993; Glenn and Eckhart, 1995). In addition, inhibition of PP2A activity with okadaic acid prevents formation of both the MT-PP2A and MT-pp60^{c-src} complexes (Glover et al, manuscript in preparation). This again suggests the two interactions are linked, and may mean that the phosphatase activity is required for MT to associate with PP2A, or alternatively, a structural change in PP2A may occur as a result of okadaic acid binding which prevents interaction. Finally, when the MT-pp60^{c-src} complex is isolated through the use of site specific monoclonal antibodies, the resulting complex has a 1:1:1 stoichiometry between MT, pp60^{c-src}, and PP2A. Therefore, an interaction between MT and pp60^{c-src} probably does not occur in the absence of PP2A.

It is not yet clear why a MT/PP2A complex is required for interaction with pp60^{c-src}. Antibodies to pp60^{c-src} co-precipitate PP2A only when MT is also present, indicating that they are present in the same complex, and so do not interact with the same region of MT (Pallas et al., 1990; Ulug et al., 1992). Recently, a site in MT required for association with pp60^{c-src}, but not PP2A, has been identified. Monoclonal antibodies that react with amino acids 200 to 220 of MT immunoprecipitate MT-PP2A, but not MT-pp60^{c-src} (Dilworth and Horner, 1993). Deletion mutants have since shown that the area between residues 185 and 210 is required for MT to bind pp60^{c-src}, but not PP2A (Brewster et al., 1997). This is the first separation of PP2A and pp60^{c-src} binding, and suggests that pp60^{c-src} may contact MT at this site, though a direct interaction has yet to be demonstrated. Point mutagenesis within this region identified two motifs, each consisting of a cluster of basic amino acids followed by a serine/threonine residue (Figure 6), as being required for pp60^{c-src} binding.

Replacement of either the serine or threonine residue with an acidic species inhibits pp60^{c-src} interaction with MT, suggesting that association occurs when the site is unphosphorylated. This interpretation has been confirmed by the demonstration that replacement of threonine 203 with a cysteine residue (which cannot be phosphorylated) has no effect on the interaction. It is tempting to link the observations that a MT sequence functions in an unphosphorylated state to bind pp60^{c-src}, and that PP2A is required for the interaction. PP2A, therefore, may be required to remove inhibitory phosphates from the residues 195S and 203T. Direct confirmation of this model has not yet been found, however. In the absence of PP2A, either through mutation of the MT or treatment with okadaic acid, this region does not appear to be phosphorylated (unpublished observations), as would be predicted were the phosphatase necessary to remove a dominant phosphate moiety. However, MT without bound PP2A is also not found in the same location as wild type MT, so this may not necessarily be conclusive. This site, then, is required for pp60^{c-src} binding, but whether phosphorylation here regulates pp60^{c-src} binding to MT remains to be determined.

As well as the possibility (described above) that pp60^{c-src} binds directly to residues 185 to 210 of MT, and PP2A is required to keep this region dephosphorylated, some other models can be postulated to account for the properties of the MT/PP2A/pp60^{c-src} interaction. A PP2A trimer has recently been shown to associate with casein kinase 2α

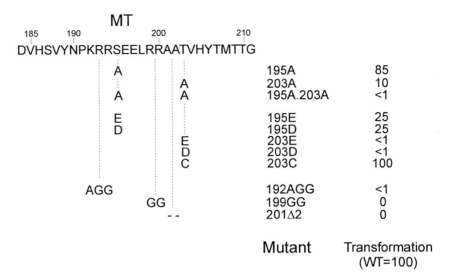

Fig. 6. Mutations in the pp60^{c-src} Binding Region of MT. The sequence of amino acids 185 to 210 in MT is shown at the top, together with the residues altered in a series of transformation-defective mutants below. The identification of the mutant, together with its transforming efficiency relative to wild type MT, is shown on the right. In each case, the transforming efficiency has been shown to exactly parallel the amount of pp60^{c-src} bound to the MT species.

and Ca^{2+}-calmodulin-dependent protein kinase IV, and this regulates kinase activity (Heriche et al., 1997; Westphal et al., 1998). Intriguingly, then, it is possible that replacement of the cellular B-subunits in PP2A by MT could change the binding properties of PP2A to promote a direct association with $pp60^{c-src}$. In this model, no direct interaction between MT and $pp60^{c-src}$ exists, and the MT unique sequences required for association with $pp60^{c-src}$ act to change the binding properties of PP2A. This would make MT a direct viral analogue of a cellular B subunit, which directs not only substrate specificity, but binding activity as well. If this theory is correct, it is possible that a B subunit may exist that promotes association between PP2A and *src*-family kinases within the cell, and MT works by mimicking this activity. A combination of direct interaction between $pp60^{c-src}$ and both MT and PP2A is also possible. In this case, two weak associations, $pp60^{c-src}$/PP2A and $pp60^{c-src}$/MT, could create a high affinity, bipartite interaction. There are a number of possible models to account for the interaction between MT/PP2A and $pp60^{c-src}$, then, but no firm evidence yet to indicate which is correct.

$pp60^{c-src}$ *site recognized by MT.* Src-family kinases have a common structure, consisting of an N-terminal myristylation site that directs membrane association, a unique region that defines the individual family members, and three *src*-homology (SH) domains. SH3 domains interact with proline-rich sequences, SH2 domains with phosphotyrosine, and the SH1 domain is the catalytic region (reviewed in Thomas and Brugge, 1997). The kinase activity of pp60$^{c\text{-}src}$ is regulated by a series of phosphorylations and intramolecular interactions. Phosphorylation of a tyrosine residue in the C-terminal region of the polypeptide (Y527 in chicken pp60$^{c\text{-}src}$) by the kinase *csk*, promotes an interaction between this site and the SH2 domain of the same molecule. This creates an interaction between the SH3 domain and the SH2 to kinase domain linker region. This causes these residues to contact the kinase domain and induce a conformation change in the substrate binding cleft, so inactivating the catalytic site (Xu et al., 1997; reviewed in Mayer, 1997). Inhibition of pp60$^{c\text{-}src}$ kinase activity can be relieved by dephosphorylating tyrosine 527, or by other binding proteins interacting with the SH2 or SH3 domains of pp60$^{c\text{-}src}$, so preventing intramolecular interaction. Once the internal associations are inhibited, tyrosine 416 in the catalytic region of pp60$^{c\text{-}src}$ is phosphorylated, possibly by autophosphorylation, to form a fully active kinase.

MT associated pp60$^{c\text{-}src}$ is unphosphorylated at Y527, and phosphorylated at Y416 (Cartwright et al. 1986; Courtneidge 1985), indicating the kinase is activated. Direct measurements show the kinase associated with MT has a specific activity approximately 20 times higher than free pp60$^{c\text{-}src}$ (Bolen et al. 1984; Cartwright et al. 1985; Courtneidge 1985). Using pp60$^{c\text{-}src}$ mutants, it has been shown that the extreme C-terminal tail of pp60$^{c\text{-}src}$ is not required for binding MT, but residues between 518 and 525 are (Cartwright et al. 1987; Cheng et al. 1988b). Y527 is not involved in MT binding, then, but a region immediately N-terminal to it. The sequence of this area is highly conserved between all *src*-family members (Figure 7), and plays a role in activation of pp60$^{c\text{-}src}$ (Cobb et al., 1991).

Two possible models can account for the stimulation of pp60$^{c\text{-}src}$ activity by MT binding, depending on which form of pp60$^{c\text{-}src}$ is initially recognized. Firstly, MT may interact with inactive pp60$^{c\text{-}src}$, and, by binding near to Y527 break the intramolecular interaction between the SH2 domain and Tyr527, enabling access of a phosphatase. It is tempting to suggest that the PP2A present in the MT complex that binds pp60$^{c\text{-}src}$ may be involved in this dephosphorylation, but there is no evidence to support this possibility yet. Alternatively, the MT/PP2A complex may interact with already active pp60$^{c\text{-}src}$, and maintain it in this state by preventing intramolecular interaction and access by *csk*, or again promoting access of a phosphatase. It is not clear which of these possibilities is correct.

The SH2 and SH3 domains of pp60$^{c\text{-}src}$ are not required for interaction with MT and may even have an inhibitory effect (Dunant et al., 1996). In addition, the kinase activity of pp60$^{c\text{-}src}$ is not required (Cheng et al. 1988b). However, interaction between MT-PP2A and pp60$^{c\text{-}src}$ involves more than the C-terminal region of pp60$^{c\text{-}src}$. Disruption of the kinase domain structure of pp60$^{c\text{-}src}$ also inhibits MT binding, and the C-terminal tail region does not interact with MT in isolation (unpublished observations). The kinase domain and a few C-terminal residues of pp60$^{c\text{-}src}$, then, are all that are required for association with MT. A number of cellular proteins are known to interact with pp60$^{c\text{-}src}$,

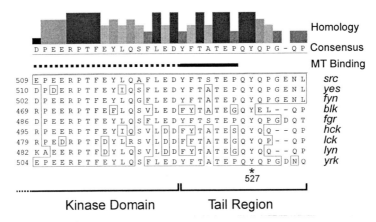

Fig. 7. *Sequence Homology at the C-Terminal End of* src-*Family Kinases. The sequences of the C-terminal end of nine members of the* src-*family of tyrosine kinases are shown aligned for maximum homology. The residues required for MT binding are indicated by a solid line above the sequences, those that are thought to be required are marked with a dashed line. A consensus sequence, and the level of homology, is also shown.*

but so far, these all bind either the SH2 or SH3 domains, or both (Erpel and Courtneidge, 1995; Taylor and Shalloway, 1996). Therefore, this interaction with MT does not seem to have any known parallels within the normal cell. It is unlikely, though, that the mechanism by which pp60^{c-src} is recognized by MT is unique to the virus. Instead, it is more probable that MT is mimicking the way a cellular protein, as yet unknown, binds to and regulates pp60^{c-src} activity, in the same way that the other polypeptides that interact with MT associate with host cell proteins by analogous mechanisms. That this speculation is probably correct is indicated by the observation that pp56^{c-lck} binds and activates the interleukin 2 receptor β (Hatakeyama et al., 1991). This interaction involves the kinase domain of *lck*, so this method of regulation may be more general than previously recognized. It is also possible that the interaction between MT and the kinase domain of *src*-family kinases is mediated via PP2A in the same way that PP2A binds to the catalytic domain of other kinases (see above). In this case the cellular homologue of MT may be a B-subunit of PP2A. This B-subunit may be expressed in only a few cells (e.g. neuronal cells), explaining why an interaction between PP2A and pp60^{c-src} may have been overlooked.

Effects of Association. Once activated, MT-associated pp60^{c-src} phosphorylates MT itself at a number of sites, notably tyrosines 250, 315 and 322 (Harvey et al. 1984; Hunter et al. 1984; Oostra et al. 1983; Schaffhausen and Benjamin 1981). A major breakthrough in signalling research has been the realisation that phosphotyrosine can be recognized by the SH2 and phosphotyrosine binding (PTB) domains found in a number of proteins (Pawson, 1995). The tyrosines in MT phosphorylated by pp60^{c-src} are all in the C-terminal half of the molecule (unpublished observation), and are known to act as binding sites for at least three important signalling molecules, Shc, PI3K and PLCγ-1 (see below). It is not clear yet whether other polypeptides outside the MT complex are also phosphorylated. Some proteins such as FAK show an increase in phosphotyrosine levels in MT transformed cells (Bachelot et al., 1996; Yonemoto et al. 1987), but the total amount of phosphotyrosine in the cell does not change (Sefton et al. 1980).

HSC70

MT that fails to associate with PP2A, interacts with a 73kDa polypeptide, which has been identified as Hsc70 (Pallas et al. 1989; Walter et al. 1987). This association is usually observed when MT does not bind PP2A because of mutation, or is over-expressed to a level that exceeds the amount of PP2A present in the cell. It is not clear whether the interaction forms only in the absence of PP2A association because binding to PP2A masks the site recognized by Hsc70, or if Hsc70 interaction indicates that the MT is unable to fold correctly, and this exposes a cryptic binding site. The HPDKGG sequence that is highly conserved between all ST species (see above) is required for Hsc70 interaction. As with ST, the area surrounding these sequences has similarity to a DnaJ domain in bacteria, and so may act as a molecular chaperone. This property may indicate that this region facilitates assembly of the multi-protein complex based on MT. In which case, association with Hsc70 may be an intermediate in the formation of the MT/PP2A interaction that becomes trapped when association with PP2A is inhibited. However, deletion of the HPDKGG sequence has no, or only minor, effects on MT transformation of cultured cells (Campbell et al., 1995; Glenn and Eckhart, 1995). The effect on cellular phenotype of Hsc70 binding to MT, remains unclear.

SHC/GRB2

Site recognized in MT. Tyrosine 250 (Y250) in MT is one of the residues phosphoryl-ated by the MT bound $pp60^{c-src}$, and mutation of Y250 to phenylalanine reduces the transforming efficiency of MT to approximately 10% of wild type (Markland et al. 1986b). Sequences N-terminal to Y250, notably an NPTY motif, are also required for MT-induced transformation (Druker et al., 1990; Druker et al., 1992), but have no effect on the amount of $pp60^{c-src}$ or PI3K (see later) bound to MT. Together, these results suggested that another polypeptide may interact with this site. Using an approach involving immunoprecipitation followed by western blotting with another antibody, the p66 and p52 forms of the Shc oncogene products were shown to be associated with the NPTY motif when Y250 in MT was phosphorylated (Campbell et al., 1994; Dilworth et al., 1994). As phosphorylation by $pp60^{c-src}$ is required for the interaction, Shc is not bound to MT that does not associate with $pp60^{c-src}$.

Site recognized in Shc. Initially, association was thought to involve interaction between the SH2 domain of Shc and phosphotyrosine 250 in MT. However, SH2 domains usually recognize sequences C-terminal to the phosphotyrosine (reviewed in Pawson, 1995), so it was unclear why the NPTY sequence involving residues N-terminal to the tyrosine was important. This problem was solved when it was discovered that Shc contains an additional phosphotyrosine binding (PTB) domain which recognizes an N-terminal NPXY motif (Blaikie et al., 1994; Gustafson et al., 1995; Kavanaugh and Williams, 1994; van der Geer et al., 1995). Interaction with the PTB domain of Shc is vital for MT-induced transformation of cells in culture; alteration of P248, or mutation of Y250 to phenylalanine, abolishes Shc binding, and decreases transformation by MT to low, though not zero, levels. Over expression of the PTB domain of Shc can block MT induced transformation, presumably by acting as a competitive inhibitor and preventing wild type Shc interaction (Blaikie et al., 1997). *In vitro* binding studies indicate that Y250 of MT can also associate with the SH2 domain of Shc (Dilworth et al., 1994; and unpublished data), but it is unclear whether this has a role in cells. p52 Shc consists of an N-terminal PTB domain, followed by a region with homology to the $\alpha 1$ chain of collagen (CH1), and at its C-terminus, an SH2 domain (Pelicci et al., 1992). The p46 form is generated by a second translation initiation methionine in the same message, which impinges slightly on the PTB domain. This may explain why the p46 form of Shc is seen to associate less well with MT in some experiments (Dilworth et al., 1994). The p66 form of Shc is thought to arise by an alternative splicing event, and contains an additional CH domain (CH2) N-terminal to the PTB domain.

Effects of Association. Shc also associates with activated growth factor receptors (GFR) via its PTB domain, and is phosphorylated by the active receptor at tyrosine residues 317 (Salcini et al., 1994) and 239/240 (Gotoh et al., 1997; van der Geer et al., 1996). Both of these sites are within the CH1 domain and act as recognition sequences for the SH2 domain of the adapter molecule, Grb2 (Rozakis Adcock et al., 1992; van der Geer et al., 1996). This brings mSos, a *ras* guanine nucleotide exchange factor (reviewed in McCormick, 1993; Schlessinger, 1993) to a membrane location, which is sufficient to activate p21*ras* (Aronheim et al., 1994). Through association with Raf-1, and phosphorylation of MEK, p21*ras* activates the ERK family of MAP Kinases, so providing a mitogenic signal. Shc interaction with MT stimulates a very similar series of events. MT-bound Shc is phosphorylated on at least four tyrosines, including Y239, 240 and 317 (unpublished observation), presumably by action of the *src*-family kinase. Phosphorylated Shc then binds Grb2, thus relocating it to a membrane site with the rest of the MT complex, where it also becomes tyrosine phosphorylated (unpublished data). *ras* activity is required for MT transformation (Jelinek and Hassell, 1992; Raptis et al., 1991), and MT activates MAP kinase (Urich et al., 1995), so it is likely that Grb2 binding to Shc in the MT complex activates *ras*, and eventually MAP Kinase.

Over-expression of the PTB domain of Shc only blocks MT transformation if the 239/240 phosphorylation site in Shc is not present, suggesting that phosphorylation of these two tyrosines is important for transformation (Blaikie et al., 1997). Interestingly, there appears to be more phosphorylated Shc present in cells than is associated with MT (Campbell et al., 1994; Dilworth et al., 1994). *V-src* transformed cells also contain tyrosine phosphorylated Shc, though the two proteins do not seem to interact directly (McGlade et al., 1992). This free phosphorylated form probably exerts some effect as Shc overexpression can transform fibroblasts (Pelicci et al., 1992), and induce *ras*-dependent neurite outgrowth in PC12 cells (Rozakis Adcock et al., 1992). The PTB domain of Shc can also interact with acidic phospholipids such as the products of PI3K, so directing Shc binding molecules to other subcellular sites (Ravichandran et al., 1997). The demonstration that Shc associates with membrane structures in cells, and undergoes re-distribution on activation by a growth factor receptor (Lotti et al., 1996), suggests this may play a role in Shc action. Interestingly, the level of PI3K products phosphatidylinositol (3,4) phosphate (PI (3,4)P_2) and phosphatidylinositol (3,4,5) phosphate (PI(3,4,5)P_3) are not raised by MT when interaction with Shc is inhibited (Ling et al., 1992). Therefore, the pathways stimulated by the Shc and PI3K-bound to MT probably interact at some level. p66 Shc has an extra CH domain, and becomes tyrosine-phosphorylated in MT-transformed cells (Dilworth et al., 1994). Recent work, however, suggests that this polypeptide is not involved in MAP Kinase activation, but may actually inhibit aspects of the pathway (Migliaccio et al., 1997). The role of p66 Shc in MT transformation has not yet been examined.

14-3-3 PROTEINS

2D gel separations of immunoprecipitates formed with antibodies directed against MT contain two polypeptides with molecular weights of 27 and 29kDa (Pallas et al. 1988). Partial amino acid sequences derived from purified polypeptides showed that the 29kDa MT-associated protein is the epsilon (ε) form of the 14-3-3 group of proteins (Aitken, 1995), and the 27kDa polypeptide a mixture of the other family members (Pallas et al., 1994). The 14-3-3 polypeptides are now known to interact with phosphoserine in the motif RSXSXP (Muslin et al., 1996; Yaffe et al., 1997), and to be dimerize. Consequently, they may act as adapter molecules for various signalling events. MT contains a good consensus sequence for a 14-3-3 binding site, centred around serine 257 (S257), and this region has been shown to interact with the 14-3-3 polypeptides (Cullere et al., 1998). It is not clear yet which kinase phosphorylates S257 in MT, or whether it is regulated. S257 is also involved in MT multimerisation, but is not required for transformation (Senften et al., 1997). Removal of S257 makes no difference to MT-induced cell transformation, but interestingly, alters the spectrum of tumors initiated in animals (Cullere et al., 1998). Alteration of S257 causes a dramatic decrease in the proportion of salivary gland tumors induced by PyV. The molecular basis for this observation remains to be established. The beta and zeta isoforms of the 14-3-3 proteins also interact with, and activate, Raf-1 (Fantl et al., 1994; Freed et al., 1994a; Freed et al., 1994b; Fu et al., 1994), suggesting MT may be influencing signalling at this level. No demonstration of a direct effect of MT on Raf-1 activity has yet been shown, however.

PI3K

MT becomes heavily phosphorylated by the *src*-family kinases when immunoprecipi-tates formed with anti-MT antibodies are incubated with radio-labelled ATP. These *in vitro* phosphorylation events are probably similar to those occurring *in vivo*, and additional polypeptides also get phosphorylated by the pp60$^{c\text{-}src}$ in these precipitates. The most prominent of these is an 80 to 85kDa polypeptide (Dilworth 1982) which is absent when some non-transforming mutants of MT are examined (Courtneidge and Heber 1987; Kaplan et al. 1987). A phosphatidylinositol kinase (PIK) activity is also found in MT immunoprecipitates (Kaplan et al. 1986; Whitman et al. 1985), and a correlation has been observed between the presence of PIK activity and the 85kDa polypeptide (Courtneidge and Heber 1987; Kaplan et al. 1987). This PIK activity has since been shown to be a novel type which phosphorylates the 3' OH of the inositol moiety, and so is now called PI3K (Whitman et al. 1988). Purified PI3K contains two polypeptides, the 85kDa component plus a 110kDa species (Carpenter et al., 1990; Morgan et al., 1990). Cloning and expression of the gene encoding the 85kDa polypeptide (Escobedo et al., 1991; Otsu et al., 1991; Skolnik et al., 1991) indicated that it did not possess PI3K activity itself. Instead, the 110kDa polypeptide was found to be the catalytic subunit, and the gene for this has also now been cloned (Hiles et al., 1992; Hu et al., 1993). Since then, many different types of PI3K subtypes have been isolated (reviewed in Vanhaesebroeck et al., 1997), but we will continue to refer to the MT bound original form as PI3K here.

Site recognized in MT. PI3K association with MT occurs mainly through tyrosine 315 (Y315) in the MT sequence (Talmage et al. 1989). Mutation of this tyrosine to the non-phosphorylatable phenylalanine reduces the amount of PI3K bound, although some studies show it is not abolished completely (Cohen et al., 1990a; Dilworth et al., 1994). *In vitro*, at least, phosphorylation of Y315 is required for PI3K association with MT (Auger et al., 1992; Cohen et al., 1990b), and it is possible that phosphorylated tyrosine 322 can also contribute to the interaction (Yoakim et al., 1992). As phosphorylation is required for the complex between MT and PI3K to form, any inhibition of pp60[c-src] binding to MT (see above), which is responsible for this phosphorylation, also abolishes PI3K association.

Site recognized in PI3K. The PI3K 85kDa subunit contains two SH2 and an SH3 domain. Not surprisingly, the SH2 domains have been shown to be responsible for the interaction with MT (Yoakim et al., 1992). The involvement of two phosphotyrosines in MT, and two SH2 domains in PI3K suggests that a bipartite recognition process may occur, for which there is some evidence (Yoakim et al., 1992). However, the identification of another protein bound to tyrosine 322 in MT suggests this residue may have a more important role (see below).

Effects of association. **PI3K Activation.** The PI3K 85kDa subunit associated with MT can be found both tyrosine and serine phosphorylated (Carpenter et al., 1993b), although it has been reported that the tyrosine phosphorylation may not occur *in vivo* (Roche et al., 1994). The 110kDa subunit is usually not tyrosine phosphorylated, either *in vivo* or *in vitro* (Roche et al., 1994), though phosphorylation has been observed *in vitro* in some experiments (Auger et al., 1992). Serine phosphorylation of the 85kDa subunit may be catalysed by an intrinsic activity of the 110kDa species (Carpenter et al., 1993b; Dhand et al., 1994), and this is thought to inhibit PI3K activity. It is possible, then, that the PP2A associated with MT dephosphorylates these serine residues, and so activates PI3K activity to some extent. Although it is tempting to speculate that tyrosine phosphorylation of the 85kDa subunit also activates PI3K, this is probably not the case. Instead, interaction between the SH2 domains and a phosphotyrosine site seems to stimulate activity (Backer et al., 1992; Carpenter et al., 1993a; Giorgetti et al., 1993; Myers et al., 1992; Shoelson et al., 1993). It is also possible that a bipartite binding of the two SH2 domains to two phosphotyrosines is required for full activation (reviewed in Kapeller and Cantley, 1994). Association with MT translocates PI3K from an essentially cytoplasmic site to a membrane location (Cohen et al., 1990b). This re-distribution of PI3K to a site where its substrates are present could be another means of stimulating product formation. The finding that addition of a membrane targeting sequence to the 110kDa subunit of PI3K is sufficient to promote its activity adds weight to this idea (Didichenko et al., 1996; Klippel et al., 1996; Reif et al., 1996). There is evidence that a number of factors could be involved in stimulating the activity of PI3K on association with MT, and it is not clear which is the most important.

Association with PI3K and stimulation of its activity is essential to the transforming actions of MT. PI3K phosphorylates the D-3 position of the inositol ring of phosphatidylinositol (4,5) phosphate ($PI(4,5)P_2$) to generate $PI(3,4,5)P_3$, which is then dephosphorylated by a 5' phosphatase to give $PI(3,4)P_2$. $PI(3)P$ is constitutively present in all cells, but $PI(3,4)P_2$, and $PI(3,4,5)P_3$ increase significantly on MT expression (Gorga et al., 1990; Serunian et al., 1990; Ulug et al., 1990). Reduction in the amount of PI3K bound to MT abolishes this increase, and decreases transformation efficiency to low levels. However, the increase in PI3K products may not be just a direct effect of the interaction between PI3K and MT, as some MT mutants that still bind and phosphorylate PI3K do not show raised levels of $PI(3,4)P_2$ and $PI(3,4,5)P_3$ (Ling et al., 1992). The observation that Shc-induced pathways contribute to the increase in the levels of $PI(3,4)P_2$ and $PI(3,4,5)P_3$ in cells is probably related to the ability of PI3K to bind activated *ras* (Kodaki et al., 1994; Rodriguez Viciana et al., 1996; Rodriguez-Viciana et al., 1994). Binding through SH2 domains to membrane bound tyrosine phosphorylated proteins seems not to be sufficient to stimulate PI3K product formation, indicating that interaction with *ras* is also required. Therefore, PI3K seems to be involved at a number of different points in the signalling pathways activated by MT. As with Shc, the amount of tyrosine phosphorylated PI3K in cells is higher than the quantity associated with MT, so transformation induces an increase in the total level of tyrosine phosphorylated PI3K in the cell (Cohen et al., 1990a). Once produced, the PI3K products are not substrates for another polypeptide bound by MT, PLC-γ1 (Lips et al. 1989; Serunian et al. 1989), instead, the lipids themselves act as signalling intermediates.

ROLE OF PI3K PRODUCTS

PKCζ, which has a role in mitogenic signalling (Berra et al., 1993) possibly through an ability to inactivate IκB, and so release NFκB (Diaz Meco et al., 1994), is directly activated by $PI(3,4,5)P_3$ (Nakanishi et al., 1993). PI3K products have also been implicated in activating other PKC family members (Toker et al., 1994), although there is no agreement in the literature about the *in vivo* significance of this, as yet. This may explain why ST, which also has an effect on PKC activation (see above), can promote MT transformation.

PI3K stimulates the activity of the kinases PDK1 and PKB (or Akt or RAC)(reviewed in Alessi and Cohen, 1998; Bos, 1995; Hemmings, 1997; Marte and Downward, 1997). PDK1 phosphorylates PKB on threonine 308, and an unknown kinase phosphorylates serine 473. These phosphorylations together activate PKB kinase activity, which then phosphorylates a number of substrates, either directly or indirectly. These substrates include the kinase GSK3, the transcription factor E2F and an apoptosis regulating protein, Bad. As a consequence, PI3K, followed by PKB, activation can influence transcriptional processes, and suppress apoptosis induction by a number of stimuli. MT stimulates PKB activity (Meili et al., 1998), and blocks apoptosis, at least partially, through activation of PI3K (Dahl et al., 1998). Suppression of apoptosis by MT may have a role in the virus life cycle, preventing the defence mechanisms of the cell interrupting the infective cycle. MT also stimulates phosphorylation and activation of pp70S6kinase by PDK1 (Dahl et al., 1996), which is involved in cell cycle progression. Both PDK1 and PKB contain a pleckstrin homology (PH) domain, and these bind to the lipid products of PI3K, resulting in both proteins being re-located to a membrane site. It is not yet clear whether binding of lipids to either, or both, PH domains also has a direct role in activation of the kinases, or merely serves to re-distribute both molecules to the same area. PKB may also be translocated to the nucleus to achieve some of its actions.

PI3K is also linked to actin filament re-organisation and membrane ruffling through the action of *rho* and *rac* (Hawkins et al., 1995; Kotani et al., 1994; Nobes et al., 1995; Rodriguez Viciana et al., 1997; Wennstrom et al., 1994), whilst MT transformation depends on *rac1* and CDC42 activity (Urich et al., 1997). PI3K activation induces actin polymerisation, the formation of actin cables, membrane ruffles, and focal adhesions in most other situations. However, transformation by MT results in the disruption of the cell's actin cable network and focal adhesions. This may indicate that all of the events stimulated by PI3K in other systems are not involved in MT induced transformation. Recently, it has been shown that *rho* is required to suppress p21Waf1/Cip1 activity after *ras* stimulation (Olson et al., 1998). As MT transformation is dependent on *ras* activity, it seems likely that this is also involved in MT transformation. The actin alterations induced by PI3K through *rho* and *rac* activity, then, may not be relevant to MT action. PI3K clearly mediates a complex series of events in the cell (Toker and Cantley, 1997), making it difficult to determine which are involved in MT transformation, and those that are unrelated. In addition, there is evidence that SH2 and PTB domains bind PI(3,4,5)P3 and this may modulate other interactions within the membrane (Rameh et al., 1995). It is not even clear, therefore, that we have yet identified all of the events invoked by binding PI3K to MT, or even uncovered those that are required for transformation.

PLCγ-1

Phosphorylation of tyrosine 322 creates a site that conforms to the consensus sequence recognized by the SH2 domain of phospholipase Cγ-1 (PLCγ-1). MT immunoprecipitates have been shown to contain PLCγ-1, which is lost when tyrosine 322 is mutated to phenylalanine (Y322F)(Su et al., 1995). Disruption of this site has only minor effects on transformation in high serum levels, but decreases the number of foci induced in low serum (Su et al., 1995). This residue could also be involved in binding PI3K (see above), but no difference in p85 association with Y322F MT was observed in these experiments. The 145kDa PLCγ-1 associated with MT is phosphorylated on tyrosines, both *in vitro* and *in vivo*, presumably by the action of the *src*-family kinases also bound to MT. The lipase activity of PLCγ-1 is stimulated by tyrosine phosphorylation (Goldschmidt Clermont et al., 1991; Nishibe et al., 1990), though the PI(3,4,5)P$_3$ produced by PI3K may also be involved in fully activating the enzyme (reviewed in Scharenberg and Kinet, 1998). It is likely, therefore, that PLCγ-1 action plays a role in MT induced transformation. On activation, PLCγ-1 cleaves phosphatidylinositol (4,5)P$_2$ to produce diacylglycerol (DAG), and inositol-1,4,5-P$_3$ (IP$_3$). DAG activates some subtypes of PKC, and transformation by MT has been shown to increase PKC activity (Delage et al., 1993; Marcellus et al., 1991), though it has not been reported yet whether removal of Y322 prevents this activation. IP$_3$ production releases Ca^{2+} from intracellular stores, which has a role in mitogenic signalling (reviewed in Berridge, 1995). The importance of this effect to MT induced cell transformation is not yet known.

OTHERS

MT interacts with a number of the polypeptides that associate with activated GFR, but there are some notable differences. Many receptors also bind the GTPase activating protein, GAP, and the tyrosine phosphatase, PTP1B. No association between MT and either of these two molecules has been observed. It is possible that these constitute negative pathways responsible for rapidly inactivating the signals arising from GFR activation when the external stimulus is removed. Clearly, there would be no selective advantage for PyV to inactivate the signalling pathways it has stimulated, so these polypeptides are not targeted.

Despite many studies, and the number of polypeptides already found associated with MT, it is feasible that there are additional, as yet unidentified, binding partners. Previously, MT mutants defective in transforming ability have identified the sequences required for association with cellular polypeptides. At least one transformation defective mutant, dl1015 (Magnusson et al. 1981), still has an unexplained defect. Some reports suggest dl1015 MT does not activate pp60$^{c\text{-}src}$ fully, has lowered Shc binding, or reduced PI3K association. However, we can find no good evidence that any of the polypeptides bound to MT associate less well with dl1015 (unpublished). There is good evidence, though, that despite binding PI3K, the levels of PI(3,4)P$_2$ and PI(3,4,5)P$_3$ are not raised in dl1015-expressing cells (Ling et al., 1992). Consistent with this, it has also been reported that dl1015 MT does not activate PKB (Meili et al., 1998), which is dependent on the presence of PI3K products. Whether there is another binding partner required for the full activation of PI3K, and which interacts with the region of MT affected by dl1015, remains to be determined. It is worth noting that the dl1015 deletion removes a run of proline residues (Magnusson et al. 1981) that may constitute an SH3 domain binding region. However, deletion of just these proline residues does not produce the full defective phenotype of dl1015, so the other altered residues are also involved (Empereur et al, manuscript in preparation).

MT immunoprecipitates analysed by 2D gel electrophoresis exhibit a number of polypeptides that have not yet been unidentified (unpublished observations). As every protein found associated with MT to date has been involved in some aspect of transformation, and most are involved in signal transduction, it is likely that these other proteins are involved in both processes. These may be new, undiscovered species, or components not previously thought to be involved in MT induced transformation. MT, then, may yet provide further insights into tumorigenesis and signal transduction.

Conclusions

MT consists of a number of interdependent binding sites that assembles a large complex within the cell membrane (Figure 5). PP2A binds first, possibly with the assistance of Hsc70, and this is required for subsequent association with a member of the src-family of tyrosine kinases. The kinase activity of $pp60^{c-src}$ is de-regulated by this interaction, and phosphorylates MT itself at a number of sites. These phosphotyrosines then bind at least three proteins containing SH2 or PTB domains, and these polypeptides in turn get phosphorylated on tyrosine residues. It is not immediately clear how the src-family kinase is able to contact at least three sites in MT, then proteins associated with these residues, and in one case (Grb2 bound to Shc), yet another protein. It certainly suggests that the MT structure must possess a large degree of flexibility to allow each polypeptide to contact the kinase active site. Once phosphorylated, not all of the protein remains bound to MT, but some may dissociate to exert an effect elsewhere.

The model described above suggests that the signals emerging from each of these sites are separate, and so these areas need not necessarily be linked in a single molecule. However, we have so far been unable to demonstrate complementation between mutants affected in different binding sites in co-transfection assays, as would be expected to occur if they could function on separate molecules. It is feasible, then, that the three phosphotyrosines need to be linked in order to generate a transforming signal. It is also not clear whether all of these phosphotyrosine sites function at the same time in one molecule. Some reports suggest there is a linkage between the three MT phosphotyrosine bound polypeptides (Campbell et al., 1994; Su et al., 1995), but this does not indicate whether this is necessary for activity. All of these binding interactions take place at a membrane location specified by the C-terminus of MT, and possibly by interaction with PP2A. The observation that membrane location can be used to control activity is becoming a general consensus from a number of studies. Activation by membrane association is observed in the case of Sos, PI3K, Raf, PKB, and PDK1, at least. Therefore, the specificity of membrane interaction is probably an important factor in MT induced transformation.

The realisation that RNA tumor virus oncogenes had cellular counterparts, i.e., proto-oncogenes, suggested that MT may have derived from the host genome. Efforts to find a host gene homologue for MT have been made, but without success (Griffin et al. 1980). Recently, however, we have begun to realise that it is possible that MT evolved small, independent, regions to mimic host protein function, rather than directly acquiring a host protein. Like most viruses of the polyoma group, an ancestor probably expressed only a ST species, comprising a cytoplasmic PP2A binding, protein. However, as the RNA encoding this protein was spliced, a separate C-terminal segment attached to ST could easily be generated. A membrane binding domain, or the ability to bind *src*-family kinases, evolved first, either by gain of small DNA segments from the host genome, or by gradual mutation. In this regard, it may be significant that the *src*-family kinase-binding site in MT is encoded immediately after the splice point in the mRNA, suggesting it may have been acquired first. Both of these interactions could stimulate cell replication to some degree, so providing the virus with a significant advantage. Only small changes in additional sequences would then be required to generate the sites recognized by SH2/PTB domains. It is not difficult to see that each one of these gave the virus an advantage, so could be acquired separately. Consequently, instead of MT having to evolve as a single protein, it could adapt one site at a time, gradually refining its effects. In each case the protein was mimicking the actions of host regulatory mechanisms to stimulate growth in the infected cell, and to prevent the host defence mechanism acting to terminate infection. This process need not happen in the same way in different viruses. The hamster polyoma virus MT also binds pp59^{c-fyn}, but by a different mechanism (Dunant et al., 1997), and the only significant homologies in the C-terminal region of the two MTs occurs at the protein binding sites and the membrane associating region. Thus, these two molecules may have evolved separately to perform the same actions.

The events stimulated by MT are clearly similar to those initiated by activated tyrosine kinase-associated growth factor receptors (GFR). In receptors, the kinase activity is triggered by receptor occupancy, and this results in phosphorylation of tyrosines in a scaffold molecule (which may be the cytoplasmic portion of the receptor or some other molecule) and recruitment of a series of SH2/PTB domain-containing molecules. These then also become phosphorylated on tyrosines. In the case of MT, these signalling pathways become permanently activated. In addition, the inhibitory processes required to inactivate the signals rapidly when the external stimulus is removed, or to modulate a sustained signal, are probably not present, or may even be actively repressed. MT, then, can be considered as a permanently active homologue of a growth factor receptor (Dilworth, 1995). GFRs, however, can initiate more responses than just mitogenesis, including differentiation induction and apoptosis promotion or suppression. There is mounting evidence that MT can also initiate these events in appropriate cells. Infection of the phaechromocytoma cell line PC12 with PyV promotes effects similar to those observed following the addition of NGF, including growth arrest and neurite outgrowth (unpublished observations). MT expression also makes the haemopoetic progenitor cell line FDC-P1 growth factor independent (Metcalf et al. 1987; Muser et al. 1989), and initiates T-cell receptor dependent transcription in T-cell lines (Kennedy et al., 1998). In HL60 cells, MT accelerates differentiation (Platko et al., 1998), and in fibroblasts can suppress some aspects of apoptosis in a similar manner to a survival factor (Dahl et al., 1998). However, MT expression often induces secretion of additional growth factors, so it is possible that MT effects are not always direct, but could be supplemented by additional pathways stimulated by other secreted growth factors. PyV, and MT in particular, then, has not only proven its worth as a tool for studying transformation, but can also be used to probe the processes behind signal transduction from GFRs.

Transformation

Cell Culture Work

The development of cell transformation assays that correlated well with the ability of cells to produce tumors in animals made studies of oncogene function considerably easier. A number of different techniques are now used to measure " cell transformation", so the original meaning has become somewhat diluted and confused. However, most assays rely on the cells gaining one of two major new properties. Firstly, transformed cells continue to grow at confluency, and lose any contact inhibition of growth or movement. This means transformed cells, unlike so-called "normal" ones, continue to grow at confluency and pile up on top of one another to form a "focus". The second property of cells used as a transformation assay is the ability to grow without attachment to a surface. Most non-haemopoetic cells need to attach to a solid surface in order to survive and grow, suggesting that signals produced when surface integrins interact with their ligands are required for cell survival. Transformed cells frequently lose this requirement, and grow when attachment is prevented, for instance after suspension in a semi-solid media such as agar or methocel. A number of other properties can be used for assessing transformation, such as reduced serum requirement, but these give more variable results.

Non-permissive cells infected with PyV go through an "abortive" transformation stage, where the T-antigens are synthesised, and the properties of the cell altered (Stoker 1968). Most of these cells regain their normal phenotype after only a few cell divisions as T-antigen synthesis is lost. When the viral genome is stably acquired by integration into the cellular DNA, however, and the T-antigens are continually expressed, the cells become permanently transformed. MT alone is sufficient to transform established cell lines to a state where they display all the above properties, including tumorigenesis (Treisman et al. 1981). Primary cultures are not transformed by MT (Rassoulzadegan et al. 1982), but require expression of the N-terminal 30% of LT, and ST. LT expression can "immortalise" primary cells (Rassoulzadegan et al. 1983), and this is dependent upon its continued synthesis. This led to the realisation that at least two genes are required for primary cell transformation in culture, which has been extended to include cellular oncogenes (Land et al. 1983; Ruley 1983). Many different aspects of cell behaviour are involved in this phenomenon, including suppression of senescence, with which LT is probably involved, and inhibition of an apoptotic response for which both ST and MT seem to be required. MT expression in an established cell line, then, is sufficient in most cases to induce transformation to a fully tumorigenic phenotype. The vast majority of PyV work has used rodent fibroblasts, though epithelial cells can be transformed by MT, particularly in co-operation with ST (Noda et al. 1987). Human cells can also be transformed when suitable promoters are employed (Strauss et al., 1990).

Some MT mutants show a complete absence of transformation induction. However, others can bring about transformation with varying degrees of defect compared to wild type MT, including lower numbers of foci formed, or reduced growth rate of the cells. This suggests that some activities are absolutely required for transformation, whereas others only contribute to the overall phenotype. In addition, where an interaction is weakened, but not abolished, by mutation, a threshold of activity is probably required. This results in lowered transformation efficiency, as only cells synthesising high levels of MT induce sufficient changes to be measured. MT transformation, then, is not an "all or nothing" response, but exhibits a full range of phenotype changes depending on the properties of the MT species used, its expression level, the recipient cells, and the conditions under which the assay is performed. Not surprisingly, there have been some problems in measuring MT-induced transformation in the past, with some notable disagreements between groups. These have usually been resolved by further experiments, however, and understanding how different mutants can induce varying results has frequently aided our overall understanding of how MT functions to induce the transformed phenotype. However, it does mean that results in one system, especially negative ones, may not be representative of the overall picture.

Animal Work

VIRAL INFECTIONS

PyV has the ability to initiate a wide variety of tumors in new-born mice. Early experiments using filtrates from leukaemic mice induced mainly parotid gland tumors, but as much higher titre viral preparations were obtained using tissue culture methods, a wide variety of tumors were observed (reviewed in Gross 1983). Whether the virus gained potency as it was passaged through tissue culture cells, or higher doses caused this increase in tumor types, has yet to be determined. Tumor induction by PyV varies between strains of mice, so the mouse genotype influences an animal's sensitivity to tumor induction. Interestingly, a gene that may be required for PyV tumorigenesis has recently been identified (Lukacher et al., 1995). Thymectomy performed within 24 hours of birth increases sensitivity to PyV tumor formation, so the host immune system also has a significant influence on tumor induction. Related to this, prior immunisation with killed polyoma transformed cells can protect against subsequent tumor formation (Dalianis et al. 1984). MT immunisation can perform at least part of this Transplantation Specific Tumor Antigen (TSTA) role (Ramqvist et al. 1988; Reinholds-son Ljunggren et al., 1992). In addition, the cells the virus can infect and replicate in have a profound influence on tumor formation. Mutants with an altered replication host range, therefore, can influence the number and type of tumors induced. As a wide range of factors influence tumor induction by PyV in the animal, interpretation of experiments is necessarily complicated. Tumors are also induced by injection of the virus into new-born hamsters and rats, but different types of tumor are produced compared to those formed in the mouse are formed. Interestingly, however, despite the wide variety of other tumors induced, leukaemias have never been observed.

MT is required for PyV-induced oncogenesis (Freund et al., 1992b), though assessing its role is complicated by the observation that MT mutants also exhibit a deficiency in viral replication. All PyV-induced tumors express MT, and the integration site seems to play little role in tumorigenesis. Both the PI3K and Shc binding sites in MT are involved in tumor formation, though neither is essential for all tumor types (Bronson et al., 1997; Freund et al., 1992a; Yi et al., 1997). Profound effects on tumor induction can be produced by changes to MT that seem to have no effect in cultured cells. For example, removal of the 14-3-3 binding site has little effect on transformation of cells in culture, but prevents the formation of salivary gland tumors (Cullere et al., 1998). The molecular basis for this difference remains to be determined.

All three early viral genes seem to be involved in tumor induction to some degree, although it not clear whether LT effects reflect its replicative role, its requirement for DNA integration, or if a direct function in tumorigenesis exists. Dawe et al (1987) tested four different strains of PyV for tumor induction and showed quite different potencies, despite all of them transforming equally well in culture. This difference is probably caused by alterations in the non-coding regions (Freund et al. 1987), and in the virion-coding regions, particularly VP-1 (Freund et al., 1991), but does not seem to be a consequence of alterations in the MT sequence (Freund et al. 1988). The ability to induce a high number of tumors also correlates with the ability to establish disseminated productive infection, with the kidney as a major site of amplification (Dubensky et al., 1991). The ability to disrupt specific pathways stimulated by MT, LT and ST, though, makes PyV a good model for studying how these complex interactions function within the organism as a whole.

MT ALONE

As other aspects of the virus are found to influence tumorigenesis through indirect mechanisms, other methods were sought to provide T-antigen expression in animals in the absence of other viral effects (reviewed in Kiefer et al., 1994b). The first approach used was to inject naked DNA into animals, and this indicated that a combination of MT and either ST or LT was required to generate tumors in rats, whereas MT alone was tumorigenic in new born hamsters (Asselin et al. 1984). Retroviral constructs were then used to express MT in young chickens (Kornbluth et al. 1986), resulting in the rapid induction of endothelial tumors that rapidly developed into cavernous haemangiomas. The finding that primary cells required MT and a complementing immortalising gene to become transformed in culture seems to have no corollary in animals, as MT expressed from a strong promoter can initiate tumors in a single step.

Transgenic mice expressing PyV T-antigens have also been studied extensively. Animals containing MT expressed from its own promoter develop multi-focal haemangiomas within 4-10 weeks of birth, probably caused by transformation of vascular endothelial cells (Bautch et al. 1987). Interestingly, though, only the tumor cells and the testis show MT expression. It is not clear why the polyoma promoter should exhibit such restricted expression, or why the testicular tissues are resistant to the transforming effects of MT. Expression of the entire early region of PyV induced a different set of alterations, including bone tumors, lymphangiomas, and fibrosarcomas (Wang and Bautch, 1991). As the viral early promoter showed restricted expression, other promoters were then used to control MT production. The first of these experiments used the thymidine kinase promoter in a retrovirus construct (Williams et al. 1988). Infection of new-born mice resulted in the rapid development of haemangiomas, whereas infection of embryos was lethal. This virus was then used to produce ES stem cell lines expressing MT. Surprisingly, MT has little effect on the growth of ES cells in culture, nor on their ability to take part in early development when injected into blastocysts to form chimeric mice. However, at mid-gestation, blood vessel formation is disrupted and development arrests. Once again, endothelial cell transformation is the probable cause, which occurs as a one step process with no requirement for a co-operating oncogene. Inoculation of $pp60^{c\text{-}src}$ null or $pp62^{c\text{-}yes}$ null new born mice with a MT expressing retrovirus also indicates that endothelial cell transformation and formation of haemangiomas is more dependent on the activity of $pp62^{c\text{-}yes}$ than $pp60^{c\text{-}src}$ (Kiefer et al., 1994a; Thomas et al., 1993).

All of the above experiments suggest that endothelial cells are particularly sensitive to MT-induced transformation, and that death of the animal/embryo occurs before effects on other cell types can be observed. To overcome this problem, a number of studies have expressed MT under the control of tissue specific promoters. Transgenic mice containing MT whose expression is controlled by the IgE heavy chain promoter (Rassoulzadegan et al., 1990) develop tumors mainly in the females. Salivary and thyroid gland tumors are frequently observed, in addition to mammary tumors, adenocarcinomas and liver haemangiomas. MT is expressed in the tumor tissue and the brain, which is not the usual profile of IgE heavy chain expression. Further work has shown that MT is also expressed in myeloid cells, but does not cause any abnormalities (Kiefer et al., 1994b). Animals with MT expression driven by the insulin promoter exhibit very little pathology, nor does simultaneous LT expression show any co-operation (Bautch 1989). Once again, this illustrates that within the organism, different cell types respond in quite separate ways to MT expression, probably depending on the signalling pathways present, and the consequences of stimulating those that are expressed. In particular, testis, ovary, neuronal and bone marrow cells seem refractory to MT-induced transformation.

Insertion of MT into the mouse genome under the control of the murine mammary tumor virus (MMTV) hormone-responsive promoter produced mice strains that exhibit a rapid induction of mammary tumors at maturation when MT expression is switched on (Guy et al., 1992). In contrast to the observations with haemangioma formation, mammary tumor development seems to depend on $pp60^{c\text{-}src}$ expression, as *src* null mice show little tumor formation (Guy et al., 1994). The availability of defined MT mutants has been used to examine the signalling pathways required to induce these breast carcinomas. Disrupting either the PI3K or Shc binding sites in MT reduces the number of tumors formed, suggesting both of these pathways are involved (Webster et al., 1998). This system has proven itself as an ideal tool for examining the molecular details of breast carcinogenesis.

MT has developed as an important model in examining how tumors form *in vivo*, therefore. In an interesting divergence to cell culture results, co-operation between MT and LT or other oncogenes is not required. In the animal, MT seems to act as a single step oncogene.

Future

PyV, and MT in particular, has proved repeatedly to be an important tool in attempts to decipher the molecular events occurring during carcinogenesis. In particular, the transgenic mouse model containing MT expressed under hormonal control in breast cells will undoubtedly provide considerably more information about the events occurring during breast carcinoma formation. In addition, the ease with which MT can activate signal transduction pathways involving tyrosine phosphorylation in a permanent fashion makes it a useful system for studying the consequences of these events as well. However, MT itself may still have some more new, unexpected, lessons to teach us. High resolution 2D gel electrophoresis of the proteins associated with MT indicate that there are a number of polypeptides bound to MT that have yet to be identified. As all the previously identified MT bound proteins are involved in growth control in some manner, it would be surprising if these other proteins were not. We have learnt a lot from studying MT, and these lessons are not yet over!

Acknowledgements

We would like to thank all our colleagues who have helped with comments on the manuscript, particularly, at the ICSM, Dr Nina Krauzewicz and Dr Nick Dibb, and in Vienna, Dr Egon Ogris. The Cancer Research Campaign, UK, and the European Community fund work in the authors' laboratory.

References

Aitken, A., 1995. 14-3-3 proteins on the MAP. *Trends in Biochem. Sci.* 20:95-97.

Alessi, D. R., and P. Cohen., 1998. Mechanism of activation and function of protein kinase B. *Curr. Opin. Genet. Dev.* 8, 55-62.

Arany, Z., W. R. Sellers, D. M. Livingston, and R. Eckner., 1994. E1A-associated p300 and CREB-associated CBP belong to a conserved family of coactivators [letter]. *Cell* 77, 799-800.

Aronheim, A., D. Engelberg, N. Li, N. Al-Alawi, J. Schlessinger, and M. Karin., 1994. Membrane targeting of the nucleotide exchange factor Sos is sufficient for activating the ras signaling pathway. *Cell* 78, 949-961.

Asselin, C., C. Gelinas, P. E. Branton, and M. Bastin. 1984. Polyoma middle T antigen requires cooperation from another gene to express the malignant phenotype in vivo. *Mol. Cell. Biol.* 4, 755-760.

Auger, K. R., C. L. Carpenter, S. E. Shoelson, H. Piwnica Worms, and L. C. Cantley., 1992. Polyoma virus middle T antigen-pp60c-src complex associates with purified phosphatidylinositol 3-kinase in vitro. *J. Biol. Chem.* 267, 5408-5415.

Azarnia, R., and W. R. Loewenstein. 1987. Polyomavirus middle T antigen downregulates junctional cell-to-cell communication. *Mol. Cell. Biol.* 7, 946-950.

Bachelot, C., L. Rameh, T. Parsons, and L. C. Cantley., 1996. Association of phosphatidylinositol 3-kinase, via the SH2 domains of p85, with focal adhesion kinase in polyoma middle t-transformed fibroblasts. *Biochim. Biophys. Acta* 1311, 45-52.

Backer, J. M., M. G. Myers, Jr., S. E. Shoelson, D. J. Chin, X. J. Sun, M. Miralpeix, P. Hu, B. Margolis, E. Y. Skolnik, J. Schlessinger, and et al., 1992. Phosphatidylinositol 3'-kinase is activated by association with IRS-1 during insulin stimulation. *EMBO. J.* 11, 3469-3479.

Bautch, V. L. 1989. Effects of polyoma virus oncogenes in transgenic mice. *Mol. Biol. Med.* 6, 309-317.

Bautch, V. L., S. Toda, J. A. Hassell, and D. Hanahan. 1987. Endothelial cell tumors develop in transgenic mice carrying polyoma virus middle T oncogene. *Cell* 51, 529-537.

Berger, H., and E. Wintersberger. 1986. Polyomavirus small T antigen enhances replication of viral genomes in 3T6 mouse fibroblasts. *J. Virol.* 60, 768-770.

Berra, E., M. T. Diaz Meco, I. Dominguez, M. M. Municio, L. Sanz, J. Lozano, R. S. Chapkin, and J. Moscat., 1993. Protein kinase C zeta isoform is critical for mitogenic signal transduction. *Cell* 74, 555-563.

Berridge, M. J., 1995. Calcium signalling and cell proliferation. *Bioessays* 17, 491-500.

Bikel, I., T. M. Roberts, M. T. Bladon, R. Green, E. Amann, and D. M. Livingston. 1983. Purification of biologically active simian virus 40 small tumor antigen. *Proc. Natl. Acad. Sci. USA.* 80, 906-910.

Blaikie, P., D. Immanuel, J. Wu, N. Li, V. Yajnik, and B. Margolis., 1994. A region in Shc distinct from the SH2 domain can bind tyrosine-phosphorylated growth factor receptors. *J. Biol. Chem.* 269, 32031-32034.

Blaikie, P. A., E. Fournier, S. M. Dilworth, D. Birnbaum, J. P. Borg, and B. Margolis., 1997. The role of the Shc phosphotyrosine interaction/phosphotyrosine binding domain and tyrosine phosphorylation sites in polyoma middle T antigen-mediated cell transformation. *J. Biol. Chem.* 272, 20671-20677.

Bolen, J. B., C. J. Thiele, M. A. Israel, W. Yonemoto, L. A. Lipsich, and J. S. Brugge. 1984. Enhancement of cellular src gene product associated tyrosyl kinase activity following polyoma virus infection and transformation. *Cell* 38, 767-777.

Bos, J. L., 1995. A target for phosphoinositide 3-kinase: Akt/PKB. *Trends Biochem. Sci.* 20, 441-442.

Brewster, C. E., H. R. Glover, and S. M. Dilworth., 1997. pp60c-src binding to polyomavirus middle T-antigen (MT) requires residues 185 to 210 of the MT sequence. *J. Virol.* 71, 5512-5520.

Bronson, R., C. Dawe, J. Carroll, and T. Benjamin., 1997. Tumor induction by a transformation-defective polyoma virus mutant blocked in signaling through Shc. *Proc. Natl. Acad. Sci. USA.* 94, 7954-7958.

Campbell, K. S., K. R. Auger, B. A. Hemmings, T. M. Roberts, and D. C. Pallas., 1995. Identification of regions in polyomavirus middle T and small t antigens important for association with protein phosphatase 2A. *J. Virol.* 69, 3721-3728.

Campbell, K. S., K. P. Mullane, I. A. Aksoy, H. Stubdal, J. Zalvide, J. M. Pipas, P. A. Silver, T. M. Roberts, B. S. Schaffhausen, and J. A. DeCaprio., 1997. DnaJ/hsp40 chaperone domain of SV40 large T antigen promotes efficient viral DNA replication. *Genes Dev* 11, 1098-110.

Campbell, K. S., E. Ogris, B. Burke, W. Su, K. R. Auger, B. J. Druker, B. S. Schaffhausen, T. M. Roberts, and D. C. Pallas., 1994. Polyoma middle tumor antigen interacts with SHC protein via the NPTY (Asn-Pro-Thr-Tyr) motif in middle tumor antigen. *Proc. Natl. Acad. Sci USA.* 91, 6344-6348.

Carmichael, G. G., B. S. Schaffhausen, D. I. Dorsky, D. B. Oliver, and T. L. Benjamin. 1982. Carboxy terminus of polyoma middle-sized tumor antigen is required for attachment to membranes, associated protein kinase activities, and cell transformation. *Proc. Natl. Acad. Sci. USA.* 79, 3579-3583.

Carpenter, C. L., K. R. Auger, M. Chanudhuri, M. Yoakim, B. Schaffhausen, S. Shoelson, and L. C. Cantley., 1993a. Phosphoinositide 3-kinase is activated by phosphopeptides that bind to the SH2 domains of the 85-kDa subunit. *J. Biol. Chem.* 268, 9478-9483.

Carpenter, C. L., K. R. Auger, B. C. Duckworth, W. M. Hou, B. Schaffhausen, and L. C. Cantley., 1993b. A tightly associated serine/threonine protein kinase regulates phosphoinositide 3-kinase activity. *Mol. Cell. Biol.* 13, 1657-1665.

Carpenter, C. L., B. C. Duckworth, K. R. Auger, B. Cohen, B. S. Schaffhausen, and L. C. Cantley., 1990. Purification and characterization of phosphoinositide 3-kinase from rat liver. *J. Biol. Chem.* 265, 19704-19711.

Cartwright, C. A., W. Eckhart, S. Simon, and P. L. Kaplan. 1987. Cell transformation by pp60c-src mutated in the carboxy-terminal regulatory domain. *Cell* 49, 83-91.

Cartwright, C. A., M. A. Hutchinson, and W. Eckhart. 1985. Structural and functional modification of pp60c-src associated with polyoma middle tumor antigen from infected or transformed cells. *Mol. Cell. Biol.* 5, 2647-2652.

Cartwright, C. A., P. L. Kaplan, J. A. Cooper, T. Hunter, and W. Eckhart. 1986. Altered sites of tyrosine phosphorylation in pp60c-src associated with polyomavirus middle tumor antigen. *Mol. Cell. Biol.* 6, 1562-1570.

Cayla, X., K. Ballmer Hofer, W. Merlevede, and J. Goris., 1993. Phosphatase 2A associated with polyomavirus small-T or middle-T antigen is an okadaic acid-sensitive tyrosyl phosphatase. *Eur. J. Biochem.* 214, 281-286.

Cheng, S. H., R. Harvey, P. C. Espino, K. Semba, T. Yamamoto, K. Toyoshima, and A. E. Smith. 1988a. Peptide antibodies to the human c-fyn gene product demonstrate pp59c-fyn is capable of complex formation with the middle-T antigen of polyomavirus. *EMBO. J.* 7, 3845-3855.

Cheng, S. H., H. Piwnica Worms, R. W. Harvey, T. M. Roberts, and A. E. Smith. 1988b. The carboxy terminus of pp60c-src is a regulatory domain and is involved in complex formation with the middle-T antigen of polyomavirus. *Mol. Cell. Biol.* 8, 1736-1747.

Cherington, V., B. Morgan, B. M. Spiegelman, and T. M. Roberts. 1986. Recombinant retroviruses that transduce individual polyoma tumor antigens: effects on growth and differentiation. *Proc. Natl. Acad. Sci. USA.* 83, 4307-11.

Cobb, B.S., D.M. Payne, A.B. Reynolds, and J.T. Parsons., 1991. Regulation of the oncogenic activity of the cellular src protein requires the correct spacing between the kinse domain and C-terminal phosphorylated tyrosine (Tyr-527). *Mol. Cell. Biol.* 11, 5832-5838.

Cohen, B., Y. X. Liu, B. Druker, T. M. Roberts, and B. S. Schaffhausen., 1990a. Characterization of pp85, a target of oncogenes and growth factor receptors. *Mol. Cell. Biol.* 10, 2909-2915.

Cohen, B., M. Yoakim, H. Piwnica Worms, T. M. Roberts, and B. S. Schaffhausen., 1990b. Tyrosine phosphorylation is a signal for the trafficking of pp85, an 85-kDa phosphorylated polypeptide associated with phosphatidylinositol kinase activity. *Proc. Natl. Acad. Sci. USA.* 87, 4458-62.

Courtneidge, S. A. 1985. Activation of the pp60c-src kinase by middle T antigen binding or by dephosphorylation. *EMBO. J.* 4, 1471-1477.

Courtneidge, S. A., and A. Heber. 1987. An 81 kd protein complexed with middle T antigen and pp60c-src: a possible phosphatidylinositol kinase. *Cell* 50, 1031-1037.

Courtneidge, S. A., and A. E. Smith. 1983. Polyoma virus transforming protein associates with the product of the c-src cellular gene. *Nature* 303, 435-439.

Courtneidge, S. A., and A. E. Smith. 1984. The complex of polyoma virus middle-T antigen and pp60c-src. *EMBO. J.* 3, 585-591.

Cullere, X., P. Rose, U. Thathamangalam, A. Chatterjee, K. P. Mullane, D. C. Pallas, T. L. Benjamin, T. M. Roberts, and B. S. Schaffhausen., 1998. Serine 257 phosphorylation regulates association of polyomavirus middle T antigen with 14-3-3 proteins. *J. Virol.* 72, 558-563.

Dahl, J., R. Freund, J. Blenis, and T. L. Benjamin., 1996. Studies of partially transforming polyomavirus mutants establish a role for phosphatidylinositol 3-kinase in activation of pp70 S6 kinase. *Mol. Cell. Biol.* 16, 2728-2735.

Dahl, J., A. Jurczak, L.A. Cheng, D.C. Baker, and T.L. Benjamin., 1998. Evidence of a role for phosphatidylinositol 3-kinase activation in the blocking of apoptosis by polyomavirus middle T antigen. *J. Virol.* 72, 3221-3226.

Dahl, J., U. Thathamangalam, R. Freund, and T. L. Benjamin., 1992. Functional asymmetry of the regions juxtaposed to the membrane-binding sequence of polyomavirus middle T antigen. *Mol. Cell. Biol.* 12, 5050-5058.

Dalianis, T., T. Ramqvist, and G. Klein. 1984. Studies on the polyoma-virus-induced tumor-specific transplantation antigen (TSTA)--does middle or large T-antigen play a role? *Int. J. Cancer* 34, 403-406.

Dawe, C. J., R. Freund, G. Mandel, K. Ballmer Hofer, D. A. Talmage, and T. L. Benjamin. 1987. Variations in polyoma virus genotype in relation to tumor induction in mice. Characterization of wild type strains with widely differing tumor profiles. *Am. J.Pathol.* 127, 243-261.

Delage, S., E. Chastre, S. Empereur, D. Wicek, D. Veissiere, J. Capeau, C. Gespach, and G. Cherqui., 1993. Increased protein kinase C alpha expression in human colonic Caco-2 cells after insertion of human Ha-ras or polyoma virus middle T oncogenes. *Cancer Res.* 53, 2762-2770.

Dhand, R., I. Hiles, G. Panayotou, S. Roche, M. J. Fry, I. Gout, N. F. Totty, O. Truong, P. Vicendo, K. Yonezawa, and et al., 1994. PI 3-kinase is a dual specificity enzyme: autoregulation by an intrinsic protein-serine kinase activity. *EMBO. J.* 13, 522-533.

Diaz Meco, M. T., I. Dominguez, L. Sanz, P. Dent, J. Lozano, M. M. Municio, E. Berra, R. T. Hay, T. W. Sturgill, and J. Moscat., 1994. zeta PKC induces phosphorylation and inactivation of I kappa B-alpha in vitro. *EMBO. J.* 13, 2842-2848.

Didichenko, S. A., B. Tilton, B. A. Hemmings, K. Ballmer Hofer, and M. Thelen., 1996. Constitutive activation of protein kinase B and phosphorylation of p47phox by a membrane-targeted phosphoinositide 3-kinase. *Curr. Biol.* 6, 1271-1278.

Dilworth, S. M. 1982. Protein kinase activities associated with distinct antigenic forms of polyoma virus middle T-antigen. *EMBO. J.* 1, 1319-1328.

Dilworth, S. M., 1995. Polyoma virus middle T antigen: meddler or mimic? *Trends Microbiol.* 3, 31-35.

Dilworth, S. M., C. E. Brewster, M. D. Jones, L. Lanfrancone, G. Pelicci, and P. G. Pelicci., 1994. Transformation by polyoma virus middle T-antigen involves the binding and tyrosine phosphorylation of Shc. *Nature* 367, 87-90.

Dilworth, S. M., and B. E. Griffin. 1982. Monoclonal antibodies against polyoma virus tumor antigens. *Proc. Natl. Acad. Sci. USA.* 79, 1059-1063.

Dilworth, S. M., H. A. Hansson, C. Darnfors, G. Bjursell, C. H. Streuli, and B. E. Griffin. 1986. Subcellular localisation of the middle and large T-antigens of polyoma virus. *EMBO. J.* 5, 491-499.

Dilworth, S. M., and V. P. Horner., 1993. Novel monoclonal antibodies that differentiate between the binding of pp60c-src or protein phosphatase 2A by polyomavirus middle T antigen. *J. Virol.* 67, 2235-2244.

Druker, B. J., L. E. Ling, B. Cohen, T. M. Roberts, and B. S. Schaffhausen., 1990. A completely transformation-defective point mutant of polyomavirus middle T antigen which retains full associated phosphatidylinositol kinase activity. *J. Virol.* 64, 4454-4461.

Druker, B. J., L. Sibert, and T. M. Roberts., 1992. Polyomavirus middle T-antigen NPTY mutants. *J. Virol.* 66, 5770-5776.

Dubensky, T. W., R. Freund, C. J. Dawe, and T. L. Benjamin., 1991. Polyomavirus replication in mice: influences of VP1 type and route of inoculation. *J. Virol.* 65, 342-349.

Dunant, N. M., A. S. Messerschmitt, and K. Ballmer Hofer., 1997. Functional interaction between the SH2 domain of Fyn and tyrosine 324 of hamster polyomavirus middle-T antigen. *J Virol* 71, 199-206.

Dunant, N. M., M. Senften, and K. Ballmer Hofer., 1996. Polyomavirus middle-T antigen associates with the kinase domain of Src-related tyrosine kinases. *J. Virol.* 70, 1323-1330.

Eckner, R., M. E. Ewen, D. Newsome, M. Gerdes, J. A. DeCaprio, J. B. Lawrence, and D. M. Livingston., 1994. Molecular cloning and functional analysis of the adenovirus E1A-associated 300-kD protein (p300) reveals a protein with properties of a transcriptional adaptor. *Genes. Dev.* 8, 869-884.

Eddy, B.E., S.E. Stewart, and W. Berkeley. 1958. Cytopathogenicity in tissue cultures by a tumor virus form mice. *Proc. Soc. Exp. Biol. and Med.* 98, 848-851.

Elliott, J., M.D. Jones, B.E. Griffin, and N. Krauzewicz., 1998. Regulation of cytoskeletal association by a basic amino acid motif in polyoma virus middle T antigen. *Oncogene* 17, 1797-1806.

Erpel, T., and S. A. Courtneidge., 1995. Src family protein tyrosine kinases and cellular signal transduction pathways. *Curr. Opin. Cell. Biol.* 7, 176-182.

Escobedo, J. A., S. Navankasattusas, W. M. Kavanaugh, D. Milfay, V. A. Fried, and L. T. Williams., 1991. cDNA cloning of a novel 85 kd protein that has SH2 domains and regulates binding of PI3-kinase to the PDGF beta-receptor. *Cell* 65, 75-82.

Fantl, W. J., A. J. Muslin, A. Kikuchi, J. A. Martin, A. M. MacNicol, R. W. Gross, and L. T. Williams., 1994. Activation of Raf-1 by 14-3-3 proteins. *Nature* 371, 612-614.

Freed, E., F. McCormick, and R. Ruggieri., 1994a. Proteins of the 14-3-3 family associate with Raf and contribute to its activation. *Cold Spring Harb. Symp. Quant. Biol.* 59, 187-93.

Freed, E., M. Symons, S. G. Macdonald, F. McCormick, and R. Ruggieri., 1994b. Binding of 14-3-3 proteins to the protein kinase Raf and effects on its activation. *Science* 265, 1713-6.

Freund, R., A. Calderone, C. J. Dawe, and T. L. Benjamin., 1991. Polyomavirus tumor induction in mice: effects of polymorphisms of VP1 and large T antigen. *J. Virol.* 65, 335-41.

Freund, R., C. J. Dawe, and T. L. Benjamin. 1988. The middle T proteins of high and low tumor strains of polyomavirus function equivalently in tumor induction. *Virology* 167, 657-659.

Freund, R., C. J. Dawe, J. P. Carroll, and T. L. Benjamin., 1992a. Changes in frequency, morphology, and behavior of tumors induced in mice by a polyoma virus mutant with a specifically altered oncogene. *Am. J. Pathol.* 141, 1409-1425.

Freund, R., G. Mandel, G. G. Carmichael, J. P. Barncastle, C. J. Dawe, and T. L. Benjamin. 1987. Polyomavirus tumor induction in mice: influences of viral coding and noncoding sequences on tumor profiles. *J. Virol.* 61, 2232-2239.

Freund, R., A. Sotnikov, R. T. Bronson, and T. L. Benjamin., 1992b. Polyoma virus middle T is essential for virus replication and persistence as well as for tumor induction in mice. *Virology* 191, 716-723.

Frost, J. A., A. S. Alberts, E. Sontag, K. Guan, M. C. Mumby, and J. R. Feramisco., 1994. Simian virus 40 small t antigen cooperates with mitogen-activated kinases to stimulate AP-1 activity. *Mol. Cell. Biol.* 14, 6244-6252.

Fu, H., K. Xia, D. C. Pallas, C. Cui, K. Conroy, R. P. Narsimhan, H. Mamon, R. J. Collier, and T. M. Roberts., 1994. Interaction of the protein kinase Raf-1 with 14-3-3 proteins [see comments]. *Science* 266, 126-129.

Garcea, R. L., K. Ballmer Hofer, and T. L. Benjamin. 1985. Virion assembly defect of polyomavirus hr-t mutants: underphosphorylation of major capsid protein VP1 before viral DNA encapsidation. *J. Virol.* 54, 311-316.

Garcea, R. L., and T. L. Benjamin. 1983. Host range transforming gene of polyoma virus plays a role in virus assembly. *Proc. Natl. Acad. Sci. USA.* 80, 3613-3617.

Garcea, R. L., D. A. Talmage, A. Harmatz, R. Freund, and T. L. Benjamin. 1989. Separation of host range from transformation functions of the hr-t gene of polyomavirus. *Virology* 168, 312-319.

Giorgetti, S., R. Ballotti, A. Kowalski Chauvel, S. Tartare, and E. Van Obberghen., 1993. The insulin and insulin-like growth factor-I receptor substrate IRS-1 associates with and activates phosphatidylinositol 3-kinase in vitro. *J. Biol. Chem.* 268, 7358-7364.

Glenn, G. M., and W. Eckhart., 1993. Mutation of a cysteine residue in polyomavirus middle T antigen abolishes interactions with protein phosphatase 2A, pp60c-src, and phosphatidylinositol-3 kinase, activation of c-fos expression, and cellular transformation. *J. Virol.* 67, 1945-1952.

Glenn, G. M., and W. Eckhart., 1995. Amino-terminal regions of polyomavirus middle T antigen are required for interactions with protein phosphatase 2A. *J. Virol.* 69, 3729-3736.

Goldschmidt Clermont, P. J., J. W. Kim, L. M. Machesky, S. G. Rhee, and T. D. Pollard., 1991. Regulation of phospholipase C-gamma 1 by profilin and tyrosine phosphorylation. *Science* 251, 1231-1233.

Gorga, F. R., C. E. Riney, and T. L. Benjamin., 1990. Inositol trisphosphate levels in cells expressing wild-type and mutant polyomavirus middle T antigens: evidence for activation of phospholipase C via activation of pp60c-src. *J. Virol.* 64, 105-112.

Gotoh, N., M. Toyoda, and M. Shibuya., 1997. Tyrosine phosphorylation sites at amino acids 239 and 240 of Shc are involved in epidermal growth factor-induced mitogenic signaling that is distinct from Ras/mitogen-activated protein kinase activation. *Mol. Cell. Biol.* 17, 1824-1831.

Graessmann, A., M. Graessmann, R. Tjian, and W. C. Topp. 1980. Simian virus 40 small-t protein is required for loss of actin cable networks in rat cells. *J. Virol.* 33, 1182-1191.

Griffin, B.E., and S.M. Dilworth. 1983. Polyomavirus: an overview of its unique properties. In *Advances in Cancer Research*, edited by G. Klein and S. Weinhouse. New York: Academic Press.

Griffin, B. E., S. M. Dilworth, Y. Ito, and U. Novak. 1980. Polyoma virus: some considerations on its transforming genes. *Proc R Soc Lond B Biol Sci* 210, 465-76.

Gross, L. 1953. A filterable agent, recovered from Ak leukemic extracts, causing salivary gland carcinomas in C3H mice. *Proc. Soc. Exp. Biol. and Med.* 83, 414-421.

Gross, L. 1983. The polyoma virus. In *Oncogenic Viruses*, edited by L. Gross. Oxford: Pergamon Press.

Grussenmeyer, T., A. Carbone Wiley, K. H. Scheidtmann, and G. Walter. 1987. Interactions between polyomavirus medium T antigen and three cellular proteins of 88, 61, and 37 kilodaltons. *J. Virol.* 61, 3902-3909.

Grussenmeyer, T., K. H. Scheidtmann, M. A. Hutchinson, W. Eckhart, and G. Walter. 1985. Complexes of polyoma virus medium T antigen and cellular proteins. *Proc. Natl. Acad. Sci. USA.* 82, 7952-7954.

Gustafson, T. A., W. He, A. Craparo, C. D. Schaub, and O. Neill TJ., 1995. Phosphotyrosine-dependent interaction of SHC and insulin receptor substrate 1 with the NPEY motif of the insulin receptor via a novel non-SH2 domain. *Mol. Cell. Biol.* 15, 2500-2508.

Guy, C. T., R. D. Cardiff, and W. J. Muller., 1992. Induction of mammary tumors by expression of polyomavirus middle T oncogene: a transgenic mouse model for metastatic disease. *Mol. Cell. Biol.* 12, 954-961.

Guy, C. T., S. K. Muthuswamy, R. D. Cardiff, P. Soriano, and W. J. Muller., 1994. Activation of the c-Src tyrosine kinase is required for the induction of mammary tumors in transgenic mice. *Genes Dev.* 8, 23-32.

Hansra, G., F. Bornancin, R. Whelan, B.A. Hemmings, and P.J. Parker., 1996. 12-O-Tetradecanoylphorbol-13-acetate-induced dephosphorylation of protein kinase Cα correlates with the presence of a membrane - associated protein phosphatase 2A heterotrimer. *J. Biol. Chem.* 271, 32785-32788.

Harvey, R., B. A. Oostra, G. J. Belsham, P. Gillett, and A. E. Smith. 1984. An antibody to a synthetic peptide recognizes polyomavirus middle-T antigen and reveals multiple in vitro tyrosine phosphorylation sites. *Mol. Cell. Biol.* 4, 1334-1342.

Hatakeyama, M., T. Kono, N. Kobayashi, A. Kawahara, S.D. Levin, R.M. Perlmutter, and T. Taniguchi., 1991. Interaction of the IL-2 receptor with the src-fmaily kinase p56lck: identification of novel intermolecular association. *Science* 252, 1523-1528.

Hawkins, P.I., A. Eguinoa, D. Stokoe, F.I. Cooke, R. Walters, S. Wennstrom, T. Evans, and M. Symons., 1995. PDGF stimulates an increase in GTP-rac via the activation of phosphoinositide 3-kinase. *Curr. Biol.* 5, 393-403.

Heiser, W. C., and W. Eckhart. 1985. Hormonal regulation of a polyoma virus middle-size T-antigen gene linked to growth hormone control sequences. *J. Gen. Virol.* 66, 2147-2160.

Hemmings, B. A., 1997. Akt signaling: linking membrane events to life and death decisions [comment]. *Science* 275, 628-630.

Heriche, J-K., F. Lebrin, T. Rabilloud, D. Leroy, E.M. Chambaz, and Y. Goldberg., 1997. Regulation of protein phosphatase 2A by direct interaction with casein kinase 2alpha. *Science* 276, 952-955.

Hiles, I. D., M. Otsu, S. Volinia, M. J. Fry, I. Gout, R. Dhand, G. Panayotou, F. Ruiz Larrea, A. Thompson, N. F. Totty, and et al., 1992. Phosphatidylinositol 3-kinase: structure and expression of the 110 kd catalytic subunit. *Cell* 70, 419-429.

Horak, I. D., T. Kawakami, F. Gregory, K. C. Robbins, and J. B. Bolen. 1989. Association of p60fyn with middle tumor antigen in murine polyomavirus-transformed rat cells. *J. Virol.* 63, 2343-2347.

Hu, P., A. Mondino, E. Y. Skolnik, and J. Schlessinger., 1993. Cloning of a novel, ubiquitously expressed human phosphatidylinositol 3-kinase and identification of its binding site on p85. *Mol. Cell. Biol.* 13, 7677-7688.

Hunter, T., M. A. Hutchinson, and W. Eckhart. 1984. Polyoma middle-sized T antigen can be phosphorylated on tyrosine at multiple sites in vitro. *EMBO. J.* 3, 73-79.

Hutchinson, M. A., T. Hunter, and W. Eckhart. 1978. Characterization of T antigens in polyoma-infected and transformed cells. *Cell* 15, 65-77.

Ito, Y., J. R. Brocklehurst, and R. Dulbecco. 1977a. Virus-specific proteins in the plasma membrane of cells lytically infected or transformed by polyoma virus. *Proc. Natl. Acad. Sci. USA.* 74, 4666-70.

Ito, Y., and N. Spurr. 1980. Polyoma virus T antigens expressed in transformed cells: significance of middle T antigen in transformation. *Cold Spring Harb. Symp. Quant. Biol.* 44, 149-157.

Ito, Y., N. Spurr, and R. Dulbecco. 1977b. Characterization of polyoma virus T antigen. *Proc. Natl. Acad. Sci. USA.* 74, 1259-1263.

Ito, Y., N. Spurr, and B. E. Griffin. 1980. Middle T antigen as primary inducer of full expression of the phenotype of transformation by polyoma virus. *J. Virol.* 35, 219-232.

Jelinek, M. A., and J. A. Hassell., 1992. Reversion of middle T antigen-transformed Rat-2 cells by Krev-1: implications for the role of p21c-ras in polyomavirus-mediated transformation. *Oncogene* 7, 1687-1698.

Kapeller, R., and L. C. Cantley., 1994. Phosphatidylinositol 3-kinase. *Bioessays* 16 (8):565-576.

Kaplan, D. R., M. Whitman, B. Schaffhausen, D. C. Pallas, M. White, L. Cantley, and T. M. Roberts. 1987. Common elements in growth factor stimulation and oncogenic transformation: 85 kd phosphoprotein and phosphatidylinositol kinase activity. *Cell* 50, 1021-1029.

Kaplan, D. R., M. Whitman, B. Schaffhausen, L. Raptis, R. L. Garcea, D. Pallas, T. M. Roberts, and L. Cantley. 1986. Phosphatidylinositol metabolism and polyoma-mediated transformation. *Proc. Natl. Acad. Sci. USA*. 83, 3624-3628.

Kavanaugh, W. M., and L. T. Williams., 1994. An alternative to SH2 domains for binding tyrosine-phosphorylated proteins. *Science* 266, 1862-1865.

Kelley, W. L., and C. Georgopoulos., 1997. The T/t common exon of simian virus 40, JC, and BK polyomavirus T antigens can functionally replace the J-domain of the Escherichia coli DnaJ molecular chaperone. *Proc. Natl. Acad. Sci. USA*. 94, 3679-3684.

Kennedy, A.P., A. Sekulic, B.J. Irvin, A.E. Nilson, S.M. Dilworth, and R.T. Abraham., 1998. Polyomavirus-derived middle-T antigen as a probe for T-cell antigen receptor-coupled signaling pathways. *J. Biol. Chem.* 273, 11505-11513.

Kiefer, F., I. Anhauser, P. Soriano, A. Aguzzi, S. A. Courtneidge, and E. F. Wagner., 1994a. Endothelial cell transformation by polyomavirus middle T antigen in mice lacking Src-related kinases. *Curr. Biol.* 4, 100-109.

Kiefer, F., S. A. Courtneidge, and E. F. Wagner., 1994b. Oncogenic properties of the middle T antigens of polyomaviruses. *Adv. Cancer Res.* 64, 125-157.

Klippel, A., C. Reinhard, W. M. Kavanaugh, G. Apell, M. A. Escobedo, and L. T. Williams., 1996. Membrane localization of phosphatidylinositol 3-kinase is sufficient to activate multiple signal-transducing kinase pathways. *Mol. Cell. Biol.* 16, 4117-4127.

Kodaki, T., R. Woscholski, B. Hallberg, P. Rodriguez Viciana, J. Downward, and P. J. Parker., 1994. The activation of phosphatidylinositol 3-kinase by Ras. *Curr. Biol.* 4, 798-806.

Kornbluth, S., F. R. Cross, M. Harbison, and H. Hanafusa. 1986. Transformation of chicken embryo fibroblasts and tumor induction by the middle T antigen of polyomavirus carried in an avian retroviral vector. *Mol. Cell. Biol.* 6, 1545-1551.

Kornbluth, S., M. Sudol, and H. Hanafusa. 1987. Association of the polyomavirus middle-T antigen with c-yes protein. *Nature* 325, 171-173.

Kotani, K., K. Yonezawa, K. Hara, H. Ueda, Y. Kitamura, H. Sakaue, A. Ando, A. Chavanieu, B. Calas, F. Grigorescu, and et al., 1994. Involvement of phosphoinositide 3-kinase in insulin- or IGF-1-induced membrane ruffling. *EMBO. J.* 13, 2313-2321.

Kremmer, E., K. Ohst, J. Kiefer, N. Brewis, and G. Walter., 1997. Separation of PP2A core enzyme and holoenzyme with monoclonal antibodies against the regulatory A subunit: abundant expression of both forms in cells. *Mol. Cell. Biol.* 17, 1692-1701.

Kypta, R. M., A. Hemming, and S. A. Courtneidge. 1988. Identification and characterization of p59fyn (a src-like protein tyrosine kinase) in normal and polyoma virus transformed cells. *EMBO. J.* 7, 3837-3844.

Land, H., L. F. Parada, and R. A. Weinberg. 1983. Tumorigenic conversion of primary embryo fibroblasts requires at least two cooperating oncogenes. *Nature* 304, 596-602.

Lill, N. L., M. J. Tevethia, R. Eckner, D. M. Livingston, and N. Modjtahedi., 1997. p300 family members associate with the carboxyl terminus of simian virus 40 large tumor antigen. *J. Virol.* 71, 129-137.

Ling, L. E., B. J. Druker, L. C. Cantley, and T. M. Roberts., 1992. Transformation-defective mutants of polyomavirus middle T antigen associate with phosphatidylinositol 3-kinase (PI 3-kinase) but are unable to maintain wild-type levels of PI 3-kinase products in intact cells. *J. Virol.* 66, 1702-1708.

Lips, D. L., P. W. Majerus, F. R. Gorga, A. T. Young, and T. L. Benjamin. 1989. Phosphatidylinositol 3-phosphate is present in normal and transformed fibroblasts and is resistant to hydrolysis by bovine brain phospholipase C II. *J. Biol. Chem.* 264, 8759-8763.

Lotti, L. V., L. Lanfrancone, E. Migliaccio, C. Zompetta, G. Pelicci, A. E. Salcini, B. Falini, P. G. Pelicci, and M. R. Torrisi., 1996. Shc proteins are localized on endoplasmic reticulum membranes and are redistributed after tyrosine kinase receptor activation. *Mol. Cell. Biol.* 16, 1946-1954.

Lukacher, A. E., Y. Ma, J. P. Carroll, S. R. Abromson Leeman, J. C. Laning, M. E. Dorf, and T. L. Benjamin., 1995. Susceptibility to tumors induced by polyoma virus is conferred by an endogenous mouse mammary tumor virus superantigen. *J. Exp. Med.* 181, 1683-1692.

Magnusson, G., M. G. Nilsson, S. M. Dilworth, and N. Smolar. 1981. Characterization of polyoma mutants with altered middle and large T-antigens. *J. Virol.* 39, 673-683.

Marcellus, R., J. F. Whitfield, and L. Raptis., 1991. Polyoma virus middle tumor antigen stimulates membrane-associated protein kinase C at lower levels than required for phosphatidylinositol kinase activation and neoplastic transformation. *Oncogene* 6, 1037-1040.

Markland, W., S. H. Cheng, B. A. Oostra, and A. E. Smith. 1986a. In vitro mutagenesis of the putative membrane-binding domain of polyomavirus middle-T antigen. *J. Virol.* 59, 82-89.

Markland, W., B. A. Oostra, R. Harvey, A. F. Markham, W. H. Colledge, and A. E. Smith. 1986b. Site-directed mutagenesis of polyomavirus middle-T antigen sequences encoding tyrosine 315 and tyrosine 250. *J. Virol.* 59, 384-391.

Markland, W., and A. E. Smith. 1987. Mutants of polyomavirus middle-T antigen. *Biochim. Biophys. Acta* 907, 299-321.

Marte, B. M., and J. Downward., 1997. PKB/Akt: connecting phosphoinositide 3-kinase to cell survival and beyond. *Trends Biochem. Sci.* 22, 355-358.

Martens, I., S. A. Nilsson, S. Linder, and G. Magnusson. 1989. Mutational analysis of polyomavirus small-T-antigen functions in productive infection and in transformation. *J. Virol.* 63, 2126-2133.

Mayer, B. J., 1997. Signal transduction: clamping down on Src activity. *Curr. Biol.* 7, R295-298.

McCormick, F., 1993. Signal transduction. How receptors turn Ras on [news; comment]. *Nature* 363, 15-16.

McGlade, J., A. Cheng, G. Pelicci, P. G. Pelicci, and T. Pawson., 1992. Shc proteins are phosphorylated and regulated by the v-Src and v-Fps protein-tyrosine kinases. *Proc. Natl. Acad. Sci. USA.* 89, 8869-8873.

Meili, R., P. Cron, B. A. Hemmings, and K. Ballmer Hofer., 1998. Protein kinase B/Akt is activated by polyomavirus middle-T antigen via a phosphatidylinositol 3-kinase-dependent mechanism. *Oncogene* 16, 903-907.

Metcalf, D., T. M. Roberts, V. Cherington, and A. R. Dunn. 1987. The in vitro behavior of hemopoietic cells transformed by polyoma middle T antigen parallels that of primary human myeloid leukemic cells. *EMBO. J.* 6, 3703-3709.

Migliaccio, E., S. Mele, A. E. Salcini, G. Pelicci, K. M. Lai, G. Superti Furga, T. Pawson, P. P. Di Fiore, L. Lanfrancone, and P. G. Pelicci., 1997. Opposite effects of the p52shc/p46shc and p66shc splicing isoforms on the EGF receptor-MAP kinase-fos signalling pathway. *EMBO. J.* 16, 706-716.

Morgan, S. J., A. D. Smith, and P. J. Parker., 1990. Purification and characterization of bovine brain type I phosphatidylinositol kinase. *Eur. J. Biochem.* 191, 761-767.

Mumby, M., 1995. Regulation by tumor antigens defines a role for PP2A in signal transduction. *Seminars in Cancer Biology* 6, 229-237.

Mungre, S., K. Enderle, B. Turk, A. Porras, Y. Q. Wu, M. C. Mumby, and K. Rundell., 1994. Mutations which affect the inhibition of protein phosphatase 2A by simian virus 40 small-t antigen in vitro decrease viral transformation. *J. Virol.* 68, 1675-1681.

Murakami, Y., T. Eki, M. Yamada, C. Prives, and J. Hurwitz. 1986. Species-specific in vitro synthesis of DNA containing the polyoma virus origin of replication. *Proc. Natl. Acad. Sci. USA.* 83, 6347-6351.

Muser, J., S. Kaech, C. Moroni, and K. Ballmer Hofer. 1989. Stimulation of pp60c-src kinase activity in FDC-P1 cells by polyoma middle-T antigen and hematopoietic growth factors. *Oncogene* 4, 1433-1439.

Muslin, A. J., J. W. Tanner, P. M. Allen, and A. S. Shaw., 1996. Interaction of 14-3-3 with signaling proteins is mediated by the recognition of phosphoserine. *Cell* 84, 889-897.

Myers, M. G., Jr., J. M. Backer, X. J. Sun, S. Shoelson, P. Hu, J. Schlessinger, M. Yoakim, B. Schaffhausen, and M. F. White., 1992. IRS-1 activates phosphatidylinositol 3'-kinase by associating with src homology 2 domains of p85. *Proc. Natl. Acad. Sci. USA.* 89, 10350-10354.

Nakanishi, H., K. A. Brewer, and J. H. Exton., 1993. Activation of the zeta isozyme of protein kinase C by phosphatidylinositol 3,4,5-trisphosphate. *J. Biol. Chem.* 268, 13-16.

Nishibe, S., M. I. Wahl, S. M. Hernandez Sotomayor, N. K. Tonks, S. G. Rhee, and G. Carpenter., 1990. Increase of the catalytic activity of phospholipase C-gamma 1 by tyrosine phosphorylation. *Science* 250, 1253-1256.

Nobes, C. D., P. Hawkins, L. Stephens, and A. Hall., 1995. Activation of the small GTP-binding proteins rho and rac by growth factor receptors. *J. Cell Sci.* 108, 225-233.

Noda, T., M. Satake, T. Robins, and Y. Ito. 1986. Isolation and characterization of NIH3T3 cells expressing polyomavirus small T antigen. *J. Virol.* 60, 105-113.

Noda, T., M. Satake, Y. Yamaguchi, and Y. Ito. 1987. Cooperation of middle and small T antigens of polyomavirus in transformation of established fibroblast and epithelial-like cell lines. *J. Virol.* 61, 2253-2263.

Novak, U., and B. E. Griffin. 1981. Requirement for the C-terminal region of middle T-antigen in cellular transformation by polyoma virus. *Nucleic Acids Res.* 9, 2055-2073.

Ogris, E., I. Mudrak, and E. Wintersberger., 1992. Polyomavirus large and small T antigens cooperate in induction of the S phase in serum-starved 3T3 mouse fibroblasts. *J. Virol.* 66, 53-61.

Olson, M.F., H.F. Paterson, and C.J. Marshall., 1998. Signals from Ras and Rho GTPases interact to regulate expression of p21Waf1/Cip1. *Nature* 394, 295-299.

Oostra, B. A., R. Harvey, R. K. Ely, A. F. Markham, and A. E. Smith. 1983. Transforming activity of polyoma virus middle-T antigen probed by site-directed mutagenesis. *Nature* 304, 456-459.

Otsu, M., I. Hiles, I. Gout, M. J. Fry, F. Ruiz Larrea, G. Panayotou, A. Thompson, R. Dhand, J. Hsuan, N. Totty, and et al., 1991. Characterization of two 85 kd proteins that associate with receptor tyrosine kinases, middle-T/pp60c-src complexes, and PI3-kinase. *Cell* 65, 91-104.

Pallas, D. C., V. Cherington, W. Morgan, J. DeAnda, D. Kaplan, B. Schaffhausen, and T. M. Roberts. 1988. Cellular proteins that associate with the middle and small T antigens of polyomavirus. *J. Virol.* 62, 3934-3940.

Pallas, D. C., H. Fu, L. C. Haehnel, W. Weller, R. J. Collier, and T. M. Roberts., 1994. Association of polyomavirus middle tumor antigen with 14-3-3 proteins. *Science* 265, 535-537.

Pallas, D. C., W. Morgan, and T. M. Roberts. 1989. The cellular proteins which can associate specifically with polyomavirus middle T antigen in human 293 cells include the major human 70-kilodalton heat shock proteins. *J. Virol.* 63, 4533-4539.

Pallas, D. C., L. K. Shahrik, B. L. Martin, S. Jaspers, T. B. Miller, D. L. Brautigan, and T. M. Roberts., 1990. Polyoma small and middle T antigens and SV40 small t antigen form stable complexes with protein phosphatase 2A. *Cell* 60, 167-176.

Pallas, D. C., W. Weller, S. Jaspers, T. B. Miller, W. S. Lane, and T. M. Roberts., 1992. The third subunit of protein phosphatase 2A (PP2A), a 55-kilodalton protein which is apparently substituted for by T antigens in complexes with the 36- and 63-kilodalton PP2A subunits, bears little resemblance to T antigens. *J. Virol.* 66, 886-893.

Pawson, T., 1995. Protein modules and signalling networks. *Nature* 373, 573-580.

Pelicci, G., L. Lanfrancone, F. Grignani, J. McGlade, F. Cavallo, G. Forni, I. Nicoletti, F. Grignani, T. Pawson, and P. G. Pelicci., 1992. A novel transforming protein (SHC) with an SH2 domain is implicated in mitogenic signal transduction. *Cell* 70, 93-104.

Pipas, J.M., 1992. Common and unique features of T antigens encoded by the polyomavirus group. *J. Virol.* 66, 3979-3985.

Pitcher, J.A., E.S. Payne, C. Csortos, A.A. DePaoli-Roach, and R.J. Lefkowitz., 1995. The G-protein-coupled receptor phosphatase: a protein phosphatase type 2A with a distinct subcellular distribution and substrate specificity. *Proc. Natl. Acad. Sci. USA.* 92, 8343-8347.

Platko, J. D., M. E. Forbes, S. Varvayanis, M. N. Williams, S. C. Brooks, 3rd, V. Cherington, and A. Yen., 1998. Polyoma middle T antigen in HL-60 cells accelerates hematopoietic myeloid and monocytic cell differentiation. *Exp. Cell Res.* 238, 42-50.

Porras, A., J. Bennett, A. Howe, K. Tokos, N. Bouck, B. Henglein, S. Sathyamangalam, B. Thimmapaya, and K. Rundell., 1996. A novel simian virus 40 early-region domain mediates transactivation of the cyclin A promoter by small-t antigen and is required for transformation in small-t antigen-dependent assays. *J. Virol.* 70, 6902-6908.

Rameh, L.E., C-S. Chen, and L.C. Cantley., 1995. Phosphatidylinositol (3,4,5)P3 interacts with SH2 domains and modulates PI 3-kinase association with tryosine-phosphorylated proteins. *Cell* 83, 821-830.

Ramqvist, T., D. O. Pallas, J. DeAnda, L. Ahrlund Richter, G. Reinholdsson, T. M. Roberts, B. S. Schaffhausen, and T. Dalianis. 1988. Immunization against the polyoma tumor-specific transplantation antigen (TSTA) with polyoma T-antigens. *Int.J. Cancer* 42, 123-128.

Raptis, L., H. Lamfrom, and T. L. Benjamin. 1985. Regulation of cellular phenotype and expression of polyomavirus middle T antigen in rat fibroblasts. *Mol. Cell. Biol.* 5, 2476-2486.

Raptis, L., R. Marcellus, M. J. Corbley, A. Krook, J. Whitfield, S. K. Anderson, and T. Haliotis., 1991. Cellular ras gene activity is required for full neoplastic transformation by polyomavirus. *J. Virol.* 65, 5203-5210.

Rassoulzadegan, M., S. A. Courtneidge, R. Loubiere, P. el Baze, and F. Cuzin., 1990. A variety of tumors induced by the middle T antigen of polyoma virus in a transgenic mouse family. *Oncogene* 5, 1507-1510.

Rassoulzadegan, M., A. Cowie, A. Carr, N. Glaichenhaus, R. Kamen, and F. Cuzin. 1982. The roles of individual polyoma virus early proteins in oncogenic transformation. *Nature* 300, 713-718.

Rassoulzadegan, M., Z. Naghashfar, A. Cowie, A. Carr, M. Grisoni, R. Kamen, and F. Cuzin. 1983. Expression of the large T protein of polyoma virus promotes the establishment in culture of "normal" rodent fibroblast cell lines. *Proc. Natl. Acad. Sci. USA* 80, 4354-4358.

Ravichandran, K.S., M-M. Zhou, J.C. Pratt, J.E. Harlan, S.F. Walk, S.W. Fesik, and S.J. Burakoff., 1997. Evidence for a requirement for both phospholipid and phosphotyrosine binding via the Shc phosphotyrosine-binding domain in vivo. *Mol. Cell. Biol.* 17, 5540-5549.

Reif, K., C. D. Nobes, G. Thomas, A. Hall, and D. A. Cantrell., 1996. Phosphatidylinositol 3-kinase signals activate a selective subset of Rac/Rho-dependent effector pathways. *Curr. Biol.* 6, 1445-1455.

Reinholdsson Ljunggren, G., T. Ramqvist, L. Ahrlund Richter, and T. Dalianis., 1992. Immunization against polyoma tumors with synthetic peptides derived from the sequences of middle- and large-T antigens. *Int. J. Cancer* 50, 142-146.

Roche, S., R. Dhand, M. D. Waterfield, and S. A. Courtneidge., 1994. The catalytic subunit of phosphatidylinositol 3-kinase is a substrate for the activated platelet-derived growth factor receptor, but not for middle-T antigen-pp60c-src complexes. *Biochem. J.* 301, 703-711.

Rodriguez Viciana, P., P. H. Warne, A. Khwaja, B. M. Marte, D. Pappin, P. Das, M. D. Waterfield, A. Ridley, and J. Downward., 1997. Role of phosphoinositide 3-OH kinase in cell transformation and control of the actin cytoskeleton by Ras. *Cell* 89, 457-467.

Rodriguez Viciana, P., P. H. Warne, B. Vanhaesebroeck, M. D. Waterfield, and J. Downward., 1996. Activation of phosphoinositide 3-kinase by interaction with Ras and by point mutation. *EMBO. J.* 15, 2442-2451.

Rodriguez-Viciana, P., P.H. Warne, R. Dhand, B. Vanhaesebroeck, I. Gout, M.J. Fry, M.D. Waterfield, and J. Downward., 1994. Phosphatidylinositol-3-OH kinase as a direct target of Ras. *Nature* 370, 527-532.

Rose, P. E., and B. S. Schaffhausen., 1995. Zinc-binding and protein-protein interactions mediated by the polyomavirus large T antigen zinc finger. *J. Virol.* 69, 2842-2849.

Rozakis Adcock, M., J. McGlade, G. Mbamalu, G. Pelicci, R. Daly, W. Li, A. Batzer, S. Thomas, J. Brugge, P. G. Pelicci, and et al., 1992. Association of the Shc and Grb2/Sem5 SH2-containing proteins is implicated in activation of the Ras pathway by tyrosine kinases. *Nature* 360, 689-692.

Ruediger, R., M. Hentz, J. Fait, M. Mumby, and G. Walter., 1994. Molecular model of the A subunit of protein phosphatase 2A: interaction with other subunits and tumor antigens. *J. Virol.* 68, 123-129.

Ruediger, R., D. Roeckel, J. Fait, A. Bergqvist, G. Magnusson, and G. Walter., 1992. Identification of binding sites on the regulatory A subunit of protein phosphatase 2A for the catalytic C subunit and for tumor antigens of simian virus 40 and polyomavirus. *Mol. Cell. Biol.* 12, 4872-4882.

Ruley, H. E. 1983. Adenovirus early region 1A enables viral and cellular transforming genes to transform primary cells in culture. *Nature* 304, 602-606.

Salcini, A. E., J. McGlade, G. Pelicci, I. Nicoletti, T. Pawson, and P. G. Pelicci., 1994. Formation of Shc-Grb2 complexes is necessary to induce neoplastic transformation by overexpression of Shc proteins. *Oncogene* 9, 2827-2836.

Schaffhausen, B., and T. L. Benjamin. 1981. Comparison of phosphorylation of two polyoma virus middle T antigens in vivo and in vitro. *J. Virol.* 40, 184-196.

Schaffhausen, B. S., H. Dorai, G. Arakere, and T. L. Benjamin. 1982. Polyoma virus middle T antigen: relationship to cell membranes and apparent lack of ATP-binding activity. *Mol. Cell. Biol.* 2, 1187-1198.

Schaffhausen, B. S., J. E. Silver, and T. L. Benjamin. 1978. Tumor antigen(s) in cell productively infected by wild-type polyoma virus and mutant NG-18. *Proc. Natl. Acad. Sci. USA.* 75, 79-83.

Scharenberg, A.M., and J-P. Kinet., 1998. PtdIns-3,4,5-P3: a regulatory nexus between tyrosine kinases and sustained calcium signals. *Cell* 94, 5-8.

Scheidtmann, K.H., M.C. Mumby, K. Rundell, and G. Walter., 1991. Dephosphorylation of simian virus 40 large-T antigen and p53 protein by protein phosphatase 2A: inhibition by small-t antigen. *Mol. Cell. Biol.* 11, 1996-2003.

Schlessinger, J., 1993. How receptor tyrosine kinases activate Ras. *Trends in Biochemistry* 18, 273-275.

Sefton, B. M., T. Hunter, K. Beemon, and W. Eckhart. 1980. Evidence that the phosphorylation of tyrosine is essential for cellular transformation by Rous sarcoma virus. *Cell* 20, 807-816.

Senften, M., S. Dilworth, and K. Ballmer Hofer., 1997. Multimerization of polyomavirus middle-T antigen. *J. Virol.* 71, 6990-6995.

Serunian, L. A., K. R. Auger, T. M. Roberts, and L. C. Cantley., 1990. Production of novel polyphosphoinositides in vivo is linked to cell transformation by polyomavirus middle T antigen. *J. Virol.* 64, 4718-4725.

Serunian, L. A., M. T. Haber, T. Fukui, J. W. Kim, S. G. Rhee, J. M. Lowenstein, and L. C. Cantley. 1989. Polyphosphoinositides produced by phosphatidylinositol 3-kinase are poor substrates for phospholipases C from rat liver and bovine brain. *J. Biol. Chem.* 264, 17809-17815.

Shoelson, S. E., M. Sivaraja, K. P. Williams, P. Hu, J. Schlessinger, and M. A. Weiss., 1993. Specific phosphopeptide binding regulates a conformational change in the PI 3-kinase SH2 domain associated with enzyme activation. *EMBO. J.* 12, 795-802.

Silver, J., B. Schaffhausen, and T. Benjamin. 1978. Tumor antigens induced by nontransforming mutants of polyoma virus. *Cell* 15, 485-496.

Skolnik, E. Y., B. Margolis, M. Mohammadi, E. Lowenstein, R. Fischer, A. Drepps, A. Ullrich, and J. Schlessinger., 1991. Cloning of PI3 kinase-associated p85 utilizing a novel method for expression/cloning of target proteins for receptor tyrosine kinases. *Cell* 65, 83-90.

Smits, P. H., H. L. Smits, R. P. Minnaar, B. A. Hemmings, R. E. Mayer Jaekel, R. Schuurman, J. van der Noordaa, and J. ter Schegget., 1992. The 55 kDa regulatory subunit of protein phosphatase 2A plays a role in the activation of the HPV16 long control region in human cells with a deletion in the short arm of chromosome 11. *EMBO. J.* 11, 4601-4606.

Sontag, E., S. Fedorov, C. Kamibayashi, D. Robbins, M. Cobb, and M. Mumby., 1993. The interaction of SV40 small tumor antigen with protein phosphatase 2A stimulates the map kinase pathway and induces cell proliferation. *Cell* 75, 887-897.

Sontag, E., J. M. Sontag, and A. Garcia., 1997. Protein phosphatase 2A is a critical regulator of protein kinase C zeta signaling targeted by SV40 small t to promote cell growth and NF-kappaB activation. *EMBO. J.* 16, 5662-5671.

Srinivasan, A., A. J. McClellan, J. Vartikar, I. Marks, P. Cantalupo, Y. Li, P. Whyte, K. Rundell, J. L. Brodsky, and J. M. Pipas., 1997. The amino-terminal transforming region of simian virus 40 large T and small t antigens functions as a J domain. *Mol. Cell. Biol.* 17, 4761-4773.

Stoker, M. 1968. Abortive transformation by polyoma virus. *Nature* 218 (138):234-238.

Strauss, M., S. Hering, L. Lubbe, and B. E. Griffin., 1990. Immortalization and transformation of human fibroblasts by regulated expression of polyoma virus T antigens. *Oncogene* 5, 1223-1229.

Su, W., W. Liu, B. S. Schaffhausen, and T. M. Roberts., 1995. Association of Polyomavirus middle tumor antigen with phospholipase C-gamma 1. *J. Biol. Chem.* 270, 12331-12334.

Talmage, D. A., R. Freund, A. T. Young, J. Dahl, C. J. Dawe, and T. L. Benjamin. 1989. Phosphorylation of middle T by pp60c-src: a switch for binding of phosphatidylinositol 3-kinase and optimal tumorigenesis. *Cell* 59 (1):55-65.

Taylor, S. J., and D. Shalloway., 1996. Src and the control of cell division. *Bioessays* 18, 9-11.

Templeton, D., and W. Eckhart. 1984. Characterization of viable mutants of polyomavirus cold sensitive for maintenance of cell transformation. *J. Virol.* 49 (3):799-805.

Templeton, D., S. Simon, and W. Eckhart. 1986. Truncated forms of the polyomavirus middle T antigen can substitute for the small T antigen in lytic infection. *J. Virol.* 57, 367-370.

Templeton, D., A. Voronova, and W. Eckhart. 1984. Construction and expression of a recombinant DNA gene encoding a polyomavirus middle-size tumor antigen with the carboxyl terminus of the vesicular stomatitis virus glycoprotein G. *Mol. Cell. Biol.* 4, 282-289.

Thomas, J. E., A. Aguzzi, P. Soriano, E. F. Wagner, and J. S. Brugge., 1993. Induction of tumor formation and cell transformation by polyoma middle T antigen in the absence of Src. *Oncogene* 8, 2521-2529.

Thomas, S.M., and J.S. Brugge., 1997. Cellular functions regulated by src family kinases. *Ann. Rev. Cell Dev. Biol.* 13, 513-609.

Toker, A., and L.C. Cantley., 1997. Signalling through the lipid products of phosphoinositide-3-OH kinase. *Nature* 387, 673-676.

Toker, A., M. Meyer, K. K. Reddy, J. R. Falck, R. Aneja, S. Aneja, A. Parra, D. J. Burns, L. M. Ballas, and L. C. Cantley., 1994. Activation of protein kinase C family members by the novel polyphosphoinositides PtdIns-3,4-P2 and PtdIns-3,4,5-P3. *J. Biol. Chem.* 269, 32358-32367.

Tooze, J. 1980. *DNA Tumor Viruses.* 2nd ed. Vol. 2. New York: Cold Spring Harbor Laboratory, Cold Spring Harbor, NY.

Treisman, R., U. Novak, J. Favaloro, and R. Kamen. 1981. Transformation of rat cells by an altered polyoma virus genome expressing only the middle-T protein. *Nature* 292, 595-600.

Turk, B., A. Porras, M. C. Mumby, and K. Rundell., 1993. Simian virus 40 small-t antigen binds two zinc ions. *J. Virol.* 67, 3671-3673.

Ulug, E. T., A. J. Cartwright, and S. A. Courtneidge., 1992. Characterization of the interaction of polyomavirus middle T antigen with type 2A protein phosphatase. *J. Virol.* 66 (3), 1458-1467.

Ulug, E. T., P. T. Hawkins, M. R. Hanley, and S. A. Courtneidge., 1990. Phosphatidylinositol metabolism in cells transformed by polyomavirus middle T antigen. *J. Virol.* 64, 3895-3904.

Urich, M., M. Y. el Shemerly, D. Besser, Y. Nagamine, and K. Ballmer Hofer., 1995. Activation and nuclear translocation of mitogen-activated protein kinases by polyomavirus middle-T or serum depend on phosphatidylinositol 3-kinase. *J. Biol. Chem.* 270, 29286-29292.

Urich, M., M. Senften, P. E. Shaw, and K. Ballmer Hofer., 1997. A role for the small GTPase Rac in polyomavirus middle-T antigen-mediated activation of the serum response element and in cell transformation. *Oncogene* 14, 1235-1241.

van der Geer, P., S. Wiley, G. D. Gish, and T. Pawson., 1996. The Shc adaptor protein is highly phosphorylated at conserved, twin tyrosine residues (Y239/240) that mediate protein-protein interactions. *Curr. Biol.* 6, 1435-1444.

van der Geer, P., S. Wiley, V. K. Lai, J. P. Olivier, G. D. Gish, R. Stephens, D. Kaplan, S. Shoelson, and T. Pawson., 1995. A conserved amino-terminal Shc domain binds to phosphotyrosine motifs in activated receptors and phosphopeptides. *Curr. Biol.* 5, 404-412.

Vanhaesebroeck, B., S. J. Leevers, G. Panayotou, and M. D. Waterfield., 1997. Phosphoinositide 3-kinases: a conserved family of signal transducers. *Trends Biochem. Sci.* 22, 267-272.

Walter, G., A. Carbone, and W. J. Welch. 1987. Medium tumor antigen of polyomavirus transformation-defective mutant NG59 is associated with 73-kilodalton heat shock protein. *J. Virol.* 61, 405-410.

Walter, G., A. Carbone Wiley, B. Joshi, and K. Rundell. 1988. Homologous cellular proteins associated with simian virus 40 small T antigen and polyomavirus medium T antigen. *J. Virol.* 62, 4760-4762.

Walter, G., F. Ferre, O. Espiritu, and A. Carbone Wiley. 1989. Molecular cloning and sequence of cDNA encoding polyoma medium tumor antigen-associated 61-kDa protein. *Proc. Natl. Acad. Sci. USA.* 86, 8669-8672.

Walter, G., R. Ruediger, C. Slaughter, and M. Mumby., 1990. Association of protein phosphatase 2A with polyoma virus medium tumor antigen. *Proc. Natl. Acad. Sci. USA.* 87, 2521-2525.

Wang, E. H., and C. Prives., 1991. DNA helicase and duplex DNA fragment unwinding activities of polyoma and simian virus 40 large T antigen display similarities and differences. *J. Biol. Chem.* 266, 12668-12675.

Wang, H. G., Y. Rikitake, M. C. Carter, P. Yaciuk, S. E. Abraham, B. Zerler, and E. Moran., 1993. Identification of specific adenovirus E1A N-terminal residues critical to the binding of cellular proteins and to the control of cell growth. *J. Virol.* 67, 476-488.

Wang, R., and V. L. Bautch., 1991. The polyomavirus early region gene in transgenic mice causes vascular and bone tumors. *J. Virol.* 65, 5174-5183.

Webster, M.A., J.N. Hutchinson, M.J. Rauh, S.K. Muthuswamy, M. Anton, C.G. Tortorice, R.D. Cardiff, F.L. Graham, J.A. Hassell, and W.J. Muller., 1998. Requirement for both Shc and phosphatidylinositol 3' kinase signaling pathways in polyomavirus middle T-mediated mammary tumorigenesis. *Mol. Cell. Biol.* 18, 2344-2359.

Wennstrom, S., P. Hawkins, F. Cooke, K. Hara, K. Yonezawa, M. Kasuga, T. Jackson, L. Claesson Welsh, and L. Stephens., 1994. Activation of phosphoinositide 3-kinase is required for PDGF-stimulated membrane ruffling. *Curr. Biol.* 4, 385-393.

Westphal, R.S., K.A. Anderson, A.R. Means, and B.E. Wadzinski., 1998. A signalling complex of Ca2+-calmodulin-dependent protein kinase IV and protein phosphatase 2A. *Science* 280, 1258-1261.

Wheat, W. H., W. J. Roesler, and D. J. Klemm., 1994. Simian virus 40 small tumor antigen inhibits dephosphorylation of protein kinase A-phosphorylated CREB and regulates CREB transcriptional stimulation. *Mol. Cell. Biol.* 14, 5881-5890.

Whitman, M., C. P. Downes, M. Keeler, T. Keller, and L. Cantley. 1988. Type I phosphatidylinositol kinase makes a novel inositol phospholipid, phosphatidylinositol-3-phosphate. *Nature* 332, 644-646.

Whitman, M., D. R. Kaplan, B. Schaffhausen, L. Cantley, and T. M. Roberts. 1985. Association of phosphatidylinositol kinase activity with polyoma middle-T competent for transformation. *Nature* 315, 239-242.

Williams, R. L., S. A. Courtneidge, and E. F. Wagner. 1988. Embryonic lethalities and endothelial tumors in chimeric mice expressing polyoma virus middle T oncogene. *Cell* 52, 121-131.

Xu, W., S.C. Harrison, and M.J. Eck., 1997. Three-dimensional structure of the tyrosine kinase c-src. *Nature* 385, 595-602.

Yaciuk, P., M. C. Carter, J. M. Pipas, and E. Moran., 1991. Simian virus 40 large-T antigen expresses a biological activity complementary to the p300-associated transforming function of the adenovirus E1A gene products. *Mol. Cell. Biol.* 11, 2116-2124.

Yaffe, M. B., K. Rittinger, S. Volinia, P. R. Caron, A. Aitken, H. Leffers, S. J. Gamblin, S. J. Smerdon, and L. C. Cantley., 1997. The structural basis for 14-3-3:phosphopeptide binding specificity. *Cell* 91, 961-971.

Yang, S-I., R.L. Lickteig, R. Estes, K. Rundell, G. Walter, and M.C. Mumby., 1991. Control of protein phosphatase 2A by simian virus 40 small-t antigen. *Mol. Cell. Biol.* 11, 1988-, 1995.

Yi, X., J. Peterson, and R. Freund., 1997. Transformation and tumorigenic properties of a mutant polyomavirus containing a middle T antigen defective in Shc binding. *J. Virol.* 71, 6279-6286.

Yoakim, M., W. Hou, Y. Liu, C. L. Carpenter, R. Kapeller, and B. S. Schaffhausen., 1992. Interactions of polyomavirus middle T with the SH2 domains of the pp85 subunit of phosphatidylinositol-3-kinase. *J. Virol.* 66, 5485-5491.

Yonemoto, W., A. J. Filson, A. E. Queral Lustig, J. Y. Wang, and J. S. Brugge. 1987. Detection of phosphotyrosine-containing proteins in polyomavirus middle tumor antigen-transformed cells after treatment with a phosphotyrosine phosphatase inhibitor. *Mol. Cell. Biol.* 7, 905-913.

Zhu, Z. Y., G. M. Veldman, A. Cowie, A. Carr, B. Schaffhausen, and R. Kamen. 1984. Construction and functional characterization of polyomavirus genomes that separately encode the three early proteins. *J. Virol.* 51, 170-180.

PATHOBIOLOGY OF HUMAN PAPILLOMAVIRUSES

Margaret A Stanley

Department of Pathology, Cambridge, UK

Introduction

Papillomaviruses (pvs) are small double stranded DNA viruses which cause a spectrum of epithelial proliferative lesions ranging from warts to cancer (Table 1). These viruses have two special properties which define their biology – exquisite species specificity and tissue tropism. The species specificity is such that the host range is absolutely restricted, thus rabbit pvs only infect rabbits, human pvs only infect humans and so on. Irrespective of the species the viral infectious cycle is expressed only during keratinocyte differentiation or in cells with the capacity for squamous maturation. Although some pvs infect fibroblasts, only a sub-set of viral genes are expressed in these cells and the infection is semi-permissive. There is no tissue culture system, at the present, which supports a complete infectious cycle and the viruses are not classified as serotypes but as genotypes. In humans, probably because there has been an intense search for viral genomes in many tissues, there is a remarkable plurality of papillomavirus types with 130 HPV genotypes identified (de Villiers, 1997). Within a species the individual viruses show a predilection for either cutaneous or mucosal surfaces and within the groups of skin or mucosal viruses they can be separated into high or low risk types depending upon their oncogenic potential. The DNA of more than 80 genotypes has now been sequenced (Delius et al., 1998) and overall there is a high degree of conservation of genomic organisation (Fig 1.) The HPV genome can be divided into 3 domains: a non-coding upstream regulatory region (URR) of approximately 1kb, an early region with open reading frames (ORFs) E6, E7, E1, E2, E4 and E5, and a late region encoding two genes, L1 (the major capsid protein) and L2 (the minor capsid protein). The functions of these ORFs is described in Table 2.

In this review I shall describe what is known of the infectious cycle of the high and low risk HPVs with an emphasis on those types which infect the genital tract and their interactions with the target cell for infection, the keratinocyte.

Infectious Cycle of the Papilloma Virus

The infectious cycle of the papillomaviruses is absolutely dependent upon the differentiation programme of the keratinocyte. Only keratinocytes or cells with the potential for squamous maturation (such as the reserve cell of the squamocolumnar junction in the cervix) are permissive for viral gene expression and only in terminally differentiated keratinocytes are viral capsid proteins synthesised and viral particles assembled. This

Table 1. Clinical lesions associated with different HPV types

Lesion	HPV type	
	Frequent	Infrequent
Skin Warts		
Plantar warts	1	2, 4, 63
Common warts	2,27	1, 4, 7, 26, 28, 29, 57, 60, 65
Flat warts	3, 10	2, 26, 27, 28, 29, 41, 49
Erythrodysplasia verruciformis specific skin lesions	5, 8, 17, 20	9, 12, 14, 15, 19, 21-25, 36, 38, 46, 47, 50
Malignant and premalignant skin lesions		
Bowens disease of the skin	2, 16, 34	
Skin cancers in patients with Erythro-dysplasia verruciformis	5, 8	14, 17, 20, 47
Skin cancers in renal transplant patients	1-6, 8, 10, 11, 14-16, 18-20, 23-25, 27, 29, 36, 38, 41, 47, 48 plus unknown types	
SCC of the finger	16	
Benign head and neck lesions		
Oral papillomas and leukoplakias	2, 6, 11, 16	7
Focal epithelial hyperplasia	13, 32	
Laryngeal papillomas (RRP patients)	6, 11	
Conjunctival papillomas	6, 11	
Nasal papillomas		6, 11, 57
Malignant Head and Neck lesions		
Laryngeal cancer		6, 11, 16, 18, 35
Oral cancer		3, 6, 11, 16, 18, 57
Tonsillar/pharyngeal cancer		16, 18, 33
Oesophageal cancer		6, 11, 16, 18
Nasal cancer		16, 57
Benign Anogenital lesions		
Condylomata acuminata	6, 11	30, 34, 33, 40, 41, 42, 44, 45, 54, 55, 61
Malignant and premalignant anogenital lesions		
CIN, VAIN, VIN, PAIN, PIN	6, 11, 16, 18, 31	30, 34, 35, 39, 40, 42-45, 51, 52, 56-59, 61, 62, 64, 66, 67, 69
Cervical cancer	16, 18, 31, 45	6, 10, 11, 26, 33, 35, 39, 51, 52, 55, 56, 58, 59, 66, 68 plus unclassified types
Non-cervical anogenital cancers	6, 16, 18	11, 31, 33
Buschke-Lowenstein tumours	6, 11	

Abbreviations: RRP = recurrent respiratory papillomatosis, SCC = squamous cell carcinoma, CIN = cervical intraepithelial neoplasia, VAIN = vaginal intraepithelial neoplasia, VIN = vulval intraepithelial neoplasia, PAIN = perianal intraepithelial neoplasia, PIN = penile intraepithelial neoplasia.

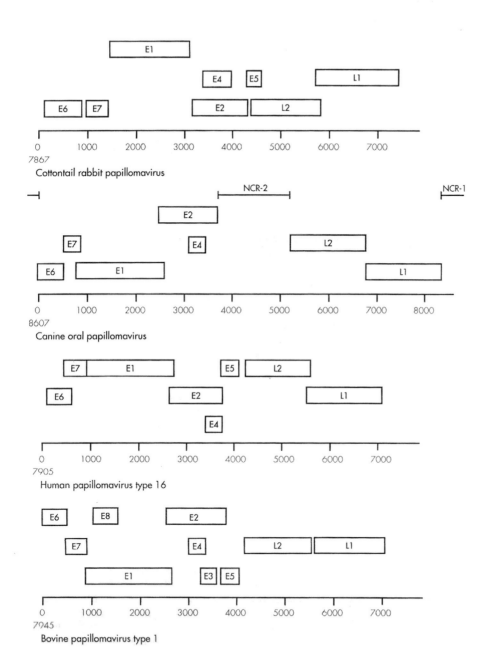

Figure 1. Genomic organisation of CRPV, COPV, HPV 16 and BPV 1. NCR = non coding region.

Table 2. Functions of HPV ORFs

ORF	Functions
E1	Essential for viral DNA replication, only viral enzyme (helicase, ATPase)
E2	Viral DNA replication - binds to E1 forming a complex which allows E1 to bind with high affinity to the ori
	Transactivation - transcriptional repressor of the early promoter
	Genome encapsidation
E6	Transactivation
	High risk HPV E6 binds to and degrades p53, cooperates with E7 to immortalise primary human cells, induces expression of telomerase
E7	Binds pRB, induces unscheduled DNA synthesis in differentiated keratinocytes
	High risk HPV E7 cooperates with E6 to immortalise primary keratinocytes
E5	Interacts with growth factor receptors and has weak transforming activity. Complexes with the 16Kda component of the vacuolar H+-ATPase complex inhibiting endosome acidification with retention non-degraded epidermal growth factor receptor and upregulation of receptor density
E4	Induces cytoskeletal changes
	Binds to keratins or keratin binding proteins
L1	Major capsid protein
L2	Minor capsid protein

absolute dependence upon the epithelial environment for infection, replication and assembly was first shown (Kreider and Bartlett, 1981) for the cotton tail rabbit papillomavirus (CRPV). In CRPV-induced papillomas viral DNA cannot be detected by DNA:DNA in situ hybridisation (ISH) in the basal layers of the papilloma but high copy numbers of viral genomes are present in the upper layers of the stratum spinosum and granulosum. Viral capsid antigen and viral particles are detectable only in the extreme superficial differentiated layers of the papilloma. This pattern of viral DNA expression is characteristic also of productive HPV infections of both skin and mucosa and has been shown in many studies using ISH of clinical biopsies. These are only cross sectional studies and do not give information on the temporal aspects of viral gene expression and our knowledge of this is still heavily dependent upon animal models of infection such as the rabbit, ox and dog and upon rodent xenograft models.

A. *Rodent xenograft models*

The original xenograft model was developed by Kreider and colleagues (Kreider et al., 1985). In this model, small fragments of human foreskin are incubated with virus for 1-

2 hours in vitro. The foreskin fragments are then implanted under the renal capsule of the nude mouse, where, after a variable period depending upon the virus type, condylomatous transformation of the graft epithelium occurs with the production of large amounts of virions. Using this system the Hershey strain of HPV 11 was isolated and its organotropism demonstrated (Kreider et al., 1987) and HPV-1 serially passaged (Kreider et al., 1990). Variations of this using SCID mice have resulted in isolation of new genital HPVs (Brown et al., 1998) and new isolates of HPV 16 (Bonnez et al., 1998).

HPV 11 gene expression during the infectious cycle was examined using the nude mouse model and RNA:RNA ISH with exon specific probes (Stoler et al., 1990). In the first 4 weeks after infection and implantation of foreskin fragments no viral activity could be detected. Viral DNA sequences could not be detected, which suggests that viral copy number was below 50 copies per cell, the sensitivity of the ISH technology used in that study. The first detectable RNA signals in the experimental condyloma were seen 4 weeks post implantation with expression detected when probes spanning the early region of the genome in general and E4/E5 in particular were used. In the 4-8 week period post-implantation, the grafts underwent condylomatous transformation with an increase in the proliferative compartment of the epithelium and koilocytosis and parakeratosis in the superficial layers of the condyloma. Viral DNA sequences became easily detectable in the upper spinous layers with intense signals in some cells of the stratum granulosum. Transcripts for E6/E7 were not detected in the basal layers of the condyloma but appeared in the parabasal layers at week 6 becoming progressively more abundant with time. Maximal E6/E7 signals were detected in the upper spinous and lower granulosum layers. Transcripts for the capsid proteins L1 and L2 did not appear until week 8 and were confined to the most superficial differentiated cells. Immunohistochemistry using anti-sera to the type common epitope in L1 revealed that L1 mRNA expressing cells were also antigen positive.

This pattern of gene expression is true also for the high risk genital viruses in productive infections (Durst et al., 1992; Higgins et al., 1992) with weak barely detectable transcription in the basal and parabasal layers of low grade squamous intra-epithelial lesions (LGSIL) but strong signals in the upper layers. The temporal regulation of HPV 16 gene expression has been examined using the W12 cell line (Stanley et al., 1989): an immortal cervical keratinocyte line derived from a LGSIL and containing around 50 copies of episomal HPV 16 per cell. In monolayer culture these cells undergo limited stratification, express basal keratins but no markers of keratinocyte differentiation such as filaggrin or keratin 10/13. The E6 and E7 genes of HPV 16 are transcribed and the proteins expressed at low level but no late transcripts or proteins are made. Transplantation of these cells to a skin pocket on the flank of the nude mouse results in the formation of a differentiated epithelium by W12 cells and dramatic changes in HPV 16 gene expression (Sterling et al., 1990). Ten days after grafting W12 cells have reformed a stratified epithelium morphologically identical to normal ectocervical epithelium but viral DNA sequences cannot be detected by ISH. At 4 weeks post grafting the epithelium has thickened and morphologically is comparable to a LGSIL. Large numbers (100's) of viral genomes can be detected in the upper spinous and lower granulosum

layers together with strong signals for E6/E7 transcripts and isolated cells in the granulosum are positive for L1 protein. At 6 weeks post grafting many cells are positive for
L1 protein and E4 protein is expressed throughout the stratum granulosum, viral particles can be detected in the degenerating nuclei of the stratum granulosum (Sterling et
al., 1990) and immunostaining confirms that these are HPV 16 (Sterling et al., 1993).
Early region transcripts are weakly expressed in the basal layers of grafts after 2 weeks
but maximum signal intensity for E6/E7 and E1/E2/E4 transcripts co-localise with
maximum signal for viral DNA sequences in the upper spinous and lower granulosum
layers. Histologically the 4 and 6 week grafts resemble LGSIL but differ in that they
exhibit extensive hyperkeratosis. Clinical, cervical LGSIL HPV 16 positive lesions
rarely contain detectable viral particles, they do not exhibit hyperkeratosis and it seems
probable that productively infected squames are exfoliated in the natural infection releasing infectious particles into cervical and vaginal secretions.

B. *Natural animal infections*

A detailed evaluation of the papillomavirus life cycle can be obtained from natural infections in animals where a chronological series of biopsies can be taken from animals
experimentally infected with known virus doses. The canine oral papillomavirus
(COPV) infection in the dog is a valuable model for this type of study. COPV infects
the oral mucosa of dogs inducing florid warts which regress within 4-8 weeks
(Chambers and Evans, 1959). In a recent study (Nicholls and Stanley, unpublished
data), beagles were infected with COPV by oral scarification and the sites of infection
marked by tattoo. Weekly biopsies were taken thereafter throughout wart progression
and regression and analysed for viral DNA by DNA:DNA ISH and viral gene expression by RNA:RNA ISH using digoxigenin-labelled exon specific probes. No viral DNA
was detected in pre-infection sections or in those taken at 1,2, and 3 weeks post infection. Viral DNA was first detected at 4 weeks in scattered foci at the lower tips of the
rete ridges and was present in tight clusters of cells suggesting a clonal origin. As infection progressed, in weeks 5 and 6, more DNA positive cells appeared within the basal
and suprabasal layers until nearly every cell within a full thickness epithelial column
was positive. The areas where viral DNA was abundant were also those areas in which
the epithelial thickness was increased and mitoses were frequent. As the papilloma progressed toward maturity (weeks 7 and 8) only certain keratinocytes in the upper spinous
layer permitted an amplification of viral DNA to high copy number in contrast to the
situation in the lower layers in which every cell was positive for about 50-100 copies of
viral DNA. As the papilloma began to regress (weeks 9-12) less DNA was detected in
the lower layers of the epithelium until no signal could be detected (week 12).

E7 mRNA expression paralleled that of viral DNA throughout the papilloma life cycle. E7 was expressed in numerous superficial cells at 8 weeks but was completely absent by 10 weeks. L1 and L2 transcripts were only detected in the keratinocytes of the
stratum granulosum and in the uppermost layer of the stratum spinosum. Transcripts
were not detectable until week 7, were abundant at week 8 and absent at weeks 10-12.
E4 expression was determined by immunohistochemistry using an anti-E4 polyclonal

antibody. A strong cytoplasmic signal was detected in the experimental papillomas from week 4 onwards and, interestingly, paralleled viral DNA expression with signal in both the basal and superficial cells. The detection of COPV genomes and expression of early genes in basal cells contrasts with some studies in other animal models such as the ox and in the rodent xenograft model (Stoler et al., 1990) and in many clinical studies. These discrepancies may reflect technical differences in the optimisation of the ISH or it may be that only some low risk pv types such as COPV permit replication in basal layers at levels detectable by ISH. It is also possible particularly in studies using clinical biopsies that the time at which the biopsy was taken is the point in the life cycle when basal layer replication has been reduced.

C. The target cell for infection

The dependence upon the keratinocyte lineage for viral gene expression extends to the target cell for infection. In experimental CRPV infections, viral gene transcription is detected first in the hair follicle (Schmitt et al., 1996), in cells which have the characteristics of stem cells (Miller et al., 1993). This is also true in COPV where viral DNA amplification and early gene transcription are first detected at the extreme tips of the rete ridges, thought to be the site of interfollicular keratinocyte stem cells (Morris et al., 1985). The stem cell as a target is supported by the evidence that the $\alpha_6\beta_4$ integrin is a receptor for the HPVs (Evander et al., 1997) since keratinocytes freshly isolated from foreskin and expressing $\alpha_6\beta_4$ at high level have stem cell characteristics in vitro (Li et al., 1998). If the target cell for infection is the stem cell then this does offer an explanation for some interesting aspects of papillomavirus biology. There is, for example, the phenomenon of the lag phase between infection and the first detection of viral DNA and early gene expression. The length of this lag in experimental models such as the rabbit (Kreider and Bartlett, 1985), the dog (Nicholls and Stanley, 1999), and rodent xenografts of HPV 11 (Stoler et al., 1990) and HPV 16 (Sterling et al., 1990) is consistently between 3-5 weeks. Anecdotal evidence in man suggests a similar time lag for genital warts (Oriel, 1971). One attractive explanation for this is that the virus infects a stem cell which is out of cycle in G_0. The 3-5 week delay before viral gene expression is detectable would then reflect the time for the stem cell to enter G_1, divide and for committed daughter cells to enter the transit amplifying population (which includes both basal and parabasal cells) permissive for viral gene expression.

Another phenomenon observed in the COPV experimental infection supports this. Thus if COPV is injected intradermally rather than applied by scarification the lag period is significantly extended by 2-3 weeks (Nicholls and Stanley 1999). This delay is particularly marked with low doses of infectious virus. Little epithelial wounding is associated with injection as compared to scarification and therefore little stimulus for epithelial wound healing during which keratinocyte stem cells transiently increase their replication rate. A dose effect might be expected, if it is assumed that at low doses only a few stem cells in a given area are infected. In the absence of trauma these cells are recruited into cycle less frequently with a resulting increase in the length of the lag phase.

D. *Viral Latency*

Dependence upon the stem cell milieu for infection and immediate early viral gene expression would also, partly, explain the phenomenon of latency. HPV is frequently present as a latent infection in the female genital tract (Toon et al., 1986) and the frequent lesion recurrence observed in respiratory papillomatosis is generally believed to reflect reactivation of latent infection rather than reinfection (Abramson et al., 1987) This is supported by the observation that histologically normal, but HPV positive, laryngeal tissues express low abundance transcripts coding for E1 and E2(Maran et al., 1995). Similarly in the rabbit low doses of CRPV lead to viral persistence and expression of truncated E1 and E2 transcripts but no lesion unless, and until, reactivation is induced by skin irritation (Amella et al., 1994). Furthermore CRPV can persist at the site of regressed papillomas in 60% of cases with occasional lesion recurrence (Selvakumar et al., 1997) and similar phenomena are seen in BPV infections (Campo et al., 1994). Relatively little is known about squamous mucosal epithelial stem cells but it is clear from studies on intestinal epithelium (Loeffler et al., 1993) that at any one time the majority of the stem cell fraction is quiescent and out of the cell cycle. They can be recruited back into the cycle after wounding or as part of the normal self renewal process of the epithelium. The frequency with which this happens is likely to be variable and if there is a keratinocyte stem cell hierarchy, as there is in the gut (Winton and Ponder, 1990), it will also depend upon the position of the stem cell in the hierarchy so that the most primitive stem cells may cycle only once in 6 months. Latency is a poorly understood aspect of papillomavirus biology but clearly of importance for therapeutic and prophylactic intervention strategies.

In Vitro Culture of HPV

Our understanding of the infectious cycle of the high risk HPVs and of the regulation of viral gene expression has been significantly enhanced by the use of organotypic culture systems which permit keratinocyte differentiation. The regulation of keratinocyte differentiation is extremely complex but depends very significantly on signals from the extracellular matrix of the sub-epithelial stroma or dermis (Leary et al., 1992). Culture systems which partially reproduce this connective tissue matrix have been developed. In essence, all these systems consist of a collagen matrix seeded with murine or human fibroblasts. Keratinocytes are inoculated onto the matrix in submerged culture and when confluent the collagen:keratinocyte sandwich is raised to the air/liquid interface where the keratinocytes stratify and differentiate (Stanley, 1994). Cell lines containing episomal HPV, such as the HPV 16 positive W12 line (Stanley et al., 1989)or the HPV 31b positive CIN 612 line (Bedell et al., 1991), when grown in such cultures stratify and differentiate, with viral DNA amplification and late gene expression in the upper layers of stratified cells (Stanley, 1994; Bedell et al., 1991). Treatment of such cultures with activators of protein kinase C such as the phorbol ester TPA results in an abrupt spinous to granular transition in the upper cell layers, induction of capsid protein synthesis and the production of virions (Meyers et al., 1992) Transcriptional analysis of HPV 31b in the CIN 612 line in organotypic culture shows significant differences compared to monolayer cultures (Hummel et al., 1992). Transcripton of HPV 31b late genes is regulated primarily from a differentiation specific promoter (p_{742}) located in the E7 ORF and controls the expression of the capsid proteins L1 and L2 as well as the E1^E4 fusion proteins. Comparison of monolayer organotypic and TPA-treated organotypic cultures of CIN 612 reveals a highly complex transcriptional pattern (Ozbun and Meyers, 1998). The major HPV 31b early promoter precisely maps to P_{99} but a transcriptional start site for both early and late transcripts mapped to P_{77}. Both these promoters were used constitutively throughout the HPV 31b life cycle but initiation from P_{99} was much stronger than P_{77}. Mapping of the major late promoter P_{742} revealed multiple start sites detectable with ease only in organotypic culture, particularly after TPA treatment. A constitutively active promoter P_{3320} responsible for the transcription of unspliced and spliced mRNAs for E5a, E5b, L2 and L1 ORFs was also identified.

The organotypic systems have been valuable in characterising the distribution of viral transcripts in differentiating epithelia but they are dependent upon rare cell lines containing episomal HPV and do not permit a genetic analysis of HPV functions during the normal viral life cycle. This barrier has been overcome, at least for the high risk HPVs, by the demonstration that recircularised HPV 31b genomes transfected together with a drug selection marker into primary foreskin keratinocytes results in cell lines which stably maintain the episome. Growth of these lines in organotypic culture resulted in the amplification of viral DNA, expression of late genes and production of viral particles (Frattini et al., 1996). Data obtained using this system clearly shows that the induction of late gene expression requires that the viral genomes be maintained as extrachromosomal elements and that the induction of terminal differentiation alone is insufficient. Using this approach some insight into the rigorous regulation required for the stable maintenance of HPV episomes has been obtained in experiments using mutants of the splice acceptor nt3295 for the polycistronic mRNAs E1^E4 and E5 (Klumpp et al., 1997). These mutations did not significantly alter the ability of HPV 31b genomes to function in transient replication assays or alter their immortalisation potential. Cell lines generated by these mutants expressed transcripts similar to those with wt genomes but contained multiple integrated copies of HPV 31b. Overall these findings suggest that there are stringent requirements for the stable maintenance of HPV genomes and these are defined by the major splice acceptor nt3295.

An important observation from the genetic analysis of HPV function has been the role of E2 in the life cycle of HPV 31b. The E2 protein exhibits sequence specific DNA binding and was first described as a transcriptional regulator either stimulating or repressing promoter activity depending upon the promoter context (Romanczuk and Howley, 1992). E2 is also directly involved in viral DNA replication forming a complex with E1 which dramatically increases the binding of E1 to the viral *ori* (Ustav and Stenlund, 1991), (Yang et al., 1991). This phenomenon is dependent upon the relative affinity of highly conserved E2 binding sites (E2BS) which flank the single E1 binding site in the URR (Seo et al., 1993; Ustav et al., 1993). The role of the conserved E2 binding sites in the HPV 31b life cycle was examined by Stubenrauch and colleagues

(Stubenrauch et al., 1998b) using viral genomes mutated in the individual E2BS. Interestingly no single E2BS was found to be necessary for replication but mutation of 3 of the 4 sites resulted in the integration of transfected genomes and loss of episomal maintenance. Overall the conclusion from these experiments was that the specific arrangement of E2BS within the URR was of more importance than the number of sites. The transcriptional properties of E2 were first described for BPV-1 (Spalholz et al., 1985) and all major early promoters of BPV-1 are activated by and highly dependent upon E2 (Spalholz et al., 1987). Transient transfection and biochemical studies have shown that the major early promoters of the genital HPVs are repressed by E2 (Bernard et al., 1989; Romanczuk et al., 1990; Dong et al., 1994). However genetic analysis of E2 function in the organotypic culture model using mutants in the N' of E2 which are replication competent but transactivation defective reveals that the mutants are permissive for a normal viral infectious cycle (Stubenrauch et al., 1998a). These data certainly bring into question the role of E2 transactivation function in the life cycle of the oncogenic HPVs and suggest that if E2 transactivation plays a role it is a relatively minor one augmenting late functions. One should, however, be cautious in totally excluding the transactivation role of E2 on the basis of these data. The organotypic culture systems are good models for the stages of the viral life cycle occurring in committed and differentiating cells in the stratum spinosum and granulosum but they do not model the immediate early events of the life cycle after infection. These events occur, it is widely suspected, in the self renewing or stem cell compartment of the epithelium (Schmitt et al., 1996). Organotypic cultures do not support self renewing or clonogenic keratinocytes (Anderson and Stanley, unpublished data) and therefore the immediate early events of the viral life cycle are not analysable with these systems at the present.

The success of the Frattini system seems to depend upon the ability of the high risk viruses to immortalise primary keratinocytes. However this precludes the use of this approach for the low risk genital HPVs although permissive growth of HPV6a in the immortalised keratinocyte line SCC-13 has been reported (Meyers personal communication). Further since the E6 and E7 genes of the high risk HPVs are essential for immortalisation this puts limitations on the genetic analysis of the functions of these genes using this approach. To circumvent these problems investigators have used retrovirus-mediated gene transfer into primary human keratinocytes combined with organotypic culture systems (Chow and Broker, 1997). Using this approach it has been shown that the HPV 18 and HPV 11 enhancer promoter located in the URR is repressed in the basal layers but upregulated in the differentiated layers of such cultures (Parker et al., 1997; Zhao et al., 1997) observations consistent with the abundant viral gene expression in these layers. The abundant expression of E6 and E7 in what are non cycling differentiated cells is of considerable interest. All the evidence indicates that the function of E6 and E7 of the pv's is to induce cellular DNA synthesis and the expression of cellular genes required for viral DNA replication. One such cellular gene is proliferating cell nuclear antigen (PCNA), an accessory protein for DNA polymerase δ. In raft cultures derived from HPV 11-induced condylomas and permissive for HPV viral replication PCNA is induced in differentiating layers in parallel with viral DNA replication (Demeter et al., 1994). This expression in vitro parallels observations in vivo in LGSIL spinous layer. Extensive host chromosomal DNA synthesis is induced in the spinous layer. Extensive host chromosomal DNA synthesis is induced in the differentiated cells of LGSIL and condylomata (Cheng et al., 1995) and it has been shown using retrovirus-mediated transduction of HPV 18 E7 under the control of the HPV 18 URR that E7 alone induces this. The function of E7 would appear to be to reactivate the host DNA replication machinery to support viral DNA replication in post mitotic cells.

The viral E6 protein is also expressed at high levels in post mitotic cells. The E6 protein of the high risk viruses binds to p53 targeting it for destruction via ubiquination (Scheffner et al., 1990; Lechner et al., 1992). In response to signals such as DNA damage or inappropriate DNA synthesis p53 induces cell cycle arrest or apoptosis. The importance of the co-ordinate expression of E6 and E7 in post mitotic cells has been shown in elegant experiments with transgenic mice in which these genes are expressed in the lens under the control of the α crystallin promoter (Griep et al., 1993). The expression of E7 alone induced cell proliferation in spatially inappropriate regions of the lens and apoptosis of these cells before differentiation could occur. Transgenics expressing a mutant defective in Rb binding had normal lens proliferation and differentiation. E6 expressing transgenics exhibited delayed apoptosis in the lens and micropthalmia. Co-expression of E6 and E7 in this system resulted in the abrogation of E7 induced apoptosis and tumour development (Pan and Griep, 1994). The E6 mediated abrogation of apoptosis was mediated both by p53 dependent and p53 independent mechanisms (Pan and Griep, 1995). The abrogation of p53 mediated apoptosis may not be the only function of p53 which needs down regulating for the viral life cycle since there is evidence from transient replication assays that p53 suppresses both HPV and BPV amplificational DNA replication (Lepik et al., 1998)

The interplay between viral gene expression and the regulation of keratinocyte differentiation has been highlighted by studies examining $p21^{WAF1/CIP1}$ in HPV infections. $p21^{WAF1/CIP1}$ is a cyclin dependent kinase (cdk) inhibitor, it is transcriptionally activated by p53 and mediates G1 arrest in DNA damage. This protein inhibits cell growth and, in some circumstances, promotes differentiation via p53-independent mechanisms. Interestingly in many tissues p21 expression in vivo correlates with the onset or commitment to but not establishment of the differentiated phenotype (Gartel et al., 1996). This is particularly relevant to squamous epithelium since this is one of the tissues in which this phenomenon occurs. In the hair follicles of the skin, p21 is highly expressed in a narrow zone of post mitotic cells of the lower bulb region whereas little or no p21 is expressed in the differentiated keratinocytes of the upper region. In primary mouse keratinocytes forced into differentiation by Ca^{++}, increased expression of p21 occurs 4-8 hours after exposure to Ca^{++} together with inhibition of CDK and cell cycle block at G1 (Missero et al., 1995). After 24 hours, despite a sustained increase in p21 mRNA, p21 protein levels return to base values (Missero et al., 1996). Forced expression of p21 in differentiated keratinocytes inhibits terminal differentiation but these events are unrelated to CDK inhibition (Di Cunto et al., 1998).

In organotypic cultures of keratinocytes transduced by recombinant retroviruses expressing HPV 18 E7, $p21^{WAF1/CIP1}$ protein is induced via p53 independent post- transcriptional mechanisms. Interestingly in these cultures, E7 induction of unscheduled DNA synthesis and p21 expression were mutually exclusive (Jian et al., 1998), observations which paralleled those made in condyloma acuminata (Schmidt Grimminger et al., 1998). These data have been interpreted as suggesting that p21$^{WAF1/CIP1}$ induction blocks E7-induced unscheduled DNA synthesis by competing for binding to key replication factors such as PCNA. In view of the data from Di Cunto and colleagues (Di Cunto et al., 1998) an alternative explanation is that E7 expression delays the entry of cells from the commitment phase (p21 high) to established differentiation (p21 low). However a subset of E7 transduced keratinocytes proceed to the p21 low state and this is compatible with E7 induction of unscheduled DNA synthesis.

Future Directions

There are a number of key aspects of the papillomavirus infectious cycle which are poorly understood. In particular the early events of the viral life cycle represent a black hole in our knowledge. Although the target cell for infection is widely suspected to be a primitive keratinocyte or stem cell there is no unequivocal evidence that this is the case. Recent developments in stem cell biology with the prospect of in vitro systems which maintain self renewal raises expectations that this issue can be addressed. The immediate early events after infection are also obscure. The only papillomavirus which can infect cells in vitro is BPV-1 which can undergo a semi-permissive infection in murine C127 cells. In this system BPV-1 infects at low copy number and immediately undergoes a round of DNA amplification raising the copy number to 50 copies per cell. This round of episomal amplification is independent of the cell cycle but subsequently cell and viral episome replicate in tandem and there is episomal maintenance. No in vitro system supports productive infection of keratinocytes so the question of whether the BPV-1/C127 model truly represents immediate early events in permissive infection in epithelia remains open. The mechanisms which regulate the switch to the late or differentiation dependent promoter and vegetative viral growth are also poorly understood but these are of immense importance in understanding papillomavirus oncogenicity. However these are questions which can be addressed using currently available in vitro culture systems for keratinocytes and further insights into this process can be expected with confidence.

References

Abramson, A.L., Steinberg, B.M. and Winkler, B. (1987) Laryngeal papillomatosis: clinical, histopathologic and molecular studies. Laryngoscope 97, 678-685.

Amella, C.A., Lofgren, L.A., Ronn, A.M., Nouri, M., Shikowitz, M.J. and Steinberg, B.M. (1994) Latent infection induced with cottontail rabbit papillomavirus. A model for human papillomavirus latency. Am. J. Pathol 144, 1167-1171.

Bedell, M.A., Hudson, J.B., Golub, T.R., Turyk, M.E., Hosken, M., Wilbanks, G.D. and Laimins, L.A. (1991) Amplification of human papillomavirus genomes in vitro is dependent on epithelial differentiation. J. Virol. 65, 2254-2260.

Bernard, B.A., Bailly, C., Lenoir, M.C., Darmon, M., Thierry, F. and Yaniv, M. (1989) The human papillo-mavirus type 18 (HPV18) E2 gene product is a repressor of the HPV18 regulatory region in human kerati-nocytes. J. Virol. 63, 4317-4324.

Bonnez, W., DaRin, C., Borkhuis, C., de Mesy Jensen, K., Reichman, R.C. and Rose, R.C. (1998) Isolation and propagation of human papillomavirus type 16 in human xenografts implanted in the severe combined immunodeficiency mouse. J. Virol. 72, 5256-5261.

Brown, D.R., McClowry, T.L., Bryan, J.T., Stoler, M., Schroeder Diedrich, J.M. and Fife, K.H. (1998) A human papillomavirus related to human papillomavirus MM7/LVX82 produces distinct histological ab-normalities in human foreskin implants grown as athymic mouse xenografts. Virology 249, 150-159.

Campo, M.S., Jarrett, W.F., O'Neil, W. and Barron, R.J. (1994) Latent papillomavirus infection in cattle. Res Vet Sci 56, 151-7.

Chambers, V.C. and Evans, C.A. (1959) Canine oral papillomatosis. I. Virus assay and observations on the various stages of the experimental infection. Cancer Res. 19, 1188-1195.

Cheng, S., Schmidt Grimminger, D.C., Murant, T., Broker, T.R. and Chow, L.T. (1995) Differentiation-dependent up-regulation of the human papillomavirus E7 gene reactivates cellular DNA replication in su-prabasal differentiated keratinocytes. Genes-Dev. 9, 2335-2349.

Chow, L.T. and Broker, T.R. (1997) In vitro experimental systems for HPV: epithelial raft cultures for inves-tigation of viral reproduction and pathogenesis and for genetic analyses of viral proteins and regulatory elements. Clin. Dermatol. 15, 217-227.

de Villiers, E.M. (1997) Papillomavirus and HPV typing. Clin Dermatol 15, 199-206.

Delius, H., Saegling, B., Bergmann, K., Shamanin, V. and de Villiers, E.M. (1998) The genomes of three of four novel HPV types, defined by differences of their L1 genes, show high conservation of the E7 gene and the URR. Virology 240, 359-365.

Demeter, L.M., Stoler, M.H., Broker, T.R. and Chow, L.T. (1994) Induction of proliferating cell nuclear antigen in differentiated keratinocytes of human papillomavirus infected lesions. Hum. Pathol. 25, 343-348.

Di Cunto, F., Topley, G., Calautti, E., Hsiao, J., Ong, L., Seth, P. and Dotto, G.P. (1998) Inhibitory function of p21Cip1/WAF1 in differentiation of primary mouse keratinocytes independent of cell cycle control. Science 280, 1069-1072.

Dong, G., Broker, T.R. and Chow, L.T. (1994) Human papillomavirus type 11 E2 proteins repress the ho-mologous E6 promoter by interfering with the binding of host transcription factors to adjacent elements. J. Virol. 68, 1115-1127.

Durst, M., Glitz, D., Schneider, A. and zur Hausen, H. (1992) Human papillomavirus type 16 (HPV 16) gene expression and DNA replication in cervical neoplasia: analysis by in situ hybridization. Virology 189, 132-140.

Evander, M., Frazer, I.H., Payne, E., Qi, Y.M. and McMillan, N.A. (1997) Identification of the alpha 6 in-tegrin as the candidate receptor for papillomaviruses. J. Virol. 71, 2449-2456.

Frattini, M.G., Lim, H.B. and Laimins, L.A. (1996) In vitro synthesis of oncogenic human papillomaviruses requires episomal genomes for differentiation dependent late expression. Proc. Natl. Acad. Sci. USA 93, 3062-3067.

Gartel, A.L., Serfas, M.S., Gartel, M., Goufman, E., Wu, G.S., El Deiry, W.S. and Tyner, A.L. (1996) p21 (WAF1/CIP1) expression is induced in newly non dividing cells in diverse epithelia and during differen-tiation of the Caco-2 intestinal epithelial cell line. Exp. Cell Res. 227, 171-181.

Griep, A.E., Herber, R., Jeon, S., Lohse, J.K., Dubielzig, R.R. and Lambert, P.F. (1993) Tumorigenicity by human papillomavirus type 16 E6 and E7 in transgenic mice correlates with alterations in epithelial cell growth and differentiation. J. Virol. 67, 1373-1384.

Higgins, G.D., Uzelin, D.M., Phillips, G.E., McEvoy, P., Marin, R. and Burrell, C.J. (1992) Transcription patterns of human papillomavirus type 16 in genital intraepithelial neoplasia: evidence for promoter usage within the E7 open reading frame during epithelial differentiation. J. Gen. Virol. 73, 2047-2057.

Hummel, M., Hudson, J.B. and Laimins, L.A. (1992) Differentiation induced and constitutive transcription of human papillomavirus type 31b in cell lines containing viral episomes. J. Virol. 66, 6070-6080.

Jian, Y., Schmidt-Grimminger, D.C., Chien, W.M., Wu, X., Broker, T.R. and Chow, L.T. (1998) Post-transcriptional induction of p21 cip1 protein by human papillomavirus E7 inhibits unscheduled DNA synthesis reactivated in differentiated keratinocytes. Oncogene 17, 2027-2038.

Klumpp, D.J., Stubenrauch, F. and Laimins, L.A. (1997) Differential effects of the splice acceptor at nucleotide 3295 of human papillomavirus type 31 on stable and transient viral replication. J. Virol. 71, 8186-8194.

Kreider, J.W. and Bartlett, G.L. (1981) The Shope papilloma-carcinoma complex of rabbits: a model system of neoplastic progression and spontaneous regression. Adv. Cancer. Res. 35, 81-110.

Kreider, J.W. and Bartlett, G.L. (1985) Shope rabbit papilloma carcinoma complex. A model system of HPV infections. Clin. Dermatol. 3, 20-26.

Kreider, J.W., Howett, M.K., Leure Dupree, A.E., Zaino, R.J. and Weber, J.A. (1987) Laboratory production in vivo of infectious human papillomavirus type 11. J. Virol. 61, 590-593.

Kreider, J.W., Howett, M.K., Wolfe, S.A., Bartlett, G.L., Zaino, R.J., Sedlacek, T. and Mortel, R. (1985) Morphological transformation in vivo of human uterine cervix with papillomavirus from condylomata acuminata. Nature 317, 639-6341.

Kreider, J.W., Patrick, S.D., Cladel, N.M. and Welsh, P.A. (1990) Experimental infection with human papillomavirus type 1 of human hand and foot skin. Virology 177, 415-417.

Leary, T., Jones, P.L., Appleby, M.W., Blight, A., Parkinson, E.K. and Stanley, M.A. (1992) Epidermal keratinocyte self renewal is dependent upon dermal integrity. J. Invest. Dermatol. 99, 422-430.

Lechner, M.S., Mack, D.H., Finicle, A.B., Crook, T., Vousden, K.H. and Laimins, L.A. (1992) Human papillomavirus E6 proteins bind p53 in vivo and abrogate p53 mediated repression of transcription. EMBO J. 11, 3045-3052.

Lepik, D., Ilves, I., Kristjuhan, A., Maimets, T. and Ustav, M. (1998) p53 protein is a suppressor of papillomavirus DNA amplificational replication. J. Virol. 72, 6822-6831.

Li, A., Simmons, P.J. and Kaur, P. (1998) Identification and isolation of candidate human keratinocyte stem cells based on cell surface phenotype. Proc. Natl. Acad. Sci. USA 95, 3902-397.

Loeffler, M., Birke, A., Winton, D. and Potten, C. (1993) Somatic mutation, monoclonality and stochastic models of stem cell organisation in the intestinal crypt. J. Theor. Biol. 160, 471-491.

Maran, A., Amella, C.A., Di Lorenzo, T.P., Auborn, K.J., Taichman, L.B. and Steinberg, B.M. (1995) Human papillomavirus type 11 transcripts are present at low abundance in latently infected respiratory tissues. Virology 212, 285-294.

Meyers, C., Frattini, M.G., Hudson, J.B. and Laimins, L.A. (1992) Biosynthesis of human papillomavirus from a continuous cell line upon epithelial differentiation. Science 257, 971-973.

Miller, S.J., Sun, T.-T. and Lavker, R.M. (1993) Hair follicles, stem cells and skin cancer. J. Invest. Dermatol. 100, 289s-294s.

Missero, C., Calautti, E., Eckner, R., Chin, J., Tsai, LH., Livingston, M. and Dotto, G.P. (1995) Involvement of the cell cycle inhibitor Cip1/WAF1 and the E1A associated p300 protein in terminal differentiation. Proc. Natl. Acad. Sci. USA 92, 5451-5455.

Missero, C., Di Cunto, F., Kiyokawa, H., Koff, A. and Dotto G.P. (1996) The absence of p21Cip1/WAF1 alters keratinocyte growth and differentiation and promotes ras-tumor progression. Genes Dev. 10, 3065-3075.

Morris, R.J., Fischer, S.M. and Slaga, T.J. (1985) Evidence that the centrally and peripherally located cells in the murine epidermal proliferative unit are two distinct populations. J. Invest. Dermatol. 84, 277-281.

Oriel, J.D. (1971) Natural history of genital warts. British Journal of Venereal Diseases 47, 1-13.

Ozbun, M.A. and Meyers, C. (1998) Temporal usage of multiple promoters during the life cycle of human papillomavirus type 31b. J. Virol. 72, 2715-2722.

Pan, H. and Griep, A.E. (1994) Altered cell cycle regulation in the lens of HPV 16 E6 or E7 transgenic mice: implications for tumor suppressor gene function in development. Genes Dev. 8, 1285-1299.

Pan, H. and Griep, A.E. (1995) Temporally distinct patterns of p53 dependent and p53 independent apoptosis during mouse lens development. Genes Dev 9, 2157-69.

Parker, J.N., Zhao, W., Askins, K.J., Broker, T.R. and Chow, L.T. (1997) Mutational analyses of differentiation-dependent human papillomavirus type 18 enhancer elements in epithelial raft cultures of neonatal foreskin keratinocytes. Cell Growth Differ. 8, 751-762.

Romanczuk, H. and Howley, P.M. (1992) Disruption of either the E1 or the E2 regulatory gene of human papillomavirus type 16 increases viral immortalization capacity. Proc. Natl. Acad. Sci. USA 89, 3159-3163.

Romanczuk, H., Thierry, F. and Howley, P.M. (1990) Mutational analysis of cis elements involved in E2 modulation of human papillomavirus type 16 P97 and type 18 P105 promoters. J. Virol. 64, 2849-2859.

Scheffner, M., Werness, B.A., Huibregtse, J.M., Levine, A.J. and Howley, P.M. (1990) The E6 oncoprotein encoded by human papillomavirus types 16 and 18 promotes the degradation of p53. Cell 63, 1129-1136.

Schmidt Grimminger, D.C., Wu, X., Jian, Y., Broker, T.R. and Chow, L.T. (1998) Post-transcriptional induction of p21cip1 protein in condylomata and dysplasias is inversely related to human papillomavirus activities. Am. J. Pathol. 152, 1015-1024.

Schmitt, A., Rochat, A., Zeltner, R., Borenstein, L., Barrandon, Y., Wettstein, F.O. and Iftner, T. (1996) The primary target cells of the high-risk cottontail rabbit papillomavirus colocalize with hair follicle stem cells. J. Virol. 70, 1912-1922.

Selvakumar, R., Schmitt, A., Iftner, T., Ahmed, R. and Wettstein, FO. (1997) Regression of papillomas induced by cotton tail rabbit papillomavirus is associated with infiltration of CD8+cells and persistence of viral DNA after regression. J. Virol. 5540-5548.

Seo, Y.S., Muller, F., Lusky, M., Gibbs, E., Kim, H.Y., Phillips, B. and Hurwitz, J. (1993) Bovine papilloma virus (BPV)-encoded E2 protein enhances binding of E1 protein to the BPV replication origin [published erratum appears in Proc. Natl. Acad. Sci. USA 90, 2865-2869.

Spalholz, B.A., Lambert, P.F., Yee, C.L. and Howley, P.M. (1987) Bovine papillomavirus transcriptional regulation: localization of the E2-responsive elements of the long control region. J. Virol. 61, 2128-2137.

Spalholz, B.A., Yang, Y.C. and Howley, P.M. (1985) Transactivation of a bovine papillomavirus transcriptional regulatory element by the E2 gene product. Cell 42, 183-191.

Stanley, M.A. (1994) Replication of human papillomaviruses in cell culture. Antiviral Res. 24, 1-15.

Stanley, M.A., Browne, H.M., Appleby, M. and Minson, A.C. (1989) Properties of a non tumorigenic human cervical keratinocyte cell line. Int. J. Cancer 43, 672-676.

Sterling, J., Stanley, M., Gatward, G. and Minson, T. (1990) Production of human papillomavirus type 16 virions in a keratinocyte cell line. J. Virol. 64, 6305-6307.

Sterling, J.C., Skepper, J. and Stanley, M.A. (1993) Immunoelectronmicroscopic localisation of HPV 16 L1 and E4 proteins in cervical keratinocytes cultured in vivo. J. Invest. Dermatol 100, 154-158.

Stoler, M.H., Whitbeck, A., Wolinsky, S.M., Broker, T.R., Chow, L.T., Howett, M.K. and Kreider, J.W. (1990) Infectious cycle of human papillomavirus type 11 in human foreskin xenografts in nude mice. J. Virol. 64, 3310-3318.

Stubenrauch, F., Colbert, A.M. and Laimins, L.A. (1998a) Transactivation by the E2 protein of oncogenic human papillomavirus type 31 is not essential for early and late viral functions. J. Virol. 72, 8115-8123.

Stubenrauch, F., Lim, H.B. and Laimins, L.A. (1998b) Differential requirements for conserved E2 binding sites in the life cycle of oncogenic human papillomavirus type 31. J. Virol. 72, 1071-1077.

Toon, P.G., Arrand, J.R., Wilson, L.P. and Sharp, D.S. (1986) Human papillomavirus infection of the uterine cervix of women without cytological signs of neoplasia. Br. Med.J. Clin. Res. 293, 1261-1264.

Ustav, E., Ustav, M., Szymanski, P. and Stenlund, A. (1993) The bovine papillomavirus origin of replication requires a binding site for the E2 transcriptional activator. Proc. Natl. Acad. Sci. U S A 90, 898-902.

Ustav, M. and Stenlund, A. (1991) Transient replication of BPV-1 requires two viral polypeptides encoded by the E1 and E2 open reading frames. EMBO J. 10, 449-457.

Winton, D.A. and Ponder, B.A. (1990) Stem cell organisation in mouse small intestine. Proc. Roy. Soc. Lond. B Biol. Sci. 241, 13-18.

Yang, L., Mohr, I., Li, R., Nottoli, T., Sun, S. and Botchan, M. (1991) Transcription factor E2 regulates BPV-1 DNA replication in vitro by direct protein-protein interaction. Cold Spring Harb. Symp. Quant. Biol. 56, 335-346.

Zhao, W., Chow, L.T. and Broker, T.R. (1997) Transcription activities of human papillomavirus type 11 E6 promoter-proximal elements in raft and submerged cultures of foreskin keratinocytes. J. Virol. 71, 8832-8840.

THE FUNCTION OF THE HUMAN PAPILLOMAVIRUS ONCOGENES

David Pim, Miranda Thomas and Lawrence Banks

International Centre for Genetic Engineering and Biotechnology, Trieste, Italy

Introduction

Human papillomaviruses (HPVs) are small double stranded DNA viruses which are widespread in the human population. They are strictly epitheliotropic, and infect cutaneous and mucosal epithelium in a variety of anatomical sites. Over a hundred different viral types have now been identified and they are associated with a variety of clinically important conditions (de Villiers et al., 1997). Perhaps the most important of these is the association with the development of ano-genital malignancies, in particular cervical cancer (zur Hausen and Schneider, 1987; zur Hausen, 1991). A very high percentage of women developing the disease harbor the viral DNA, the most frequently found types being HPV-16 and HPV-18, and tumors, and tumor-derived cell lines, continue to express a subset of the viral oncoproteins, suggesting a continued involvement of these proteins in the development of the malignancy (Schwarz, et al., 1985; Smotkin and Wettstein, 1986; Androphy et al., 1987; Banks et al., 1987). In addition to cervical carcinoma, HPVs are also associated with several other human malignancies. The viral types which have been linked to cervical cancer have also been found associated with the development of squamous cell carcinomas (SCCs) of the anus (Scheurlen et al., 1986; Palmer et al., 1987). HPVs have also been linked with the development of SCC at cutaneous sites in patients with the rare skin disorder, epidermodysplasia verruciformis, and have been associated with the development of SCC in patients undergoing immunosuppression following transplant surgery (Sheil et al., 1985; Dyall-Smith et al., 1991). Again, a subset of virus types is associated with the development of these malignancies, in particular HPV-5 and HPV-8 (Orth et al., 1978).

In the following pages we shall address those studies which have attempted to clarify the mechanism of action of the viral oncoproteins. Recent advances in organotypic raft culture systems have allowed us to examine the link between the differentiation status of keratinocytes and human papillomavirus gene expression, and, in turn, the effects of HPV proteins on keratinocyte differentiation. These systems are now approaching a tissue culture system for normal viral productive infection, yet in the past the lack of such a system necessitated the dissection and expression of the viral open reading frames, generally from heterologous promoters, either *in vitro* or in various cell lines. Such an approach for investigating the functions of the viral proteins has proved to be extremely powerful, and has furthered our understanding of how this group of viruses replicate and how, under certain circumstances, they induce the cellular changes which ultimately lead to malignancy. One disadvantage to this approach, however, is that these viral proteins are often considered to function in isolation rather than as a complementary group. In reality, the viral proteins are translated from a complex selection of spliced, polycistronic transcripts, the control of which is, as yet, poorly understood, but whose function is to replicate, package, and ultimately release infectious virus. This is particularly true for the E5, E6 and E7 proteins which have evolved complementary, yet interacting, systems for avoiding host cell-cycle controls and apoptotic responses in order to facilitate viral replication. It should also be emphasised that the loss of the virus-infected cell's ability to differentiate, which accompanies immortalisation and transformation, is non permissive for viral replication. Hence, although this chapter is intended to deal mainly with aspects of viral oncoprotein function relating to transformation, all the associations and activities of the viral oncoproteins that will be discussed should also be viewed in the light of viral replication, since it is in this context that their functions have evolved.

Much of the work to date has focussed on the identification of important cellular targets of the viral oncoproteins and, as will be seen, these studies have not only provided us with vital information concerning the mechanisms of viral mediated cell transformation, but have also provided insights into the regulation of cell proliferation, differentiation and apoptosis under normal circumstances. As a prelude to these discussions, it will first be necessary to review the different transformation systems that have been used to identify the different viral oncoproteins and the relevance of each system to the transforming effects of the virus *in vivo*.

HPV Transformation Assays

Assays for assessing the transforming activity of the different viral oncoproteins fall into three broad categories: transformation of established rodent cells, transformation of primary rodent cells in the presence of a cooperating oncogene, and immortalisation of primary human cells. Obviously the last system is the most relevant with respect to the normal target cells of the virus in vivo, but much useful information has also been provided by the rodent cell systems and, with a few notable exceptions, most of the biochemical activities of the viral oncoproteins which correlate with transformation in one assay are relevant to the others.

Transformation of established rodent cells

The association between HPV and human tumors has divided the virus types into those classified as 'high risk' and 'low risk' depending upon their association with neoplastic disease. Thus HPV-16 and HPV-18 which are the most frequently found viral types in cervical tumors, are classified as high risk. In contrast, HPV-6 and HPV-11 are largely found in benign genital lesions and are thus referred to as low risk (zur Hausen and Schneider, 1987). Some of the earliest work carried out on human papillomaviruses attempted to differentiate between the so-called high risk and low risk mucosal types in terms of their ability to transform established rodent cells. The first analyses, using entire viral early regions expressed in mouse NIH3T3 cells, demonstrated that the HPV-

16 genome encodes proteins with transforming potential, giving rise to rapidly proliferating foci capable of forming tumors in nude mice (Tsunokawa et al., 1986; Yasumoto
et al., 1986; Matlashewski et al., 1987a). Since the region of the HPV-16 and HPV-18
genomes that is retained and expressed in cervical tumors contains the E6 and E7 open
reading frames, attention naturally shifted to the analysis of these two proteins in the
transformation assays. The most potent transforming activity was found to be encoded
by the E7 open reading frame (Kanda et al., 1988; Vousden et al., 1988) and cells transfected with HPV-16 E7 expressed from a retroviral promoter formed rapidly growing
colonies in semi-solid medium (Yutsudo et al., 1988). E7 shares some sequence homology with both Adenovirus E1a and the SV40 large T antigen and, as will be discussed
later, is also able to bind to the product of the Retinoblastoma susceptibility gene, pRb.
This interaction is deemed essential for the ability of E7 to transform NIH3T3 cells,
since mutations in E7 within this region of homology with SV40/E1a that abolish pRb
binding also abolish transformation (Edmonds and Vousden, 1989).

Although both HPV-16 E6 (Sedman et al., 1991) and HPV-18 E6 (Bedell et al.,
1989) proteins can bring about the transformation of NIH3T3 and Rat-1 cells, the efficiency with which this occurs is much lower than that of E7. This may in part be due to
levels of expression since constructs which remove the splice donor sites on the E6 open
reading frame, and hence make only full length E6 protein, are significantly more effective in these assays (Sedman et al., 1991). Nonetheless, it is reasonable to assume that
transformation of established rodent cells by the E6 oncoproteins is weak in comparison
to that by the E7 proteins.

Since the region of the genome encoding the E5 gene is frequently deleted during
the development of cervical tumors, this gene was neglected for a considerable time.
However, the first studies that indicated that E5 might have transforming potential came
from experiments in which a transforming activity was detected in the HPV-18 genome
outside the region encoding E6 and E7 (Bedell et al., 1989). Indeed, these authors
speculated that this activity might be due to the presence of the E5 gene. Surprisingly it
was studies with HPV-6 E5 which first directly demonstrated transforming activity
associated with this protein (Chen and Mounts, 1990). This is in marked contrast to the
E6 and E7 genes derived from the low risk viruses, which exhibit extremely weak activity in any of the transformation assays that have so far been analysed. Further analysis of
the HPV-16 E5 protein also revealed transforming activity in established murine keratinocytes (Leptak et al., 1991), and in NIH3T3 cells where the activity was found to be
stimulated by the presence of Epidermal Growth Factor (EGF) (Pim et al., 1992;
Leechanachai et al., 1992). These studies thus defined E5 as the third oncoprotein to be
encoded by HPVs.

Transformation of primary rodent cells

Although the use of established cells has yielded important information about the transforming potential of the different viral oncoproteins, the use of primary rodent cells is
considered to be a more relevant assay for the transforming potential of the virus in
vivo. These studies have been performed on primary baby rat kidney cells (BRK), pri-

mary baby mouse kidney cells (BMK) and rat embryo fibroblasts (REF). Although the results obtained with each group of cells are similar, BRK and BMK are preferable since the target cells are principally epithelial in origin. Despite sharing some sequence homology with adenovirus E1a, E7, unlike E1a, does not encode a function allowing the establishment of primary rodent cells in culture, and all assays must be carried out in the presence of a cooperating, activated oncogene. Therefore, the first study demonstrating that HPV-16 could contribute to the immortalisation and transformation of primary BRKs required co-transfection of EJ-ras (Matlashewski et al., 1987b). This study also localised the transforming activity on the HPV-16 genome to the region encoding the E6 and E7 oncoproteins. Although in most of these studies EJ-ras was the oncogene of choice, Crook et al., (1988) also showed that HPV-16 could cooperate with v-fos to transform primary BMKs. Further analysis of the HPV-16 genome demonstrated that, as with established rodent cells, the principal activity was encoded by the E7 gene (Phelps et al., 1988; Storey et al., 1988). Where analysis of early gene co-transforming capacity was undertaken on the low risk group of HPVs, the studies demonstrated a marked reduction in efficiency. (Storey et al., 1988, 1990). Mutations made in the region homologous to E1a, which destroyed E7's ability to bind pRb, were also found to destroy E7's activity in these co-transformation assays.

In primary cell transformation assays the E6 gene exhibits quite different activities depending upon the species of origin of the cells. Thus, with one exception (Liu et al., 1994), very little transforming activity has ever been detected in BRK assays (Storey et al., 1988; Phelps et al., 1988). In contrast, cooperating with EJ-ras in BMK cells, HPV-16 and HPV-18 E6 proteins have a transforming capacity close to or equivalent to that of HPV-16 E7 (Storey and Banks, 1993; Pim et al., 1994). Based on these studies, it is tempting to speculate that differences between BRK and BMK cells might be a reflection of differences in the cellular targets of E6 between rat and mouse cell lines, although confirmation of this remains elusive.

The HPV-16 E5 gene is quite different from E6 and E7 in that there are no reports of it cooperating with cellular oncogenes to bring about the immortalisation of primary rodent cells. However an important demonstration of the cooperativity of the HPV oncoproteins was provided by studies demonstrating that E5 and E7 could cooperate in inducing proliferation of primary BRK cells (Bouvard et al., 1994). Under normal circumstances the proliferative capacity of primary BRK cells is quite limited and transfection with either E7 or E5 alone results in very few proliferating colonies. However, when E5 and E7 were transfected in combination a dramatic increase in the number of proliferating colonies was observed, and this was further augmented by the addition of EGF (Bouvard et al., 1994). These cells are not truly immortalised, so this assay is largely a measure of increased cellular proliferation. Rarely, however, cells do become immortalised in these assays and in these cases they are capable of anchorage independent growth (Faulkner Valle and Banks, 1995). As is the case in established rodent cells, HPV-6 E5 can also cooperate with E7 in these cell proliferation assays (Faulkner Valle and Banks, 1995). Thus, although the effects of E5 do not appear to be as potent as those of E6 or E7 in primary rodent cells, its activity appears to be common to proteins derived from both high and low risk virus types. As will also be seen below, E7 has also been reported to be able to cooperate with insulin-like growth factor in inducing cellular DNA synthesis (Morris et al., 1993); the observation that E7 also cooperates with the E5 protein, which is intimately involved in growth-factor signalling, provides a good explanation for these findings.

Immortalisation of primary human cells

The immortalisation system which most closely resembles the natural sequence of events in vivo is that using primary human keratinocytes. These are the natural host cells for human papillomavirus infection and are much more difficult to immortalise than cells of rodent origin. Recent studies have also made use of human mammary epithelial cells for dissecting the immortalising activities of E6 and E7.

The keratinocyte immortalisation studies have been done in keratinocytes derived from a variety of anatomical sites, including genital tract and oral mucosa, with highly consistent results. Several studies have shown that transfection of the HPV-16 or HPV-18 genome into foreskin, cervical or oral keratinocytes greatly extends the lifespan of these cells in culture (Dürst et al., 1987; Pirisi et al., 1987; Kaur and McDougall, 1988; Schlegel et al., 1988; Pecoraro et al., 1989; Woodworth et al., 1989; Park et al., 1991). In parallel with the situation in primary rodent cells, only high risk HPV types have been found to be effective in these assays, again providing a correlation with the high and low risk assessment of these viruses in vivo. When assays are performed with HPV-6 or HPV-11 only small colonies form. These cannot be propagated and senesce at an early passage (Woodworth et al., 1989; Pecoraro et al., 1989).

It should be noted that although results between laboratories are broadly in agreement, significant differences exist in how the immortalisation assays are performed. Cells can be transfected with HPV DNA sequences and selected for prolonged growth by inclusion of a selectable marker (McCance et al., 1988). Alternatively, differentiation-resistant cells can be selected by switching the cells from low to high Ca^{2+} after transfection (Schlegel et al., 1988). Whichever method is chosen immortalised cells can be obtained, albeit at a low frequency. However, for comparative mutational analysis of the HPV oncoproteins it is important to be aware of which immortalisation system is being used for the assays.

Dissection of the HPV genome defined both E6 and E7 as being essential for keratinocyte immortalisation (Barbosa and Schlegel 1989; Hawley-Nelson et al., 1989; Münger et al., 1989a). Although primary human keratinocyte immortalisation parallels the rodent systems in the way that the E6 and E7 proteins from the high risk, but not the low risk group of viruses will lead to immortalisation, there are also substantial differences between the two systems. First, the cooperation between E6 and E7 removes the necessity of using a cooperating, activated oncogene. This point is potentially very interesting since it implies that either the viral proteins interact more effectively with target proteins present in human cells than with those in rodent cells or, alternatively, that there are activities of these proteins in human cells which are not detected in rodent assay systems. Secondly, although frequently referred to as 'transformed', keratinocytes expressing both E6 and E7 have an extended life span, but are not tumorigenic in nude mice. Only after extended passage in culture or transfection with activated oncogenes do these immortalised keratinocytes become fully transformed (Dürst et al., 1989; DiPaolo et al., 1989; Hurlin et al., 1991; Pei et al., 1993). Thirdly, and perhaps most importantly, there is evidence to suggest that the regions of both E6 and E7 required for primary rodent cell transformation differ from those required for primary human cell immortalisation. For example, a mutant of E7 has been described that fails to bind pRb, is defective in primary rodent cell transformation assays, and yet retains the ability to cooperate with E6 in the immortalisation of primary human keratinocytes (Jewers et al., 1992). In addition, it has also been reported that E7 alone can induce the immortalisation of human keratinocytes in the absence of E6, albeit at a low frequency (Hudson et al., 1990; Halbert et al., 1991).

There are now several reports of E5 activity in primary human keratinocytes. A number of studies using full length HPV genomes have noted higher frequencies of immortalisation than when just the E6 and E7 genes were present (Romanczuk et al., 1991; Stöppler et al., 1996). This provides circumstantial evidence that E5 may have a role in the immortalisation of primary human keratinocytes. More direct evidence came from studies in which both the HPV-6 and HPV-16 E5 genes were shown to stimulate mitogenesis in primary human keratinocytes (Straight et al., 1993; Venuti et al., 1998) which was also enhanced by the addition of EGF. This is similar to the situation in rodent cells where the E5 proteins derived from both high and low risk virus types have been found to be similarly active. However the clearest demonstration of HPV-16 E5 contributing to the immortalisation of human keratinocytes was obtained from studies where the whole HPV-16 genome, mutated only in the E5 gene, gave a reduced level of immortalisation, equivalent to that seen with E6 and E7 alone. Addition of wild type HPV-16 E5 sequences greatly increased the frequency of immortalisation, strongly supporting the notion that, although E5 has no intrinsic immortalising activity in primary human cells, it can effectively cooperate with E6 and E7 (Stöppler et al., 1996).

The only other system of primary human cells which has been used extensively to analyse HPV oncoprotein activity is that of mammary epithelial cells. Both HPV-16 and HPV-18 have been shown to immortalise these cells (Band et al., 1990) and the principal activity appeared to reside within the E6 open reading frame (Band et al., 1991). More recent studies have however shown that both E6 and E7 can independently bring about immortalisation of these cells and this would appear to be dependent on the lineage of the target cell. Thus, late passage cells were immortalised by HPV-16 E6, whereas early passage cells were immortalised by HPV-16 E7 (Wazer et al., 1995). However, a note of caution should be added about the interpretation of these studies, since immortalisation by the low risk HPV-6 E6 and the Bovine Papillomavirus type 1 (BPV-1) E6 proteins has also been reported in these cells, albeit at a low frequency (Band et al., 1993).

Biochemical Properties of the HPV Oncoproteins

In the following pages we shall discuss some of the biochemical properties of the HPV oncoproteins which account for the observed biological activities of these proteins. Naturally, some aspects are more defined than others and, although a large number of cellular targets for E5, E6 and E7 have been described, we shall attempt to highlight those activities which have a defined biological consequence, whether this be for viral replication and/or cell transformation.

The HPV E5 Protein

During the development of cervical tumors, deletions frequently occur in the region of the genome encoding the E5 protein. Therefore it is generally assumed that E5 has no role in the later stages of malignancy, and for this reason it has not attracted the level of interest attached to the E6 and E7 oncoproteins. However, as should be clear from the above discussion, HPV E5 proteins have very interesting properties relating to cell proliferation and mitogenesis, and E5 may well play a role in the early stages of malignant conversion, prior to the events leading up to viral integration into the cellular genome. Due to the weak intrinsic transforming activity of the HPV E5 proteins, most of the early work on E5 has been done on the BPV-1 E5 protein which has a far higher transforming potential than the HPV equivalent. Therefore, although this chapter deals mainly with HPV, it will be necessary in this section to refer to some of the studies which have been done with the BPV-1 E5 since this has been the prototype for this group of proteins for many years.

INTERACTIONS WITH GROWTH FACTOR RECEPTORS

The E5 proteins are approximately 10kd in size, are extremely hydrophobic and localise to the Golgi apparatus, endoplasmic reticulum and nuclear membranes (Conrad et al., 1993). The first link between the E5 proteins and growth factor receptors was provided by studies with BPV-1 E5 where increased transforming efficiency was observed in the presence of activated EGFR (Martin et al., 1989). Most interestingly, these studies indicated that E5 was perturbing the processing of the activated receptor, thus increasing its half life and hence the duration of the mitogenic signal (Martin et al.,1989). In a separate series of studies, BPV-1 E5 was also shown to activate the platelet-derived growth factor receptor (PDGFR). This represents a different activity of BPV-1 E5 since, instead of increasing receptor half life as in the case of EGFR, E5 appears to be directly activating the PDGFR (Petti et al., 1991; Petti and DiMaio 1992). Interestingly, BPV-1 E5 appears to activate the PDGFR β in preference to the closely related PDGFR α and, when both EGFR and PDGFR are present, the PDGFR appears to be the preferred target (Petti and DiMaio, 1994). In the case of the HPV-16 E5 protein, most of its activity appears to be via the EGFR, although HPV-6 E5 has been reported to complex with EGFR, c-erb B2 and PDGFR (Conrad et al., 1994). In a manner analogous to that of BPV-1 E5, HPV-16 E5 has also been shown to perturb EGFR processing in human keratinocytes (Straight et al., 1993). This appears to be mediated by a reduction in the acidification of endosomes which are involved in receptor processing (Straight et al., 1995). The most likely mechanism by which this occurs is through the ability of E5 proteins to complex with the 16kD component of the vacuolar H^+ ATPases (Goldstein et al., 1991; Conrad et al., 1993). These are complexes of proteins involved in the processing of internalised growth factor receptors and contribute to the acidification of the endosomes. BPV-1, HPV-6, HPV-11 and HPV-16 E5 proteins exhibit binding to this protein and it is believed that this complex formation blocks 16kD function, resulting in the observed reduction in endosome acidification (Straight et al., 1995). In addition, mutants of the 16kD protein itself have been reported to possess transforming activity (Andresson et al., 1995). Studies with BPV-1 E5 have associated its ability to transform cells with its ability to complex with the 16kD ATPase (Goldstein and Schlegel, 1990), although mutants of BPV-1 E5 have been described which retain wild type levels of binding to the 16kD ATPase, yet are still defective for transformation (Goldstein et al., 1992). In the case of the HPV E5 proteins the situation is similar. Two studies have reported a lack of correlation between 16kD binding and transforming activity (Faulkner Valle and Banks, 1995; Chen et al., 1996) and other functions of E5 clearly exist.

The consequences of increased receptor activation are not difficult to envisage. Several studies have now shown that, as a consequence of E5's ability to stimulate signalling from receptors, there is increased activation of MAP Kinase (MAPK) (Gu and Matlashewski, 1995; Crusius et al., 1997) and a concomitant increase in the levels of expression of the early response genes c-fos and c-jun (Bouvard et al., 1994). In addition to EGFR stimulation, there is also evidence to suggest that E5 may activate the Protein Kinase C (PKC) pathway, also giving rise to an increase in early gene expression (Crusius et al., 1997). Therefore E5 can be viewed as activating those processes within the cell at the very early part of the G1 phase of the cell cycle. In terms of viral replication, this will most probably prime the cell for the stimulatory effects of E7 which, as will be discussed below, upregulates the cellular DNA replication machinery.

An additional consequence of the increased c-fos and c-jun expression induced by HPV-16 E5, is upregulation of the viral upstream regulatory region (URR). The HPV-16 URR contains a complex series of recognition motifs for a variety of transcription factors, including three AP-1 recognition sites which have been shown to be essential for viral gene expression (Chan et al., 1990). In a series of studies designed to investigate the effects of HPV-16 E5 upon viral gene expression, HPV-16 E5 was shown to be able to upregulate the viral major early promoter in human keratinocytes, and this was further enhanced by the addition of EGF (Bouvard et al., 1994). Thus E5 function links directly back to the regulation of viral gene expression and it is not too difficult to envisage a scenario where E5 might increase E6 and E7 gene expression and, as a result, contribute to the early steps of cell immortalisation. Finally, it is also worth noting that although E5 sequences are often lost during the progression to malignancy, the EGFRs are frequently amplified in cervical tumors (Bauknecht et al., 1989; Köhler et al., 1989). Thus, loss of E5 could be compensated for by receptor amplification during the development of cervical tumors.

PERTURBATION OF GAP JUNCTIONS BY E5 PROTEINS

Although most of the information concerning E5 function has come from studies on its effects on growth factor signal transduction pathways, there is also evidence that E5 has additional activities. One of the most interesting studies is the demonstration that E5 impairs the function of gap junctions, thus reducing cell-cell communication (Oelze et al., 1995). In the HaCat cells analysed in this study, connexin 43 is the major component of the gap junctions. Interestingly, although there were no differences in the level of expression of connexin 43, there was a marked decrease in its levels of phosphorylation in the presence of E5 compared with control cells. Since de-phosphorylation of the connexins is related to a decrease in gap junction activity, this would appear to be the explanation for these observations, although the mechanism by which E5 brings this about remains to be determined.

The HPV E6 Protein

During the development of cervical tumors and in the cell lines derived from them, the E6 gene is retained and continually expressed. In addition, a number of studies have shown that expression of the E6 gene is required for continued cell proliferation and for maintenance of the transformed phenotype (von Knebel Doeberitz et al., 1988; Storey et al., 1995; Alvarez-Salas et al., 1998). For these reasons it has long been assumed that E6 plays an important role in the development of cervical tumors. In addition, the fact that inhibition of E6 function results in a cessation of cell growth highlights the potential of this protein as a therapeutic target.

The HPV E6 proteins are polypeptides of approximately 150 amino acids with an apparent molecular weight of 18kD. Although there is a certain variation in the sequences of E6 proteins derived from different HPV types, all retain the strict conservation of four metal binding Cys-X-X-Cys motifs which allow the formation of two zinc fingers (Cole and Danos, 1987; Barbosa et al., 1989). Mutants that cannot form these fingers are, perhaps not surprisingly, compromised in the majority of assays performed (Kanda, et al., 1991; Sherman and Schlegel, 1996) thus emphasising the importance of the three-dimensional structure of the protein. A schematic diagram showing the major structural motifs and some of the known sites of protein interactions of the HPV E6 protein, which will be discussed in this section, is shown in Figure 1.

Owing to the very low levels of the protein found in the cell (Androphy et al., 1987; Banks et al., 1987), the determination of the intracellular location of endogenous E6 has been difficult. When expressed in baculovirus, HPV-18 E6 localised to the nuclear matrix and to non-nuclear membranes (Grossman et al., 1989). Subsequent assays performed on BPV and HPV E6 proteins also found them to be localised in nuclear and membraneous compartments (Androphy et al., 1985; Kanda et al., 1991; Chen et al., 1995; Sherman and Schlegel, 1996). It is also possible that the intracellular localisation of E6 might change, depending upon the differentiation status of the cell, or in response to various exogenous stimuli.

As will be apparent from the following discussion, a large number of cellular targets of the high risk HPV E6 proteins has now been described. However, the most widely

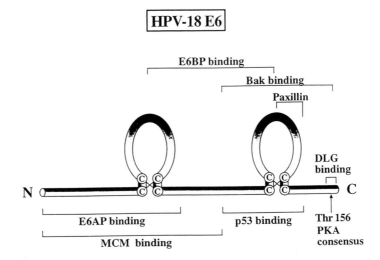

Fig. 1. The E6 protein. A schematic diagram showing the E6 protein with the zinc finger structures, together with the regions involved in interacting with its various cellular protein targets.

studied interaction is that between E6 and the cellular tumor suppressor protein p53. As will also be apparent from the section dealing with E7, the pathways that are affected by E6 and E7 frequently connect to p53. Therefore, prior to a more detailed description of E6 function, it will be necessary to review some of the literature relating to p53 so that the activities of the viral oncoproteins can be viewed in the correct context.

THE P53 TUMOR SUPPRESSOR

p53 is a short-lived nuclear phosphoprotein and it is one of the most frequently mutated genes in human tumors (Hollstein et al., 1991; Levine et al., 1991), indicating the importance of its anti-oncogenic function. Interestingly, p53 does not appear to be necessary for the normal processes of development since p53-null mice develop normally to sexual maturity (Donehower et al., 1992). However, such mice are highly susceptible to the development of tumors after a few months (Donehower et al., 1992; Kemp et al., 1993). This, together with the Li-Fraumeni syndrome, in which one p53 allele is deleted and p53 tumor-suppressor function is consequently more likely to be lost due to the acquisition of inactivating mutations in the remaining allele (Srivastava et al 1990; Malkin et al., 1990), led to the suggestion that p53 acts as a monitor of genomic integrity (Lane 1992). p53 normally has a half-life of approximately 30 minutes (An et al., 1998), however, a genotoxic insult, such as γ-irradiation, ultra-violet irradiation or chemically induced DNA damage, activates p53 causing it to become stabilised. This appears to be mediated in part by inhibition of mdm2 binding to p53, which normally maintains low levels of p53 protein by targeting p53 for ubiquitin-mediated degradation (Haupt et al., 1997; Kubbutat et al., 1997). Activated p53 is a powerful transcriptional activator of genes which possess a p53-responsive element in their promoters. A number of such sequences have been identified (Kern et al., 1991, Funk et al., 1992; El-Deiry et al., 1992; Harper et al., 1993) and it has been shown that the ability of p53 to function as a suppressor of cell growth correlates closely with its ability to act as a transcriptional activator (Vogelstein and Kinzler, 1992; Kern et al., 1992, Crook et al., 1994). Interestingly different genotoxic insults appear to result in differing patterns of p53 phosphorylation which may, in turn, affect its stability and/or its affinity for different p53-responsive elements (Shieh et al., 1997; Kapoor and Lozano, 1998; An et al., 1998). One of the most important targets of p53 is p21/WAF1 (El-Deiry et al., 1993). The p21 gene product is critical for the induction of a cell cycle arrest in G1 through the inhibition of cyclin dependent kinases (CDKs) which are necessary for the G1/S transition. It has also been reported that p53 can induce a growth arrest in G2/M (Stewart et al., 1995; Agarwal et al., 1995). Although the precise mechanism by which this is brought about is still unclear, a number of potential mediators of this activity of p53 have recently been identified. These include p21 (Dulic et al., 1998; Niculescu et al., 1998), cyclin G (Shimizu et al., 1998) and the 14-3-3 sigma gene (Hermeking et al., 1997), all of which are upregulated by p53. Overexpression of 14-3-3 sigma results in a G2 arrest and, interestingly, the fission yeast homologues rad24 and rad25 mediate a similar effect (Hermeking et al., 1997).

The other major biological effect of p53 activation is its ability to induce apoptosis; this is more likely to occur if the cell is beyond the G1 restriction point, or if there are the conflicting signals of DNA damage plus continued stimulation of cell proliferation (Clarke et al., 1993; Lowe et al., 1993; 1994; Wu and Levine, 1994). A classic example of this is provided by the Adenovirus E1a and HPV-16 E7 genes which, although inducing cell proliferation, also activate p53, resulting in apoptosis (Howe et al., 1994; Lowe et al., 1994; Qin et al., 1994). These observations clearly provide one of the explanations for the necessity of the Adenovirus E1b-p53 and HPV E6-p53 interactions to allow viral replication. It has also been shown by analysis with oligomerisation-defective mutants and their interactions with HPV-18 E6 that the growth arrest and apoptosis-inducing functions of p53 are separable (Slingerland et al., 1993; Crook et al., 1994; Thomas et al., 1996). In fact, the apoptosis-inducing functions of p53 may also be subdivisible since there are reports that p53 can induce apoptosis in the absence of additional transcription (Caelles et al., 1994), whereas other reports indicate that induction of apoptosis correlates with p53's ability to repress transcription from the MAP4 promoter (Murphy et al., 1996) and activate the Bax and PIG3 promoters (Miyashita and Reed, 1995; Polyak et al., 1997). Thus it is clear that p53's induction of apoptosis is complex and may involve several different and quite separate pathways.

INTERACTIONS BETWEEN E6 AND P53

p53 was initially identified through its association with another DNA tumor virus protein, SV40 TAg (Lane and Crawford, 1979; Linzer and Levine, 1979), and it was also found in association with the adenovirus E1b 55k protein (Sarnow et al., 1982); both of these interactions resulted in stable inactive complexes between the viral proteins and p53. In contrast, p53 protein could not be detected in HPV-transformed cell lines, such as HeLa, despite there being high levels of the mRNA present (Matlashewski et al.,1986, Scheffner et al., 1991). Investigation of this anomaly led to the finding that in vitro translated HPV-16 and HPV-18 E6 proteins are indeed able to bind to in vitro translated p53 (Werness et al., 1990), and this binding was found to promote the degradation of p53 via the ubiquitin pathway (Scheffner et al., 1990). The ability of oncogenic type E6 proteins to stimulate the degradation of p53 provides a clear reason for the very low levels of p53 found in HPV-transformed cell lines (Band et al., 1991). It also provides a logical explanation for the fact that p53 is wild type in such lines, and, indeed, in almost all HPV-positive cervical tumors (Crook et al 1991b; Scheffner et al., 1991). If the protein is only present in vanishingly low amounts, below the threshold level where its activity becomes apparent, there would be no selective pressure in favour of acquired inactivating mutations.

Cells expressing E6 lose the G1 checkpoint activity very early, presumably due to the degradation of p53 (Dulic et al.,1994) and are resistant to p53-induced growth arrest and apoptosis as a result of DNA damage (Kessis, et al., 1993; Foster et al., 1994; Pan and Griep, 1995; Thomas et al.,1996; Cai et al., 1997). The G2 checkpoint is initially unaffected (Paules et al., 1995) but there is increased chromosomal instability in E6-expressing cells over time, and this appears to be associated with concurrent attenuation of the G2 checkpoint function (White et al., 1994 ; Kaufmann et al.,1997), possibly by E6 alteration of cyclin/cdk complexes (Xiong et al., 1996). It is not yet clear whether this relates to the ablation of the G2/M checkpoint that is regulated by p53 (Stewart et al., 1995; Hermeking et al., 1997), or whether E6 has additional targets at this stage of the cell cycle. HPV-16 E6 has recently been shown to affect G2/M checkpoint controls in a number of ways (Thompson et al., 1997). In IMR-90 cells stably expressing E6, the G2 delay in response to ionising radiation is considerably reduced due to an increase in the concentrations and activities of cdc2, cyclin A and cyclin B. In these cells okadaic acid and caffeine can induce premature chromosome condensation, indicating that the checkpoint which couples entry into mitosis to completion of DNA replication has also been overcome. In addition such cells accumulate a DNA content of greater than 4N in the presence of nocodazole, indicating that the mitotic spindle checkpoint is also disregulated. Abrogation of the mitotic spindle checkpoint has also been reported in E6-expressing human foreskin keratinocytes (HFKs) (Thomas and Laimins, 1998) and these cells, not surprisingly, have very low p53 levels. However, this study also found that HFKs expressing E7 exhibited an abrogation of mitotic spindle checkpoint activity, despite expressing high levels of transcriptionally active p53. This correlates with data suggesting that the mitotic spindle checkpoint does not act effectively in cells which are null for either p53 or pRb (Di Leonardo et al., 1997), and it also demonstrates that the complementary activities of p53 and pRb are mirrored by the complementarity between E6 and E7 functions.

The degradation of p53 in the presence of HPV-16 and HPV-18 E6 is dependent upon a cellular protein (Huibregtse et al., 1991, 1993a, Scheffner et al., 1993). This

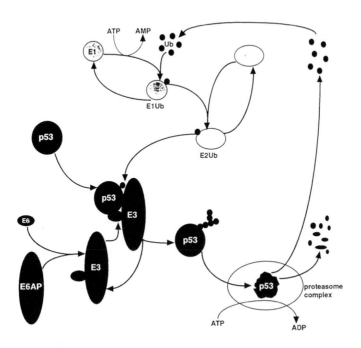

Fig. 2. The Ubiquitination pathway in the degradation of p53. The E1 ubiquitin activating enzyme activates the ubiquitin (Ub); the E2 ubiquitin conjugating enzyme then transfers the activated Ub to the E3 ubiquitin-protein ligase. HPV E6 binds E6-AP to form an E3 enzyme which specifically binds and ubiquitinates p53. The poly-ubiquitinated p53 is then degraded by the proteasome complex.

protein, called E6-AP (for E6-Associated Protein), is a monomeric protein of approximately 100kD which was found to be an E3 ubiquitin-protein ligase. In the ubiquitination pathway (see Figure 2), a ubiquitin-activating enzyme (E1) activates the ubiquitin which is then transferred by a ubiquitin conjugating enzyme (E2) to a ubiquitin-protein ligase (E3), to which the substrate protein is specifically bound (Hershko and Ciechanover, 1992). The finding that HPV-18 E6*I can bind to E6-AP (Pim et al., 1997, and see below), maps the binding site to within the first 43 amino acids of E6. The region of E6-AP which is involved in the interaction has also been mapped by deletion analysis to an 18 amino acid region in the central part of the protein (Huibregtse et al., 1993b). However, loss of this region also ablates p53 binding (Huibregtse et al., 1993b) and mutant p53s which are unable to bind E6 are not susceptible to ubiquitin-mediated degradation (Scheffner et al., 1992). No study has yet shown any association between p53 and E6-

AP in the absence of HPV E6, and indeed it has been shown that the antisense inhibition of E6-AP results in increased p53 levels only in those cells which express E6 (Beer-Romero et al., 1997). This tends to suggest that E6-AP is not normally involved in the control of p53 levels, but that E6 may have hijacked the E6-AP in order to circumvent the accumulation of activated p53. The E6:E6-AP complex has also been detected in the degradation of a number of other cellular proteins, including c-Myc and Bak (Gross-Mesilety et al., 1998; Thomas and Banks 1998), and these will be discussed in more detail below. However, E6-AP does not require E6 in order to function as a ubiquitin-protein ligase, since it has recently been shown that E6-AP alone is capable of ubiquitinating itself and a number of other cellular proteins (Nuber et al., 1998) and E6-AP, in fact, belongs to a family of closely related ubiquitin ligases (Huibregtse et al., 1995; Schwarz et al., 1998).

It is widely assumed that the degradation of p53 contributes to the oncogenic potential of the high risk group of viruses. However, a note of caution is necessary. Several studies have shown that mutants of E6 defective in their ability to induce the degradation of p53 can still immortalise human embryonic cells (Ishiwatari et al., 1994; Nakagawa et al., 1995), can co-transform primary BMK cells (Pim et al., 1994) and can transform established murine cells (Inoue et al., 1998). Thus, although it seems extremely unlikely that E6-induced degradation of p53 will have no role in the development of HPV associated malignancies, other functions of E6 are also likely to be involved.

An important question which arises is why do the high risk virus type E6s interact so effectively with p53 compared with the low risk types, since one would expect that both groups of viruses have to overcome similar cellular restrictions for an effective round of replication. The answer to this most probably lies in their respective sites of replication. HPVs infect keratinocyte stem cells in the basal layers of the epidermis, but can only replicate in terminally differentiating keratinocytes and the virus requires the cell's DNA replication machinery in order to replicate its own DNA. Since a defining feature of terminal differentiation is the cessation of DNA replication, and the response of a healthy cell to inappropriate DNA replication is p53 induced apoptosis, the virus has to walk a physiological tightrope; stimulating DNA replication whilst inhibiting apoptosis. There is however, a spatial and temporal difference between the low and high risk HPVs in their sites of DNA replication within the differentiating epithelium (Doorbar et al., 1997). The replication of the low risk HPVs is generally restricted to the lower levels of the stratified epithelium where the keratinocytes are still undergoing cell division. In contrast, the high risk HPVs replicate their genomes in the higher levels of the epithelium where the keratinocytes are undergoing terminal differentiation; in these cells DNA replication would normally have been switched off and the cells would have exited from the cell cycle. As a consequence, the low risk viruses perturb the normal differentiation pathways of the cell causing highly visible proliferations of infected tissue. In contrast, infection by the high risk viruses leads to less perturbation of the normal differentiation pattern of the host cell, thus producing smaller, less obvious, lesions. It is tempting to view the tumor-associated virus types as having to keep cells in the cell cycle in a more unnatural environment, hence the more effective induction of DNA synthesis observed with oncogenic associated virus type E7 proteins (see below) and hence the requirement for a more effective ablation of the responding p53 by the oncogenic E6 proteins.

E6 BINDING TO P53 WITHOUT DEGRADATION

The finding that the E6 proteins from high and low risk HPVs could bind to p53 in the absence of degradation (Crook et al., 1991a; Lechner and Laimins, 1994,) suggested that E6 might have additional activities with respect to p53. This was confirmed by studies which indicated that E6 proteins could relieve p53's transcriptional repression of promoters containing TATA elements without the degradation of p53 (Lechner et al., 1992). It has also been shown that HPV-18 E6 mutants unable to stimulate the degradation of p53 were nevertheless wild type in their ability to repress p53's transactivation of promoters containing p53-responsive elements (Pim et al., 1994), and recent studies indicate that E6 can perturb p53 localisation to the nucleus independently of degradation (Mantovani and Banks, 1999). Further, E6's binding to p53 in the absence of degradation can prevent p53 from binding to a range of recognition sequences, and thus prevent its activating transcription (Lechner and Laimins, 1994; Thomas et al.,1995).

An interesting analysis by Li and Coffino (1996) showed that two regions of p53 can be bound by E6: a region in the C terminus between amino acids 376-384 is bound by both HPV-6 and HPV-16 E6s, but this binding has no effect upon p53 stability; while HPV-16 but not HPV-6 E6 can bind to the core region, (amino acids 66-326) which correlates with the induction of p53 degradation. There has been considerable controversy over the years about which regions of the E6 protein are necessary for interactions with p53 (Crook et al., 1991a; Mietz et al., 1992; Pim et al., 1994). This has also been compounded by the fact that many of these data were originally generated by in vitro assays, which have been since shown to be not altogether representative of the in vivo situation (Foster et al., 1994, Crook et al., 1996, Gardiol and Banks, 1998). Li and Coffino (1996) also refer to their use of chimæric E6 proteins (Crook et al., 1991a) to demonstrate that the C-terminal half of E6 can bind to p53 but that the N-terminal half is required to induce degradation. This is not surprising in the light of more recent data showing that the N-terminal 43 amino acids of E6 are required for binding to E6-AP (Pim et al., 1997).

P53 POLYMORPHISMS AND E6

When human wild type p53 cDNAs were originally cloned, a sequence polymorphism was found in the general population that resulted in either a proline (p53Pro) or an arginine (p53Arg) residue at position 72 (Matlashewski et al., 1987c) which causes a mobility difference on SDS-PAGE. These two polymorphic forms appeared to be functionally equivalent with respect to their interaction with SV40TAg (Moreau and Matlashewski, 1992) and there appeared to be no clear association of either type with any increased cancer risk. However, the finding that the polymorphism lies in a region of p53 which is necessary for the induction of apoptosis (Walker and Levine, 1996; Sakamuro et al.,1997) gave rise to renewed interest, particularly since the p53Arg polymorphism ablates one of the five PxxP SH3-binding domains (Yu et al., 1994) found in this region. It has recently been shown that p53Arg is considerably more susceptible than p53Pro to the degradation induced in vivo by HPV-18 E6 and HPV-16 E6 (Storey et al., 1998). In addition, HPV-11 E6 was also shown to be able to induce the degradation of p53Arg, but not p53Pro. This suggests that although the division of mucosal HPVs into high-risk and low-risk types may be relevant clinically, in molecular terms there is likely to be more of a spectrum of differences between types rather than a clear cut-off.

POLYMORPHIC VARIANTS OF E6
It should be emphasised here that, in addition to differences between HPV types, many intratypic variants have also been identified. The frequency of detection of these variants differs markedly depending upon geographical location (Yamada et al., 1997), and their DNA sequences may differ by up to 2% in certain open reading frames (Bernard et al., 1994). The majority of the studies of E6 function have been performed upon the prototype protein, but it is possible that certain variants may differ significantly in their activities. Indeed, one study recently found that although the prototype HPV-16 E6 was present in 44% of CINIII lesions, it was found in less than 10% of invasive cervical carcinomas (Zehbe et al., 1998). It has also been found that a number of HPV-16 E6 variants, from different geographical locations, show a range of abilities to cooperate with E7 in the immortalisation of keratinocytes (Conrad-Stöppler et al., 1996) and this correlates, in part, with their ability to induce the degradation of p53 in vitro. Thus it seems probable that there may be clinically important biochemical differences between the variant and prototype E6 proteins, and this needs bearing in mind when considering the respective activities of the E6 proteins. A systematic study of the different E6 variants with respect to their different cellular target proteins is obviously a high priority.

E6 AND E6BP
The next cellular protein which was defined as being a target of E6 is E6BP (E6 Binding Protein). This was identified using HPV-16 E6 in a yeast two-hybrid screen of cDNAs from HeLa cells (Chen et al., 1995). HPV-31 E6 and, to a lesser extent, HPV-18 E6, but neither HPV-6 E6 nor HPV-11 E6, were also shown to bind to E6BP in vitro. The oncogenic BPV-1 E6 also binds to E6BP, and mutants of BPV-1 E6 unable to bind were also defective in transformation assays. Therefore, at least for BPV E6, binding to E6BP correlates with transforming potential. The E6BP cDNA encodes a 210 amino acid protein with four potential calcium-binding motifs which is homologous to the calcium-binding protein, ERC-55. The exact function of ERC-55 is not clear but its mouse homologue appears to be a Vitamin D Receptor (VDR)-associated factor (Imai et al., 1997). The VDR is a member of the nuclear receptor superfamily and has been shown to mediate vitamin D3's growth suppressive effects: in keratinocytes, disruption of the VDR:RXR complex has been shown to be equivalent to ras-transformation in its effects upon cell growth (Solomon et al., 1998). In addition, the post-transcriptional activation of VDR expression in the epidermis has been linked to cellular differentiation (Zineb et al.,1998). Taken together, it seems possible that the association of E6 with ERC-55 may prevent the VDR from exerting such growth suppressive effects. However, the exact function of ERC-55 has not yet been clarified and the effect of E6 upon it is, as yet, unknown, although it does not appear to result in the

degradation of E6BP (Chen et al.,1995). More recently it has been shown that E6 can induce resistance to calcium- and serum-induced differentiation of human keratinocytes, and this may well be related to its interaction with E6BP (Chen et al., 1995; Sherman and Schlegel, 1996).

E6 INDUCTION OF TELOMERASE

Telomeres are repetitive nucleotide sequences (TTAGGG, in mammalian cells) that are found on the ends of each chromosome (Ishikawa, 1997, for review). They form complexes with DNA-binding proteins which position the chromosomes within the nucleus, protect the chromosomal ends and prevent the end-to-end associations and fusions between chromosomes that would result in dicentric chromosomes which are vulnerable to breakage during the segregation of daughter chromosomes (Blackburn, 1991; Coquelle et al., 1997). Normal diploid cells lose up to 100bp of these repetitive sequences with each round of replication and it has been suggested that this shortening results, eventually, in the onset of senescence (Harley et al., 1990). The activation of telomerase, which adds the repetitive sequences to the chromosomal ends (Greider and Blackburn, 1985) is thought to occur normally only in embryonic cells and in adult germ cells (Noble et al., 1996) and it has been suggested that the activation of telomerase is a critical event during immortalisation. Using human cervical keratinocyes infected with retroviral constructs expressing HPV-16 E6 and E7, either separately or together, Klingelhutz et al. (1996) showed that only those cells expressing both E6 and E7 became immortalised. However, when assayed for telomerase activity, the cells expressing E6 and E7, or E6 alone, exhibited high levels of telomerase activity both before and after crisis: cells expressing E7 alone showed no increase in telomerase activity. However, in this study, and in others (Stöppler et al.,1997, Filatov et al.,1998), the E6 alone-expressing cells showed no additional stability in telomere length compared with controls, while the cells expressing E7 showed an increase in chromosome length despite having no detectable telomerase activity (Stöppler et al.,1997). Thus, telomeric truncation alone is not sufficient to prevent immortalisation, since the E6 plus E7 cells had shorter telomeres than senescing control-transfected cells; conversely, neither is telomerase activity alone sufficient to cause immortalisation. It is probable that other mechanisms exist to restore telomere length upon immortalisation, and, thus, the induction of telomerase activity by E6 may have an additional, as yet unknown, function in the replication of the virus.

INHIBITION OF APOPTOSIS BY E6

The interaction of E6 with p53, leading to its ubiquitination and degradation, prevents p53 from inducing apoptosis and hence from exercising its tumor-suppressive activities. Recent work using transgenic mice expressing HPV-16 E6 in the ocular lens (Pan and Griep, 1995) confirmed that E6 prevents apoptosis in vivo. Furthermore, in p53-null mice, HPV-16 E6 is still able to prevent the induction of apoptosis (Pan and Griep, 1995). It has also been shown that E6 will inhibit drug-induced apoptosis in cells lacking p53 (Steller et al., 1996). These studies have demonstrated that the E6 protein of oncogenic HPV types is able to prevent the apoptosis induced by both p53-dependent and p53-independent pathways. Recent studies have identified c-Myc and Bak as being targets for E6 mediated degradation, and both proteins are intimately associated with the events leading to apoptosis.

The c-Myc protein is a cellular oncogene which has a well-established association with tumorigenesis (Bouchard et al., 1998) but whose unscheduled expression gives rise to high levels of apoptosis (Askew et al., 1991; Evan et al., 1992). In keratinocytes, the downregulation of c-Myc expression appears to be necessary to inhibit cell proliferation and to promote differentiation (Pietenpol et al., 1990; Freytag et al., 1990). c-Myc's ability to activate transcription is dependent upon its heterodimerisation with the Max protein (Amati et al., 1992; Kretzner et al., 1992). However, heterodimers of Max and Mad repress transcription from the same target promoters (Ayer et al., 1993; 1995). Therefore, the equilibrium between these two complexes may be a common mechanism for controlling the transcription of genes involved in differentiation (Hurlin et al., 1995). A recent study showed that HPV-16 E6 is able to enhance the normal rate of c-Myc degradation by the proteasome and, moreover, does so in an E6-AP-dependent manner (Gross-Mesilaty et al., 1998). The authors of this study were concerned by the apparent anomaly of an oncogenic virus causing the degradation of a proto-oncogene, particularly as a small number of invasive HPV-associated cancers have HPV sequences integrated such that c-Myc is induced (Couturier et al., 1991). However, since c-Myc levels must be low to allow differentiation and, presumably, to inhibit apoptosis, and since HPV absolutely requires differentiation in order to produce viable progeny virions, the acceleration of c-Myc degradation is a logical step as part of viral replication. As we have attempted to emphasise throughout this chapter, oncogenesis is an unfortunate side-effect, as destructive of the virus as it is of the host. When integration of the virus occurs, this may confer a growth advantage on the cells which harbor HPV sequences, but this is a late event during tumor development and by that stage the virus, as a replicating organism, is effectively dead.

An important point in the apoptosis pathway, downstream of the initial signalling, is the Judgement phase which forms a second major controlling point, either ameliorating or reinforcing upstream signals before the irrevocable entry into the apoptotic process (Reed, 1994; Nagata, 1997, for reviews). It has also been shown that the adenovirus E1b 19k protein can act as an anti-apoptotic member of the bcl-2 family of apoptosis control proteins (Huang et al., 1997). Since there is a tendency for a conservation of function between DNA tumor viruses, and the Bak protein is highly expressed in the upper epithelial layers where HPV replicates (Krajewski et al., 1996), it was tempting to investigate possible associations between E6 and the bcl-2 family of proteins. Indeed, HPV-18 E6 has been shown to stimulate the degradation of Bak via E6-AP and the ubiquitin pathway, resulting in a reduction of Bak protein levels in the cell (Thomas and Banks, 1998). This activity was found to correlate with a reduction in the numbers of cells entering apoptosis and an increase in the length of cell survival. The E6 protein is a very scarce protein and degradation is therefore an extremely effective method to control the levels of more abundant cellular proteins, particularly those like p53 and Bak which are not dangerous to the virus at low levels but become so when more highly expressed. In the case of Bak, unlike p53, it appears that the levels of protein within the cell are normally regulated through E6-AP and the interaction with E6 increases the rate of degradation of Bak.

Until quite recently, the only significant activity which had been described for E6-AP was its participation in the E6-mediated degradation of p53 and, as we have seen, E6-AP would normally not appear to be involved in this pathway in the absence of E6. Therefore it was very interesting when recent studies showed that point mutations in E6-AP are associated with Angelman syndrome (Kishino et al., 1997; Matsuura et al., 1997) indicating that the syndrome may be associated with abnormality in ubiquitin-mediated degradation during brain development. Given the importance of apoptosis in development and the fact that Bak is found at high levels in the frontal cortex (Krajewski et al., 1996), it is tempting to speculate that the association between E6-AP and Bak may partly explain the biochemical basis of this serious developmental disease.

E6 AND DLG

During this discussion we have tried to emphasise the importance of epidermal differentiation in the life cycle of the virus. It was therefore particularly interesting when recent studies showed an interaction between E6 proteins and hDlg/SAP97 (DLG) protein (Lee et al., 1997; Kiyono et al., 1997). This protein is a PDZ domain-containing protein and is the mammalian homologue of the Drosophila discs large protein (dlg). The PDZ domains recruit plasma membrane and cytoskeletal proteins to regions of cell-cell contact; PDZ-containing proteins, such as DLG also possess other protein motifs, such as SH3 domains, through which they may mediate association between cytoskeletal and signalling molecules. Thus it is thought that they may function as components of signal transduction pathways, transmitting growth inhibitory signals from regions of cell-cell contact to downstream effectors and may act to block cell proliferation and migration, in a temporally defined manner (Goode and Perrimon, 1997). Drosophila null for dlg exhibit aberrant organisation of the cytoskeleton and, most interestingly, their columnar epithelial cells are altered to an apolar morphology. Lee et al (1997) found that DLG is bound by a number of viral oncogenes, including adenovirus 9ORF1, HTLV-1 Tax and HPV-18 E6, via consensus PDZ binding motifs. A mutational analysis of the DLG protein has shown that the role of DLG in maintaining cell polarity is separable from its role in controlling cellular proliferation (Woods et al., 1996). It seems clear that it would be of advantage for HPV replication to increase proliferation without losing polarity, however, recent work indicates that the binding of E6 to DLG results in its degradation (Gardiol et al.,1999) which obviously ablates both functions. The binding site for DLG is at the extreme carboxy terminus of E6; mutations within this region abolish degradation of DLG but the ability of E6 to degrade p53 is retained, indicating that quite different pathways are involved. In addition, low risk HPV E6 proteins lack this binding motif, and are incapable of degrading DLG (Gardiol et al., 1999). Interestingly, the association with DLG and the adenovirus 9ORF1 protein results in DLG forming insoluble aggregates (R. Javier, personal communication). Thus, once again, there is a fascinating conservation of function between the DNA tumor viruses, yet the precise pathways by which the activities are mediated are different.

E6 AND PAXILLIN

In view of E6's ability to bind and degrade DLG, it is also interesting that BPV-1 E6 and HPV-16 E6 have been shown to interact with paxillin (Tong and Howley, 1997). Paxillin is a protein which is involved in signal transduction of messages from the plasma membrane to focal adhesions and to the actin cytoskeleton. Paxillin is activated by tyrosine phosphorylation in response to a number of stimuli, including treatment with growth factors (Rankin and Rosengurt, 1994). The cytoskeleton is also important in the cell cycle and in response to cell-cell contact (Ridley, 1995, for review), presumably at least partly through the mediation of paxillin. In BPV E6-expressing cells the focal adhesions are morphologically normal and the tyrosine phosphorylation of paxillin is unaffected, but the actin cytoskeleton is completely disrupted, apparently in an E6 dose-dependent manner (Tong and Howley, 1997). Mutational analysis of E6 showed that this actin disruption correlates with the ability to bind to paxillin, and with the trans-forming activity of the mutant. This correlation with transforming ability is further confirmed by the finding that the oncogenic HPV-16 E6 can bind paxillin, at least in vitro, but the E6 proteins of the non-oncogenic HPV types 6 and 11 cannot. Presumably the disruption of the actin cytoskeleton and the consequent interference with signal transduction releases the cell from certain cell cycle controls and prevents the growth inhibition caused, for example, by cell-cell contact. It is not yet clear how E6 causes this effect, since the interaction with paxillin does not appear to result in its degradation nor in any change to its tyrosine phosphorylation.

MCM BINDING BY E6

During cellular DNA replication a complex of proteins known as the licensing system binds to each origin of replication before the G1/S transition. The presence of the licensing system complex is essential to allow the initiation from that origin and it is displaced during DNA replication, thus preventing a second initiation of replication (Thommes and Blow, 1997, for review). The MCM family of proteins has at least six members, all of which are involved in the formation of the replication licensing system (Thommes et al., 1997). Thus it was extremely interesting that a yeast two-hybrid assay identified hCDC47, an MCM protein, as a potential target for HPV-16 E6 binding (Fujita et al., 1996). Two other yeast two-hybrid screens also identifed MCM7 as a target of the E6 proteins derived from both benign and oncogenic HPV types (Kukimoto et al., 1998; Kühne and Banks, 1998), indicating that this interaction is related to the normal DNA replication requirements of the virus. Although the biological consequences of this interaction remain to be determined, it is conceivable that, by disturbing the normal function of the licensing system, E6 could increase the rate of cellular, and hence, viral DNA replication. Alternatively, E6 could relocate the licensing factor from cellular to viral origins of replication; this might be partly responsible for the massive increase in episomal numbers in infected cells as they begin to differentiate. It is also possible that the disturbance of the replication licensing system might contribute to the chromosomal instability seen in long term E6-expressing cells (White et al., 1994 ; Kaufmann et al.,1997).

E6 BINDING MOTIFS

It is clear that HPV E6 proteins are capable of interacting with a large number of cellular proteins; the question which arises is: how? This has been partly answered by a recent study which has identified a conserved E6-binding motif in several of the protein targets of E6 (Elston et al., 1998). This motif is **E/D-L/I/F-L/V-G** (ELLG, for convenience), together with an upstream requirement for hydrophobic residues. Such motifs have been identified within the previously defined 18-amino acid E6 binding domain in E6-AP (Huibregtse et al., 1993b) and in the E6BP protein sequence. Similar motifs are also present within the PDZ domain of DLG (Lee et al., 1997) and in the C-terminal E6-binding domain of Bak (Thomas and Banks, 1998) and MCM7 (Kühne and Banks, 1998). An additional study has indicated that the structure of this motif, an alpha helix, is vital to the integrity of binding through this region (Chen et al., 1998). Thus it appears that the interaction of E6 with various cellular proteins may occur through a similar mechanism. The conservation of this motif implies that it has some functional significance for the proteins which possess it; it also implies very strongly that it is a fairly widespread sequence and thus the ability of E6 to bind to a protein in vitro does not necessarily mean that it will do so in vivo.

The range of cellular proteins to which E6 is reported to bind is continually increasing; and the question which arises is, under what circumstances, if at all, do these interactions take place in the infected cell?. As we have pointed out, the induction of degradation, as in the cases of p53, c-Myc, Bak, and DLG seems to be a logical method for a protein in low abundance to decrease the amounts of more highly abundant control proteins, thus disabling potentially harmful cellular activities, or inducing conditions which are more favourable to viral replication. However, during infection the levels of E6 protein produced are very low and it is clear that E6 would in no way be capable of binding all its putative targets simultaneously. It is possible that the differentiation state of the cell may dictate which cellular proteins are targeted by E6, as might post translational modifications of E6 itself. During differentiation it is unlikely that all the target proteins of E6 will be simultaneously available, hence this alone would provide a degree of specificity for these interactions. Another scenario is also possible: the immediately apparent effect of E6 activity upon p53, Myc or Bak is degradation of the protein. However, from the homeostatic point of view, what actually occurs is an alteration in the equilibria, of p53 with mdm2, of Myc with Max and Mad and of Bak with bcl-XL, in favour of survival. It is conceivable that the binding of E6 to its cellular targets, however transiently, is sufficient to alter various equilibria in favour of survival and cell cycle progression. An accumulation of small changes in key biochemical equilibria might lead to the observed effects of E6 upon the cell. In addition, the extreme carboxy terminal region of E6 has a consensus recognition motif for cAMP-directed protein kinase A (PKA) phosphorylation (Kühne et al., submitted for publication). Interestingly, this lies immediately within the core PDZ-binding domain which is involved in the interaction with DLG and possibly with other PDZ domain containing proteins. In the case of the K+ channel Kir2.3 binding to PSD-95 (a PDZ containing protein) the C terminal serine of Kir2.3 is critical for the interaction. This serine residue is a substrate for PKA phosphorylation which negatively regulates the association with PSD-95

(Cohen et al., 1996). Thus, by analogy, phosphorylation at the equivalent site within E6 could negatively regulate the ability of E6 to interact with DLG. Therefore, post translational modifications of E6 will probably be found to be involved in directing the specificity of the E6 proteins during viral replication and transformation.

The E6* Proteins

Although this chapter is intended to discuss the function of the viral oncoproteins, it is necessary at this stage to diverge somewhat and address the E6* family of proteins. As will be seen from the following discussion, these proteins have no intrinsic transforming activity, yet recent studies suggest that they may play an important role in regulating the activity of E6 during both viral replication and virus-associated neoplasia. As we have said, an important point is the question of specificity, and the E6* proteins would appear to be another means of providing this with respect to the E6 protein.

The transcription patterns of HPVs in general are extremely complex and little is yet known about the controls which dictate how the viral pre-mRNAs from either early or late promoters are spliced. In general terms however, early transcripts tend to be polycistronic, encoding several viral polypeptides. In recent years the use of riboprobes on sections of infected mucosal tissue, or the use of RT-PCR in cell lines which harbor episomal HPVs, has led to accurate quantitation and mapping of viral transcripts (Bohm et al., 1993; Doorbar et al., 1990). It has became apparent that E6 and E7 are transcribed differently by the high risk and low risk mucosal HPVs (Smotkin et al., 1989). HPV-6 and 11 transcribe E6 and E7 as two separate mRNAs, whereas HPV-16 and 18 transcribe E6 as a linear transcript linked to E7, and E7 also as a transcript linked to one or more alternatively spliced E6 ORFs (Figure 3). These spliced E6 transcripts are referred to as E6*. What is striking about them is, first, that they are exclusive to the high risk mucosal HPVs, and, second, that the splice donor site is found at almost precisely the same point in all of them. There is a series of, generally four, downstream splice acceptors which all change the reading frame of the transcripts so that the E6* polypeptides terminate at the first available termination codon. Many of these downstream splice acceptors lie in sequences which are lost upon viral integration, so that in cell lines derived from cervical tumors the number of E6* species tends to be limited. It would perhaps be accurate to suggest that all the E6* mRNA species, in addition to encoding downstream polypeptides, are a means of producing a truncated E6 protein.

E6* FUNCTION

Despite the abundance of transcripts encoding E6*, the E6* proteins are elusive. The HPV-16 and 18 E6* proteins have been translated in vitro (Seedorf et al., 1987; Shalley et al., 1996; Pim et al., 1997), and the HPV-16 E6* I-IV proteins have been expressed in COS cells when driven by a heterologous promoter (Sherman and Schlegel 1996) and where they are predominantly localised to the cytoplasm. However, there is only one example of E6* protein detection in HPV transformed cells, when cervical tumor cells containing HPV-18 sequences were grown in nude mice (Schneider-Gädicke et al.,

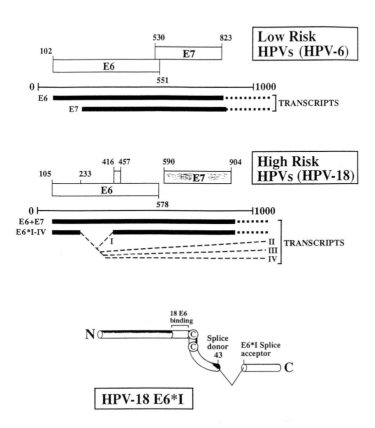

Fig. 3. *Alternative splicing of the E6-E7 mRNA transcripts. A schematic diagram showing the differences in the transcription of the E6 and E7 genes between high and low risk viruses. The low risk HPV genes are transcribed linearly while the high risk HPV genes are spliced, resulting in at least five different mRNA species. A schematic diagram shows the structure of one of the alternatively spliced protein products, the HPV-18 E6*I, together with the region of the protein involved in binding to full-length HPV-18 E6. The first 43 amino acid residues of HPV-18 E6*I are identical to those of the full-length protein while the remaining 12 residues come from the alternative splicing into a different reading frame.*

1988). The difficulty in detecting E6* protein implies that either translation of the protein is strictly controlled, or it has an extremely short half-life. When translated in vitro HPV-16 E6* proteins are generally unstable (Shalley et al., 1996; D. Pim, personal observations), which suggests that E6* proteins are probably turned over extremely rapidly in vivo. It has been suggested that E6* proteins have no intrinsic role and that the existence of the splice functions to facilitate translation of other encoded transcripts such as E7 (Sedman et al., 1991). However, other studies have shown that E7 is translated with equal efficiency from spliced and unspliced transcripts (Stacey et al., 1995). In addition, mutation of the splice donor site within the E6 open reading frame does not decrease the level of PCNA induced by E7 in differentiating keratinocytes, suggesting indirectly that E7 levels are not affected by this splicing event (Cheng et al., 1995). One of the first studies to show that E6* may have a function came from Shalley et al., (1996) who showed that in vitro translated HPV-16 E6* can inhibit the E6-directed, ubiquitin-mediated degradation of p53 in vitro. This important observation was followed by the demonstration that HPV-18 E6*I can inhibit E6 mediated degradation of p53 both in vitro and in vivo (Pim et al., 1997). In transient assays in p53-null cells, the degradation of exogenous p53 in the presence of HPV-18 E6 was inhibited upon co-expression of HPV-18 E6*I. E6* overexpression also causes an upregulation of p53 responsive promoters in the E6-expressing CaSKi and HeLa cell lines, leading to a reduction in cell proliferation (Pim et al., 1997). In contrast, E6* overexpression in cells lacking either wild-type p53 or HPV E6 sequences has no significant effect on cell proliferation. An explanation for this activity of E6* was provided by the demonstration that HPV-18 E6*I binds both to in vitro translated E6-AP, the cellular ubiquitin ligase involved in E6-directed p53 degradation, and to full-length E6 protein, but not to p53 itself. Mutational analysis of HPV-18 E6*I has shown that, although the binding sites for E6-AP and E6 partially overlap, the antiproliferative effects of E6* appear to correlate with its ability to interact with the full length E6 protein (Pim and Banks, 1999). Whether the association between E6* and E6-AP has a biological function remains to be determined.

These studies suggest that one of the functions of E6* involves the modulation of the interaction between p53 and the full-length E6 protein. This might be an important factor during the viral life-cycle since the inhibition of the apoptotic function of p53 by E6 is thought to pre-dispose HPV-infected cells to the subsequent genetic changes which can lead to immortalisation. Therefore in terms of inhibition of p53 degradation, E6* might be considered to function as a kind of 'fail safe' to reduce the risk of immortalisation. E6* proteins are likely to have an important role during the viral life cycle and, although most of the work to date has focussed on their effects on the E6-p53 interaction, it is possible that they may also affect E6's interaction with other cellular targets.

The HPV E7 Protein

As is the case with the E6 proteins, E7 is also retained and expressed in cervical tumors and in cell lines derived from them (Smotkin and Wettstein, 1986; Seedorf et al., 1987). In addition, inhibition of E7 function, either by blocking expression (von Knebel Doeberitz et al., 1988; Crook et al., 1989; Alvarez-Sales et al., 1998) or the use of single chain antibodies (Wang-Johanning et al., 1998) results in a cessation of transformed cell growth. Therefore E7 also represents an ideal target for potential therapeutic intervention.

The E7 proteins from all the HPV types are small, highly conserved, multifunctional proteins, of approximately 100 amino acids. They have a zinc-binding cysteine loop towards the C-terminus (Barbosa et al., 1989; McIntyre et al., 1993), which is remarkably similar to the cysteine loop within E6, suggesting that there may have been a gene duplication at some stage of viral evolution (Cole and Danos, 1987). This cysteine loop structure also contributes to the ability of the E7 protein to form homodimers (McIntyre et al., 1993; Zwerschke et al., 1996). The E7 protein is normally phosphorylated (Smotkin and Wettstein, 1987) and has been found in a variety of locations within the cell, including the cytoplasm (Smotkin and Wettstein, 1987), nucleus (Sato et al., 1989a; Greenfield et al., 1991) and nucleoli (Zatsepina et al., 1997). An intriguing possibility is that shuttling of E7 between these different parts of the cell may be related to cell differentiation and/or post translational modification of the E7 protein. Phosphorylation of E7 is largely by casein kinase II (CKII) (Barbosa et al., 1990), which interestingly, has also been reported to be more active in keratinocytes (Hashida and Yasumoto, 1990).

HPV E7 shares homology with Adenovirus E1a and SV40 large T antigen, and has been shown to interact with many of the same cellular targets, such as cyclin A, cyclin E, the AP-1 family of transcription factors, and members of the 'pocket protein' family such as pRb, p107 and p130 (Tommasino et al., 1993; McIntyre et al., 1996; Antinore et al., 1996; Davies et al., 1993; Dyson et al., 1989; Dyson et al., 1992). It will become apparent that, as a consequence of these interactions, E7 function is intimately linked to deregulation of the normal cell cycle. Several studies have shown that E7 expression in keratinocytes results in a substantial increase in DNA synthesis without inducing a marked alteration in the normal pattern of keratinocyte differentiation (Blanton et al., 1992; Cheng et al., 1995). Therefore E7 has, to some extent, uncoupled DNA synthesis from differentiation in these cells. In an attempt to explain how E7 can achieve this uncoupling, we will, in the following pages, examine interactions between E7 and the cellular proteins which regulate the cell division cycle.

A summary of the major functional domains of the HPV-16 E7 protein, together with some of the important sites of protein interactions, is shown in Figure 4.

'POCKET PROTEIN' INTERACTIONS OF E7

The first cellular target of E7 to be identified was the pRb tumor suppressor protein (Dyson et al., 1989). These studies were mainly driven by the observation that residues within the region of Adenovirus E1a necessary for binding pRb were also largely conserved within the HPV-16 E7 protein (Figure 4). The demonstration that E7 could interact with pRb was particularly exciting, since pRb had been shown to play a vital role in the control of the cell cycle (Buchkovich et al., 1989; DeCaprio et al., 1989). The E7 proteins derived from HPV-16 and HPV-18 exhibit stronger interaction with pRb than E7 proteins derived from HPV-6 and HPV-11 (Münger et al., 1989b), and this may account, in part, for differences in their respective transforming activities. The interac-

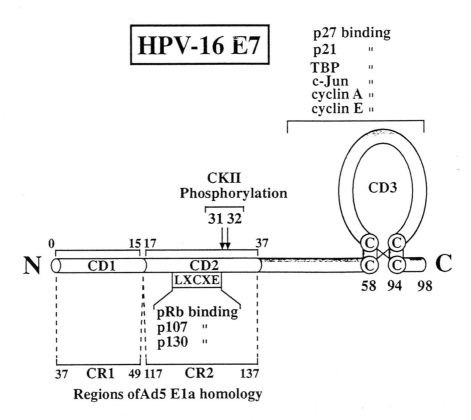

Fig. 4. The E7 protein. A schematic diagram showing the structure of the E7 protein, together with its regions of homology with the adenovirus 5 E1a protein and the regions of the protein involved in interactions with cellular proteins.

tion occurs primarily with the active, underphosphorylated form of pRb (Imai et al., 1991), and it is interesting to note that this is the form of pRb predominantly found in differentiating keratinocytes (Nead et al., 1998) and which is bound to the E2F family of proteins (Chellappan et al., 1991). As a consequence of the interaction between E7 and pRb, the transcriptionally active proteins of the E2F family are released from pRb (Chellappan et al., 1992; Pagano et al., 1992; Morris et al., 1993).

The E7 proteins bind to the 'pocket domain' of pRb encompassing residues 394-571 and 649-772 (Hu et al., 1990; Kaelin et al., 1990) and mutations in this region of pRb are found in many tumors. Interestingly, this is not the case in cervical tumors (Scheffner et al., 1991) suggesting that E7 function with respect to pRb is analogous to an inactivating mutation. The region of E7 which binds to pRb lies between residues 20-30. The principal element consists of the "LXCXE" motif which is sufficient for binding to pRb (Münger et al., 1989b; Dyson et al., 1992) and recent studies have defined the crystal structure of a nine-residue E7 peptide containing the "LXCXE" motif bound to the retinoblastoma pocket (Lee et al., 1998). However, binding of the conserved domain 2 (CD2) of E7 to pRb is, alone, insufficient for both the release of free E2F and inhibition of pRb DNA binding activity (Jones et al 1990; 1992). Indeed, sequences within the carboxy terminal half of E7 appear to be required for high affinity binding to pRb, resulting in a release of free E2F (Huang et al., 1993; Patrick et al., 1994) which then upregulates a variety of genes involved in cell-cycle control and DNA synthesis (Phelps et al., 1991; Bandara et al., 1991). These include DNA polymerase α (Pol α), thymidine kinase (TK) and dihydrofolate reductase (DHFR) (Nevins, 1992 for review). Proliferating cell nuclear antigen (PCNA) is also upregulated in an E7 dependent manner (Cheng et al., 1995) but it is not clear at present whether this is a direct result of transcriptional activation by E2F or by another protein (Huang and Prystowsky, 1996).

HPV-16 E7 expression alone will stimulate DNA replication in growth-arrested rodent cells in the absence of any additional stimuli (Sato et al., 1989b; Banks et al., 1990), and this activity correlates with the ability of E7 to bind pRb (Banks et al., 1990) and release E2F (Pagano et al., 1992; Morris et al., 1993). Interestingly, as was mentioned previously, HPV-16 E7 induction of DNA synthesis in quiescent cells can be stimulated by certain growth factors (Morris et al., 1993), and this is the most likely explanation for the reported cooperativity between E5 and E7. It has also been shown that E7 can overcome the G1 cell-cycle arrest induced by either growth factor withdrawal or DNA damage (Demers et al., 1994; Hickman et al., 1994; Slebos et al., 1994), thus suggesting that E7 can independently overcome one aspect of p53 function, although unlike E6, it does not inhibit p53 induced apoptosis.

Mutations made in the pRb-binding domain of HPV-16 E7 destroy the transforming activity of the protein in a variety of assay systems (Edmonds and Vousden, 1989; Watanabe et al., 1990; Barbosa et al., 1990; Banks et al., 1990), yet they do not affect the ability of E7 to cooperate with E6 in immortalising primary human keratinocytes (Jewers et al., 1992). The cotton tail rabbit papillomavirus (CRPV) E7 protein also interacts with pRb in a manner similar to that of HPV-16 E7 (Haskell et al., 1993), and mutational analysis of CRPV E7 also indicates that viruses which have been mutated such that E7 no longer binds pRb, nonetheless induce wart formation in the infected rabbits (Defeo-Jones et al., 1993). In addition, the interaction of HPV-16 E7 with pRb, and the subsequent induction of DNA synthesis, were found to be insufficient for efficient transformation of NIH3T3 cells (Banks et al., 1990). Thus mutations in other regions of E7, particularly in the extreme amino terminus of the protein (CD1), lead to a loss or reduction of transforming ability even while retaining wild type levels of interaction with pRb (Banks et al., 1990; Barbosa et al., 1990; Watanabe et al., 1990). Taken together, these observations demonstrate that, although the pRb interaction is vital for a number of E7's activities, interactions with other cellular proteins play a part in E7 function, and these will be discussed below.

Prevailing views on cell-cycle control suggest that members of the pocket protein family control cell cycle progression, not merely by sequestering members of the E2F family of transcription factors, but by actively suppressing the transcription of genes required for the G1 to S-phase transition (Nevins, 1992). Two recent reports suggest that when cells are still in the G1 phase of the cell cycle, pRb actively represses genes required during G2 by recruiting a histone deacetylase (HDAC1) (Brehm et al., 1998; Magnaghi-Jaulin et al., 1998). Thus, G2 phase specific E2F1 responsive promoters are suppressed during G1 by the E2F:pRb:HDAC1 complex at the promoter. Although the mechanism of action is not clear it is thought that HDAC1 might convert surrounding chromatin from a transcriptionally active (hyperacetylated) to a transcriptionally re-pressed (hypoacetylated) state. Most interestingly, HPV-16 E7 was shown to be capable of disrupting this complex (Brehm et al., 1998). This suggests that stimulation of E2F responsive promoters by HPV E7 is not solely due to the release of free E2F, but that removal of HDAC1 from the vicinity of the promoter may also be required. Recent studies have also demonstrated that the other two members of the pocket protein family, p107 and p130, also recruit histone de-acetylases to suppress E2F transcription (Ferreira et al., 1998), and it will be particularly interesting to determine whether E7 also has a role in these complexes.

Recent observations suggest that there is an additional consequence of the interac-tion between the HPV-16 E7 protein and pRb. Using recombinant retroviruses for ex-pressing HPV-16 E7 in human keratinocytes, it was found that expression of E7 pro-duced a reduction in pRb levels, suggesting that E7 could in some way lead to a de-stabilization of the pRb protein (Demers et al., 1994). In support of this, Wazer et al., (1995) also demonstrated that, in E7 immortalised human mammary epithelial cells, the pRb protein levels were reduced even though pRb mRNA levels remained constant. Subsequently it has been shown in both mammary epithelial cells and human keratino-cytes that E7 induces the degradation of pRb, and also possibly p107, through the ubiq-uitin proteasome pathway (Boyer et al., 1996; Jones and Munger, 1997; Jones et al., 1997a). Although the mechanism by which this takes place has not been defined, it is interesting to note that E7 has been reported to interact with S4 subunit of the 26S pro-teasome (Berezutskaya and Bagchi, 1997) and, as a consequence, increases the ATPase activity of S4 enzyme, which is involved in the assembly of the 26S proteasome. There-fore it would appear that E7 links directly to the proteasome, and it may be through this route that pRb destabilisation is attained. It is also intriguing that the region of E7 which is involved in the complex formation with S4 is also required for the release of E2F from pRb (Patrick et al., 1994). Whether the two observations are directly connected remains to be determined.

As well as binding pRb, the oncogenic HPV E7 proteins also form complexes with two other pocket proteins, p130 and p107 (Dyson et al., 1992). Both proteins are also involved in the regulation of cell cycle progression and interact with the E2F family of proteins in a manner similar to pRb (Dyson et al., 1992; Schwarz et al., 1993; Cobrinik et al., 1993). Since the region of E7 which interacts with p107 and p130 is very similar to that which binds pRb, it has been very difficult to perform mutational analyses on the E7 protein in order to determine which interactions are relevant for the transforming activity of E7, although the indications are that pRb binding is more important for cell transformation than the interaction with p107 (Davies et al., 1993). This may not be too surprising since there is no evidence that p107 is a tumor suppressor protein.

An interesting aspect of the E7-p107 interaction is that this forms part of the cyclin-cdk complex (see below), which can be found during G1/S phase transition or S phase, depending on whether cyclin E or cyclin A is part of the complex. Unlike the situation with pRb, the association between E7 and p107 does not dissociate E2F (Arroyo et al., 1993; Lam et al., 1994). In addition, p107 is one of the targets of the associated kinase activity found within these complexes, suggesting that altered phosphorylation of p107 may be one of the mechanisms by which E7 may alter p107 function.

INTERACTION OF E7 WITH P21 AND P27

As we have already noted, one of the most important questions is how E7 can promote DNA synthesis while maintaining keratinocyte differentiation. A clue as to how this might be achieved came from reports demonstrating how E7 proteins can affect the function of the cyclin/cdk2 inhibitors. We have already seen how degradation of p53 may result in lower levels of p21 protein, yet this is only part of the story. Serum withdrawal or loss of cell adhesion are often accompanied by increased levels of p27 and both antiproliferative states can be overcome by E7. In addition, both p27 and p21 are transiently upregulated during keratinocyte differentiation and this is independent of p53 (Missero et al., 1996). Most interestingly, E7 expression antagonises the ability of p27 to inhibit cyclin E associated kinase activity and, in addition, E7 can overcome p27 inhibition of cyclin A gene expression (Zerfass-Thome et al., 1996). These activities of E7 correlate with its ability to interact with p27 through sequences in the carboxy terminal half of the E7 protein (Zerfass-Thome et al., 1996). A similar interaction also seems to take place with respect to p21. Induction of p21 protein can occur in response to DNA damage in a p53-dependent manner (El-Deiry et al., 1993) or, as mentioned above, in a p53-independent manner (Missero et al., 1995; Butz et al., 1998) in response to TGF-β or other differentiation related signals. A number of studies have demonstrated that when p21 is induced it can inhibit both cdk2/cyclin activity and PCNA-dependent DNA replication, by binding both to cyclin/cdk complexes and to PCNA via two separate domains (Chen et al., 1995; Luo et al., 1995). Interestingly, it has been shown that HPV-16 E7 expression blocks p21-mediated growth arrest in vivo, despite there being high levels of p21 protein after induction of DNA-damage. This activity of E7 appears to be mediated by preventing p21 inhibition of cyclin E/cdk2 activity and blocking p21 inhibition of PCNA-dependent DNA replication (Funk et al., 1997; Jones et al., 1997b). Both reports showed that the HPV-16 E7 protein exerts this inhibitory activity by binding directly to p21 protein. It was also found that HPV-6 E7 can bind to p21, but less strongly than HPV-16 E7. This might explain why the E7 proteins derived from the low risk group of HPVs have a much reduced ability to relieve p21-mediated cell-cycle arrest in vivo (Demers et al., 1994).

It should be clear at this stage that there is an apparent complementarity between the ability of E7 to block p53-independent p21 function and the ability of E6 to inhibit p53-dependent p21 function. The most likely explanation for this is that E7 has to overcome p21 activity for effective entry into the cell cycle, whereas E6 is probably targeting the apoptotic functions of p53; the apparent inhibition of p21 expression is simply a by-product of the E6 mediated degradation of p53.

INTERACTION OF E7 WITH CYCLINS AND CYCLIN/CDK COMPLEXES

As well as inhibiting the function of cyclin/cdk inhibitors, E7 has also been shown to sequentially activate both the cyclin E and the cyclin A promoters (Zerfass et al., 1995). Using BRK cells transformed with EJ-ras and HPV-16 E7 under the control of an inducible promoter they showed that E7 expression led to an increase in the levels of cyclins E and A, but not cyclin D1. Increased levels of cyclin E expression required sequences within the CD2 domain of E7, and this is probably related to the ability of E7 to bind pRb and release transcriptionally active E2F. In contrast, cyclin A upregulation required additional protein synthesis (other than that of cyclin E) and furthermore, sequences in both CD1 and CD2 domains of E7 were also necessary. This is an interesting observation, since it has been demonstrated that E7 mutants disrupted in the CD1 domain are defective for transformation (Banks et al., 1990; Watanabe et al., 1990) yet have wild type levels of pRb binding activity. Thus although cyclin A upregulation may be somewhat dependent on cyclin E expression, it is interesting to note that in serum starved cells, where cyclin E levels are low, E7 expression alone can lead to upregulation of the cyclin A promoter, suggesting the existence of at least two routes by which E7 can exert its activity. It is also clear that the increases in the levels of both cyclins are associated with increases in their associated kinase activities. The situation is made even more complex by observations which show that E7 can become associated both with the S-phase-specific E2F/cyclin A/p107/cdk2 complex (Arroyo et al., 1993) and the G1-specific E2F/cyclin E/p107/cdk2 complex (McIntyre et al., 1996). The first study shows that, unlike Adenovirus E1a, which dissociates the cyclin A complex to release free E2F, E7 does not dissociate the complex but becomes part of it (Arroyo et al., 1993). This appears consistent with the requirement of Adenovirus for free E2F to transactivate its own E2 gene, whereas no such requirement exists for HPVs. Interestingly, b-myb which is regulated by S-phase specific p107/cyclin A/E2F complexes, was found to be constitutively activated in E7 expressing cells (Lam et al., 1994), which is probably a consequence of E7's overriding the cell cycle control of this complex. Although it has been demonstrated that E7 can bind directly to cyclin A (Tommasino et al., 1993), it is difficult to rule out the possibility that E7 interacts with this complex via p107. As with so many of these associations, the non-oncogenic HPV-6 E7 protein fails to demonstrate any significant degree of association with the E2F/cyclin A/p107/cdk2 complex. In the case of the G1-specific E2F/cyclin E/p107/cdk2 complex, no direct interaction between E7 and cyclin E was observed, again suggesting that the interaction occurs via p107.

INTERACTION OF E7 WITH ELEMENTS OF THE CELLULAR TRANSCRIPTIONAL MACHINERY

Although the principal transcriptional activity that has been associated with E7 is related to its ability to induce E2F transcriptional activation, E7 also possesses intrinsic transcriptional activities independent of pRb binding (Zwerschke et al., 1996). As part of a series of studies to investigate such activities it was found that E7 could bind to the core component of the TFIID transcription factor complex, the TATA Box Binding Protein (TBP) (Massimi et al., 1996) and to a TBP associated factor (TAF), TAF110 (Mazzerelli et al., 1995). Most interestingly, the association with TBP appears to be regulated by CKII phosphorylation of the E7 protein. Previous studies had shown that mutants of

E7 defective for CKII phosphorylation were reduced in their ability to transform cells, although no explanation was then available for these observations (Barbosa et al., 1990; Banks et al., 1990). The phosphorylation of the E7 protein by CKII occurs on serine residues at positions 31 and 32 (Barbosa et al., 1990), however the basic interaction with TBP appears to be mediated by a domain in the cysteine loop of E7. Mutational analysis of the E7 within the cysteine loop identified a region responsible for the basic E7-TBP interaction, and mutations within this region result in a significantly reduced level of transforming activity (Massimi et al., 1997). These observations indicate that the interaction between E7 and TBP may alter the transcriptional levels of genes involved in transformation other than those which are up-regulated by E2F. An alternative possibility is that the TBP interaction plays a role in the activation of promoters by p107-E2F-E7 complexes, since E7 has also been found in these complexes at the appropriate E2F-driven promoters (Arroyo et al., 1993).

A point which we have attempted to emphasise throughout the chapter is the provision of specificity to the viral protein-cellular protein interactions. As should be apparent, E7 also has a very large number of cellular targets, and it is unlikely that all could be bound simultaneously. Therefore the finding that the interaction between E7 and TBP can be regulated by CKII phosphorylation of E7 is extremely encouraging. This means that only when E7 is phosphorylated will it form an effective complex with TBP, freeing non-phosphorylated E7 for other roles. Indeed, recent studies indicate that E7 may be differentially phosphorylated by CKII during the cell cycle (Massimi and Banks, in press), suggesting that there is a specific window when E7 will effectively bind TBP. Thus, by analogy with E6 and PKA phosphorylation, CKII may also provide specificity to E7 function.

As well as being associated with the basal elements of the cellular transcriptional machinery, E7 has also been reported to interact with the AP-1 family of transcription factors. It has been shown that HPV-16 E7 can bind c-Jun, JunB, JunD and c-Fos in vitro, and the interaction between E7 and c-Jun has also been shown in vivo by coprecipitation experiments and the yeast two-hybrid assay (Antinore et al, 1996). This study also demonstrated that mutations in the zinc-binding CD3 domain, but not in the pRb-binding pocket of E7, abolished the interaction with c-Jun. One of the consequences of this interaction would appear to be the upregulation of c-Jun responsive promoters (Antinore et al., 1996). This is particularly interesting in the light of the induction of c-Fos and c-Jun expression by the HPV E5 proteins, and the subsequent cooperation between E5 and E7 in mitogenesis. The relevance of the E7-c-Jun interaction for E7 mediated transformation was demonstrated indirectly by the use of dominant negative c-Jun. This effectively abolished cooperation between E7 and EJ-ras in primary rodent cell transformation assays (Antinore et al., 1996), and recent studies have shown that expression of dominant negative c-Jun in HPV transformed keratinocytes can suppress the anchorage independent growth of these cells (Li et al., 1998). These studies therefore indicate that upregulation of c-Jun responsive promoters by HPV-16 E7 contributes to the transforming potential of the protein.

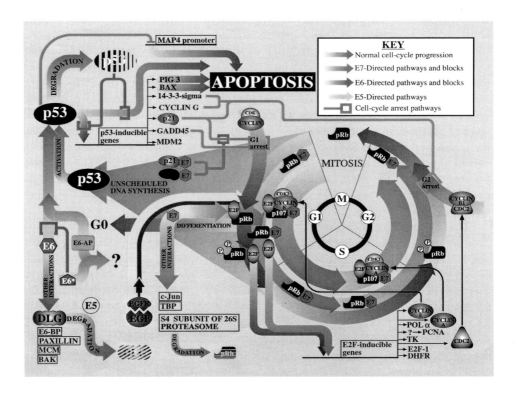

Fig. 5. The E5, E6 and E7 proteins act in a complementary fashion to drive the cell through the cell cycle, to override cell cycle arrest, and to prevent the induction of apoptosis.

Synergism between E5, E6 and E7

From the above discussion it is clear that the viral oncoproteins have very diverse effects upon the pathways regulating cell growth and diferentiation. Figure 5 shows a schematic diagram of how these different pathways might interconnect, since it is through these connections that efficient viral replication is obtained. The fundamental nature of the pathways which are being perturbed offers a clear explanation of why these viruses are associated with the development of a number of human tumors.

Perhaps the most critical phase of the cell cycle is that of G1. It is the phase through which cells have to pass on either entering or exiting the cell cycle. In addition, many of the restriction points regulated by the pocket proteins and cdk inhibitors also lie within this phase of the cell cycle. Therefore it is not surprising that the majority of the pathways through which the viral oncoproteins exert their activities converge at this point in the cell cycle. The E5 protein in particular, by effectively amplifying the normally diminishing cellular response to mitogenic signalling, contributes to 'restarting' the cell cycle through AP-1 transcriptional regulators, which may also additionally upregulate the HPV E6 and E7 genes. The E7 protein overrides the normal cell cycle controls through its interactions with the cell cycle machinery, resulting in an upregulation of the genes required for the transition into S phase. In so doing, despite the presence of signals for cellular differentiation, this E7-directed induction of unscheduled DNA synthesis provokes a p53 mediated apoptotic response. Although E6 clearly has additional roles, the most well-characterised is its ability to abrogate this p53-mediated apoptotic response by inducing the ubiquitin-mediated degradation of p53. At later stages during keratinocyte differentiation, when Bak protein levels increase, E6 may also block this apoptotic pathway by decreasing the stability of the Bak protein. Perturbing these complex pathways of regulation is dangerous, and it is not surprising that this process may on occasion break down, with fatal consequences for both virus and host.

Although this array of interactions and pathways is somewhat daunting, from the point of view of dissecting out the role of each individual interaction during viral replication and/or transformation, it does offer some hope for an effective form of therapeutic intervention. The fact that the molecular basis behind many of these interactions is constantly being more accurately defined should allow the specific targeting of some of these viral protein-cellular protein interactions. Needless to say, papillomaviruses will also continue to teach us a great deal about the processes which regulate normal and malignant cell proliferation.

Acknowledgements

We would like to thank Christian Kühne for comments on the manuscript and we gratefully acknowledge the research support provided by the European Union BioMed 2 program and the Associazione Italiana per la Ricerca sul Cancro.

References

Agarwal, M. L., Agarwal, A., Taylor, W. R. and Stark, G. R. (1995). p53 controls both the G2/M and the G1 cell cycle checkpoints and mediates reversible growth arrest in human fibroblasts. Proc. Natl. Acad. Sci USA, 92, 8493-8497.

Alvarez-Salas, L. M., Cullinan, A. E., Siwkowski, A., Hampel, A. and DiPaolo, J. A. (1998). Inhibition of HPV-16 E6/E7 immortalisation of normal keratinocytes by hairpin ribozymes. Proc. Natl. Acad. Sci. USA., 95, 1189-1194.

Amati, B., Dalton, S., Brooks, M., Littlewood, T., Evan, G. and Land, H. (1992). Transcriptional activation by the human c-Myc oncoprotein in yeast requires interaction with Max. Nature, 359, 423-426.

An, W., Kanekal, M., Simon, C., Maltepe, E., Blagosklonny, M and Neckers, L. (1998). Stabilisation of wild type p53 by hypoxia-inducible factor 1α. Nature, 392, 405-408.

Andresson, T., Sparkowski, J., Goldstein, D. J. and Schlegel, R. (1995). Vacuolar H(+)- ATPase mutants transform cells and define a binding site for the papillomavirus E5 oncoprotein. J. Biol. Chem., 270, 6830-6837.

Androphy, E., Schiller, J. and Lowy, D. (1985). Identification of the protein encoded by the E6 transforming gene of bovine papillomavirus. Science, 230, 442-445

Androphy, E., Hubbert, N., Schiller, J. and Lowy, D. (1987). Identification of the HPV 16 E6 protein from transformed mouse cells and human cervical carcinoma cells. EMBO J., 6, 989-992.

Antinore, M., Birrer, M., Patel, D., Nader, L., and McCance, J. (1996). The human papillomavirus type 16 E7 gene product interacts with and trans-activates the AP-1 family of transcription factors. EMBO J. 15, 1950-1960.

Arroyo, M., Bagchi, S., and Raychaudhuri, P. (1993). Association of the human papillomavirus type 16 E7 protein with the S-phase-specific E2F-cyclin A complex. Mol. Cell Biol., 13, 6537-6546.

Askew, D., Ashmun, R., Simmons, B and Cleveland, J. (1991). Constitutive c-myc expression in an IL-3-dependent myeloid cell line suppresses cell cycle arrest and accelerates apoptosis. Oncogene, 6, 1915-1922.

Ayer, D., Kretzner, L and Eisenman, R. (1993) Mad: a heterodimeric partner for Max that antagonises Myc transcriptional activity. Cell, 72, 211-222.

Ayer, D., Lawrence, Q. and Eisenman, R. (1995). Mad-Max transcriptional repression is mediated by ternary complex formation with mammalian homologues of yeast repressor Sin3. Cell, 80, 767-776.

Band, V., Zajchowshi, D., Kulesa, V. and Sager, R. (1990). Human papillomavirus DNAs immortalise normal human mammary epithelial cells and reduce growth factor requirements. Proc. Natl. Acad. Sci. USA., 87, 463-467.

Band, V., DeCaprio, J., Delmolino, L., Kulesa, V. and Sager, R. (1991) Loss of p53 protein in human papillomavirus type 16 E6-immortalised human mammary epithelial cells. J. Virol., 65, 6671-6676

Band, V., Dalal, S., Delmolino, L. and Androphy, E. (1993). Enhanced degradation of p53 protein in HPV-6 and BPV-1 E6-immortalised human mammary epithelial cells. EMBO J., 12, 1847-1852.

Bandara, L. R., Adamczewski, J. P., Hunt, T., and LaThangue, N. B. (1991). Cyclin A and the retinoblastoma gene product complex with a common transcription factor. Nature, 352, 249-251.

Banks, L., Spence, P., Androphy, E., Hubbert, N., Matlashewski, G., Murray, A. and Crawford, L. (1987). Identification of human papillomavirus type 18 E6 polypeptide in cells derived from human cervical carcinomas. J. Gen. Virol., 68, 1351-1359.

Banks, L., Edmonds, C., and Vousden, K. H. (1990). Ability of the HPV16 E7 protein to bind RB and induce DNA synthesis is not sufficient for efficient transforming activity in NIH3T3 cells. Oncogene, 5, 1383-1389.

Barbosa, M. S. and Schlegel, R. (1989) The E6 and E7 genes of HPV-18 are sufficient for inducing two-stage in vitro transformation of human keratinocytes. Oncogene, 4, 1529-1532.

Barbosa, M. S., Lowy, D. and Schiller, J. (1989) Papillomavirus polypeptides E6 and E7 are zinc-binding proteins. J. Virol., 63, 1404-1407

Barbosa, M. S., Edmonds, C., Fisher, C., Schiller, J. T., Lowy, D. R., and Vousden, K. H. (1990). The region of the HPV E7 oncoprotein homologous to adenovirus E1a and SV40 large T antigen contains separate domains for Rb binding and casein kinase II phosphorylation. EMBO J., 9, 153-160.

Bauknecht, T., Kohler, M., Janz, I. and Pfleiderer, A. (1989). The occurrence of epidermal growth factor receptors and the characterisation of EGF-like factors in human ovarian, endometrial, cervical and breast cancer. J. Cancer Res. Clin. Oncol., 115, 193-199.

Bedell, M., Jones, K., Grossman, S. and Laimins, L. (1989). Identification of human papillomavirus type 18 transforming genes in immortalised and primary cells. J. Virol., 63, 1247-1255.

Beer-Romero, P., Glass, S. and Rolfe, M. (1997) Antisense targeting of E6AP elevates p53 in HPV-infected cells but not in normal cells. Oncogene, 14, 595-602.

Berezutskaya, E., and Bagchi, S. (1997). The human papillomavirus E7 oncoprotein functionally interacts with the S4 subunit of the 26 S proteasome. J. Biol Chem., 272, 30135-30140.

Bernard, H., Chan, S., Manos, M., Ong, C., Villa, L., Delius, H., Peyton, C., Bauer, H. and Wheeler, C. (1994) Identification and assessment of known and novel human papillomaviruses by polymerase chain reaction amplification, restriction fragment length polymorphisms, nucleotide sequence, and phylogenetic algorithms. J. Infect. Dis., 170, 1077-1085.

Blackburn, E. (1991) Structure and function of telomeres. Nature, 350, 569-573;

Blanton, R. A., Coltrera, M. D., Gown, A. M., Halbert, C. L., and McDougall, J. K. (1992). Expression of the HPV16 E7 gene generates proliferation in stratified squamous cell cultures which is independent of endogenous p53 levels. Cell Growth Diff., 3, 791-802.

Bohm, S., Wilczynsnki, S. P., Pfister, H., and Iftner, T. (1993). The predominant mRNA class in HPV16-infected genital neoplasias does not encode the E6 or the E7 protein. Int. J. Cancer, 55, 791-798.

Bouchard, C., Staller, P., Eilers, M. (1998). Control of cell proliferation by Myc. Trends Cell Biol. 8, 202-206.

Bouvard, V., Matlashewski, G., Gu, Z., Storey, A. and Banks, L. (1994). The human papillomavirus type 16 E5 gene cooperates with the E7 gene to stimulate proliferation of primary cells and increase viral gene expression. Virology, 203, 73-80.

Boyer, S. N., Wazer, D. E., and Band, V. (1996). E7 protein of human papilloma virus-16 induces degradation of retinoblastoma protein through the ubiquitin-proteasome pathway. Cancer Res., 56, 4620-4624.

Brehm, A., Miske, E., McCance, D., Reid, J., Bannister, A. and Kouzarides, T. (1998). Retinoblastoma protein recruits histone deacetylase to repress transcription. Nature, 391, 597-601.

Buchkovich, K., Duffy, L. and Harlow, E. (1989). The retinoblastoma protein is phosphorylated during specific phases of the cell cycle. Cell, 58, 1097-1105.

Butz, K., Geisen, C., Ullman, A., Zentgraf, H. and Hoppe-Seyler, F. (1998). Uncoupling of p21WAF1/CIP1/SDI1 mRNA and protein expression upon genotoxic stress. Oncogene, 17, 781-787.

Cai, Z., Capoulade, C., Moyret-Lalle, C., Amor-Gueret, M., Feunteun, J., Larson, A. K., Paillerets, B. B. and Chouaib, S. (1997). Resistance of MCF7 human breast carcinoma cells to TNF-induced cell death is associated with loss of p53 function. Oncogene, 15, 2817-2826.

Caelles, C., Helmberg, A. and Karin, M. (1994) p53 dependent apoptosis in the absence of transcriptional activation of p53 target genes. Nature, 370, 220-223.

Chan, W-K., Chong, T. Bernard, H-U. and Klock, G. (1990). Transcription of the transforming genes of the oncogenic human papillomaviru-16 is stimulated by tumor promoters through AP1 binding sites. Nuc. Acid Res., 18, 763-769.

Chellappan, S. P., Hiebert, S., Mudryj, M., Horowitz, J. M. and Nevins, J. R. (1991). The E2F transcription factor is a cellular target for the RB protein. Cell, 65, 1053-1061.

Chellappan, S., Kraus, V. B., Kroger, B., Münger, K., Howley, P. M., Phelps, W. C. and Nevins, J. R. (1992). Adenovirus E1A, simian virus 40 tumor antigen, and human papillomavirus E7 protein share the capacity to disrupt the interaction between transcription factor E2F and the retinoblastoma gene product. Proc. Natl. Acad. Sci. USA., 89, 4549-4553.

Chen, J., Reid, C., Band, V. and Androphy, E. (1995). Interaction of papillomavirus E6 oncoproteins with a putative calcium-binding protein. Science, 269, 529-531.

Chen, J., Jackson, P. K., Kirschner, M. W. and Dutta, A. (1995). Separate domains of p21 involved in the inhibition of cdk kinase and PCNA. Nature, 374, 386-388.

Chen, J., Hong, Y., Rustumzadeh, E., Baleja, J and Androphy, E. (1998) Identification of an alpha helical motif sufficient for association with papillomavirus E6. J. Biol. Chem., 273, 13537-13544.

Chen, S. and Mounts, P. (1990). Transforming activity of E5a protein of human papillomavirus type 6 in NIH3T3 and C127 cells. J. Virol., 64, 3226-3233.

Chen, S. L., Tsai, T. Z. and Tsao, Y. P. (1996). Mutational analysis of human papillomavirus type 11 E5a oncoprotein. J. Virol., 70, 3502-3508.

Cheng, S., Schmidt-Grimminger, D. C., Murant, T., Broker, T. R., and Chow, L. T. (1995). Differentiation-dependent up-regulation of the human papillomavirus E7 gene reactivates cellular DNA replication in suprabasal differentiated keratinocytes. Genes Dev., 9, 2335-2638.

Clarke, A., Purdie, C., Harrison, D., Morris, R., Bird, C., Hooper, M. and Wyllie, A. (1993) Thymocyte apoptosis induced by p53-dependent and independent pathways. Nature, 362, 849-852.

Cobrinik, D., Whyte, P., Peeper, D., Jacks, T., Weinberg, R. (1993). Cell cycle-specific association of E2F with p130 E1A-binding protein. Genes Dev., 7, 2392-2404.

Cohen, N., Brenman, J., Snyder, S. and Bredt, D. (1996) Binding of the inward rectifier K+ channel Kir2.3 to PSD-95 is regulated by protein kinase A phosphorylation. Neuron, 17, 759-767.

Cole, S. T. and Danos, O. (1987). Nucleotide sequence and comparative analysis of the human papillomavirus type 18 genome. Phylogeny of papillomaviruses and repeated structure of the E6 and E7 gene products. J. Mol. Biol., 193, 599-608.

Conrad, M., Bubb, V. and Schlegel, R. (1993). The human papillomavirus type 6 and 16 E5 proteins are membrane-associated proteins which associate with the 16-kilodalton pore-forming protein. J. Virol., 67, 6170-6178.

Conrad, M., Goldstein, D., Andresson, T. and Schlegel, R. (1994). The E5 protein of HPV 6, but not HPV 16, associates efficiently with cellular growth factor receptors. Virology, 200, 796-800.

Conrad-Stöppler, M., Ching, K., Stöppler, H., Clancy, K., Schlegel, R. and Icenogle, J. (1996) Natural variants of the human papillomavirus type 16 E6 protein differ in ther abilities to alter keratinocyte differentiation and to induce p53 degradation. J. Virol., 70, 6987-6993.

Coquelle, A., Pipiras, E., Toledo, F., Buttin, G. and Debatisse, M. (1997) Expression of fragile sites triggers intrachromasomal mammalian gene amplification and sets boundaries to early amplicons. Cell, 89, 215-225

Couturier, J., Sastre-Garau, X., Schneider-Manoury, S., Labib, A. and Orth, G. (1991).Integration of papillomavirus DNA near myc genes in genital carcinomas and its consequence for proto-oncogene expression. J. Virol., 65, 4534-4538.

Crook, T., Storey, A., Almond, N., Osborn, K., and Crawford, L. (1988). Human papillomavirus type 16 cooperates with activated ras and fos oncogenes in the hormone-dependent transformation of primary mouse cells. Proc. Natl. Acad. Sci. USA., 85, 8820-8824.

Crook, T., Morgenstern, J. P., Crawford, L. and Banks, L. (1989). Continued expression of the HPV-16 E7 protein is required for maintenance of the transformed phenotype of cells transformed by HPV-16 E7 plus EJ-ras. EMBO J., 8, 513-519.

Crook, T., Tidy, J. and Vousden ,K. (1991a). Degradation of p53 can be targeted by HPV sequences distinct from those required for p53 binding and transactivation. Cell, 67,547-556.

Crook, T., Wrede, D. and Vousden K. (1991b) p53 point mutation in HPV negative human cervical carcinoma cell lines. Oncogene, 6, 873-875.

Crook,T., Marston, N., Sara, E. and Vousden, K. (1994) Transcriptional activation by p53 correlates with suppression of growth but not transformation. Cell, 79, 817-827

Crook, T., Ludwig, R., Marston, N., Willkomm, D. and Vousden, K. (1996). Sensitivity of p53 lysine mutants to ubiquitin-directed degradation targeted by human papillomavirus E6. Virology, 217, 285-292.

Crusius, K., Auvinen, E. and Alonso, A. (1997). Enhancement of EGF- and PMA-mediated MAP kinase activation in cells expressing the human papillomavirus type 16 E5 protein. Oncogene, 15, 1437-1444.

Davies, R., Hicks, R., Crook, T., Morris, J. and Vousden, K. H. (1993). Human papillomavirus type 16 E7 associates with a histone H1 kinase and with p107 through sequences necessary for transformation. J. Virol., 67, 2521-2528.

DeCaprio, J., Ludlow, J., Lynch, D., Furukawa, Y., Griffin, J., Piwnica-Worms, H., Huang, C. and Livingstone, D. (1989). The product of the retinoblastoma susceptibility gene has properties of a cell cycle regulatory element. Cell, 58, 1085-1095.

Defeo-Jones, D., Vuocolo, G. A., Haskell, K. M., Hanobik, M. G., Kiefer, D. M., McAvoy, E. M., Ivey-Hoyle, M., Brandsma, J. L., Oliff, A. and Jones, R. E. (1993). Papillomavirus E7 protein binding to the retinoblastoma protein is not required for viral induction of warts. J. Virol., 67, 716-725.

Demers, G. W., Foster, S. A., Halbert C. L., and Galloway, D. A. (1994). Growth arrest by induction of p53 in DNA damaged keratinocytes is bypassed by human papillomavirus 16E7. Proc. Natl. Acad. Sci. USA., 91, 4382-4386.

de Villiers, E. M., Lavergne, D., McLaren, K. and Benton, C. (1997). Prevailing papillomavirus type in non-melanoma carcinomas of the skin in renal allograft recipients. Int. J. Cancer, 73, 356-361.

Di Leonardo, A., Khan, S., Linke, S., Greco, V., Seidita, G. and Wahl, G. (1997) DNA replication in the presence of mitotic spindle inhibitors in human and mouse fibroblasts lacking either p53 or pRb function. Cancer Res., 57, 1013-1019.

DiPaolo, J., Woodworth, C., Popescu, M. C., Notario, V. and Doniger, J. (1989). Induction of human cervical squamous cell carcinoma by sequential transfection with human papillomavirus 16 DNA and viral Harvey ras. Oncogene, 4, 395-399.

Donehower, L., Harvey, M., Slagle, B., McArthur, M., Montgomery, C., Butel, J and Bradley, A. (1992) Mice deficient for p53 are developmentally normal but susceptible to spontaneous tumors. Nature, 356, 215-221.

Doorbar, J., Parton, A., Hartley, K., Banks, L., Crook, T., Stanley, M., and Crawford, L. (1990). Detection of novel splicing patterns in a HPV16-containing keratinocyte cell line. Virology, 178, 254-262.

Doorbar, J., Foo, C., Coleman, N., Medcalf, L., Hartley, O., Prospero, T., Napthine, S., Sterling, J., Winter, G. and Griffin, H. (1997) Characterisation of events during the late stages of HPV16 infection in vivo using high affinity synthetic Fabs to E4. Virology, 238, 40-52.

Dulic, V., Kaufmann, W., Wilson, S., Tlsty, T., Lees, E., Harper, J., Elledge, S. and Reed, S. (1994) p53-dependent inhibition of cyclin-dependent kinase activities in human fibroblasts during radiation-induced G1 arrest. Cell, 76, 1013-1023.

Dulic, V., Stein, G. H., Far, D. F. and Reed, S. I. (1998). Nuclear accumulation of p21/Cip1 at the onset of mitosis: a role at the G2/M-phase transition. Mol. Cell. Biol., 18, 546-557.

Dürst, M., Dzarlieva-Petrusevska, R., Boukamp, P., Fusenig, N. and Gissmann, L. (1987). Molecular and cytogenetic analysis of immortalised human primary keratinocytes obtained after transfection with human papillomavirus type 16 DNA. Oncogene, 1, 251-256.

Dürst, M., Gallahan, D., Gilbert, J. and Rhim, J. S. (1989). Glucocorticoid enhanced neoplastic transformation of human keratinocytes by human papillomavirus type 16 and an activated ras oncogene. Virology, 173, 767-771.

Dyall-Smith, D., Trowell, H., Mark, A. and Dyall-Smith, M. (1991). Cutaneous squamous cell carcinomas and papillomaviruses in renal transplant recipients: a clinical and molecular biological study. J. Dermatol. Sci., 2, 139-146.

Dyson, N., Howley, P. M., Münger, K., and Harlow E. (1989). The human papillomavirus-16 E7 oncoprotein is able to bind to the retinoblastoma gene product. Science, 243, 934-936.

Dyson, N., Guida, P., Münger, K. and Harlow, E. (1992). Homologous sequences in adenovirus E1A and human papillomavirus E7 proteins mediate interaction with the same set of cellular proteins. J. Virol., 66, 6893-6902.

Edmonds, C., and Vousden, K. H. (1989). A point mutational analysis of human papillomavirus type 16 E7 protein. J. Virol., 63, 2650-2656.

El-Deiry, W., Kern, S., Pietenpol, J., Kinzler, K and Vogelstein, B. (1992) Definition of a consensus binding site for p53. Nature Genet., 1, 45-49.

El-Deiry, W., Tokino, T., Velculescu, V., Levy, D., Parsons, R., Trent,J., Lin, D., Mercer, W., Kinzler, K. and Vogelstein, B. (1993). WAF-1, a potential mediator of p53 tumor suppression. Cell, 75, 817-825.

Elston, R., Napthine, S. and Doorbar, J. (1998). The identification of a conserved binding motif within human papillomavirus binding peptides. J. Gen. Virol., 79, 371-374.

Evan, G., Wyllie, A., Gilbert, C., Littlewood, T., Land, H., Brooks, M., Waters, C., Penn, L. and Hancock, D. (1992) Induction of apoptosis in fibroblasts by c-myc protein. Cell, 69, 119-128.

Faulkner Valle, G. and Banks, L. (1995). The human papillomavirus (HPV)-6 and HPV-16 E5 proteins co-operate with HPV-16 E7 in the transformation of primary rodent cells. J. Gen. Virol., 76, 1239-1245.

Ferreira, R., Magnagi-Jaulin, L., Robin, P., Harel-Bellan, A. and Trouche, D. (1998). The three members of the pocket protein family share the ability to repress E2F activity through recruitment of a histone de-acetylase. Proc. Natl. Acad. Sci. USA., 95, 10494-10498.

Filatov, L., Golubovskaya, V., Hurt, J., Byrd, L., Phillips, J and Kaufmann, W. (1998) Chromosomal instability is correlated with telomere erosion and inactivation of G2 checkpoint function in human fibroblasts expressing human papillomavirus type 16 E6 oncoprotein. Oncogene, 16, 1825-1838.

Foster, S., Demers, W., Etscheid, B. and Galloway, D. (1994). The ability of human papillomavirus E6 proteins to target p53 for degradation in vivo correlates with their ability to abrogate actinomycin D-induced growth arrest. J. Virol., 68, 5698-5705.

Freytag, S., Dang, C and Lee, W. (1990) Definition of the activities and properties of c-myc required to inhibit cell differentiation. Cell Growth Differ., 1, 339-343.

Fujita, M., Kiyono, T., Hayahi, Y and Ishibashi, M. (1996) hCDC47, a human member of the MCM family, J. Biol. Chem., 271, 4349-4354.

Funk,W., Pak, D., Karas, R., Wright, W. and Shay,J. (1992) A transcriptionally active DNA-binding site for human p53 protein complexes. Mol. Cell. Biol., 12, 2866-2871.

Funk, J. O., Waga, S., Harry, J. B., Espling, E., Stillman, B., and Galloway, D. A. (1997). Inhibition of CDK activity and PCNA-dependent DNA replication by p21 is blocked by interaction with the HPV-16 E7 oncoprotein. Genes Dev., 11, 2090-2100.

Gardiol, D. and Banks, L. (1998) Comparison of human papillomavirus type 18 (HPV-18) E6-mediated degradation of p53 in vitro and in vivo reveals significant differences based on p53 structure and cell type but little difference with respect to mutants of HPV-18 E6. J. Gen. Virol., 79, 1963-1970.

Gardiol, D., Kühne, C., Glaunsinger, B., Lee, S.S., Javier, R. and Banks, L. (1999). Oncogenic Human Papillomavirus E6 proteins target the discs large tumour suppressor for proteasome-mediated degradation. Oncogene 18, 5487-5496,

Goldstein, D. J. and Schlegel, R. (1990). The E5 oncoprotein of bovine papillomavirus binds to a 16kd cellular protein. EMBO J., 137-146.

Goldstein, D. J., Finbow, M. E., Andresson, T., McLean, P., Smith, K., Bubb, V. and Schlegel, R. (1991). Bovine papillomavirus E5 oncoprotein binds to the 16K component of vacuolar H^+-ATPase. Nature, 352, 347-349.

Goldstein, D. J., Reinhard, K., DiMaio, D. and Schlegel, R. (1992). A glutamic residue in the membrane-associating domain of the bovine papillomavirus type 1 E5 oncoprotein mediates its binding to a transmembrane component of the vacuolar H^+ -ATPase. J. Virol., 66, 405-413.

Goode, S. and Perrimon, N. (1997). Inhibition of patterned cell shape change and cell invasion by discs large during Drosophila oogenesis. Genes Dev., 11, 2532-2544.

Greenfield, I., Nickerson, J., Penman, S. and Stanley, M. (1991). Human papillomavirus 16 E7 protein is associated with the nuclear matrix. Proc. Natl. Acad. Sci. USA, 88, 11217-11221.

Greider, C. and Blackburn, E. (1985) Identification of a specific telomere terminal transferase activity in Tetrahymena extracts. Cell, 43, 405-413

Gross-Mesilaty, S., Reinstein, E., Bercovich, B., Tobias, K., Schwartz, A., Kahana, C. and Ciechanover, A. (1998). Basal and human papillomavirus E6 oncoprotein-induced degradation of Myc proteins by the ubiquitin pathway. Proc. Natl. Acad. Sci. USA, 95, 8058-8063.

Grossman, S., Mora, R. and Laimins, L. (1989). Intracellular localisation and DNA-binding properties of human papillomavirus type 18 E6 protein expressed with a baculovirus vector. J.Virol., 63, 366-374.

Gu, Z. and Matlashewski, G. (1995). Effect of human papillomavirus type 16 oncogenes on MAP kinase activity. J. Virol., 69, 8051-8056.

Halbert, C. L., Demers, G. W. and Galloway, D. A. (1991). The E7 gene of human papillomavirus type 16 is sufficient for immortalisation of human epithelial cells. J. Virol., 65, 473-478.

Harley, C. Futcher, A. and Greider, C. (1990) Telomeres shorten during ageing of human fibroblasts. Nature, 345, 458-60

Harper, J., Adami, G., Wei, N., Keyomarsi, K. and Elledge, S. (1993) The p21 cdk-interacting protein Cip-1 is a potent inhibitor of G1 cyclin-dependent kinases. Cell, 75, 805-816.

Hashida, T. and Yasumoto, S. (1990). Casein kinase II activities related to hyperphosphorylation of human papillomavirus type 16-E7 oncoprotein in epidermal keratinocytes. Biochem. Biophys. Res. Comm. 172, 958-964.

Haskell, K. M., Vuocolo, G. A., Defeo-Jones, D., Jones, R. E. and Ivey-Hoyle, M. (1993). Comparison of the binding of the human papillomavirus type 16 and cottontail rabbit papillomavirus E7 proteins to the retinoblastoma gene product. J. Gen. Virol., 74, 115-119.

Haupt, Y., Maya, R., Kazaz, A. and Oren, M. (1997). Mdm2 promotes the rapid degradation of p53. Nature, 387, 296-299.

Hawley-Nelson, P., Vousden, K., Hubbert, N., Lowy, D. and Schiller, J. (1989). HPV-16 E6 and E7 proteins cooperate to immortalise human foreskin keratinocyes. EMBO J. 8 3905-3910.

Hermeking, H., Lengauer, C., Polyak, K., He, T., Zhang, L., Thiagalingam, S., Kinsler, K and Vogelstein, B. (1997). 14-3-3 sigma is a p53 regulated inhibitor of G2/M progression. Mol. Cell., 1, 3-11.

Hershko, A. and Ciechanover, A. (1992). The ubiquitin system for protein degradation. Annu. Rev. Biochem., 61, 761-807.

Hickman, E. S., Picksley, S. M., and Vousden, K. H. (1994). Cells expressing HPV16 E7 continue cell cycle progression following DNA damage induced p53 activation. Oncogene, 9, 2177-2181.

Hollstein, M., Sidrowsky, D., Vogelstein, B and Harris, C. (1991). p53 mutations in human cancers. Science 253, 49-53.

Howes, K. A., Ransom, N., Papermaster, D. S., Lasudry, J. G., Albert, D. M. and Windle, J. J. (1994). Apoptosis or retinoblastoma: alternative fates of photoreceptors expressing the HPV-16 E7 gene in the presence or absence of p53. Genes Dev., 8, 1300-1310.

Hu, Q., Dyson, N. and Harlow, E. (1990). The regions of retinoblastoma protein needed for binding to adenovirus E1A or SV40 large T antigen are common sites for mutations. EMBO J., 9, 1147-1155.

Huang, D. and Prystowsky, M. (1996). Identification of an essential cis-element near the transcription start site for transcriptional activation of the proliferating cell nuclear antigen gene. J. Biol. Chem., 271, 1218-1225.

Huang, D., Cory, S. and Strasser, A. (1997). Bcl-2, Bcl-XL and adenovirus protein E1B 19kD are functionally equivalent in their ability to inhibit cell death. Oncogene, 14, 405-414.

Huang, P., Patrick, D., Edwards, G., Goodhart, P., Huber, H., Miles, L., Garsky, V., Oliff, A. and Heimbrook, D. (1993). Protein domains governing interactions between E2F, the retinoblastoma gene product, and human papillomavirus type 16 E7 protein. Mol Cell. Biol., 13, 953-960.

Hudson, J., Bedell, M., McCance, D. J., Laimins, L.A. (1990). Immortalisation and altered differentiation of human keratinocytes in vitro by the E6 and E7 open reading frames of human papillomavirus type 18. J. Virol., 64, 519-526.

Huibregtse, J., Scheffner, M. and Howley, P. (1991). A cellular protein mediates association of p53 with the E6 oncoprotein of human papillomavirus types 16 or 18. EMBO J., 10, 4129-4135.

Huibregtse, J., Scheffner, M. and Howley, P. (1993a). Cloning and expression of the cDNA for E6-AP, a protein that mediates the interaction of the human papillomavirus E6 oncoprotein with p53. Mol. Cell. Biol., 13, 775-784.

Huibregtse, J., Scheffner, M. and Howley, P. (1993b). Localisation of the E6-AP regions that direct human papillomavirus E6 binding, association with p53, and ubiquitination of associated proteins. Mol. Cell. Biol., 13, 4918-4927.

Huibregtse, J., Scheffner, M., Beaudenon, S and Howley, P. (1995) A family of proteins structurally and functionally related to the E6-AP ubiquitin-protein ligase. Proc. Natl. Acad. Sci. USA., 92, 2563-2567.

Hurlin, P. J., Kaur, P., Smith, P. P., Perez-Reyes, N., Blanton, R. A. and McDougall, J. K. (1991). Progression of human papillomavirus type 18-immortalised human keratinocytes to a malignant phenotype. Proc. Natl. Acad. Sci. USA., 88, 570-574.

Hurlin, P., Foley, K., Ayer, D., Eisenman, R., Hanahan, D. and Arbeit, J. (1995). Regulation of Myc and Mad during epidermal differentiation and HPV-associated tumorigenesis. Oncogene, 11, 2487-2501.

Imai, T., Matsuda, K., Shimojima, T., Hashimoto, T., Matsuhiro, Y., Kitamoto, T., Sugita, A., Suzuki, K., Matsumoto, H., Masushige, S., Nogi, Y., Muramatsu, M., Handa, H. and Kato, S. (1997) ERC-55, a binding protein for the papillomavirus E6 oncoprotein, specifically interacts with vitamin D receptor amongst nuclear receptors. Biochem. Biophys. Res. Commun., 233, 765-769.

Imai, Y., Matsushima, Y., Sugimura, T., and Terada, M. (1991) Purification and characterization of human papillomavirus type 16 E7 protein with preferential binding to the underphosphorylated form of retinoblastoma gene product. J.Virol., 65, 4966-4972.

Inoue, T., Oka, K., Yong-Il, H., Vousden, K. H., Kyo, S., Jing, P., Hakura, A. and Yutsodu, M. (1998). Dispensability of p53 degradation for tumorigenicity and decreased serum requirement of human papillomavirus type 16 E6. Mol. Carcinog. 21, 215-222.

Ishikawa, F. (1997) Telomere crisis, the driving force in cancer cell evolution. Biochem. Biophys. Res. Commun., 230, 1-6.

Ishiwatari, H., Hayasaka, N., Inoue, H., Yutsudo, M. and Hakura, A. (1994). Degradation of p53 only is not sufficient for the growth stimulatory effect of human papillomavirus 16 E6 oncoprotein in human embryonic fibroblasts. J. Med. Virol., 44, 243-249.

Jewers, R. J., Hildebrandt, P., Ludlow, J. W., Kell, B., and McCance, D. J. (1992). Regions of human papillomavirus type 16 E7 oncoprotein required for immortalisation of human keratinocytes. J. Virol., 66, 1329-1335.

Jones, D. L., and Münger, K. (1997). Analysis of the p53-mediated G1 growth arrest pathways in cells expressing the human papillomavirus type 16 E7 oncoprotein. J. Virol., 71, 2905-2912.

Jones, D. L. , Thompson, D. A. and Münger, K. (1997a). Destabilisation of the RB tumor suppressor protein and stabilisation of p53 contribute to HPV type 16 E7-induced apoptosis. Virology, 239, 97-107.

Jones, D. L., Alani, R. M., and Münger, K. (1997b). The human papillomavirus E7 oncoprotein can uncouple cellular differentiation and proliferation in human keratinocytes by abrogating p21^{cip1}-mediated inhibition of cdk2. Genes Dev., 11, 2101-2111.

Jones, R. E., Wegrzyn, R. J., Patrick, D. R., Balishin, N. L., Vuocolo, G. A., Rieman, M. W., Defeo-Jones, D., Garsky, V. M., Heimbrook, D. C. and Oliff, A. (1990). Identification of HPV-16 E7 peptides that are potent antagonists of E7 binding to the retinoblastoma suppressor protein. J. Biol. Chem., 265, 12782-12785.

Jones, R. E., Heimbrook, D. C., Huber, H. E., Wegrzyn, R. J., Rotberg, N. S., Stauffer, K. J., Lumma, P. K., Garsky, V. M. and Oliff, A. (1992). Specific N-methylations of HPV-16 E7 peptides alter binding to the retinoblastoma suppressor protein. J. Biol. Chem., 267, 908-912.

Kaelin, W., Ewen, M. and Livingston, D. (1990). Definition of the minimal simian virus 40 large T antigen and adenovirus E1A -binding domain in the retinoblastoma gene product. Mol. Cell. Biol., 10, 3761-3769.

Kanda, T., Furuno, A, and Yoshiike, K. (1988). Human papillomavirus type 16 open reading frame E7 encodes a transforming gene for rat 3Y1 cells. J.Virol., 62, 610-613.

Kanda, T., Watanabe, S., Zanma, S., Sato, H., Furuno, A. and Yoshiike, K. (1991) Human papillomavirus type 16 E6 proteins with glycine substituted for cysteine in metal binding motifs. Virology, 185, 536-543

Kapoor, M. and Lozano, G. (1998) Functional activation of p53 via phosphorylation following DNA damage by UV but not γ-radiation. Proc. Natl. Acad. Sci. USA, 95, 2834-2837.

Kaufmann, W., Schwartz, J., Hurt, J., Byrd, L., Galloway, D., Levedakou, E. and Paules, R. (1997) Inactivation of G2 checkpoint function and chromosomal destabilisation are linked in human fibroblasts expressing human papillomavirus type 16 E6. Cell Growth Differ., 8, 1105-1114.

Kaur, P. and McDougall, J. (1988). Characterisation of primary human keratinocytes transformed by human papillomavirus type 18. J. Virol., 62, 1917-1924.

Kemp, C., Donehower, L., Bradley, A. and Balmain, A. (1993) Reduction of p53 gene dosage does not increase initiation or promotion but enhances malignant progression of chemically induced skin tumors. Cell, 74, 813-822.

Kern, S., Kinzler, K., Bruskin, A., Jarosz, D., Friedman, P., Prives, C. and Vogelstein, B. (1991) Identification of p53 as a sequence-specific DNA-binding protein. Science, 252, 1708-1711.

Kern, S., Pietenpol, J., Thiagalingam, S., Seymour, A., Kinzler, K. and Vogelstein, B. (1992) Oncogenic forms of p53 inhibit p53 regulated gene expression. Science, 256, 827-830.

Kessis, T., Slebos, R., Nelson, W., Kastan, M., Plunkett, B., Han, S., Lorincz, A., Hedrick, L. and Cho, K. (1993). Human papillomavirus 16 E6 expression disrupts the p53 mediated cellular response to DNA damage. Proc. Natl. Acad. Sci. USA, 90, 3988-3992.

Kishino, T., Lalande, M. and Wagstaff, J. (1997). UBE3A/E6-AP mutations cause Angelman syndrome. Nat. Genet., 15, 70-73.

Kiyono, T., Hiraiwa, A., Fujita, M., Hayashi, Y., Akiyama, T. and Ishibashi, M. (1997). Binding of high-risk human papillomavirus E6 oncoproteins to a human homologue of the Drosophila discs large tumor suppressor protein. Proc. Natl. Acad. Sci. USA, 94, 11612-11616.

Klingelhutz, A., Foster, S. and McDougall, J. (1996) Telomerase activation by the E6 gene product of human papillomavirus type 16. Nature, 380, 79-82.

Köhler, M., Janz, I., Wintzer, H. O., Wagner, E. and Bauknecht, T. (1989). The expression of EGF receptors, EGF-like factors and c-myc in ovarian and cervical carcinomas and their potential clinical significance. Anticancer Res. 9, 1537-1547.

Krajewski, S., Krajewska, M. and Reed, J. (1996). Immunohistochemical analysis of in vivo patterns of Bak expression, a proapoptotic member of the bcl-2 protein family. Cancer Res. 56, 2849-2855.

Kretzner, L., Backwood, E. and Eisenman, R. (1992) Myc and Max proteins possess distinct transcriptional activities. Nature, 359, 426-429.

Kubbutat, M. H., Jones, S. N. and Vousden, K. H. (1997). Regulation of p53 stability by Mdm2. Nature, 387, 299-303.

Kühne, C. and Banks, L. (1998). UBE3A/E6-AP links multicopy maintenance protein 7 to the ubiquitination pathway by a novel motif: the L2G box. J/ Biol. Chem. 273, 34302-34309.

Kukimoto, I., Aihara, S., Yoshiike, K. and Kanda, T. (1998) Human papillomavirus oncoprotein E6 binds to the C-terminal region of human minichromosome maintenance 7 protein. Biochem. Biophys. Res. Comm., 249, 258-262.

Lam, E.W. F., Morris, J. D. H., Davies, R., Crook, T., Watson ,R. J. and Vousden, K. H. (1994). HPV16 E7 oncoprotein deregulates b-myb expression: correlation with targeting of p107/E2F complexes. EMBO J., 13, 1383-1389.

Lane, D. and Crawford, L. (1979) T antigen is bound to a host protein in SV40-transformed cells. Nature, 278, 426-429.

Lane, D. (1992) p53: Guardian of the genome. Nature, 358, 15-16.

Lechner, M. and Laimins, L. (1994) Inhibition of p53 DNA binding by human papillomavirus E6 proteins. J. Virol., 68, 4262-4273.

Lechner, M., Mack, D., Finicle, A., Crook, T., Vousden, K. and Laimins, L. (1992). Human papillomavirus E6 proteins bind p53 in vivo and abrogate p53-mediated repression of transcription. EMBO J., 11, 3045-3052.

Lee, J. O., Russo, A. A. and Pavletich, N. P. (1998). Structure of the retinoblastoma tumor-suppressor pocket domain bound to a peptide from HPV E7. Nature, 391, 859-865.

Lee,S., Weiss, R. and Javier, R. (1997) Binding of human virus oncoproteins to hDlg/SAP97, a mammalian homologue of the Drosophila discs large tumor suppressor protein. Proc. Natl. Acad. Sci. USA, 94, 6670-6675.

Leechanachai, P., Banks, L., Moreau, F. and Matlashewski, G. (1992). The E5 gene from human papillomavirus type 16 is an oncogene which enhances growth factor-mediated signal transduction. Oncogene, 7, 19-25.

Leptak, C., Ramon y Cajal, S., Kulke, R., Horwitz, B., Riese, D., Dotto, G. and DiMaio, D. (1991). Tumorigenic transformation of murine keratinocytes by the E5 genes of bovine papillomavirus type 1 and human papillomavirus type 16. J. Virol., 65, 7078-7083.

Levine, A., Momand, J. and Finlay, C. (1991) The p53 tumor suppressor gene. Nature, 351, 453-456.

Li, J. J., Rhim, J. S., Schlegel, R., Vousden, K. H. and Colburn, N. H. (1998). Expression of dominant negative Jun inhibits elevated AP-1 and NF-kappaB transcription and suppresses anchorage independent growth of HPV immortalised human keratinocytes. Oncogene, 16, 2711-2721.

Li, X and Coffino, P. (1996) High risk human papillomavirus E6 protein has two distinct binding sites within p53, of which only one determines degradation. J. Virol., 70, 4509-4516.

Linzer, D. and Levine, A. (1979) Characterisation of a 54k dalton cellular SV40 tumor antigen present in SV40-transformed cells and uninfected embryonal carcinoma cells. Cell, 17, 43-52.

Liu, Z., Ghai, J., Ostrow, R., McGlennen, R. and Faras, A. (1994). The E6 gene of the human papillomavirus type 16 is sufficient for transformation of baby rat kidney cells in co-transfection with activated Ha-ras. Virology, 201, 388-396.

Lowe, S., Ruley, E. Jacks, T. and Housman, D. (1993). p53-dependent apoptosis modulates the cytotoxicity of anti-cancer agents. Cell, 74, 847-849.

Lowe, S., Jacks, T., Houseman, D. and Ruley, E. (1994). Abrogation of oncogene-associated apoptosis allows transformation of p53-deficient cells. Proc. Natl. Acad. Sci. USA, 91, 2026-2030.

Luo, Y., Hurwitz, J. and Massague, J. (1995). Cell cycle inhibition mediated by functionally independent CDK and PCNA binding domains on p21Cip1. Nature, 375, 159-161.

Magnaghi-Jaulin, L., Groisman, R., Naguibneva, I., Robin, P., Lorain, S., Le Villain, J., Troaleu, F., Trouche, D. and Harel-Bellan, A. (1998). Retinoblastoma protein represses transcription by recruiting a histone deacetylase. Nature, 391, 601-605.

Malkin, D., Li, F., Strong, L., Fraumeni, J., Nelson, C., Kim, D., Kassel, J., Gryka, M., Bischoff, F., Tainsky, M. and Friend, S. (1990) Germ line p53 mutations in a familial syndrome of breast cancer, sarcomas and other neoplasms. Science, 250, 1233-1238.

Mantovani, F. and Banks, L. (1999). Inhibition of E6 induced degradation of p53 is not sufficient for stabilisation of p53 protein in cervical tumour derived cell lines. Oncogene 18, 3309-3315.

Martin, P., Vass, W. C., Schiller, J. T., Lowy, D. R. and Velu, T. J. (1989). The bovine papillomavirus E5 transforming protein can stimulate the transforming activity of EGF and CSF-1 receptors. Cell, 59, 21-32.

Massimi, P., Pim, D., Storey, A., and Banks, L. (1996). HPV-16 E7 and adenovirus E1a complex formation with TATA box binding protein is enhanced by casein kinase II phosphorylation. Oncogene, 12, 2325-2330.

Massimi, P., Pim, D., and Banks, L.(1997). Human papillomavirus type 16 E7 binds to the conserved carboxy-terminal region of the TATA box binding protein and this contributes to E7 transforming activity. J. Gen. Virol., 78, 2607-2613.

Massimi, P. and Banks, L. (2000). Differential phosphorylation of the HPV-16 E7 oncoprotein during the cell cycle. Virology, in press.

Matlashewski, G., Banks, L., Pim, D. and Crawford, L. (1986). Analysis of human p53 proteins and mRNA levels in normal and transformed cells. Eur. J. Biochem. 154, 665-672.

Matlashewski, G. J., Osborn, K., Murray, A., Banks, L., and Crawford, L. V. (1987a). Transformation of mouse fibroblasts with HPV type 16 DNA using a heterologous promoter. In Cancer Cells, papillomaviruses, vol 5, ed. B. M. Steinberg, J. L. Brandsma, and L.B. Taichman, pp. 195-199, New York: Cold Spring Harbor.

Matlashewski, G., Schneider, J., Banks, L., Jones, N., Murray, A. and Crawford, L. (1987b). Human papillomavirus type 16 DNA cooperates with activated ras in transforming primary cells. EMBO J., 6, 1741-1746.

Matlashewski, G., Tuck, S., Pim, D., Lamb, P., Schneider, J. and Crawford, L. (1987c) Primary structure polymorphism at amino acid residue 72 of human p53. Mol. Cell. Biol., 7, 961-963

Matsuura, T., Sutcliffe, J., Fang, P., Galjaard, R., Jiang, Y., Benton, C., Rommens, J. and Beaudet, A. (1997). De novo truncating mutations in E6-AP ubiquitin-protein ligase gene (UBE3A) in Angelman syndrome. Nat. Genet., 15, 74-77.

Mazzerelli, J. M., Atkins, G. B., Geisberg, J. V. and Ricciardi, R. P. (1995). The viral oncoproteins Ad5 E1A, HPV16 E7 and SV40 TAg bind a common region of the TBP-associated factor-110. Oncogene, 11, 1859-1864.

McCance, D. J., Kopan, R., Fuchs, E. and Laimins, L. A. (1988). Human papillomavirus type 16 alters human epithelial cell differentiation in vitro. Proc. Natl. Acad. Sci. USA., 85, 7169-7173.

McIntyre, M. C., Frattini, M. G., Grossman, S. R. and Laimins, L. A. (1993). Human papillomavirus type 18 E7 protein requires intact Cys-X-X-Cys motifs for zinc binding, dimerisation and transformation but not for Rb binding. J. Virol., 67, 3142-3150.

McIntyre, M. C., Ruesch, M., and Laimins, L. (1996). Human papillomavirus E7 oncoproteins bind a single form of cyclin E in a complex with cdk2 and p107. Virology, 215, 73-82.

Mietz, J., Unger, T., Huibregtse, J. and Howley, P. (1992). The transcriptional transactivation function of wild type p53 is inhibited by SV40 large T-antigen and by HPV-16 E6 oncoprotein. EMBO J., 11, 5013-5020.

Missero, C., Calautti, E., Eckner, R., Chin, J., Tsai, L. H., Livingstone, D. M., and Dotto, G. P. (1995). Involvement of the cell-cycle inhibitor Cip1/WAF1 and the E1A-associated p300 protein in terminal differentiation. Proc. Natl. Acad. Sci. USA., 92, 5451-5455.

Missero, C., Di Cunto, F., Kiyokawa, H., Koff, A., and Dotto, G. P. (1996). The absence of p21Cip1/WAF1 alters keratinocyte growth and differentiation and promotes ras-tumor progression. Genes and Dev., 10, 3065-3075.

Miyashita, T. and Reed, J. (1995) Tumor suppressor p53 is a direct transcriptional activator of the human bax gene. Cell, 80, 293-299.

Moreau, F. and Matlashewski, G. (1992) Molecular analysis of different allelic variants of wild type human p53. Biochem. Cell. Biol., 70, 1014-1019.

Morris, J., Crook, T., Bandara, L., Davies, R., LaThangue, N. and Vousden, K. H. (1993). Human papillomavirus type 16 E7 regulates E2F and contributes to mitogenic signalling. Oncogene, 8, 893-898.

Muller, U., Steinhoff, U., Reis, L., Hemmi, S., Pavlovic, J., Zinkernagel, R. and Aguet, M. (1994). Functional role of type I and type II interferons in antiviral defence. Science, 264, 1918-1921.

Münger, K., Phelps, W., Bubb, V., Howley, P. and Schlegel, R. (1989a). The E6 and E7 genes of the human papillomavirus type 16 together are necessary and sufficient for transformation of primary human keratinocytes. J. Virol., 63, 4417-4421.

Münger, K., Werness, B. A., Dyson, N., Phelps, W. C., Harlow, E. and Howley, P. M. (1989b). Complex formation of human papillomavirus E7 proteins with the retinoblastoma tumor suppressor gene product. EMBO J., 8, 4099-4105.

Murphy, M., Hinman, A. and Levine, A. (1996) Wild type p53 negatively regulates the expression of a microtubule-associated protein. Genes Dev., 10, 2971-2980.

Nagata, S. (1997). Apoptosis by death factor. Cell, 88, 355-365.

Nakagawa, S., Watanabe, S., Yoshikawa, H., Taketani, Y., Yoshiike, K. and Kanda, T. (1995). Mutational analysis of human papillomavirus type 16 E6 protein: transforming function for human cells and degradation of p53 in vitro. Virology, 212, 535-542.

Nead, M., Baglia, L., Antinore, M., Ludlow, J., and McCance, D. (1998). Rb binds c-Jun and activates transcription. EMBO J., 17, 2342-2352.

Nevins, J. R. (1992). E2F: a link between the Rb tumor suppressor protein and viral oncoproteins. Science, 258, 424-429.

Niculescu, A. B., Chen, X., Smeets, M., Hengst, L., Prives, C. and Reed, S. I. (1998). Effects of p21Cip1/Waf1 at both the G1/S and the G2/M cell cycle transitions: pRb is a critical determinant in blocking DNA replication and in preventing endoreduplication. Mol. Cell. Biol., 18, 629-643.

Noble, J., Rogan, E., Neuman, A., Maclean, K., Bryan, T. and Reddel, R. (1996) Association of extended in vitro proliferative potential with loss of p16^{INK4} expression. Oncogene, 13, 1259-1268.

Nuber, U., Schwarz, S. and Scheffner, M. (1998). The ubiquitin-protein ligase E6-associated protein (E6-AP) serves as its own substrate. Eur. J. Biochem., 254, 643-649.

Oelze, I., Kartenbeck, J., Crusius, K. and Alonso, A. (1995). Human papillomavirus type 16 E5 protein affects cell-cell communication in an epithelial cell line. J. Virol., 69, 4489-4494.

Orth, G., Jablonska, S., Favre, M., Croissant, O., Jarzabek-Chorzelska, M. and Rzesa, G. (1978). Characterisation of two types of human papillomaviruses in lesions of epidermodysplasia verruciformis. Proc. Natl. Acad. Sci. USA., 75, 1537-1541.

Pagano, M., Dürst, M., Joswig, S., Draetta, G. and Jansen-Dürr, P. (1992). Binding of the human E2F transcription factor to the retinoblastoma protein but not to cyclin A is abolished in HPV-16-immortalised cells. Oncogene, 7, 1681-1686.

Palmer, J. G., Shepard, N. A., Jass, J. K., Crawford, L. V. and Northover, J. M. A. (1987). Human papillomavirus 16 DNA in anal squamous cell carcinoma. Lancet, 2 (8549), 42.

Pan, H, and Griep, A. (1995). Temporally distinct patterns of p53-dependent and p53-independent apoptosis during mouse lens development. Genes Dev. 9, 2157-2169.

Park, N., Min, B-M., Li, S-L., Huang, M., Cherick, H. and Doniger, J. (1991). Immortalisation of normal human oral keratinocytes with type 16 human papillomavirus. Carcinogenesis, 12, 1627-1631.

Patrick, D., Oliff, A. and Heimbrook, D. (1994). Identification of a novel retinoblastoma gene product binding site on human papillomavirus type 16 E7 protein. J. Biol. Chem., 269, 6842-6850.

Paules, R., Levedakou, E., Wilson, S., Innes, C., Rhodes, N., Tlsty, T., Galloway, D., Donehower, L., Tainsky, M. and Kaufmann, W. (1995) Defective G2 checkpoint function in cells from individuals with familial cancer syndromes. Cancer Res., 55, 1763-1773.

Pecoraro, G., Morgan, D. and Defendi, V. (1989). Differential effects of human papillomavirus type 6, 16 and 18 DNAs on immortalisation and transformation of human cervical epithelial cells. Proc. Natl. Acad. Sci. USA., 86, 563-567.

Pei, X. F., Meck, J. M., Greenhalgh, D. and Schlegel, R. (1993). Cotransfection of HPV-18 and v-fos DNA induces tumorigenicity of primary human keratinocytes. Virology, 196, 855-860.

Petti, L., Nilson, L. A. and DiMaio, D. (1991). Activation of the platelet-derived growth factor receptor by the bovine papillomavirus E5 transforming protein. EMBO J., 10. 845-855.

Petti, L. and DiMaio, D. (1992). Stable association between the bovine papillomavirus E5 transforming protein and activated platelet-derived growth factor receptor in transformed mouse cells. Proc. Natl. Acad. Sci. USA, 89, 8736-8740.

Petti, L. and DiMaio, D. (1994). Specific interaction between the bovine papillomavirus E5 transforming protein and the β receptor for platelet-derived growth factor in stably transformed and acutely transfected cells. J. Virol., 68, 3582-3592.

Phelps, W. C., Yee, C. L., Münger, K., and Howley, P. M. (1988). The human papillomavirus type 16 E7 gene encodes transactivation and transformation functions similar to adenovirus E1a. Cell, 53, 539-547.

Phelps, W. C., Bagchi, S., Barnes, J. A., Raychaudhuri, P., Kraus, V., Münger, K., Howley, P. M. and Nevins, J. R. (1991) Analysis of trans activation by human papillomavirus type 16 E7 and adenovirus 12S E1A suggests a common mechanism. J. Virol., 65, 6922-6930.

Pietenpol, J., Holt, J., Stein, R. and Moses, H. (1990) Transforming growth factor beta-1 suppression of c-Myc gene transcription: role in inhibition of keratinocyte proliferation. Proc. Natl. Acad. Sci. USA, 87, 3758-3762.

Pim, D., Collins, M., and Banks, L. (1992). Human papillomavirus type 16 E5 gene stimulates the transforming activity of the epidermal growth factor receptor. Oncogene, 7, 27-32.

Pim, D., Storey, A., Thomas, M., Massimi, P. and Banks, L. (1994). Mutational analysis of HPV-18 E6 identifies domains required for p53 degradation in vitro, abolition of p53 transactivation in vivo and immortalisation of primary BMK cells. Oncogene, 9, 1869-1876

Pim, D., Massimi, P. and Banks, L. (1997). Alternatively spliced HPV-18 E6* protein inhibits E6-mediated degradation of p53 and suppresses transformed cell growth. Oncogene, 15, 257-264.

Pim, D. and Banks, L. (1999). HPV-18 E6*I protein modulates the E6-directed degradation of p53 by binding to full-length HPV-18 E6. Oncogene 18, 7403-7408.

Pirisi, L., Yasumoto, S., Feller, M., Doniger, J. and DiPaolo, J. (1987). Transformation of human fibroblasts and keratinocytes with human papillomavirus type 16 DNA. J. Virol., 61, 1061-1066.

Polyak, K., Xia, Y., Zweier, J., Kinzler, K. and Vogelstein, B. (1997) A model for p53-induced apoptosis. Nature, 389, 300-305.

Qin, X-Q., Livingston, D. M., Kaelin, W. G. and Adams, P. D. (1994). Deregulated transcription factor E2F-1 expression leads to S-phase entry and p53-mediated apoptosis. Proc. Natl. Acad. Sci. USA., 10918-10922.

Rankin, S. and Rosengurt, E. (1994). Platelet-derived growth factor modulation of focal adhesion kinase (p125FAK) and paxillin tyrosine phosphorylation in Swiss 3T3 cells. Bell-shaped dose response and cross talk with bombesin. J. Biol. Chem. 269, 704-710.

Reed, J. (1994). Bcl-2 and the regulation of programmed cell death. J. Cell. Biol., 124, 1-6.

Ridley, A. (1995) Rho-related proteins: actin cytoskeleton and the cell cycle. Curr. Opin. Genet. Dev., 5, 24-30.

Romanczuk, H., Villa, L. L., Schlegel, R. and Howley, P. M. (1991). The viral transcriptional regulatory region upstream of the E6 and E7 genes is a major determinant of the differential immortalisation activities of human papillomavirus types 16 and 18. J. Virol., 65, 2739-2744.

Sakamuro, D., Sabbatini, P., White, E and Prendergast, G.(1997) The polyproline region of p53 is required to activate apoptosis but not growth arrrest. Oncogene, 15, 887-898.

Sarnow, P., Ho, Y., Williams, J. and Levine, A. (1982). Adenovirus E1B 58kD tumor antigen and SV40 large tumor antigen are physically associated with the same 54k cellular protein in transformed cells. Cell, 28, 387-394.

Sato, H., Watanabe, S., Furuno, A. and Yoshiike, K. (1989a). Human papillomavirus type 16 E7 protein expressed in Escherichia coli and monkey COS-1 cells: immunofluorescence detection of the nuclear E7 protein. Virology, 170, 311-315.

Sato, H., Furuno, A. and Yoshiike, K. (1989b). Expression of human papillomavirus type 16 E7 gene induces DNA synthesis of rat 3Y1 cells. Virology, 168, 195-199.

Scheffner, M., Werness, B., Huibregtse, J., Levine, A. and Howley, P. (1990). The E6 oncoprotein encoded by human papillomavirus types 16 and 18 promotes the degradation of p53. Cell, 63, 1129-1136.

Scheffner, M., Münger, K., Byrne, J. and Howley, P. (1991). The state of the p53 and retinoblastoma genes in human cervical carcinoma cell lines. Proc. Natl. Acad. Sci. USA, 88, 5523-5527.

Scheffner, M., Takahashi, T., Huibregtse, J., Minna, J. and Howley, P. (1992). Interactions of human papillomavirus type 16 E6 oncoprotein with wild type and mutant human p53. J. Virol., 66, 5100-5105.

Scheffner, M., Huibregtse, J., Vierstra, R. and Howley, P. (1993). The HPV-16 E6 and E6-AP complex functions as a ubiquitin-protein ligase in the ubiquitination of p53. Cell, 75, 495-505.

Scheurlen, W., Stremlau, A., Gissmann, L., Horn, D., Zenner, H-P. and zur Hausen, H. (1986). Rearranged HPV-16 molecules in an anal and in a laryngeal carcinoma. Int. J. Cancer, 38, 671-676.

Schlegel, R., Phelps, W., Zhang, Y. and Barbosa, M. (1988). Quantitative keratinocyte assay detects two biological activities of human papillomavirus DNA and identifies viral types associated with cervical carcinoma. EMBO J., 7, 3181-3187.

Schneider-Gädicke, A., Kaul, S., Schwarz, E., Gausepohl, H., Frank, R., and Bastert, G. (1988). Identification of the human papillomavirus type 18 E6 and E6 proteins in nuclear protein fractions from human cervical cancer cells grown in the nude mouse or in vitro. Cancer Res., 48, 2969-2974.

Schwarz, E., Freese, U., Gissmann, L., Mayer, W., Roggenbuck, B., Stremlau, A. and zur Hausen, H. (1985) Structure and transcription of human papillomavirus sequences in cervical carcinoma cells. Nature, 314, 111-114.

Schwarz, E., Rosa, J. and Scheffner, M. (1998). Characterisation of human hect domain family members and their interaction with UbcH5 and UbcH7. J. Biol. Chem., 273, 12148-12154.

Schwarz, J., Devoto, S., Smith, E., Chellappan, S., Jakoi, L. and Nevins, J. (1993). Interactions of the p107 and Rb proteins with E2F during the cell proliferation response. EMBO J., 12, 1013-1020.

Sedman, S., Barbosa, M., Vass, W., Hubbert, N., Hass, J., Lowy, D. and Schiller, J. (1991). The full-length E6 protein of human papillomavirus type 16 has transforming and transactivating activities and cooperates with E7 to immortalise keratinocytes in culture. J.Virol., 65, 4860-4866.

Seedorf, K., Olersdorf, T., Krammer, G. and Rowekamp, W. (1987). Identification of early proteins of the human papilloma viruses type 16 (HPV 16) and type 18 (HPV 18) in cervical carcinoma cells. EMBO J., 6, 139-144.

Shalley, M., Alloul, N., Jackman, A., Muller, M., Gissman, L., and Sherman, L. (1996). The E6 variant proteins E6I-E6IV of human papillomavirus 16: expression in cell free systems and bacteria and study of their interaction with p53. Virus Research, 42, 81-96.

Sheil, A., Flavel, S., Disney, A. and Mathew, T. (1985). Cancer development in patients progressing to dialysis and renal transplantation. Transplant Proc., 17, 1685-1688.

Sherman, L. and Schlegel, R. (1996) Serum- and calcium-induced differentiation of human keratinocytes is inhibited by the E6 oncoprotein of human papillomavirus type 16. J. Virol., 70 3269-3279.

Shieh, S., Ikeda, M., Taya, Y. and Prives, C. (1997). DNA damage-induced phosphorylation of p53 alleviates inhibition by MDM2. Cell, 91, 325-334.

Shimizu, A., Nishida, J., Ueoka, Y., Kato, K., Hachiya, T., Kuriaki, Y. and Wake, N. (1998). Cyclin G contributes to G2/M arrest of cells in response to DNA damage. Biochem. Biophys. Res. Comm. 242, 529-533.

Slebos, R. J., Lee, M. H., Plunkett, B. S., Kessis, T. D., Williams, B. O., Jacks, T., Hedrick, L., Kastan, M. B. and Cho, K. R. (1994). p53-dependent G1 arrest involves pRB-related proteins and is disrupted by the human papillomavirus 16 E7 oncoprotein. Proc. Natl. Acad. Sci. USA., 91, 5320-5324.

Slingerland, J., Jenkins, J. and Benchimol, S. (1993). The transforming and suppressor functions of p53 alleles: effects of mutations that disrupt phosphorylation, oligomerisation and nuclear translocation. EMBO J., 12, 1029-1037.

Smotkin, D. and Wettstein, F. (1986) Transcription of human papillomavirus type 16 early genes in a cervical cancer and a cancer-derived cell line, and identification of the E7 protein. Proc. Natl. Acad. Sci. USA, 83, 4680-4684.

Smotkin, D. and Wettstein, F.O. (1987). The major human papillomavirus protein in cervical cancer is a cytoplasmic phosphoprotein. J. Virology 61, 1686-1689.

Smotkin, D., Prokoph, H. and Wettstein, F. (1989) Oncogenic and non-oncogenic human genital papillomaviruses generate the E7 mRNA by different mechanisms. J. Virol., 63, 1441-1447.

Solomon, C., Sebag, M., White, J., Rhim, J & Kremer, R. 1998. Disruption of vitamin D receptor-retinoid X receptor heterodimer formation following ras transformation of human keratinocytes. J. Biol. Chem., 273, 17573-17578.

Srivastava, S., Zou, Z., Pirolla, K., Blattner, W. and Chang, E. (1990). Germline transmission of a mutated p53 gene in a cancer-prone family with Li-Fraumeni syndrome. Nature 348, 747-749.

Stacey, S., Jordan, D., Snijders, P., Mackett, M., Walboomers, J. and Arrand J. (1995) Translation of the human papillomavirus type 16 E7 oncoprotein from bicistronic mRNA is independent of splicing events within the E6 open reading frame. J. Virol. 69, 7023-7031.

Steller, M., Zou, Z., Schiller, J. and Baserga, R., (1996). Transformation by human papillomavirus 16 E6 and E7: role of the insulin-like growth factor receptor. Cancer Res., 56, 5087-5091.

Stewart, N., Hicks, G., Paraskevas, F and Mowat, M. (1995) Evidence for a second cell cycle block at G2M by p53. Oncogene, 10, 109-115.

Stöppler, H., Hartmann, D., Sherman, L. and Schlegel, R. (1997) The human papillomavirus type 16 E6 and E7 oncoproteins dissociate cellular telomerase activity from the maintenance of telomere length. J. Biol. Chem., 272, 13332-13337.

Stöppler, M. C., Straight, S. W., Tsao, G., Schlegel, R. and McCance, D. J. (1996). The E5 gene of HPV-16 enhances keratinocyte immortalisation by full-length DNA. Virology, 223, 251-254.

Storey, A., Pim, D., Murray, A., Osborn, K., Banks, L., and Crawford L. (1988). Comparison of the in vitro transforming activities of human papillomavirus types. EMBO J., 7, 1815-1820.

Storey, A., Osborn, K., and Crawford, L. (1990). Co-transformation by human papillomavirus types 6 and 11. J. Gen. Virol., 71, 165-171.

Storey, A. and Banks, L. (1993) Human papillomavirus type 16 E6 gene cooperates with EJ-ras to immortalise primary mouse cells. Oncogene, 8, 919-924

Storey, A. Massimi, P., Dawson, K. and Banks, L. (1995). Conditional immortalisation of primary cells by human papillomavirus type 18 E6 and EJ-ras defines an E6 activity in G_0/G_1 phase which can be substituted for mutations in p53. Oncogene, 11, 653-661.

Storey, A., Thomas, M., Kalita, A., Harwood, C., Gardiol, D., Mantovani, F., Breuer, J., Leigh, I., Matlashewski, G. and Banks, L. (1998). Role of a p53 polymorphism in the development of human papillomavirus-associated cancer. Nature, 393, 229-234.

Straight, S. W., Hinkle, P. M. Jewers, R. J. and McCance, D. J. (1993). The E5 oncoprotein in human papillomavirus type 16 transforms fibroblasts and effects the downregulation of the epidermal growth factor receptor in keratinocytes. J. Virol., 67, 4521-4532.

Straight, S. W., Herman, B. and McCance, D. J. (1995). The E5 oncoprotein of human papillomavirus type 16 inhibits the acidification of endosomes in human keratinocytes. J. Virol., 69, 3185-3192.

Thomas, J. and Laimins, L. (1998) Human papillomavirus oncoproteins independently abrogate the mitotic spindle checkpoint. J. Virol., 72, 1131-1137.

Thomas, M., Massimi, P., Jenkins J. and Banks, L. (1995). HPV-18 E6 mediated inhibition of p53 DNA binding activity is independent of E6-induced degradation. Oncogene, 10, 261-268.

Thomas, M., Matlashewski, G., Pim, D. and Banks, L. (1996). Induction of apoptosis by p53 is independent of its oligomeric state and can be abolished by HPV-18 E6 through ubiquitin-mediated degradation. Oncogene, 13, 265-273.

Thomas, M and Banks, L. (1998) Inhibition of Bak induced apoptosis by HPV-18 E6. Oncogene 17, 2943-2954.

Thommes, P and Blow, J. (1997) The DNA replication licensing system. Cancer Surv., 29, 75-90.

Thommes, P., Kubota, Y., Takisawa, H. and Blow, J. (1997) The RLF-M component of the replication licensing system forms complexes containing all six MCM/P1 polypeptides. EMBO J., 16, 3312-3319.

Tommasino, M., Adamczewski, J. P., Carlotti, F., Barth, C. F., Manetti, R., Contorni, M., Cavalieri, F., Hunt, T., and Crawford, L. (1993). HPV16 E7 protein associates with the protein kinase p33CDK2 and cyclin A. Oncogene, 8, 195-202.

Thompson, D., Belinsky, G., Chang, T., Jones, D., Schlegel, R. and Münger, K. (1997). The human papillomavirus-16 E6 oncoprotein decreases the vigilance of mitotic checkpoints. Oncogene, 15, 3025-3035.

Tong, X. and Howley, P. (1997) The bovine papillomavirus E6 oncoprotein interacts with paxillin and disrupts the actin cytoskeleton. Proc. Natl. Acad. Sci. USA, 94, 4412-4417.

Tsunokawa, Y., Takebe, N., Kasamatsu, T., Terada, M., and Sugimura, T. (1986). Transforming activity of human papillomavirus type 16 DNA sequences in cervical cancer. Proc. Natl. Acad. Sci. USA., 83, 2200-2203.

Venuti, A., Salani, D., Poggiali, F., Manni, V. and Bagnato, A. (1998). The E5 oncoprotein of human papillomavirus type 16 enhances endothelin-1-induced keratinocyte growth. Virology, 248, 1-5.

Vogelstein,B. and Kinzler,K. (1992) p53 function and dysfunction. Cell, 70, 523-526.

von Knebel Doeberitz, M., Oltersdorf, T., Schwarz, E. and Gissmann, L. (1988). Correlation of modified human papillomavirus early gene expression with altered growth properties in C4-I cervical carcinoma cells. Cancer Res., 48, 3780-3786.

Vousden , K. H., Doniger, J., DiPaolo, J. A., and Lowy D. R. (1988). The E7 open reading frame of human papillomavirus type 16 encodes a transforming gene. Oncogene Res., 3, 167-175.

Walker, K. and Levine, A. (1996) Identification of a novel p53 functional domain that is necessary for efficient growth suppression. Proc. Natl. Acad. Sci. USA, 93, 15335-15340.

Wang-Johanning, F., Gillespie, G. Y., Grim, J., Alvarez, R. D., Siegal, G. P. and Curiel, D. T. (1998). Intracellular expression of a single-chain antibody directed against human papillomavirus type 16 E7 oncoprotein achieves targeted antineoplastic effects. Cancer Res., 58, 1893-1900.

Watanabe, S., Kanda, T. and Yoshiike, K. (1990). Mutational analysis of human papillomavirus type 16 E7 functions. J. Virol., 64, 207-214.

Wazer, D. E., Liu, X. L., Chu, Q., Gao, Q., and Band, V. (1995). Immortalisation of distinct human mammary epithelial cell types by human papillomavirus 16 E6 or E7. Proc. Natl. Acad, Sci. USA., 92, 3687-3691.

Werness, B., Levine, A and Howley, P. (1990). Association of human papillomavirus types 16 and 18 E6 proteins with p53. Science, 248, 76-79.

White, A., Livanos, E. and Tlsty, T. (1994) Differential disruption of genomic integrity and cell cycle regulation in normal human fibroblasts by the HPV oncoproteins. Genes Dev., 8, 666-677.

Woods, D., Hough, C., Peel, D., Callaini, G. and Bryant, P. (1996) Dlg protein is required for junction structure, cell polarity and proliferation control in Drosophila epithelia. J. Cell. Biol., 134, 1469-1482.

Woodworth, C., Doniger, J. and DiPaolo, J. (1989). Immortalisation of human foreskin keratinocytes by various human papillomavirus DNAs corresponds to their association with cervical carcinoma. J. Virol., 63, 159-164.

Wu, X. and Levine, A. (1994). p53 and E2-F cooperate to mediate apoptosis. Proc. Natl. Acad. Sci. USA, 91, 3602-3606.

Xiong, Y., Kuppuswamy, D., Li, Y., Livanos, E., Hixon, M., White, A., Beach, D. and Tlsty, T. (1996) Alteration of cell cycle kinase complexes in human papillomavirus E6- and E7-expressing fibroblasts precedes neoplastic transformation. J. Virol., 70, 999-1008.

Yamada, T., Manos, M., Peto, J., Greer, C., Munoz, N., Bosch, F. and Wheeler, C. (1997). Human papillomavirus type 16 sequence variation in cervical cancers: a worldwide perspective. J. Virol., 2463-2472.

Yasumoto, S., Burkhardt, A. L., Doniger, J., and DiPaolo, J. A. (1986). Human papillomavirus type 16 DNA induces malignant transformation of NIH3T3 cells. J. Virol., 57, 572-577.

Yu, H., Chen, J., Feng, S., Dalgarno, D., Brauer, A. and Schreiber, S. (1994) Structural basis for the binding of proline rich peptides to SH3 domains. Cell, 76, 933-945.

Yutsudo, M., Okamoto, Y., and Hakura, A. (1988). Functional dissociation of the transforming genes of human papillomavirus type 16. Virology, 166, 594-597.

Zatsepina, O., Braspenning, J., Robberson, D., Hajibagheri, M. A. N., Blight, K. J., Ely, S., Hibma, M., Spitkovsky, D., Trendelenburg, M., Crawford, L. and Tommasino, M. (1997). The human papillomavirus type 16 E7 protein is associated with the nucleolus in mammalian and yeast cells. Oncogene, 14, 1137-1145.

Zehbe, I., Wilander, E., Delius, H. and Tommasino, M. (1998) Human papillomavirus 16 E6 variants are more prevalent in invasive cervical carcinoma than the prototype. Cancer Res., 58, 829-833.

Zerfass, K., Schulze, A., Spitkovsky, D., Friedman, V., Henglein, B., and Jansen-Dürr, P. (1995). Sequential activation of cyclin E and cyclin A gene expression by human papillomavirus type 16 E7 through sequences necessary for transformation. J. Virol., 69, 6389-6399.

Zerfass-Thome, K., Zwerschke, W., Mannhardt, B., Tindle, R., Botz, J. W., and Jansen-Dürr, P. (1996). Inactivation of the cdk inhibitor p27^{KIP1} by the human papillomavirus type 16 E7 oncoprotein. Oncogene, 13, 2323-2330.

Zineb,R., Zhor, B., Odile, W. & Marthe, R. R. (1998). Distinct tissue-specific regulation of vitamin D receptor in the intestine, kidney, and skin by dietary calcium and vitamin D. Endocrinology, 139, 1844-1852.

zur Hausen, H. and Schneider, A. (1987). The role of papillomaviruses in human anogenital cancers. In: The Papovaviridae, vol. 2, pp. 245-263. Edited by N. Salzman and P. M. Howley. New York: Plenum Press.

zur Hausen, H. (1991). Human papillomaviruses in the pathogenesis of anogenital cancer. Virology, 184, 9-13.

Zwerschke, W., Joswig, S. and Jansen-Dürr, P. (1996). Identification of domains required for transcriptional activation and protein dimerisation in the human papillomavirus type-16 E7 protein. Oncogene, 12, 213-220.

HEPATITIS B VIRUS IN EXPERIMENTAL CARCINOGENESIS STUDIES

Stephan Schaefer

Institut für Medizinische Virologie,
Justus-Liebig-Universität, Giessen, Germany

Introduction

Hepatocellular carcinoma (HCC) is the fifth most prevalent cancer in men and the eighth in women (IARC, 1998). The major risk factors for the development of HCC now are well recognized (Table 1).

Chronic infection with hepatitis B (HBV) and C virus (HCV) is associated with a very high risk for the development of HCC decades after infection. For HBV it has been estimated that chronic carriers have a 100 to 300 fold greater risk of HCC than the general population (Beasley et al., 1981; Maynard, 1990). In immune competent adults infection with HBV leads to chronic infection in less than 10% of infected immune competent adults. Liver damage is induced by cytotoxic T lymphocytes which specifically recognize HBV antigens expressed in infected hepatocytes (Chisari and Ferrari, 1995). Chronic hepatitis develops after many years into liver cirrhosis. Endpoint of chronic infection often is the development of HCC, but occurrence of HCC before cirrhosis is possible

The oncogenic potential of mammalian hepadnaviruses (genus Orthohepadnavirus) (Burrell, 1995) has been proven by experimental infection of the susceptible host with the closely related animal hepadnaviruses woodchuck hepatitis virus (WHV) and ground squirrel hepatitis virus (GSHV) (Marion et al., 1986; Popper et al., 1987). Whereas the tumorigenic effect in vivo, during chronic infection, is no longer a matter of debate, the direct contribution of viral gene products in the absence of the host immune system has remained controversial. This review will mainly focus on the results obtained in several experimental settings to clarify the contribution of HBV to HCC.

The Hepadnaviruses

The hepatitis B virus was identified as causative agent of serum hepatitis in the 1970s after B. Blumberg discovered Australia antigen (Blumberg et al., 1968). Subsequent studies revealed that HBV is a virus that is endemic in many parts of the world, with more than two billion people who had contact with the virus and more than 350 million chronic carriers of the virus (Anonymous, 1992).

Several viruses closely related to HBV were discovered in various primates, in members of the *sciuridae* in Northern America as well as in evolutionary more distantly related members of the *aves* (Table 2).

Table 1. Life time risk for the development of HCC in %

Hepatitis C Virus persistence	55
Hepatitis B Virus persistence	50
Tyrosinemia	37
Hemochromatosis	35
α_1-Antitrypsin deficiency	29
Glycogen storage disease type 1	13
Morbus Wilson	2
Alcohol induced cirrhosis	25
autoimmune hepatitis	2
primary biliary cirrhosis	5

All these (and several not yet officially acknowledged) viruses are now united in the family of hepadnaviridae (Burrell, 1995), which is divided into the genus orthohepadnavirus in mammals and the genus avihepadnavirus in birds (Table 2). In chimpanzees and gibbons putative new members of hepadnaviridae were discovered and sequenced (Vaudin et al., 1988; Mimms et al., 1993; Norder et al., 1996). Although it is not completely excluded that these primates were infected with human HBV and only represent a variant of HBV, the results of a comparison based on the DNA sequence of the whole genome seems to support the notion that both primate hepadnaviruses are indigenous to their hosts (Norder et al., 1996) and form their own genotypes of HBV.

The degree of homology of the whole viral genome between the viruses is shown in Figure 1.

Avihepadnaviruses are the most distant relatives of HBV with a nucleic acid homology of only 40% with HBV. WHV, ASHV and GSHV as mammalian hepadnaviruses are closer related to HBV. Woodchuck, ground squirrel and arctic squirrel belong to the sciuridae and their respective hepadnaviruses also appear to be evolutionarily related. Clearly different but closest to human HBV is the recently discovered hepadnavirus of the woolly monkey (WMHBV). Human HBV can be grouped into six genotypes A-F which differ by 8% (Norder et al., 1994). Genotype F, which is found in Brazil, Colombia and Polynesia is the most divergent genotype (Naumann et al., 1993). Estimating the rate of synonymous substitutions for hepatitis B virus to be 4.57×10^{-5} per site per year, DHBV should have diverged about 30,000

Table 2: Hepadnaviruses and their host

name of the virus	acronym	host
Orthohepadnaviruses		
hepatitis B virus	HBV	Man
woodchuck hepatitis virus	WHV	woodchuck
		Marmota monax
ground squirrel hepatitis virus	GSHV	Beechey ground squirrel
		Spermophilus beecheyi
arctic squirrel hepatitis virus	ASHV	Arctic squirrel
		Spermophylus parryi kennicotti
woolly monkey hepatitis B virus	WMHBV	woolly monkey
		Lagothrix lagotricha
Avihepadnaviruses		
duck hepatitis B virus	DHBV	pekin duck
		Anas domesticus
grey teal hepatitis B virus	GTHBV	grey teal
		Anas gibberifrons gracilis
heron hepatitis B virus	HHBV	grey heron
		Ardea cinerea
maned duck hepatitis B virus	MDHBV	maned duck
		Chenonetta jubata
Ross goose hepatitis B virus	RGHBV	Ross´ goose
		Anser rossi
snow goose hepatitis B virus	SGHBV	lower snow goose
		Anser caerulescens
stork hepatitis B virus	STHBV	white stork
		Ciconia ciconia

years ago from a common ancestor. GSHV and WHV may have diverged about 10,000 years ago from HBV and the HBV serotypes are separated by about 3000 years (Orito et al., 1989). It can, however, not be excluded that the hepadnaviruses of the different animal species co-evolved with their host and that the time point of separation of the viral species is of more recent origin.

Despite a considerable divergence based on DNA sequence of up to 60 % for avi-from orthohepadnaviridae the genome organization, replication mechanism and mode of transmission of hepadnaviruses are very similar and make animal hepadnaviruses a useful tool for the study of HBV.

The genome of orthohepadnaviruses codes for four groups of proteins; all on the minus strand (Fig. 2).

The four open reading frames encode:

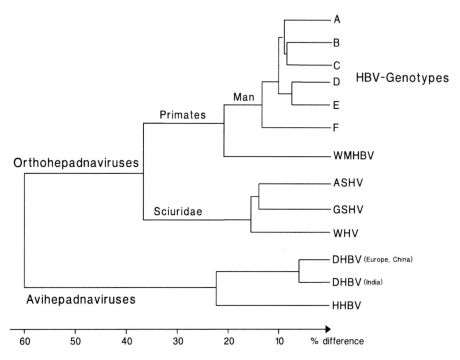

Figure 1. Alignment of the complete genomes of hepadnaviral sequences available through DNA data banks.

(1) The core protein (HBcAg) and a modified secreted form of the core protein (HBeAg) of unknown function that is produced after use of the in frame start codon situated upstream of the core start.

(2) The three carboxyterminally identical hepatitis B surface antigens (HBsAg): small surface protein (SHBs); middle HBs generated by start of translation from a start codon in frame upstream of the SHBs start (MHBs) and the large surface protein (LHBs) coding for the largest surface protein of HBV which contains all domains of S- and MHBsAg plus additional amino acids derived from usage of the third in frame start codon of the nested set of surface ORFs.

(3) The DNA polymerase which is also a reverse transcriptase with a primer function and an RNAseH domain.

(4) Protein X (HBx). A protein with unknown function for the virus and a plethora of reported properties in vitro.

The hepadnaviridae are enveloped viruses with a diameter of 40 to 47 nm and similar morphology. The viral genome is packed, together with the viral polymerase and a cellular kinase, into a capsid with a diameter of 27 to 30 nm by negative staining and 34 nm by cryoelectronmicroscopy (Crowther et al., 1994). In serum of chronic carriers the viral surface protein is found as DNA-free spherical or filamentous particles in large excess over virions.

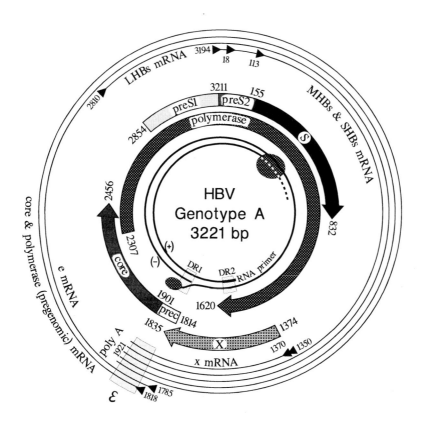

Figure 2. Schematic diagram of the HBV genome and genetic organisation. The inner circle represents the viral DNA as found in virions. The arrows represent the four different ORF. Outer circles represent the coterminal viral mRNAs as found in infected cells.

While the DNA-minus strand encapsidated in virions has full length; the length of the plus strand varies. The viral DNA is held in circular form by an overlap between plus and minus strand of ca. 240 bp for orthohepadnaviruses and ca. 60 bp for avi-hepadnaviruses. A schematic diagram of the replication cycle of HBV is given in Fig. 3.

HBV is taken up by an as yet unknown mechanism/receptor by the hepatocyte. Somewhere in the cytoplasm the viral envelope is removed such that free core particles can move to the nuclear pores (Kann et al., 1997) where – still situated on the cytoplasmic side – the HBV genome leaves the capsid and is then imported into the nucleus. In the nucleus the non-covalently closed circular DNA with the incomplete plus strand and the viral DNA polymerase attached covalently to the 5′end of the minus strand is converted by cellular enzymes to covalently closed circular double stranded DNA (cccDNA). This cccDNA serves as a nuclear template for the transcription of viral RNAs. The largest 3.5 kB mRNA is translated to give the core and the viral polymerase.

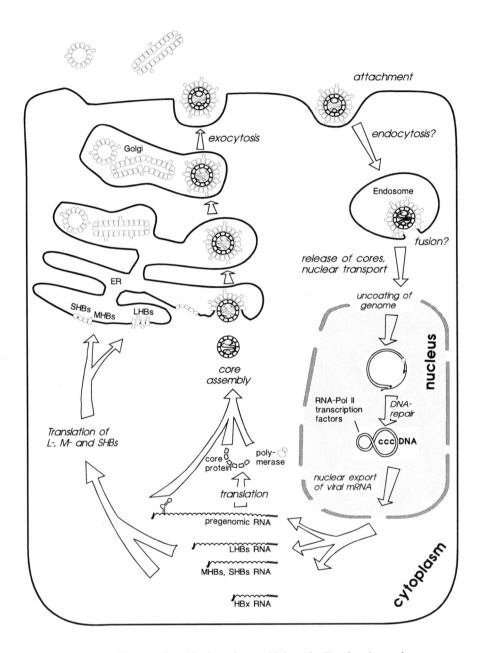

Figure. 3: Simplified model of the hepadnaviral life cycle. For details see the text.

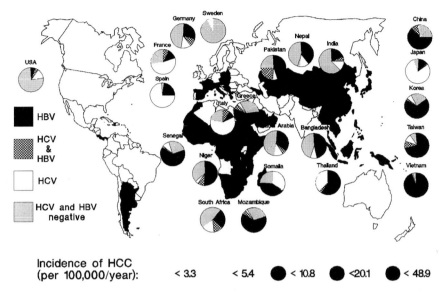

Figure 4. World-wide prevalence of HCC in males is indicated in color (IARC, 1998). The relative prevalence of viral markers in HCC patients in different countries of the world is shown. Modified from (Kiyosawa et al., 1998) with additional data from (Kaczynski et al., 1996; Abdul-Mujeeb et al., 1997; Bréchot et al., 1998; Donato et al., 1998)

These two proteins form a complex with their mRNA and are encapsidated as a viral pregenome in the cytoplasm. The encapsidated viral RNA is transcribed by the viral polymerase with reverse transcriptase activity into the complete DNA minus strand. The viral capsid is enveloped in the cytoplasm and secreted. Although integration into the cellular genome can occur early after infection (Bréchot et al., 1981) it is not needed for the completion of the replication cycle. Unlike retroviruses it leads to integrants that are not capable of supporting replication. (Detailed reviews on HBV replication can be found in: Nassal and Schaller, 1996; Kann and Gerlich, 1998).

Epidemiology of HBV Associated HCC

Worldwide more than 2 billion people have had contact with the HDV, 350 million people are chronic carriers of this virus (persistence of HBsAg in serum for more than 6 months). It is estimated that about 25 % of chronic HBV carriers, i.e. 1 million people per year, die of cirrhosis or HCC as sequelae of hepatitis B (WHO, 1998). After serologic assays for detection of HBsAg became available Palmer Beasley and coworkers could provide firm epidemiological evidence that chronic HBV carriers had an about 100 fold higher risk for developing hepatocellular cancer (HCC) than non-infected people or those with no signs of past HBV infection (Beasley et al., 1981). This correlation has been confirmed in several surveys in HBV endemic or non-endemic areas (for reviews see Bréchot et al., 1998). After the discovery of HCV in 1989 (Kuo et al., 1989) its epidemiological association to the development of HCC has been confirmed in several larger surveys (for reviews see Bréchot et al., 1998). Thus, epidemiological data on HBV association with HCC had to be reevaluated. A consideration of world wide data reveals that HBV is the prime risk factor for the development of HCC in South East Asia, China and in South Africa (fig. 4), whereas HCV seems to be the major risk factor in Japan or Spain.

In countries with low endemicity of HCV and HBV like Sweden (Kaczynski et al., 1996) these two viruses do not play a major role and nonviral factors, (e.g. alcohol) are more often associated with HCC (for details and literature see Fig. 4). Studies from several areas of the world found HBV and HCV coinfection in HCC patients (Bréchot et al., 1998; Donato et al., 1998). A meta-analysis described a synergism between HCV and HBV infection in the risk for the development of HCC (Donato et al., 1998). The effect of coinfection on HCC induction was not multiplicative and thus provided epidemiological evidence of an independent and an interfering effect. In this respect it is noteworthy that chronic HCV patients – despite serological absence of HBV markers – frequently harbor HBV DNA in liver biopsies as revealed by PCR (Koike et al., 1998; Lee et al., 1997). Thus, the contribution of HBV to HCV-associated HCC might be higher than currently anticipated. In vitro, repression of HBV replication by expression of hepatitis C virus core protein has been described (Shih et al., 1993). Interestingly, the protein reported to interfere with HBV replication – HCV core – has been reported to transform primary rat embryo fibroblasts (Ray et al., 1996). However, other groups could not support this report (Chang et al., 1998; and Schüttler et al.; unpublished results).

While development of HBV associated HCC has been thought to be invariably preceded by cirrhosis (Popper, 1988), except for development of HCC in Alaskan natives (Popper et al., 1988), newer data raise doubt in regard to the sequence of events. A large European study where patients with HCC were investigated for the presence of HBV DNA by PCR confirmed the epidemiological assciation of HBV and HCC irrespective of cirrhosis (Bréchot et al., 1998). In this report, 25/60 HBV associated tumors arose in tissue without signs of cirrhosis. These findings support the view that viral sequences/products alone are able to transform in vivo, without massive liver regeneration induced by cytotoxic T cell response to HBV proteins.

Impact of Vaccination against HBV on HCC Incidence

At the beginning of the 1980s mass vaccination programs for the prevention of HBV-related disease were started in Taiwan; the People's Republic of China and Korea. First epidemiological data show a sharp decrease of the incidence of HCC in the vaccinees (Blumberg, 1997; Chang et al., 1997; Lee et al., 1998; Zuckerman, 1997). By universal vaccination in Taiwan the carrier rate in children aged 6 years declined from 10% to 0.9% (Chang et al., 1997). Concomitantly, the incidence of HCC in 6 to 14 years old children fell significantly from 0.7 per 100,000 between 1981 and 1986 to 0.36 between 1990 and 1994. The outcome of this vaccination program (Chang et al., 1997) is an excellent confirmation of the previous investigations of the epidemiological relationship between HBV and HCC and provides further evidence for a causal relation between HBV and HCC. If preventable risk factors for the development of HCC could be eliminated (HBV and HCV infection, aflatoxin exposure and excessive alcohol consumption) ca. 60% of all HCC could be prevented (Stuver, 1997).

HBV Infection in Experimental Animals

Soon after detection of HBsAg in the 1960s, it was found that some chimpanzees were carriers of this protein (Barker et al., 1973; Blumberg et al., 1968) and that acute infection could be induced in these primates by injection of serum from human hepatitis B virus carriers (Barker et al., 1973). Beside the chimpanzee, experimental infection of gibbons, orang utans and even rhesus monkeys has been reported (Dcinhardt, 1976; Pillot, 1990; Shouval, 1994). The chimpanzee remained the experimanetal animal of choice because in contrast to the other primates they develop hepatic lesions similar to those in man and show a rise of transaminases. The histologic lesions were usually milder in chimpanzees than in man (Dienstag et al., 1976; Popper et al., 1980; Pillot, 1990; Shouval, 1994). Because HBV-infected chimpanzees also become asymptomatic carriers of HBV infection they have served as a model to study persistence of HBV (Dienstag et al., 1976; Shikata et al., 1980; Shouval et al., 1980). Although several hundred chimpanzees have served as an animal model for HBV infection for more than 20 years only two cases of HCC have been observed in them (Muchmore et al., 1988). One case appeared only two months after infection with HBV and hepatitis Delta virus containing serum, the other was attributed to serum containing non-A-non-B virus (Muchmore et al., 1988).

Intensive studies did not find any suitable substitute for chimpanzees (for review see (Deinhardt, 1976; Pillot, 1990; Schaefer et al., 1998)) until recently when the tupaia (Tupaia belangeri, tree shrew), a small animal that can be kept without difficulties in captivity, was found to be infectable by HBV (Walter et al., 1996). In a recent report even the development of HCC in HBV infected tupaias (Yan et al., 1996) was described. However, further studies with these animals are needed to confirm this finding.

HCC in Natural and Experimental Infection by Non Human Hepadnaviridae

Many data on epidemiology, pathology and course of disease in the natural hosts have been accumulated in the last two decades after the identification of animal hepadnaviruses (Table 3).

Table 3: *Mode of transmission, course of disease and pathology of different hepadnaviruses*

	vertical transmission	horizontal transmission	viral titer in serum of chronic carriers	pathology in chronic carriers	development of HCC
HBV	common, post-, perinatal 90 to 100% chronic	common, parenteral acute self limited 1-10% chronic	up to 10^{10}/ml	mild to severe hepatitis, relatively frequent beyond periportal area, cirrhosis relatively frequent	risk of HCC increased by 100 in chronic carriers (more than 40% in male carriers older than 40 years)
WHV	common, perinatal? high rate of chronicity 30 to 70% become chronic	occurs in nature 5% to 15% become chronic in experiments	up to 2×10^{11}/ml	lesions similar to those in man, rarely cirrhosis,	100% in chronic carriers
GSHV	common, postnatal? rate of chronicity high	occurs in nature 3/22 became chronic in experiments	7×10^{8}/ml - 10^{10}/ml	less severe than WHV and HBV, no cirrhosis, no hepatitis beyond portal area	7% to ca. 20% in chronic carriers
ASHV	unknown	unknown	only limited data; comparable to GSHV	drastic fatty infiltration, steatosis; lymphocytic in-filtration in portal and peri-portal area	very limited data, less common than in WHV
DHBV	Major route 100% become chronic	uncommon, only 2 cases described	10^{11}/ml to 10^{13}/ml	none or very mild hepatitis, only viremia	none or rare

Modified from (Schaefer et al., 1998) with new data from (Testut et al., 1996)

Only very limited data are available on disease in grey heron (Schödel et al., 1991) and woolly monkey (Lanford et al., 1998). All hepadnaviruses induce chronic viremia at high rate in their natural host when the virus is transmitted from mother to offspring. The respective hepadnavirus is transmitted vertically in ducks, i.e. maternal virus is present in high amounts in yolk (Urban et al., 1985), whereas transmission is peri- or postnatal in mammalian hosts (Table 3). Infection of mammals by orthohepadnaviruses at a later age leads to acute self-limited disease in about 90% of recipients. While infection of neonatal ducks (Jilbert et al., 1996) requires just one virus, the dose required to obtain acute self-limited infection at 10 to 16 months of age increases to 10^{11}/ml infectious doses. Using these high doses of inoculum only 1 out of 5 inoculated ducks acquired viral persistence (>46 d) (Jilbert et al., 1998).

The course of disease and pathology in infected woodchucks and ground squirrels is more similar to the disease spectrum in man (Marion, 1991; Paronetto and Tennant, 1990; Popper, 1988). However, there are at least two aspects of chronic disease strikingly different between man and sciuridae. In persistently infected ground squirrels, cirrhosis is absent and they seem to have the mildest disease, where hepatitis has never been observed beyond the portal area (Marion, 1991). An interesting feature of naturally and experimentally infected woodchucks is the development of hepatocellular carcinoma at a rate much higher (100%) than in persistently infected man and ground squirrel (Popper et al., 1987) (Table 3). Both hosts therefore are suitable models for the study of specific of aspects of pathogenesis of chronic and acute hepatitis in man. The hepatitis in ducks is extremely mild (Marion et al., 1984; Schödel et al., 1991). DHBV does not play a role in the development of HCC in infected ducks. HCC which has been reported in DHBV-infected ducks probably was due to aflatoxin exposure (Cova et al., 1994).

Woodchuck hepatitis virus

WHV was identified by a search for HBV related viruses in a colony of woodchucks in a zoo in Philadelphia where a high occurrence of hepatomas was observed (Summers et al., 1978). Soon after the discovery of WHV Popper and coworkers showed that woodchucks infected in the wild or in captivity soon after birth develop HCC within 2 to 4 years (Popper et al., 1987). Even under carefully controlled laboratory conditions 100% of animals developed HCC in the absence of dietary carcinogens (Popper et al., 1987). In contrast no liver tumors were observed in uninfected woodchucks for more than 10 years (Korba et al., 1989; Gerin et al., 1991). In ground squirrels infected with GSHV liver tumors develop at lower rate and after a longer latency period (Marion et al., 1986). In Alaskan squirrels infected with the recently detected ASHV liver tumors were also observed and a correlation with ASHV infection suspected (Testut et al., 1996). Although histopathologic lesions seem to be comparable in the three hosts, with only mild hepatitis and – a remarkable difference to chronic human HBV carriers – absence of cirrhosis, WHV seems to be far more oncogenic than GSHV and probably ASHV (see table 3).

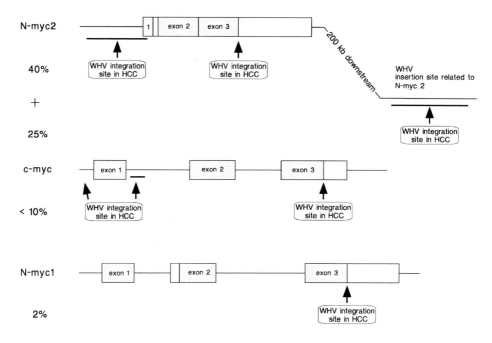

Figure 5. Integration of the WHV genomes into the woodchuck genome in WHV associated liver tumors. Modified from Buendia and Pineau, (1995).

Analysis of liver tumors from chronic carriers of WHV showed clonal integration of WHV DNA (Dejean et al., 1982; Hsu et al., 1990; Korba et al., 1989). Careful studies showed that WHV acts as an insertional mutagen that activates members of the *c-myc* family (Buendia and Pineau, 1995). Integration close to the *c-myc* ORF caused increased level of *c-myc* steady state RNA (Hsu et al., 1988; Möröy et al., 1986; Wei et al., 1992). It is now estimated that in about 80% of WHV associated HCC WHV integrates in the vicinity of members of the *myc*-family and leads to increased expression of Myc-proteins (Buendia and Pineau, 1995) (Fig. 5).

Thus, for WHV, the main mechanism for hepatocarcinogenicity appears to be the favored, clonally selected, integration close to a strong oncogene. The closely related virus of the ground squirrel is less oncogenic (Seeger et al., 1991) and although activation of members of the *c-myc* family is common, integration close to *myc* genes appears to be a much rarer event than in woodchucks (Hansen et al., 1993). Thus, even for members of nonhuman orthohepadnaviruses the mode of transformation by cis-activation of *myc* genes by WHV integration appears to be unique for woodchucks.

Table 4: Growth properties of rodent cell lines stably transfected with complete HBV genomes

cell line	transfected with	soft agar growth	tumor growth in mice	reference
FMH202	nothing	<1%	0/8	Höhne et al., 1990
FMHneo11	G418 resistance	1%	0/6	*ibid*
FMHHBV[a]	HBV dimer	48-72%	11/12	*ibid*
NIH3T3	nothing	0%	n.d.	Seifer et al., 1991
3T3neo	G418 resistance	0%	n.d.	*ibid*
3T3HBV2	HBV dimer	2.6%	n.d.	*ibid*
NIH3T3	nothing	no	0/3	Robinson et al., 1990
HBV 3T3[b]	HBV dimer	yes	10/11	*ibid*
AMLneo[c]	G418 resistance	0%	n.d.	Schaefer and
AMLHBV[d]	HBV dimer	0.3 %-6.8%	n.d.	Gerlich, 1995
LTK	nothing	5%	n.d.	Seifer and
LTK4/36	HBV dimer	23%	n.d	Gerlich, 1992

In Vitro Carcinogenesis by HBx and HBV

Several established systems for the analysis of oncogenic potential of DNAs have been used to study the transforming potential of the HBV genome. One of the classical immortalized cell lines used is the murine fibroblast line NIH3T3. This is a permanent, immortalized line that has been used in many assays to characterize oncogenes. With this cell line it was reported for the first time that HBV encodes oncogenic sequences (Shirakata et al., 1989). Later, other groups also reported successful transformation of NIH3T3 cells by HBx expression vectors or the whole HBV genome (Robinson et al., 1990; Seifer et al., 1991; Seifer et al., 1991). For review see Schaefer and Gerlich, 1995 and Tables 4 and 5.

NIH3T3 cells have several drawbacks as a transformation system for HBV. They can transform spontaneously and the cells are of fibroblast origin. The latter point might be important when examining the transforming capacity of the whole genome because, dependent on the construct, one or more viral proteins will have to be transcribed from their viral promoters which are more or less hepatocyte specific. To circumvent this point, an immortalized murine hepatocyte line FMH202 (Paul et al., 1988) has been employed to study transformation by HBV (Höhne et al., 1990; Luber et al., 1996) and

Table 5. Growth properties of rodent cell lines stably transfected with HBx expression vectors

cell line	HBx expression	soft agar growth	nude mouse tumor	ref.
NIH3T3	∅	n.d.	0/5	Shirakata et al., 1989
NpKSV	∅	n.d.	0/5	ibid.
NHBx-1	high	n.d.	5/5	ibid.
NHBx-32	high	n.d.	5/5	ibid.
NHBx-22	very low	n.d.	1/5	ibid.
FMH202	∅	< 1%	0/8	Seifer et al., 1991 and
FMHneo11	∅	1%	0/6	Schaefer et al., 1998
FMHx1	low	6%	0/5	ibid.
FMHx5	high	9%	4/4	ibid.
FMHx26	high	7%	5/5	ibid.
FMHx1443⁻ [a]	high[b]	< 1%[c]	n.d.	ibid.
NIH3T3	∅	0%	n.d.	Seifer et al., 1991
NIH3T3neo	∅	0%	n.d.	ibid.
NIH3T3x1/5	yes	1.4%	n.d.	ibid.
NIH3T3 [a]	n.d.	0%	n.d.	Rakotomahanina
NIH3T3	yes	2%	n.d.	et al., 1994
REV-2	∅	-		Gottlob et al., 1998
REV-2	yes	+++		ibid.

a) transfected with inactive HBx

b) expression of HBx mRNA with a stop codon as negative control

c) twelve different clones

HBx (Seifer et al., 1991; Schaefer et al., 1998). Because FMH202 cells are immortalized by SV40TAg further studies on the mechanism of transformation by HBV are hampered; therefore other immortalized cell lines of liver origin are preferable. So far less encouraging results have been obtained in immortalized murine and rat hepatocytes (Petzinger et al., 1994; Wu et al., 1994) with the complete HBV genome (Schaefer and Gerlich, 1995; Schaefer et al., unpublished results; Guilhot et al., 1996) (Tables 4 and 5) or HBx (Oguey et al., 1996). Several other liver cell lines immortalized with different growth promoting genes have been established in the last few years and may be used as potential models for carcinogenesis by HBV. Primary liver cells cannot be transformed by HBV sequences alone (Robinson et al., 1990; Robinson, 1994; Schuster and Schaefer, unpublished results).

```
                                                                          60
HBV     MAARLCCQLDPSRDVLCLRPVGAESRGRPLSGPLGTLSSPSPSAVPADHGAHLSLRGLPV
WMHBV   MAARLCCYLDPERDVLCLRPLQAEPSGRPFSGLSRPAETAAAAAVPAFHGAHLSLRGLPS
WHV     MAARLCCQLDSARDVLLLRPFGPQSSGPSFPRPAAGSAASSASSPSPSDESDLPLGRLPA
ASHV    MAARLCCQLDSSRDVVLLRPFGSESGGPAVSRPSAGSASRADSPLPSAAESHLPLGRLPA
GSHV    MAARLCCQLDSSRDVLLLRPLRGQPSGPSVSGTSAGSASSAASAFSSGHQADIPVGRLPA
        *******  **   ***   ***          *                        **

              RAA                                                         120
HBV     CAFSSAGPCALRFTSA--RCMETTVNAHQILPKVLHKRTLGLPAMSTTDLEA-YFKDCVFK
WMHBV   CAFSSAGPCALRFTSATWRCMETPMN----SVTCLRKRTLGLRTAPPTVMEQ-YIKDCLFE
WHV     CFASASGPCCLVFTCAELRTMDSTVN----FVSWHANRQLG---MPSKDLWTPYIKDQLLT
ASHV    CFASPSGPCCLGFTCAEFGAMVSTMN----FVTWHAKRQLG---MPTKDLWTPYVRNQLLT
GSHV    CFYSSAGPCCLGFTCADLRTMDSTVN----FVPWHAKRQLG---MMQKDFWTAYIRDQLLT
        *   *  *** *  ** *      *         *       * **             *

                    D       P
HBV     DWEELGEEIRLKVFVLGGCRHKLVCAPAPCNFFTSA.      154 aa
WMHBV   QWEEQGEEPRLKVFVLGGCRHKLVGTASPCIFFTSA.      152 aa
WHV     KWEEGSIDPRLSIFVLGGCRHKCMRLL.              141 aa
ASHV    KWEEGTIDSRLPLFVLGGCRHKYM.                 138 aa
GSHV    LWEEGIIDPRLKLFVLGGCRHKYM.                 138 aa
        ***         **  *********
```

Figure 6. Alignment of the coding sequence of X-proteins of all known orthohepadnaviruses. The start codon for putative smaller X proteins is printed in bold. The Kunitz-like domain found in all X proteins is underlined. Amino acids in italics above the protein sequences indicate amino acid exchanges in human HBx that lead to a loss of transactivation activity by more than 50%. The accession numbers for the HBV genomes used for comparison are: HBV X51970 (Genotype A); ASHV U29144; GSHV K02715; WHV M18752; WMHBV AF046996.

Functions of HBx

An open reading frame for a protein of unknown function – termed HBx for HBV – is conserved in the genome of all members of the orthohepadnaviruses. The X proteins of these mammalian hepadnaviruses share a considerable amount of homology (Fig. 6) such that activities found for one member of this protein family should be relevant for all other members.

No cellular homologue for HBx has been found which might give a hint to its function. There are two domains conserved in all orthohepadnaviral X proteins termed "Kunitz-like" domains because of similarities to functional regions of serine proteases (Arii et al., 1992) – these have been underlined in fig. 6. Expression of HBx in infected liver is low and detection by western blot in human specimens remains uncertain, whereas detection by indirect immune staining appears to give faithful results (Su et al., 1998). Detection of WHx protein in liver tissue of chronically infected animals was possible using immune precipitation and immune blot (Dandri et al., 1996; Dandri et al., 1998).

Despite numerous and highly intensive efforts to identify the function(s) of the viral protein X for the life cycle of HBV no definite clues or even hypotheses based on sound experimental evidence have been put forward. However, the following observations on HBx are generally accepted based on the use of cell culture systems:
- HBx is dispensable for viral replication in cell cultures (Blum et al., 1992).
- Hepatitis B virions derived from HBV producing cell cultures without functional HBx are indistinguishable from wt virions (Blum et al., 1992);
- WHx protein is necessary for infection of Woodchucks (Chen et al., 1993; Zoulim et al., 1994)

In vitro, a plethora of biochemical findings have been published on which several excellent and detailed reviews have appeared in the last years (Caselmann, 1995; Henkler and Koshy, 1996; Yen, 1996). Whether the reported in vitro activities of X proteins have anything to do with functions needed in vivo for viral replication is unknown.

The first function attributed to HBx was the activation of several cellular and viral promoter/enhancers (Twu and Schloemer, 1987; Spandau and Lee, 1988; Wollersheim et al., 1988; Zahm et al., 1988). Continuous studies of many groups world wide found that HBx is able to transactivate indiscriminately virtually any promoter/enhancer tested (for review: Rossner, 1992; Caselmann, 1995). Transactivation is indirect, i.e. HBx presumably does not bind to promoter/enhancer sequences. In transfected cell lines (Doria et al., 1995) and naturally infected woodchucks (Dandri et al., 1998) the protein is localized mainly in the cytoplasm although the remainder is found in the nucleus. HBx activates transcription through many different transcription factors and by the activation of many tested intracellular signaling pathways like JAK/STAT; ras-raf-signaling cascade, cyclosporine A-sensitive pathways, PKC and many others (for review: Henkler and Koshy, 1996 and recent publications: Klein and Schneider, 1997; Lara-Pezzi et al., 1998; Lee and Yun, 1998).

In vitro, HBx has been reported to bind to a large number of cellular proteins representing nearly all imaginable cellular biochemical functions from proteasome subunits (Fischer et al., 1995; Huang et al., 1996), many transcription factors, DNA polymerase subunits (Cheong et al., 1995), p53 (see below) to members of the DNA repair machinery (Wang et al., 1994). In one of the rare publications which confirmed the reports of at least one other group (Sitterlin et al., 1997) C. Transy's group confirmed that HBx binds to a protein of the DNA repair machinery called UVDDBP-C. In contrast to all other reports, binding to UVDDBP-C was even confirmed by co-immunoprecipitation from cell culture lysates (Sitterlin et al., 1997). This report is supported by further data which showed an interference of HBx with DNA repair (Becker et al., 1998; Prost et al., 1998). One function found for many viral oncogenes — the ability to override cell cycle controls at G1/S boundary, thus driving quiescent cells into cycle has also been reported for HBx (Koike et al., 1994; Benn and Schneider, 1995).

Taken together, the function of HBx for the viral life cycle is unknown. A unifying concept which explains all the reported in vitro biochemical properties of HBx is not in sight. But still there are a lot of groups that have not given up the pursuit of the elusive truth about HBx.

Interference of HBx with apoptosis and p53 functions

The tumor suppressor protein p53 was identified in 1979 as a cellular protein bound to SV40-TAg in cells transformed by the polyomavirus Simian virus 40 (SV40) (Lane and Crawford, 1979; Linzer and Levine, 1979). After clarification of p53´s role as a tumor suppressor it turned out to be inactivated by point mutations in about 70% of all human cancers (Soussi et al., 1994; Hollstein et al., 1997). This apparently central protein in the defense of multicellular organisms against unrestricted growth has been called the guardian of the genome. p53 also is a major target for oncoproteins of DNA tumor viruses which have evolved quite distinct ways to circumvent growth control by p53 (Hoppe-Seyler and Butz, 1995). SV40 TAg binds to and inactivates p53. E6 of papillomaviruses enhances ubiqitination of p53 which leads to faster degradation by proteasomes. Adenoviruses and herpesviruses found other ways to inactivate p53-regulated growth control (for details see the relevant chapters of this book).

These ongoing investigations of the interaction of p53 and oncoproteins of DNA tumor viruses were taken up by many researchers in the HBV field. We observed that in hepatocyte lines transformed by HBx (Seifer et al., 1991; Schaefer et al., 1998) p53 was visible only in the cytoplasm by immune fluorescence. The same findings of cytoplasmic localization of p53 by immune staining were later reported for the livers of mice transgenic for HBx (Ueda et al., 1995) that develop HCC (Kim et al., 1991). While pursuing our studies on HBx and p53, we found, however, that p53 in our HBx transformed cell lines was nuclear when immune precipitated from cell extracts. Three well-characterized monoclonal antibodies recognizing mainly the aminoterminus of p53 stained p53 also in the nucleus, thus, confirming the results of immune precipitation, i.e. nuclear localization of p53. However, three mabs − including those two used for our initial study − pertinently failed to stain nuclear p53 and only showed staining of the cytoplasm. We explain these findings by the masking of carboxyterminal epitopes of p53 by enhanced phosphorylation and postulated binding of cellular proteins, e.g. casein kinase II to the carboxyterminus of p53 in our HBx-transformed clones (Schaefer et al., 1998).

Several other investigators also examined the intracellular distribution of p53 in cell lines expressing HBx. Microinjection of HBx expression vectors into an immortalized rat fibroblast line did not change the − regular − nuclear localization of p53 (Gottlob et al., 1998). Wang et al., 1995 found that microinjection of HBx expression vectors along with p53 constructs into primary hepatocytes of rat origin confirmed nuclear immune staining of p53. The same group later on reported that using the identical methods in primary hepatocytes of human origin, p53 immune staining was mainly cytoplasmic (Elmore et al., 1997).

In the well differentiated human hepatocyte line HepG2 microinjection of expression vectors for HBx and p53 also induced a sequestration of p53 by HBx in the cytoplasm (Takada et al., 1997). Using the same cell line, stably transfected with HBx, p53 was found mainly in the nucleus (Fink and Schaefer, unpublished results). The different results may be explained by several relevant differences in the experimental approach. Transfection of HBx constructs and selection of G418 resistant clones results in stable transfectants with low level expression of HBx protein that is below the detection limit of immune fluorescence or immune precipitation. Expression of HBx could be detected only in our stable cell lines as HBx specific RNA which causes transactivation of transfected reporter gene constructs (Fiedler and Schaefer, unpublished results). In contrast, transient transfection of HBx constructs as done by Takada et al., 1997, leads to expression of HBx protein detectable with methods of relatively low sensitivity. Thus, the suggested sequestration of p53 in the cytoplasm as judged by immune staining, may only be observed under conditions of high level expression of HBx that may be much higher than that occurring in natural infection. Unequivocal detection of HBx protein in material from naturally infected human liver has never been reported (Su et al., 1998). Data from naturally infected woodchucks – a thoroughly investigated model for human HBV infection – only point to low level expression of the WHV homologue of HBx (Dandri et al., 1996). Schaefer et al., (1998) only observed sequestration of p53 in HBx transformed hepatocyte lines under growth arrest conditions, which induce higher expression of HBx RNA in the clones investigated (Grimmsmann et al., unpublished results). Taken together, the available data, suggest that high levels of HBx lead to immune staining of p53 at a site where it is inactive – the cytoplasm. Whether p53 positivity by immune staining in the cytoplasm means the real presence of p53 at this site or only absence of immune staining of nuclear p53 and nonspecific staining in the cytoplasm is a matter of further investigations.

Inactivation of p53 by tumor proteins of DNA viruses often is achieved by direct interaction (Hoppe-Seyler and Butz, 1995). Binding of p53 to HBx has been shown by many groups in vitro (Truant et al., 1995; Wang et al., 1995; Elmore et al., 1997; Lin et al., 1997) and has been reported in vivo (Ueda et al., 1995). Closer investigation found that the carboxyterminus of HBx is needed to bind to the carboxyterminus of p53 (Wang et al., 1995; Elmore et al., 1997; Lin et al., 1997). However, experiments in yeast using the two hybrid system and constructs that expressed HBx and p53 failed to show such an interaction (Sitterlin et al., 1997).

Damage to hepatocytes infected by HBV is not caused by the virus itself but by CD95-mediated apoptotic signals (Galle et al., 1995; Galle, 1997) from infiltrating cytotoxic T lymphocytes (Chisari and Ferrari, 1995). Thus, although HBV per se is not cytopathic, infection of hepatocytes indirectly induces apoptosis. The extent of cell death in an infected liver of a seemingly healthy chronic carrier can be enormous, without signs of liver disease in serum. It has been estimated that between 0.3% to 3% (0.3 to 3×10^9 hepatocytes) of all hepatocytes are killed per day and have to be replenished (Nowak et al., 1996).

Aside from T-cell mediated apoptosis, many reports have been published which show a direct or indirect association of HBV products with apoptosis. Most studies have been performed with only one gene, HBx. For all other genes no published data are available. While there are two reports from one group which claim that HBx counteracts apoptosis by wt p53 in primary rat (Wang et al., 1995) and human hepatocytes (Elmore et al., 1997) several other groups reported a strong induction of apoptosis using different experimental approaches (Chirillo et al., 1997; Su and Schneider, 1997; Kim et al., 1998; Terradillos et al., 1998). One out of three rat hepatocyte lines stably expressing HBV strongly underwent apoptosis after exposure to low level of tumor necrosis factor α (Su and Schneider, 1997). In support of this potential proapoptotic HBx effect, under conditions of stable expression, Chang liver lines stably expressing transactivation competent HBx were more sensitive to apoptosis induced by UV irradiation. We (Quant and Schaefer, unpublished results) and others (Kim et al., 1998) found similar effects in the transformed human hepatocyte line HepG2. However, in a murine cell line transformed by HBx (Oguey et al., 1996) stable expression of HBx supported survival of apoptosis induced by UV irradiation (Quant and Schaefer, unpublished results).

In transient transfections, HBx-induced apoptosis could be partially relieved by apoptosis inhibitors of the *bcl2*-type (Su and Schneider, 1997; Kim et al., 1998). HBx-induced apoptosis occurred independent of p53 in p53-knock-out mice (Terradillos et al., 1998). In this experimental setting HBx-induced apoptosis could only be relieved by apoptosis inhibitors unrelated to *bcl2* like crmA (M. Buendia, personal communication). HBx-induced apoptosis even prevented transformation of primary rat embryo fibroblasts (Schuster and Schaefer, unpublished results). Careful analysis using linker scanning mutants of HBx (Runkel et al., 1993) showed that apoptosis inducing domains overlapped to a great extent with transactivation domains (Schuster and Schaefer, unpublished results). In addition, all available X-proteins from non human members of the hepadnaviridae (ASHV, GSHV, WHV) also induced apoptosis in primary REFS (Schuster and Schaefer, unpublished results). Furthermore, preliminary results indicate that ASHx, WHx and GSHx might even have a stronger apoptotic effect than human HBx of genotype A and D (Schuster and Schaefer, unpublished results).

The apparent paradox, that expression of an isolated protein of a non-cytopathic virus is a strong inductor of apoptosis in vitro could not be relieved by expression of HBx from the context of the whole genome. In Chang liver cells (Su and Schneider, 1997) and in primary REF (Schuster and Schaefer, unpublished results) transient transfection of a complete HBV genome induced apoptosis as well, whereas no apoptosis was observed after transfection of an HBV genome that could not express functional HBx. One possible explanation of this paradox might be that HBx only induces apoptosis in cells undergoing cell cycling. Thus all cell lines and primary REF which divide in vitro might be prone for apoptosis induction by HBx, whereas infection of hepatocytes – which are in G_0 – by HBV is not cytopathic. This hypothesis might also explain why microinjection of HBx in primary hepatocytes prevents otherwise triggered apoptosis (Wang et al., 1995; Elmore et al., 1997). Primary hepatocytes undergo just one, maximally two cell cycles whereupon they rest. Possibly, Harris'group microinjected resting hepatocytes which according to this hypothesis are not vulnerable to HBx-induced apoptosis. If HBx induced apoptosis mainly in dividing cells, HBx would enhance hepatocyte destruction by HBV specific cytotoxic T lymphocytes and would thus contribute to HBV pathogenesis by increasing the hepatocyte turnover. Unfortunately, this hypothesis is partly in contradiction to data from Koike et al. (1994) and Benn and Schneider (1995) who reported that HBx overrides G_1/S control and drives resting cells into the cell cycle and would thus produce conditions that favor HBx induced apoptotic activity.

Transgenic Animals in HBV Research

Transgenic mice are a useful model to test specific genes for transforming activity in vivo (Christofori and Hanahan, 1994; Hanahan, 1988). In the past, several mouse lines transgenic for HBV DNA fragments have been established (Babinet et al., 1985; Farza et al., 1987; Hino et al., 1987; Yamamura et al., 1987; Burk et al., 1988; Farza et al., 1988; Araki et al., 1989). Only one of these transgenic lines showed an increased risk for the development of carcinoma (Chisari et al., 1989). Even transgenic mouse lines which contain replication competent HBV genomes (Farza et al., 1988; Araki et al., 1989; Guidotti et al., 1995) and support an active HBV replication did not show signs of tumor development.

Many transgenic mouse lines that express HBx from different liver specific promoters in several mouse strains have been established world-wide (Lee et al., 1990; Balsano et al., 1994; Terradillos et al., 1997) (M. Tripodi, personal communication, F.V. Chisari, personal communication). These HBx transgenic mice did not develop HCC spontaneously, even though the presence of HBx protein with transactivation activity was demonstrated in one line (Balsano et al., 1994). Only one mouse line transgenic for HBx was reported to develop liver tumors without administration of chemical carcinogens (Kim et al., 1991). Unfortunately in the hands of other investigators these HBx transgenic mouse lines did not develop tumors (F. Chisari and H. Schaller, personal communication). But these investigators also only noticed a very weak expression of the transgene HBx, much weaker than reported. Thus, for reasons unknown, the expression of HBx might have been downregulated below a level needed for carcinogenic action.

However, exposure of HBx transgenic mice that did not develop malignancies (Lee et al., 1990) to diethylnitrosamine induced tumors (Slagle et al., 1996). The same was found for another HBx transgenic mouse strain. After these mice were crossed with a mouse strain that was transgenic for a WHV insert near *c-myc* from a tumor (Terradillos et al., 1997), carcinoma development in these double transgenic lines was enhanced. Latency of tumor development in WHV-*c-myc* transgenic mice was reduced from 12 to 9 months, which shows again that HBx is able to promote tumor growth in vivo.

It appears possible that HBV sequences only transform in chronic inflamed liver of transgenic mice (Chisari et al., 1989) or in mouse strains which spontaneously develop liver adenoma anyway (Kim et al., 1991) (for discussion see: Chisari, 1995; Koike, 1995; Schaefer and Gerlich, 1995).

Role of hepatitis B virus surface proteins in liver cancer

A mouse line that is transgenic for the LHBs-gene under the control of the albumin promoter (Chisari et al., 1985) turned out to be an unexpected model for the development of hepatocellular carcinoma due to long-standing inflammation, Kupffer cell hyperplasia and concomitant hepatocellular regeneration (Chisari et al., 1989). This extensively examined mouse line (Hagen et al., 1994; Pasquinelli et al., 1992) is characterized by a storage of LHBs-proteins as long filaments in the endoplasmatic reticulum. These cells resemble ground glass hepatocytes in the liver of patients with chronic hepatitis B. The storage of the filaments in these transgenic mice leads to a necroinflammatory infection that has many similarities to the pathological picture seen in human HCC and surrounding tissue. However, in humans the storage of LHBs-proteins in ground glass hepatocytes could not be linked with the development of HCC (Dienes et al., 1990). In other systems a transforming effect of LHBs protein has not been shown.

Support for the hypothesis of LHBsAg as an oncogenic protein comes from the group of P.H. Hofschneider. In their investigations of viral cellular-fusion genes at the site of integration in a HCC they found that carboxyterminally truncated MHBs fused with cellular DNA sequences is transactivating (Caselmann et al., 1990; Kekulé et al., 1990). A closer investigation on the mechanisms of transactivation revealed that full length MHBs does not transactivate, whereas truncation of the carboxyterminus restored transactivation activity (Hildt et al., 1995). In unpublished studies Hildt et al. (Hofschneider and Hildt, personal communication) found that transactivating variants of MHBs bound PKC. Thus, an important tumor promoter pathway has been linked to MHBst transactivation with these studies.

Recently, LHBs was shown to be a transactivating protein too (Hildt et al., 1996). Most notably, the intracellular topology of full length LHBs-protein is similar to that of truncated transactivating MHBs variants (See fig. 7).

In full length MHBs the preS2 domain – that part of MHBs which is unique for MHBs – is found inside the ER. However, in truncated MHBs with transactivating properties (MHBst) the preS2 domain is facing the cytosol. LHBs which shares the whole carboxyterminus (i.e. SHBsAg) and the preS2 domain with MHBs can be present in both intracellular topologies (Bruss et al., 1994), i.e. the M- and LHBs specific domains are presented to the cytosol or ER.

Thus, in cells overexpressing LHBs transactivation of cellular genes may occur as has been shown for HBx. This transactivation of potentially growth regulating genes might be indispensable for the development of HCC. In this regard cells which store massive excess of LHBs – ground glass cells so called because of their opaque appearance in naturally infected human liver – might be regarded as precancerous However, careful studies did not demonstrate a correlation between the presence of ground glass cells and development to HCC (Dienes et al., 1990). There is no existing data to show that LHBs or MHBst possess a transforming potential, except for one publication where a cloned HBV integrate from HCC was found to transform an immortalized murine hepatocyte line (Luber et al., 1996). This transforming HBV

Cytosolic orientation of preS domains determines the activity of HBV surface proteins as transactivator

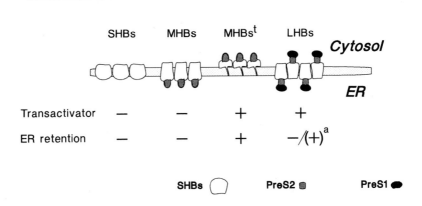

Figure 7. Intracellular orientation and properties of wildtype and variant surface proteins of HBV. ([a]Retention of LHBs in the ER is resolved in most cells by coexpression of an excess of SHBs; but if SHBs is lacking LHBs is retained and transactivates.)

integrate coded for MHBst and HBx and hence these data support the assumption that MHBst might be a cofactor in hepatocarcinogenesis by HBV.

Besides activation of cell growth, inhibition of apoptosis is an important mechanism of oncogenesis. F. Chisari´s group presented data that LHBs might have the potential to inhibit apoptosis (F. Chisari, personal communication). If these data could be confirmed, HBV as a DNA tumor virus, would have two proteins which may contribute to transformation. One of these proteins, HBx, would drive resting hepatocytes into active cell cycling by overriding restriction points (Koike et al., 1994; Benn and Schneider, 1995). This activity would be accompanied by a strong induction of apoptosis (Chirillo et al., 1997; Kim et al., 1998; Su and Schneider, 1997; Terradillos et al., 1998), Schuster and Schaefer, unpublished results). The other protein, LHBs or MHBst, would be needed to keep those cells alive that were forced into cell cycling by HBx, by preventing apoptosis. This scenario is very similar to that drawn for oncogenic adenoviruses. E1A of adenovirus 5 (Ricciardi, 1995) forces entry into the cell cycle, overriding restriction points. Such oncogenes often have an intrinsic apoptotic activity which must be counteracted by other genes as in the case of adenovirus 5 E1B which is a very strong inhibitor of apoptosis (Ricciardi, 1995). Only the balanced action of both genes efficiently transforms the host cell. Although data for the role of HBV proteins HBx and LHBs in transformation are not as convincing as those for E1A and E1B proteins of oncogenic adenoviruses, they are supported by data from Schaack et al. (1996) who showed that HBx can substitute activities of E1A needed for replication of adenoviruses.

Surprisingly, even for the smallest HBV surface protein a transforming potential has been claimed. Two independent groups reported that even small HBs can induce liver carcinoma in mice transgenic only for SHBs-constructs (Dragani et al., 1990; Ghebraniou and Sell, 1998). Development of HCC was dependent either on exposure of SHBs-transgenic mice to chemical carcinogens (Dragani et al., 1990) or choice of a mouse strain that is at high risk for the development of liver adenoma (Ghebraniou and Sell, 1998). In many other mice transgenic for SHBs that were kept without exposure to chemical caricnogens and were of genetic background with no altered tumor susceptibility, no HCC were observed (for example Babinet et al., 1985).

Functions of HBV integrates in tumor tissue

Various fragments of HBV DNA are found integrated in chromosomes of most HBV associated HCC (Robinson et al., 1987; Matsubara and Tokino, 1990; Schröder and Zentgraf, 1990). Although HBV shares some features with retroviruses and has therefore been considered as a pararetrovirus (Robinson et al., 1987), integration of the HBV genome into the host genome is not necessary for hepadnaviral replication. Quite the contrary, in that integration of HBV always leads to the disruption of structures or ORFs necessary for viral replication (Schröder and Zentgraf, 1990).

It has been speculated that integration of HBV close to growth controlling genes leads to the perturbation of cell growth control. In the woodchuck system examples for this mechanism have been frequently found (Buendia and Pineau, 1995). In human HCC, HBV has up to now been found to integrate on at least 16 chromosomes and at, at least, 25 insertion sites (Matsubara and Tokino, 1990; Schröder and Zentgraf, 1990; Koike, 1998). A clear pattern has not yet been identified.

The following integration events in human HCC have been mapped close to growth control related genes:

A single HBV integration was fused in frame with the retinoic acid receptor β (RARβ) gene (Dejean et al., 1986; Dejean and de Thé, 1990). Expression of this MHBs-RARβ chimera transformed erythrocytic progenitor cells of chicken origin (Garcia et al., 1993).

HBV DNA was found integrated in the cyclin A gene in one HCC (Wang et al., 1990). This integration led to the expression of a truncated MHBs-cyclin A fusion gene. The resulting fusion protein could not be degraded in an in vitro cyclin degradation assay (Wang et al., 1992). Thus, the expression of cyclin A is no longer controlled during cell cycle and has been found to be oncogenic in vitro (Berasain et al., 1998).

In the PLC/PRF/5 human hepatoma cell line mevalonate kinase was activated by insertion of HBV gene sequences into the upstream promoter region of the mevalonate kinase gene (Graef et al., 1994). This fusion event led to an aberrant expression of mevalonate kinase-HBV hybrid RNA and protein, which might deregulate the growth control of hepatocytes (Graef et al., 1994).

HBV DNA was found integrated close to the hst-1 and int-2 locus and amplified along with these oncogenes, but an activation has not been demonstrated in this report (Hatada et al., 1988).

Integrated HBV DNA with about 1 kb flanking cellular sequences has been cloned from a human hepatoma cell line huH-4 (Caselmann et al., 1990; Kekulé et al., 1990). No growth related ORFs have been detected in the vicinity of this single integration event. The single HBV integrate contains a full length surface gene, a complete HBx ORF and a truncated reading frame for middle HBsAg. Due to multiple rearrangements no other HBV genes have remained functionally intact. This HBV integrate was stably transfected into FMH202 cells which had been previously shown to become successfully transformed by a replication competent HBV genome (Höhne et al., 1990). FMH202 clones transfected stably with the huH-4 derived HBV DNA showed all features of transformed cells (Luber et al., 1996).

Several hypotheses for the effect of this HBV integrate that transformed the immortalized hepatocyte line FMH202 are possible. The hypothesis favored by Luber et al. (1996) is that the HBV integrate harbors two viral proteins with known transactivating function: HBx and truncated MHBs-protein (Caselmann et al., 1990; Kekulé et al., 1990). These two transactivating viral proteins have been shown to activate the promoters of several cellular protooncogenes. HBx transactivates *c-myc* (Kekulé et al., 1993), *c-jun* (Twu et al., 1993) and *c-fos* (Avantaggiati et al., 1993; Schaefer and Gerlich, 1995); truncated MHBsAg activates the *c-myc* (Kekulé et al., 1990) and the *c-fos* promoter (Meyer et al., 1992). The long standing suggestion that aberrant expression of cellular proto-oncogenes by the transactivating effect of viral proteins leads to the development of HCC (reviewed in Kekulé, 1991) gets further support by these results. Taken together, for three different HBV integrates from human hepatocellular carcinoma a transforming effect in vitro has been demonstrated (Garcia et al., 1993; Luber et al., 1996; Berasain et al., 1998).

For development of HCC in woodchucks by WHV activation of the N-*myc2* gene was found to be responsible (Buendia and Pineau, 1995). The promoter of N-*myc2* is activated over a long range by enhancer II of WHV (Fourel et al., 1994). For human HBV-associated HCC such a cis activation of cellular oncogenes has also been assumed. Activation of cellular oncogenes like *ras, fos* and *myc* has been found in a high percentage of HBV-associated HCC (Tabor, 1994). But only one recent manuscript investigated whether HBV integrates from human HCC retained the ability to act as enhancers of transcription (Pineau et al., 1998). The data of these authors not only failed to observe enhancer activities of the integrates investigated but in contrast found repression activity (Pineau et al., 1998). Thus, at least in this single case, HBV integrates might not act as activators of transcription in cis such that observed enhanced expression of oncogenes in HBV associated HCC indeed might come from trans-activating viral proteins (Kekulé, 1991).

After integration of HBV into the host chromosome not only the integrity of the HBV genome (Schröder and Zentgraf, 1990) is damaged. Integrated HBV and surrounding host DNA show a broad range of recombination events like inversions, deletions and amplification of viral and host sequences (Matsubara and Tokino, 1990;

Schröder and Zentgraf, 1990; Koike, 1998;). Recombination of chromosomal DNA is an acknowledged risk factor in the development of human cancers (Lengauer et al., 1998). The recombinaton events observed in HBV associated HCC might lead to the activation of oncogenes or the inactivation of tumor suppressors in the host DNA. Indeed, integration close to the tumor suppressor p53 by HBV has been found in two human hepatocellular carcinomas (Hino et al., 1986; Slagle et al., 1991). It has been demonstrated that HBV DNA is sufficient to increase the recombination activity in cytoplasmic extracts in vitro (Hino et al., 1991), furthermore a cellular recombination-associated protein has been shown to bind to HBV DNA (Kajino et al., 1994). A long-standing concept is that integration of foreign DNA into the host chromosome is sufficient to cause chromosomal instability that ultimately leads to oncogenic transformation of the cell (Dörfler, 1995). Indeed, in the cell line transformed by HBV (Höhne et al., 1990) we observed activated transcription of endogenous retroviruses (Schaefer and Höhne, unpublished observations). These endogenous retroviruses might reintegrate at other points in the genome and may thus enhance the chromosomal instability potentially started by the integration of HBV DNA. Furthermore, we (Höhne et al., 1990; Schaefer et al., 1998) and Luber et al. (1996) observed a rearrangement of integrated HBV DNA. However, a direct contribution of the increased rearrangements induced by HBV DNA for the pathogenesis of HCC has not been shown yet and is probably difficult to demonstrate in vitro.

In most human hepatocellular carcinomas the reading frame of HBx is integrated (Schlüter et al., 1994) but the carboxyterminus of the putative HBx protein is often deleted in this process. Such HBx ORFs fused to cellular flanking sequences have been cloned. The resulting HBx-cellular-sequence fusion-proteins retained the transactivating function of wild type HBx (Wollersheim et al., 1988; Takada and Koike, 1990; Yamamoto et al., 1993; Yamamoto et al., 1993). But none of these cloned HBx fusion proteins has ever been tested for a transforming effect so that the contribution of truncated HBx-fusion proteins in carcinogenesis remains hypothetical. However, there are recent results which might indirectly show a contribution of these HBx-fusion proteins in carcinogenesis. The group of C.H. Schröder found that there is a weak polyA-signal at the 3´-end of the HBx-ORF. This CATAAA signal is indeed used so that a truncated HBx-mRNA with a long polyA-tail is transcribed (Hilger et al., 1991). Translation results in a truncated HBx (HBx^t)with a polylysin-stretch. A large survey in HCC showed the regular expression of HBx^t which increased with duration of the disease (Kairat et al., in press). The working hypothesis of the authors has recently been extended. The integration of HBV sequences usually results in an HBx reading frame where less than the last 14 codons are deleted. By this integration process the additional poly(A)-signal is retained so that expression of truncated HBx with carboxyterminal polylysin-stretch (HBx^t -polylysin) is possible in most HCC-tissues (Rakotomahanina et al., 1994). Rakotomanahina et al. (1994) tested an expression vector for this HBx^t -polylysin for transactivating and transforming activity in NIH3T3 cells. Wildtype HBx showed a transactivation increase of 11.8 fold on the SV40-enhancer. HBx^t -polylysin only had a transactivating activity of 2 fold in the same system. Wildtype HBx transformed NIH3T3 cells with an efficiency of 2%, whereas the transforming activity of HBx^t -polylysin was much higher with 83 %. There might be several explanations for the strong transforming effect of HBx^t -polylysin: the polylysin stretch might stabilize the protein and thereby prolong the short half life of wild type HBx (about 15 minutes) (Dandri et al., 1998; Schek et al., 1991). Such a stabilized HBx protein might be more oncogenic. Or, as has been demonstrated recently, HBxt -polylysin is localized in the nucleus (Schröder, personal communication) in contrast to wild type HBx, which is predominantly localized in the cytoplasm (Doria et al., 1995; Dandri et al., 1998; Sirma et al., 1998). The altered properties of HBxt compared with wt HBx include subcellular localization, enhanced transforming effect (Rakotomahanina et al., 1994) and markedly decreased apoptotic activities (Schuster & Schaefer, unpublished results). Interestingly apoptotic activities of HBx appear to depend on cytoplasmic localization (Su and Schneider, 1997).

Résumé

Speaking of Foulds´dangerous ideas about multistep development of tumors G. Klein (Klein, 1998) writes in a recent review:

> Tumor biologists must welcome and indeed embrace complexity... Some of our clinical colleagues and most of the lay public expect us to come up with "the solution". For those who have followed in Darwin´s and Foulds´ footsteps there is no return. Even though tumor development is a tiny piece of evolution..., it is an evolutionary process, with many subtle, seemingly disconnected selective steps, based on an almost infinite cellular variability.

These words are appropriate for what is known about the contribution of HBV to hepatocarcinogenesis brought to a higher order of complexity by our missing clues as to the functions of HBx. In his consideration of multistep tumor development G. Klein reminds us of the mathematical models that indicated that most human tumors arose after five to seven mutation-like changes (Farber and Cameron, 1980). Four groups of genes are affected during tumor development, oncogenes, tumor supressors, DNA repair genes and genes controlling apoptosis. All these families of genes are affected by HBV during development of liver cancer:

- Oncogenes are activated in cis by WHV and in trans by HBV products HBx and MHBs^t.
- Tumor suppressor p53 is affected by HBx, although no unifying concept for HBx-p53 interactions has emerged yet.
- Apoptosis induction is influenced – enhanced or reduced depending on the system used – by HBx and perhaps by LHBs.
- DNA repair is impaired by HBx (Becker et al., 1998) and HBx has been shown to bind to proteins involved in DNA repair (Wang et al., 1994; Sitterlin et al., 1997)

Further progression of tumors is most probably supported by increased recombination. Thus, hepatocytes infected by HBV acquire a "mutator phenotype" (Loeb, 1998). Loss of fidelity of DNA replication by HBV products leads to mutations ranging from translocation of whole chromosomes to increased occurrence of point mutations in HBV sequences found integrated in the genomes of HCC (Bréchot, C, personal communication).

Without doubt HBV products are involved in molecular events ultimately leading to transformation of the infected hepatocyte. Several aspects related to the molelular events taking place during hepatocarcinogenesis by HBV will remain topics of primary research interest. For example:

• Whether HBx´ role as tumor promoter in vivo is as important as its role as an object of molecular biological research?

• Whether LHBs and its counterpart found in tumors – truncated MHBs^{t-} will turn out to play a prominent role in transformation?

• Whether use of a cryptic polyadenylation signal activates a strongly oncogenic truncated HBx?

• Whether new HBV products either wild type or variants found will contribute to our understanding of transformation?

Many years of research have not found "the solution" but have helped to clarify many issues. These results now enable us to ask questions more precisely so that many complexities and contradictory results will turn out to be plain and simple.

Acknowledgement

I thank Dr. W. H. Gerlich for many helpful discussions and critical reading of the manuscript.

References

Abdul-Mujeeb, S., Jamal, Q., Khanani, R., Iqbal, N., and Kaher, S. (1997). Prevalence of hepatitis B surface antigen and HCV antibodies in hepatocellular carcinoma cases in Karachi, Pakistan. Trop Doct 27, 45-6.

Anonymous (1992). Hepatitis B vaccine set for introduction into national immunization programmes. Press Release WHO 12:1.

Araki, K., Miyazaki, J., Hino, O., Tomita, N., Chisaka, O., Matsubara, K., and Yamamura, K. (1989). Expression and replication of hepatitis B virus genome in transgenic mice. Proc Natl Acad Sci U S A 86, 207-11.

Arii, M., Takada, S., and Koike, K. (1992). Identification of three essential regions of hepatitis B virus x protein for trans-activating function. Oncogene 7, 397-403.

Avantaggiati, M. L., Natoli, G., Balsano, C., Chirillo, P., Artini, M., De Marzio, E., Collepardo, D., and Levrero, M. (1993). The hepatitis B virus (HBV) pX transactivates the c-fos promoter through multiple cis-acting elements. Oncogene 8, 1567-74.

Babinet, C., Farza, H., Morello, D., Hadchouel, M., and Pourcel, C. (1985). Specific expression of hepatitis B surface antigen (HBsAg) in transgenic mice. Science 230, 1160-3.

Balsano, C., Billet, O., Bennoun, M., Cavard, C., Zider, A., Grimber, G., Natoli, G., Briand, P., and Levrero, M. (1994). Hepatitis B virus X gene product acts as a transactivator in vivo. J Hepatol 21, 103-9.

Barker, L. F., Chisari, F. V., McGrath, P. P., Dalgard, D. W., L, K. R., Almeida, J. D., Edgington, T. S., Sharp, D. G., and Peterson, M. P. (1973). Transmission of viral hepatitis type B, to chimpanzees. J. Infect. Dis. 127, 648- 662.

Beasley, R. P., Hwang, L. Y., Lin, C. C., and Chien, C. S. (1981). Hepatocellular carcinoma and hepatitis B virus. A prospective study of 22 707 men in Taiwan. Lancet 2, 1129-33.

Becker, S. A., Lee, T. H., Butel, J. S., and Slagle, B. L. (1998). Hepatitis B virus X protein interferes with cellular DNA repair. J Virol 72, 266-72.

Benn, J., and Schneider, R. J. (1995). Hepatitis B virus HBx protein deregulates cell cycle checkpoint controls. Proc Natl Acad Sci U S A 92, 11215-9.

Berasain, C., Patil, D., Perara, E., Huang, S. M., Mouly, H., and Bréchot, C. (1998). Oncogenic activation of a human cyclin A2 targeted to the endoplasmic reticulum upon hepatitis B virus genome insertion. Oncogene 16, 1277-88.

Blum, H. E., Zhang, Z. S., Galun, E., von Weizsäcker, F., Garner, B., Liang, T. J., and Wands, J. R. (1992). Hepatitis B virus X protein is not central to the viral life cycle in vitro. J Virol 66, 1223-7.

Blumberg, B. S. (1997). Hepatitis B virus, the vaccine, and the control of primary cancer of the liver. Proc. Natl. Acad. Sci., USA 94, 7121-7125.

Blumberg, B. S., Sutnick, A. I., and London, W. T. (1968). Bull. N.Y. Acad. Med. 44, 1566-1586.

Bréchot, C., Hadchouel, M., Scotto, J., Fonck, M., Potet, F., Vyas, G. N., and Tiollais, P. (1981). State of hepatitis B virus DNA in hepatocytes of patients with hepatitis B surface antigen-positive and -negative liver diseases. Proc Natl Acad Sci U S A 78, 3906-10.

Bréchot, C., Jaffredo, F., Lagorce, D., Gerken, G., Meyer zum Büschenfelde, K., Papakonstontinou, A., Hadziyannis, S., Romeo, R., Colombo, M., Rodes, J., Bruix, J., and Naoumov, N. (1998). Impact of HBV, HCV and GBV-C/HGV on hepatocellular carcinomas in Europe: results of a European concerted action. J. Hepatol. 29, 173-183.

Bruss, V., Lu, X., Thomssen, R., and Gerlich, W. H. (1994). Post-translational alterations in transmembrane topology of the hepatitis B virus large envelope protein. EMBO J. 13, 2273-79.

Buendia, M. A., and Pineau, P. (1995). The Complex Role of Hepatitis B Virus in Human Hepatocarcinogenesis. In Infectious Agents and Pathogenesis, G. Barbanti-Brodano, M. Bendinelli and H. Friedman, eds. (New York: Plenum Press), pp. 171-193.

Burk, R. D., DeLoia, J. A., el Awady, M. K., and Gearhart, J. D. (1988). Tissue preferential expression of the hepatitis B virus (HBV) surface antigen gene in two lines of HBV transgenic mice. J Virol 62, 649-54.

Burrell, C. J. (1995). Hepadnaviridae. In Classification and Nomenclature of Viruses. Sixth Report on Taxonomy of the International Committee of Viruses, Archives of Virology, Suppl. 10. F. A. Murphy, C. M. Fauquet, D. H. L. Bishop, S. A. Ghabrial, A. W. Jarvis, G. P. Martelli, M. A. Mayo and M. D. Summers, eds. (Springer, Wien), pp. 179-184.

Caselmann, W. H. (1995). Transactivation of cellular gene expression by hepatitis B viral proteins: a possible molecular mechanism of hepatocarcinogenesis. J Hepatol 22, 34-7.

Caselmann, W. H., Meyer, M., Kekulé, A. S., Lauer, U., Hofschneider, P. H., and Koshy, R. (1990). A transactivator function is generated by integration of hepatitis B virus preS/S sequences in human hepatocellular carcinoma DNA. Proc Natl Acad Sci U S A 87, 2970-4.

Chang, J., Yang, S. H., Cho, Y. G., Hwang, S. B., Hahn, Y. S., and Sung, Y. C. (1998). Hepatitis C virus core from two different genotypes has an oncogenic potential but is not sufficient for transforming primary rat embryo fibroblasts in cooperation with the H-ras oncogene. J Virol 72, 3060-5.

Chang, M.-H., Chen, C.-J., Lai, M.-S., Hsu, H.-M., Wu, T.-C., Kong, M.-S., Liang, D.-C., Shau, W.-Y., and Chen, D.-S. (1997). Universal Hepatitis B Vaccination in Taiwan and the Incidence of Hepatocellular Carcinoma in Children. New Eng J Med 336, 1855-1859.

Chen, H. S., Kaneko, S., Girones, R., Anderson, R. W., Hornbuckle, W. E., Tennant, B. C., Cote, P. J., Gerin, J. L., Purcell, R. H., and Miller, R. H. (1993). The woodchuck hepatitis virus X gene is important for establishment of virus infection in woodchucks. J Virol 67, 1218-26.

Cheong, J. H., Yi, M., Lin, Y., and Murakami, S. (1995). Human RPB5, a subunit shared by eukaryotic nuclear RNA polymerases, binds human hepatitis B virus X protein and may play a role in X transactivation. Embo J 14, 143-50.

Chirillo, P., Pagano, S., Natoli, G., Puri, P. L., Burgio, V. L., Balsano, C., and Levrero, M. (1997). The hepatitis B virus X gene induces p53-mediated programmed cell death. Proc. Natl. Acd. Sci. USA 94, 8162- 8167.

Chisari, F. V. (1995). Hepatitis B virus transgenic mice: insights into the virus and the disease. Hepatology 22, 1316-25.

Chisari, F. V., and Ferrari, C. (1995). Hepatitis B virus immunopathogenesis. Annu Rev Immunol *13*, 29-60.

Chisari, F. V., Klopchin, K., Moriyama, T., Pasquinelli, C., Dunsford, H. A., Sell, S., Pinkert, C. A., Brinster, R. L., and Palmiter, R. D. (1989). Molecular pathogenesis of hepatocellular carcinoma in hepatitis B virus transgenic mice. Cell *59*, 1145-56.

Chisari, F. V., Pinkert, C. A., Milich, D. R., Filippi, P., McLachlan, A., Palmiter, R. D., and Brinster, R. L. (1985). A transgenic mouse model of the chronic hepatitis B surface antigen carrier state. Science *230*, 1157-60.

Christofori, G., and Hanahan, D. (1994). Molecular dissection of multi-stage tumorigenesis in transgenic mice. Semin Cancer Biol *5*, 3-12.

Cova, L., Mehrotra, R., Wild, C. P., Chutimataewin, S., Cao, S. F., Duflot, A., Prave, M., Yu, S. Z., Montesano, R., and Trépo, C. (1994). Duck hepatitis B virus infection, aflatoxin B1 and liver cancer in domestic Chinese ducks. Br J Cancer *69*, 104-9.

Crowther, R. A., Kiselev, N. A., Bottcher, B., Berriman, J. A., Borisova, G. P., Ose, V., and Pumpens, P. (1994). Three-dimensional structure of hepatitis B virus core particles determined by electron cryomicroscopy. Cell *77*, 943-50.

Dandri, M., Schirmacher, P., and Rogler, C. E. (1996). Woodchuck Hepatitis Virus X Protein is Present in Chronically Infected Liver and Woodchuck Hepatocellular Carcinomas Which Are Permissive for Viral Replication. J. Virol. *70*, 5246-5254.

Dandri, M., Schirrmacher, P., and Rogler, C. E. (1996). Woodchuck Hepatitis B Virus X Protein is Present in Chronically Infected Woodchuck Liver and Hepatocellular Carcinomas Which Are Permissive for Viral Replication. J Virol *70*, 5246- 5254.

Dandri, M., Petersen, J., Stockert, R. J., Harris, T. M., and Rogler, C. E. (1998). Metabolic Labeling of Woodchuck Hepatitis Virus X Protein in Naturally Infected Hepatocytes Reveals a Bimodal Half-Life and Association with the Nuclear Framework. J Virol *72*, 9359-64.

Deinhardt, F. (1976). Hepatitis in Primates. Advances in Virus Research *20*, 113-157.

Dejean, A., Bougueleret, L., Grzeschik, K., and Tiollais, P. (1986). Hepatitis B virus DNA integration in a sequence homologous to v erb A and steroid receptor genes in a hepatocellular carcinoma. Nature *322*, 70-72.

Dejean, A., and de Thé, H. (1990). Hepatitis B virus as an insertional mutagene in a human hepatocellular carcinoma. Mol Biol Med *7*, 213-22.

Dejean, A., Vitvitski, L., Bréchot, C., Trépo, C., Tiollais, P., and Charnay, P. (1982). Presence and state of woodchuck hepatitis virus DNA in liver and serum of woodchucks: further analogies with human hepatitis B virus. Virology *121*, 195-9.

Dienes, H. P., Gerlich, W. H., Wörsdorfer, M., Gerken, G., Bianchi, L., Hess, G., and Meyer zum Büschenfelde, K. H. (1990). Hepatic expression pattern of the large and middle hepatitis B virus surface proteins in viremic and nonviremic chronic hepatitis B. Gastroenterology *98*, 1017-1023.

Dienstag, J. L., Popper, H., and Purcell, R. H. (1976). The pathology of viral hepatitis types A and B in chimpanzees. A comparison. Am J Pathol *85*, 131-48.

Donato, F., Boffetta, P., and Puoti, M. (1998). A meta-analysis of epidemiological studies on the combined effect of hepatitis B and C virus infections in causing hepatocellular carcinoma. Int J Cancer *75*, 347-354.

Dörfler, W. (1995). The insertion of foreign DNA into mammalian genomes and its consequences: a concept in oncogenesis. Adv Cancer Res *66*, 313-44.

Doria, M., Klein, N., Lucito, R., and Schneider, R. J. (1995). The hepatitis B virus HBx protein is a dual specificity cytoplasmic activator of Ras and nuclear activator of transcription factors. Embo J *14*, 4747-57.

Dragani, T. A., Manenti, G., Farza, H., Della Porta, G., Tiollais, P., and Pourcel, C. (1990). Transgenic mice containing hepatitis B virus sequences are more susceptible to carcinogen-induced hepatocarcinogenesis. Carcinogenesis *11*, 953-6.

Elmore, L. W., Hancock, A. R., Chang, S. F., Wang, X. W., Chang, S., Callahan, C. P., Geller, D. A., Will, H., and Harris, C. C. (1997). Hepatitis B virus X protein and p53 tumor suppressor interactions in the modulation of apoptosis. Proc Natl Acad Sci U S A *94*, 14707-12.

Farber, E., and Cameron, R. (1980). The sequential analysis of cancer development. Adv Cancer Res *31*, 125-226.

Farza, H., Hadchouel, M., Scotto, J., Tiollais, P., Babinet, C., and Pourcel, C. (1988). Replication and gene expression of hepatitis B virus in a transgenic mouse that contains the complete viral genome. J Virol *62*, 4144-52.

Farza, H., Salmon, A. M., Hadchouel, M., Moreau, J. L., Babinet, C., Tiollais, P., and Pourcel, C. (1987). Hepatitis B surface antigen gene expression is regulated by sex steroids and glucocorticoids in transgenic mice. Proc Natl Acad Sci U S A *84*, 1187-91.

Fischer, M., Runkel, L., and Schaller, H. (1995). HBx protein of hepatitis B virus interacts with the C-terminal portion of a novel human proteasome alpha-subunit. Virus Genes *10*, 99-102.

Fourel, G., Couturier, J., Wei, Y., Apiou, F., Tiollais, P., and Buendia, M. A. (1994). Evidence for long-range oncogene activation by hepadnavirus insertion. Embo J *13*, 2526-34.

Galle, P. R. (1997). Apoptosis in liver disease. J Hepatol *27*, 405-12.

Galle, P. R., Hofmann, W. J., Walczak, H., Schaller, H., Otto, G., Stremmel, W., Krammer, P. H., and Runkel, L. (1995). Involvement of the CD95 (Apo-1/Fas) receptor and ligand in liver damage. J Exp Med *182*, 1223- 30.

Garcia, M., de Thé, H., Tiollais, P., Samarut, J., and Dejean, A. (1993). A hepatitis B virus pre-S-retinoic acid receptor beta chimera transforms erythrocytic progenitor cells in vitro. Proc Natl Acad Sci U S A *90*, 89-93.

Gerin, J. L., Cote, P. J., Korba, B. E., Miller, R. H., Purcell, R. H., and Tennant, B. C. (1991). Hepatitis B virus and liver cancer: The woodchuck as an experimental model of hepadnavirus-induced liver cancer. In Viral Hepatitis and Liver Disease, F. B. Hollinger, S. M. Lemon and H. Margolis, eds. (Baltimore: Williams & Wilkins), pp. 556-559.

Ghebraniou, N., and Sell, S. (1998). Hepatitis B injury, male gender, aflatoxin, and p53 expression each contribute to hepatocarcinogenesis in transgenic mice. Hepatology *27*, 383-91.

Gottlob, K., Pagano, S., Levrero, M., and Graessmann, A. (1998). Hepatitis B virus X protein transcription activation domains are neither required nor sufficient for cell transformation. Cancer Res *58*, 3566- 3570.

Graef, E., Caselmann, W., Wells, J., and Koshy, R. (1994). Insertional activation of mevalonate kinase by hepatitis B virus DNA in a human hepatoma cell line. Oncogene *9*, 81-87.

Guidotti, L. G., Matzke, B., Schaller, H., and Chisari, F. V. (1995). High-level hepatitis B virus replication in transgenic mice. J Virol *69*, 6158-69.

Guilhot, S., Miller, T., Cornamn, G., and Isom, H. C. (1996). Apoptosis induced by tumor necrosis factor-alpha in rat hepatocyte cell lines expressing hepatitis B virus. Am. J. Pathol. *148*, 801-814.

Hagen, T. M., Huang, S., Curnutte, J., Fowler, P., Martinez, V., Wehr, C. M., Ames, B. N., and Chisari, F. V. (1994). Extensive oxidative DNA damage in hepatocytes of transgenic mice with chronic active hepatitis destined to develop hepatocellular carcinoma. Proc Natl Acad Sci U S A *91*, 12808-12.

Hanahan, D. (1988). Dissecting multistep tumorigenesis in transgenic mice. Annu Rev Genet *22*, 479-519.

Hansen, L. J., Tennant, B. C., Seeger, C., and Ganem, D. (1993). Differential activation of myc gene family members in hepatic carcinogenesis by closely related hepatitis B viruses. Mol Cell Biol *13*, 659-67.

Hatada, I., Tokino, T., Ochiya, T., and Matsubara, K. (1988). Co-amplification of integrated hepatitis B virus DNA and transforming gene hst-1 in a hepatocellular carcinoma. Oncogene *3*, 537-540.

Henkler, F. F., and Koshy, R. (1996). Hepatitis B virus transcriptional activators: mechanisms and possible role in oncogenesis. J Viral Hepat *3*, 109-21.

Hildt, E., Saher, G., Bruss, V., and Hofschneider, P. H. (1996). The hepatitis B virus large surface protein (LHBs) is a transcriptional activator. Virology *225*, 235-239.

Hildt, E., Urban, S., and Hofschneider, P. H. (1995). Characterization of essential domains for the functionality of the MHBst transcriptional activator and identification of a minimal MHBst activator. Oncogene *11*, 2055-2066.

Hilger, C., Velhagen, I., Zentgraf, H., and Schröder, C. H. (1991). Diversity of hepatitis B virus transcripts in hepatocellular carcinoma – a novel polyadenylation site on viral DNA. J Vir *65*, 4284- 4291.

Hino, O., Nomura, K., Ohtake, K., Kawaguchi, T., Sugano, H., and Kitagawa, T. (1987). Instability of hepatitis B virus with inverted repeat structure in transgenic mouse. Cancer Genet Cytogenet *37*, 273-278.

Hino, O., Shows, T. B., and Rogler, C. E. (1986). Hepatitis B virus integration site in hepatocellular carcinoma at chromosome 17;18 translocation. Proc Natl Acad Sci U S A *83*, 8338-42.

Hino, O., Tabata, S., and Hotta, Y. (1991). Evidence for increased in vitro recombination with insertion of human hepatitis B virus DNA. Proc Natl Acad Sci U S A *88*, 9248-52.

Höhne, M., Schaefer, S., Seifer, M., Feitelson, M. A., Paul, D., and Gerlich, W. H. (1990). Malignant transformation of immortalized transgenic hepatocytes after transfection with hepatitis B virus DNA. Embo J *9*, 1137-45.

Hollstein, M., Soussi, T., Thomas, G., von Brevern, M. C., and Bartsch, N. D. (1997). P53 gene alterations in human tumors: perspectives for cancer control. Recent Results Cancer Res *143*, 369-89.

Hoppe-Seyler, F., and Butz, K. (1995). Molecular mechanisms of virus-induced carcinogenesis: the interaction of viral factors with cellular tumor suppressor proteins. J Mol Med *73*, 529-38.

Hsu, T., Möröy, T., Etiemble, J., Louise, A., Trépo, C., Tiollais, P., and Buendia, M. A. (1988). Activation of c-myc by woodchuck hepatitis virus insertion in hepatocellular carcinoma. Cell *55*, 627-35.

Hsu, T. Y., Fourel, G., Etiemble, J., Tiollais, P., and Buendia, M. A. (1990). Integration of hepatitis virus DNA near c-myc in woodchuck hepatocellular carcinoma. Gastroenterol Jpn *2*, 43-8.

Huang, J., Kwong, J., Sun, E. C., and Liang, T. J. (1996). Proteasome complex as a potential cellular target of hepatitis B virus X protein. J Virol *70*, 5582-91.

IARC (1998). Globocan. Cancer in the world. Internet: http:\\www.iarc.fr.

Jilbert, A. R., Botten, J. A., Miller, D. S., Bertram, E. M., Hall, P. M., Kotlarski, J., and Burrell, C. J. (1998). Characterization of age- and dose-related outcomes of duck hepatitis B virus infection. Virology *244*, 273-82.

Jilbert, A. R., Miller, D. S., Scougall, C. A., Turnbull, H., and Burrell, C. J. (1996). Kinetics of duck hepatitis B virus infection following low dose virus inoculation: one virus DNA genome is infectious in neonatal ducks. Virology *226*, 338-45.

Kaczynski, J., Hansson, G., Hermodsson, S., Olsson, R., and Wallerstedt, S. (1996). Minor Role of Hepatitis B and C Virus Infection in the Etiology of Hepatocellular Carcinoma in a Low-Endemic Area. Scand J Gastroenterol *31*, 809-13.

Kairat, A., Beerheide, W., Zhou, G., Tang, Z.-Y., Edler, L., and Schröder, C.-H. (in press). Truncated hepatitis B virus RNA in human hepatocellular carcinoma: its representation in patients with advancing age. Intervirology.

Kajino, K., Hotta, Y., and Hino, O. (1994). Determination of a putative recombinogenic human hepatitis B virus sequence and its binding cellular protein. Cancer Res *54*, 3971-3973.

Kann, M., Bischof, A., and Gerlich, W. (1997). In vitro model for the nuclear transport of the hepadnavirus genome. J Virol *71*, 1310-1316.

Kann, M., and Gerlich, W. H. (1998). Hepatitis B. In Virology, B. W. J. Mahy and L. Collier, eds. (London, Sydney, Auckland: Arnold), pp. 745-773.

Kekulé, A. (1991). The "trans" hypothesis of liver carcinogenesis. In Human primary liver cancer, C. Bréchot, ed. (Boca Raton: CRC press), pp. 191-210.

Kekulé, A. S., Lauer, U., Meyer, M., Caselmann, W. H., Hofschneider, P. H., and Koshy, R. (1990). The preS2/S region of integrated hepatitis B virus DNA encodes a transcriptional transactivator. Nature *343*, 457-61.

Kekulé, A. S., Lauer, U., Weiss, L., Luber, B., and Hofschneider, P. H. (1993). Hepatitis B virus transactivator HBx uses a tumour promoter signalling pathway [see comments]. Nature *361*, 742-5.

Kim, C. M., Koike, K., Saito, I., Miyamura, T., and Jay, G. (1991). HBx gene of hepatitis B virus induces liver cancer in transgenic mice. Nature *351*, 317-20.

Kim, H., Lee, H., and Yun, Y. (1998). X-gene product of hepatitis B virus induces apoptosis in liver cells. J Biol Chem *273*, 381-5.

Kiyosawa, K., Tanaka, E., and Sodeyama, T. (1998). Hepatitis C Virus and Hepatocellular Carcinoma. In Hepatitis C Virus, H. W. Reesink, ed. (Basel: Karger), pp. 161-180.

Klein, G. (1998). Foulds´ dangerous idea revisited: the multistep development of tumors 40 years later. Adv Cancer Res *72*, 1-23.

Klein, N. P., and Schneider, R. J. (1997). Activation of src family kinases by hepatitis B virus HBx protein and coupled signalling to Ras. Mol Cell Biol *17*, 6427-6436.

Koike, K. (1995). Hepatitis B virus HBx gene and hepatocarcinogenesis. Intervirology *38*, 134-42.

Koike, K. (1998). HBV DNA Integration and Insertional Mutagenesis. In Hepatitis B Virus. Molecular Mechanisms in Disease and Novel Strategies for Therapy, R. Koshy and W. H. Caselmann, eds. (London: Imperial College Press), pp. 133-181.

Koike, K., Kobayashi, M., Gondo, M., Hayashi, I., Osuga, T., and Takada, S. (1998). Hepatitis B virus DNA is frequently found in liver biobsy samples from hepatitis C virus-infected chronic hepatitis patients. J Med Virol *54*, 249- 255.

Koike, K., Moriya, K., Yotsuyanagi, H., Iino, S., and Kurokawa, K. (1994). Induction of cell cycle progression by hepatitis B virus HBx gene expression in quiescent mouse fibroblasts. J Clin Invest *94*, 44-9.

Korba, B. E., Wells, F. V., Baldwin, B., Cote, P. J., Tennant, B. C., Popper, H., and Gerin, J. L. (1989). Hepatocellular carcinoma in woodchuck hepatitis virus-infected woodchucks: presence of viral DNA in tumor tissue from chronic carriers and animals serologically recovered from acute infections. Hepatology *9*, 461-70.

Kuo, G., Choo, Q. L., Alter, H. J., Gitnick, G. L., Redeker, A. G., Purcell, R. H., Miyamura, T., Dienstag, J. L., Alter, M. J., Stevens, C. E., and et al. (1989). An assay for circulating antibodies to a major etiologic virus of human non-A, non-B hepatitis. Science *244*, 362-4.

Lane, D. P., and Crawford, L. V. (1979). T Antigen is bound to a host protein in SV40-transformed cells. Nature *278*, 261-263.

Lanford, R. E., Chavez, D., Brasky, K. M., Burns III, R. B., and Rico-Hesse, R. (1998). Isolation of a hepadnavirus from the woolly monkey, a New World primate. Proc. Natl. Acad. Sci., USA *95*, 5757-5761.

Lara-Pezzi, E., Armesilla, A. L., Majano, P. L., Redondo, J. M., and Lopez-Cabrera, M. (1998). The hepatitis B virus X protein activates nuclear factor for activated T cells (NF-AT) by a cyclosporine A-sensitive pathway. EMBO J *17*, 7066-7077.

Lee, D. S., Huh, K., Lee, E. H., Lee, D. H., Hong, K. S., and Sung, Y. C. (1997). HCV and HBV coexist in HBsAg-negative patients with HCV viraemia: possibility of coinfection in these patients must be considered in HBV-high endemic area. J Gastroenterol Hepatol *12*, 855-61.

Lee, M. S., Kim, D. H., Kim, H., Lee, H. S., Kim, C. Y., Park, T. S., Yoo, K. Y., Park, B. J., and Ahn, Y. O. (1998). Hepatitis B vaccination and reduced risk of primary liver cancer among male adults: a cohort study in Korea. Int. J Epidemiol. *27*, 316-9.

Lee, T. H., Finegold, M. J., Shen, R. F., DeMayo, J. L., Woo, S. L., and Butel, J. S. (1990). Hepatitis B virus transactivator X protein is not tumorigenic in transgenic mice. J Virol *64*, 5939-47.

Lee, Y. H., and Yun, Y. (1998). HBx protein of hepatitis B virus activates Jak1-STAT signaling. J Biol Chem *273*, 25510-5.

Lengauer, C., Kinzler, K. W., and Vogelstein, B. (1998). Genetic instabilities in human cancers. Nature *396*, 643-649.

Lin, Y., Nomura, T., Yamashita, T., Dorjsuren, D., Tang, H., and Murakami, S. (1997). The transactivation and p53-interacting functions of hepatitis B virus X protein are mutually interfering but distinct. Cancer Res *57*, 5137-42.

Linzer, D. I. H., and Levine, A. J. (1979). Characterisation of a 54 K dalton cellular SV40 tumor antigen present in SV40 transformed cells and uninfected embryonal cells. Cell *17*, 43-52.

Loeb, L. A. (1998). Cancer cells exhibit a mutator phenotype. Adv Cancer Res *72*, 25-56.

Luber, B., Arnold, N., Stürzl, M., Höhne, M., Schirmacher, P., Lauer, U., Wienberg, J., Hofschneider, P. H., and Kekulé, A. S. (1996). Hepatoma-derived integrated HBV-DNA causes multi-stage transformation *in vitro*. Oncogene *12*, 1597-1608.

Marion, P. L. (1991). Ground Squirrel Hepatitis Virus. In Molecular Biology of the Hepatitis B Virus, A. MacLachlan, ed. (Boca Raton: CRC Press), pp. 39-51.

Marion, P. L., Knight, S. S., Ho, B. K., Guo, Y. Y., Robinson, W. S., and Popper, H. (1984). Liver disease associated with duck hepatitis B virus infection of domestic ducks. Proc Natl Acad Sci U S A *81*, 898-902.

Marion, P. L., Van Davelaar, M. J., Knight, S. S., Salazar, F. H., Garcia, G., Popper, H., and Robinson, W. S. (1986). Hepatocellular carcinoma in ground squirrels persistently infected with ground squirrel hepatitis virus. Proc Natl Acad Sci U S A *83*, 4543-6.

Matsubara, K., and Tokino, T. (1990). Integration of hepatitis B virus and its implications for hepatocarcinogenesis. Mol Biol Med *7*, 243-260.

Maynard, J. E. (1990). Hepatitis B. Global Importance and need for control. Vaccine *8*, S18- S20.

Meyer, M., Caselmann, W. H., Schlüter, V., Schreck, R., Hofschneider, P. H., and Baeuerle, P. A. (1992). Hepatitis B virus transactivator MHBst: activation of NF-kappa B, selective inhibition by antioxidants and integral membrane localization. Embo J *11*, 2991-3001.

Mimms, L. T., Solomon, L. R., Ebert, J. W., and Fields, H. (1993). Unique preS sequence in a gibbon-derived hepatitis B virus variant. Biochem Biophys Res Commun *195*, 186-91.

Möröy, T., Marchio, A., Etiemble, J., Trépo, C., Tiollais, P., and Buendia, M. A. (1986). Rearrangement and enhanced expression of c-myc in hepatocellular carcinoma of hepatitis virus infected woodchucks. Nature *324*, 276-9.

Muchmore, E., Popper, H., Peterson, D. A., Miller, M. F., and Lieberman, H. M. (1988). Non-A, non-B hepatitis related hepatocellular carcinoma in a chimpanzee. J. Med. Primatol. *17*, 235-246.

Nassal, M., and Schaller, H. (1996). Hepatitis B virus replication – an update. J Viral Hepatitis *3*, 217-226.

Naumann, H., Schaefer, S., Yoshida, C. F., Gaspar, A. M., Repp, R., and Gerlich, W. H. (1993). Identification of a new hepatitis B virus (HBV) genotype from Brazil that expresses HBV surface antigen subtype adw4. J Gen Virol *74*, 1627-32.

Norder, H., Courouce, A. M., and Magnius, L. O. (1994). Complete genomes, phylogenetic relatedness, and structural proteins of six strains of the hepatitis B virus, four of which represent two new genotypes. Virology *198*, 489-503.

Norder, H., Ebert, J. W., Filds, H., Mushawar, I. K., and Magnius, L. O. (1996). Complete Sequencing of a Gibbon Hepatitis B Virus Genome Reveals a Unique Genotype Distantly Related to the Chimpanzee Hepatitis B Virus. Virology *218*, 214-223.

Nowak, M. A., Bonhoeffer, S., Hill, A. M., Boehme, R., Thomas, H. C., and McDade, H. (1996). Viral dynamics in hepatitis B virus infection. Proc Natl Acad Sci U S A *93*, 4398-402.

Oguey, D., Dumenco, L. L., Pierce, R. H., and Fausto, N. (1996). Analysis of the tumorigenicity of the X gene of HBV in a non-transformed hepatocyte cell line and the effects of cotransfection with murine p53 mutant equivlent to human codon 249. Hepatology *24*, 1024-1033.

Orito, E., Mizokami, M., Ina, Y., Moriyama, E. N., Kameshima, N., Yamamoto, M., and Gojobori, T. (1989). Host-independent evolution and a genetic classification of the hepadnavirus family based on nucleotide sequences. Proc Natl Acad Sci U S A *86*, 7059-62.

Paronetto, F., and Tennant, B. C. (1990). Woodchuck hepatitis virus infection: a model of human hepatic diseases and hepatocellular carcinoma. Prog Liver Dis *9*, 463-83.

Pasquinelli, C., Bhavani, K., and Chisari, F. V. (1992). Multiple oncogenes and tumor suppressor genes are structurally and functionally intact during hepatocarcinogenesis in hepatitis B virus transgenic mice. Cancer Res *52*, 2823-9.

Paul, D., Höhne, M., Pinkert, C., Piasecki, A., Ummelmann, E., and Brinster, R. L. (1988). Immortalized differentiated hepatocyte lines derived from transgenic mice harboring SV40 T-antigen genes. Exp Cell Res *175*, 354-62.

Petzinger, E., Follmann, W., Blumrich, M., Walther, P., Hentschel, J., Bette, P., Maurice, M., and Feldmann, G. (1994). Immortalization of rat hepatocytes by fusion with hepatoma cells. I. Cloning of a hepatocytoma cell line with bile canaliculi. Eur J Cell Biol *64*, 328-38.

Pillot, J. (1990). [Primates in the study of hepatitis viruses]. Pathol Biol Paris *38*, 177-81.

Pineau, P., Marchio, A., Mattei, M. G., Kim, W. H., Youn, J. K., Tiollais, P., and Dejean, A. (1998). Extensive analysis of duplicated-inverted hepatitis B virus integrations in human hepatocellular carcinoma. J Gen Virol *79*, 591-600.

Popper, H. (1988). Viral versus chemical hepatocarcinogenesis. J Hepatol *6*, 229-38.

Popper, H., Dienstag, J. L., M, F. S., Alter, H. J., and Purcell, R. H. (1980). Virchows Arch. A Pathol. Anat. Histol. *387*, 91- 106.

Popper, H., Roth, L., Purcell, R. H., Tennant, D. C., and Gerin, J. L. (1987). Hepatocarcinogenicity of the woodchuck hepatitis virus. Proc Natl Acad Sci U S A *84*, 866-70.

Popper, H., Thung, S. N., McMahon, B. J., Lanier, A. P., Hawkins, I., and Alberts, S. R. (1988). Evolution of hepatocellular carcinoma associated with chronic hepatitis B virus infection in Alaskan Eskimos. Arch Pathol Lab Med *112*, 498-504.

Prost, S., Ford, J. M., Taylor, C., Doig, J., and Harrison, D. J. (1998). Hepatitis B x protein inhibits p53-dependent DNA repair in primary mouse hepatocytes. J Biol Chem *273*, 33327- 32.

Rakotomahanina, C. K., Hilger, C., Fink, T., Zentgraf, H., and Schröder, C. H. (1994). Biological activities of a putative truncated hepatitis B virus X gene product fused to a polylysin stretch. Oncogene 9, 2613-21.

Ray, R. B., Lagging, L. M., Meyer, K., and Ray, R. (1996). Hepatitis C virus core protein cooperates with ras and transforms primary rat embryo fibroblasts to tumorigenic phenotype. J Virol 70, 4438-43.

Ricciardi, R. P. (1995). Transformation and Tumorigenesis Mediated by the Adenovirus E1A and E1B Oncogenes. In DNA Tumor Viruses. Oncogenic Mechanisms, G. Brabanti-Brodano, M. Bendinelli and H. Friedman, eds. (New York and London: Plenum Press), pp. 195- 225.

Robinson, W. S. (1994). Molecular events in the pathogenesis of hepadnavirus-associated hepatocellular carcinoma. Annu Rev Med 45, 297-323.

Robinson, W. S., Klote, L., and Aoki, N. (1990). Hepadnaviruses in cirrhotic liver and hepatocellular carcinoma. J Med Virol 31, 18-32.

Robinson, W. S., Miller, R. H., and Marion, P. L. (1987). Hepadnaviruses and retroviruses share genome homology and features of replication. Hepatology 7, 64s-73s.

Rossner, M. (1992). Review: Hepatitis B Virus X-Gene Product: A Promiscuous Transcriptional Activator. Journal of Medical Virology 36, 101-117.

Runkel, L., Fischer, M., and Schaller, H. (1993). Two-codon insertion mutations of the HBx define two separate regions necessary for its trans-activation function. Virology 197, 529-36.

Schaack, J., Maguire, H. F., and Siddiqui, A. (1996). Hepatitis B virus X protein partially substitutes for E1A transcriptional function during adenovirus infection. Virology 216, 425-30.

Schaefer, S., and Gerlich, W. H. (1995). In Vitro Transformation by Hepatitis B Virus DNA. Intervirology 38, 143-154.

Schaefer, S., Seifer, M., Grimmsmann, T., Fink, L., Wenderhold, S., Höhne, M. W., and Gerlich, W. H. (1998). Properties of tumour suppressor p53 in murine hepatocyte lines transformed by hepatitis B virus X protein. J. Gen. Virol. 79, 767-777.

Schaefer, S., Tolle, T., Lottmann, S., and Gerlich, W. H. G. (1998). Animal Models and Experimental Systems in Hepatitis B Virus Research. In Hepatitis B Virus: Molecular Mechanisms in Disease and Novel Strategies for Therapy, R. Koshy and W. H. Caselmann, eds., pp. 51-74.

Schek, N., Bartenschlager, R., Kuhn, C., and Schaller, H. (1991). Phosphorylation of hepatitis B virus X-Protein expressed in HepG2 cells from a recombinant vaccinia virus. Oncogene 6, 1735-1744.

Schlüter, V., Meyer, M., Hofschneider, P. H., Koshy, R., and Caselmann, W. H. (1994). Integrated hepatitis B virus X and 3' truncated preS/S sequences derived from human hepatomas encode functionally active transactivators. Oncogene 9, 3335-44.

Schödel, F., Weimer, T., Fernholz, D., Schneider, R., Sprengel, R., Wildner, G., and Will, H. (1991). The Biology of Avian Hepatitis B Viruses. In Molecular Biology of the Hepatitis B Virus, A. MacLachlan, ed. (Boca Raton: CRC Press), pp. 53-80.

Schröder, C., and Zentgraf, H. (1990). Hepatitis B virus related hepatocellular carcinoma: chronicity of infection- the opening to different pathways of malignant transformation? Biochim et Biophys Acta 1032, 137-156.

Seeger, C., Baldwin, B., Hornbuckle, W. E., Yeager, A. E., Tennant, B. C., Cote, P., Ferrell, L., Ganem, D., and Varmus, H. E. (1991). Woodchuck hepatitis virus is a more efficient oncogenic agent than ground squirrel hepatitis virus in a common host. J Virol 65, 1673-9.

Seifer, M., and Gerlich, W. H. (1992). Increased growth of permanent mouse fibroblasts in soft agar after transfection with hepatitis B virus DNA. Arch Virol 126, 119-28.

Seifer, M., Höhne, M., Schaefer, S., and Gerlich, W. H. (1991). In vitro tumorigenicity of hepatitis B virus DNA and HBx protein. J Hepatol 13, S61-5.

Seifer, M., Höhne, M., Schaefer, S., and Gerlich, W. H. (1991). Malignant transformation of immortalized cells by hepatitis B virus DNA. In Viral Hepatitis-1990, F. Hollinger, S. Lemon and H. Margolis, eds. (New York: Williams and Wilkins), pp. 586-588.

Shih, C. M., Lo, S. J., Miyamura, T., Chen, S. Y., and Lee, Y. H. (1993). Suppression of hepatitis B virus expression and replication by hepatitis C virus core protein in HuH-7 cells. J Virol 67, 5823-32.

Shikata, T., Karasawa, T., and Abe, K. (1980). Two distinct types of hepatitis in experimental hepatitis B virus infection. Am. J. Pathol. 99, 343- 368.

Shirakata, Y., Kawada, M., Fujiki, Y., Sano, H., Oda, M., Yaginuma, K., Kobayashi, M., and Koike, K. (1989). The X gene of hepatitis B virus induced growth stimulation and tumorigenic transformation of mouse NIH3T3 cells. Jpn J Cancer Res *80*, 617-21.

Shouval, D. (1994). Hepatitis B in Chimpanzees. In The Role of the Chimpanzee in Research, G. Eder, E. Kaiser and F. A. King, eds. (Basel: Karger), pp. 175-179.

Shouval, D., Chakraborty, P. R., Ruiz Opazo, N., Baum, S., Spigland, I., Muchmore, E., Gerber, M. A., Thung, S. N., Popper, H., and Shafritz, D. A. (1980). Chronic hepatitis in chimpanzee carriers of hepatitis B virus: morphologic, immunologic, and viral DNA studies. Proc Natl Acad Sci U S A *77*, 6147-51.

Sirma, H., Weil, R., Rosmorduc, O., Urban, S., Israel, A., Kremsdorf, D., and Bréchot, C. (1998). Cytosol is the prime compartment of hepatitis B virus X protein where it colocalizes with the proteasome. Oncogene *16*, 2051-63.

Sitterlin, D., Lee, T. H., Prigent, S., Tiollais, P., Butel, J. S., and Transy, C. (1997). Interaction of the UV-damaged DNA-binding protein with hepatitis B virus X protein is conserved among mammalian hepadnaviruses and restricted to transactivation-proficient X-insertion mutants. J Virol *71*, 6194-9.

Slagle, B. L., Lee, T. H., Medina, D., Finegold, M. J., and Butel, J. S. (1996). Increased Sensititvity to the hepatocarcinogen diethylnitrosamine in transgenic mice carrying the hepatitis B virus X gene. Mol. Carcinogen *15*, 261-269.

Slagle, B. L., Zhou, Y. Z., and Butel, J. S. (1991). Hepatitis B virus integration event in human chromosome 17p near the p53 gene identifies the region of the chromosome commonly deleted in virus-positive hepatocellular carcinomas. Cancer Res *51*, 49-54.

Soussi, T., Legros, Y., Lubin, R., Ory, K., and Schlichtholz, B. (1994). Multifactorial analysis of p53 alteration in human cancer: a review. Int J Cancer *57*, 1-9.

Spandau, D. F., and Lee, C. H. (1988). Trans-activation of viral enhancers by the hepatitis B virus X protein. J Virol *62*, 427-34.

Stuver, S. O. (1997). Towards Global Control of Liver Cancer? Semin Cancer Biol *8*, 299- 306.

Su, F., and Schneider, R. J. (1997). Hepatitis B virus HBx protein sensitizes cells to apoptotic killing by tumor necrosis factor alpha. Proc. Natl. Acad. Sci. USA *94*, 8744-8749.

Su, Q., Schröder, C. H., Hofmann, W. J., Otto, G., Pichlmayr, R., and Bannasch, P. (1998). Expression of hepatitis B virus X protein in HBV-infected human livers and hepatocellular carcinomas. Hepatology *27*, 1109-20.

Summers, J., Smolec, J. M., and Snyder, R. (1978). A virus similar to human hepatitis B virus associated with hepatitis and hepatoma in woodchucks. Proc Natl Acad Sci U S A *75*, 4533-7.

Tabor, E. (1994). Tumor suppressor genes, growth factor genes, and oncogenes in hepatitis B virus-associated hepatocellular carcinoma. J Med Virol *42*, 357-65.

Takada, S., Kaneniwa, N., Tsuchida, N., and Koike, K. (1997). Cytoplasmic retention of the p53 tumor suppressor gene product is observed in the hepatitis B virus X gene-transfected cells. Oncogene *15*, 1895-1901.

Takada, S., and Koike, K. (1990). Trans-activation function of a 3' truncated X gene-cell fusion product from integrated hepatitis B virus DNA in chronic hepatitis tissues. Proc Natl Acad Sci U S A *87*, 5628-32.

Terradillos, O., Billet, O., Renard, C. A., Levy, R., Molina, T., Briand, P., and Buendia, M. A. (1997). The hepatitis B virus X gene potentiates c-myc-induced liver oncogenesis in transgenic mice. Oncogene *14*, 395-404.

Terradillos, O., Pollicino, T., Lecoeur, H., Tripodi, M., Gougeon, M. L., Tiollais, P., and Buendia, M. A. (1998). p53-independent apoptotic effects of the hepatitis B virus X protein in vivo and in vitro. Oncogene *17*, 2115-23.

Testut, P., Renard, C. A., Terradillos, O., Vitvitski Trépo, L., Tekaia, F., Degott, C., Blake, J., Boyer, B., and Buendia, M. A. (1996). A new hepadnavirus endemic in arctic ground squirrels in Alaska. J Virol *70*, 4210-9.

Truant, R., Antunovic, J., Greenblatt, J., Prives, C., and Cromlish, J. A. (1995). Direct interaction of the hepatitis B virus HBx protein with p53 leads to inhibition by HBx of p53 response element-directed transactivation. J Virol *69*, 1851-9.

Twu, J. S., Lai, M. Y., Chen, D. S., and Robinson, W. S. (1993). Activation of protooncogene c-jun by the X protein of hepatitis B virus. Virology *192*, 346-50.

Twu, J. S., and Schloemer, R. H. (1987). Transcriptional trans-activating function of hepatitis B virus. J Virol *61*, 3448-53.

Ueda, H., Ullrich, S. J., Gangemi, J. D., Kappel, C. A., Ngo, L., Feitelson, M. A., and Jay, G. (1995). Functional inactivation but not structural mutation of p53 causes liver cancer. Nat Genet *9*, 41-7.

Urban, M. K., AP, O. C., and London, W. T. (1985). Sequence of events in natural infection of Pekin duck embryos with duck hepatitis B virus. J Virol *55*, 16-22.

Vaudin, M., Wolstenholme, A. J., Tsiquaye, K. N., Zuckerman, A. J., and Harrison, T. J. (1988). The complete nucleotide sequence of the genome of a hepatitis B virus isolated from a naturally infected chimpanzee. J Gen Virol *69*, 1383-9.

Walter, E., Keist, R., Niederöst, B., Pult, I., and Blum, H. E. (1996). Hepatitis B Virus Infection of Tupaia Hepatocytes *In Vitro* and *In Vivo*. Hepatology *24*, 1-5.

Wang, J., Chenivesse, X., Henglein, B., and Bréchot, C. (1990). Hepatitis B virus integration in a cyclin A gene in a hepatocellular carcinoma. Nature *343*, 555-7.

Wang, J., Zindy, F., Chenivesse, X., Lamas, E., Henglein, B., and Bréchot, C. (1992). Modification of cyclin A expression by hepatitis B virus DNA integration in a hepatocellular carcinoma. Oncogene *7*, 1653-6.

Wang, X. W., Forrester, K., Yeh, H., Feitelson, M. A., Gu, J. R., and Harris, C. C. (1994). Hepatitis B virus X protein inhibits p53 sequence-specific DNA binding, transcriptional activity, and association with transcription factor ERCC3. Proc Natl Acad Sci U S A *91*, 2230-4.

Wang, X. W., Gibson, M. K., Vermeulen, W., Yeh, H., Forrester, K., Stürzbecher, H. W., Hoeijmakers, J. H., and Harris, C. C. (1995). Abrogation of p53-induced apoptosis by the hepatitis B virus X gene. Cancer Res *55*, 6012-6.

Wei, Y., Ponzetto, A., Tiollais, P., and Buendia, M. A. (1992). Multiple rearrangements and activated expression of c-myc induced by woodchuck hepatitis virus integration in a primary liver tumour. Res Virol *143*, 89-96.

WHO (1998). The World Health Report 1998. Life in the 21st century – A vision for all. http://www.who.org.

Wollersheim, M., Debelka, U., and Hofschneider, P. H. (1988). A transactivating function encoded in the hepatitis B virus X gene is conserved in the integrated state. Oncogene *3*, 545-52.

Wu, J. C., Merlino, G., Cveklova, K., Mosinger, B., Jr., and Fausto, N. (1994). Autonomous growth in serum-free medium and production of hepatocellular carcinomas by differentiated hepatocyte lines that overexpress transforming growth factor alpha 1. Cancer Res *54*, 5964-73.

Yamamoto, S., Mita, E., Nakatake, H., Takimoto, M., Koshy, R., and Matsubara, K. (1993). Transactivating function of integrated hepatitis B virus. Biochem Biophys Res Commun *197*, 1209-15.

Yamamoto, S., Nakatake, H., Kawamoto, S., Takimoto, M., Koshy, R., and Matsubara, K. (1993). Transactivation of cellular promoters by an integrated hepatitis B virus DNA. Biochem Biophys Res Commun *192*, 111-8.

Yamamura, K., Tsurimoto, T., Ebihara, T., Kamino, K., Fujiyama, A., Ochiya, T., and Matsubara, K. (1987). Methylation of hepatitis B virus DNA and liver-specific suppression of RNA production in transgenic mouse. Jpn J Cancer Res *78*, 681-8.

Yan, R. Q., Su, J. J., Huang, D. R., Gan, Y. C., Yang, C., and Huang, G. H. (1996). Human hepatitis B virus and hepatocellular carcinoma. II. Experimental induction of hepatocellular carcinoma in tree shrews exposed to hepatitis B virus and aflatoxin B1. J Cancer Res Clin Oncol *122*, 289-95.

Yen, T. S. B. (1996). Hepadnaviral X Protein: Review of Recent Progress. Journal of Biomedical Science *3*, 20-30.

Zahm, P., Hofschneider, P. H., and Koshy, R. (1988). The HBV X-ORF encodes a transactivator: a potential factor in viral hepatocarcinogenesis. Oncogene *3*, 169-77.

Zoulim, F., Saputelli, J., and Seeger, C. (1994). Woodchuck hepatitis virus X protein is required for viral infection in vivo. J Virol *68*, 2026-30.

Zuckerman, A. J. (1997). Prevention of Primary Liver Cancer by Immunization. New Eng J Med *336*, 1906-1907.

EPSTEIN-BARR VIRUS AND ONCOGENESIS:
FROM TUMORS TO TRANSFORMING GENES

Lawrence S. Young

CRC Institute for Cancer Studies, University of Birmingham Medical School

Background

Epstein-Barr virus (EBV) is a human herpesvirus which is found as a widespread and largely asymptomatic infection in all human communities. Primary infection with EBV usually occurs in childhood and, once infected, individuals become life-long virus carriers. The virus is the causative agent of infectious mononucleosis (IM), a self-limiting disease resulting from delayed primary EBV infection, and is also associated with the pathogenesis of a number of malignant diseases, including Burkitt's lymphoma (BL), the immunoblastic lymphomas that may arise in immunocompromised patients and nasopharyngeal carcinoma (NPC) (Rickinson and Kieff, 1996). The B lymphotropic nature of EBV is evidenced by its association with the B cell lymphoproliferative diseases and by the unique ability of the virus to immortalise normal resting B lymphocytes *in vitro*, converting them into permanently growing lymphoblastoid cell lines (LCLs) (Kieff, 1996). When peripheral blood lymphocytes from chronic virus carriers are placed in culture, the few EBV-infected B cells that are present regularly give rise to spontaneous outgrowth of EBV-transformed LCLs provided that immune T cells are either removed or inhibited by addition of cyclosporin A to the culture (Rickinson et al., 1984). This phenomenon highlights the importance of EBV-specific cytotoxic T lymphocytes (CTLs) in controlling EBV-induced B cell transformation *in vivo*.

EBV is orally transmitted and infectious virus, measured by its ability to immortalise B cells *in vitro*, can be detected in oropharyngeal secretions from IM patients, from patients who are immunosuppressed and at lower levels from healthy EBV seropositive individuals (Gerber et al., 1972; Strauch et al., 1974; Yao et al., 1985). These observations, together with the demonstration of replicating EBV in exfoliated oropharyngeal epithelial cells from IM patients (Sixbey et al., 1984) and the rampant virus replication observed in the AIDS-associated oral hairy leukoplakia lesion (Greenspan et al., 1985), suggest that EBV replicates and is shed at epithelial sites in the oropharynx or from salivary glands. The close proximity of B lymphoid tissue to oropharyngeal epithelium may provide a route of spread of EBV from epithelial cells to B cells, the latter serving to disseminate the infection via the circulation; subsequently the virus may reactivate from the B cell reservoir to re-infect epithelial sites. Whilst it has been hypothesised that epithelial cells are the site of EBV persistence, recent evidence points to a central role for B lymphocytes in mediating primary infection and in the subsequent maintenance of the asymptomatic virus carrier state (Niedobitek and Young, 1994). The

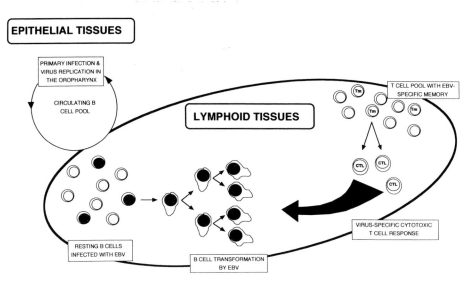

Figure 1. EBV infection in normal healthy virus carriers. Virus infection involves two cellular compartments: (i) B lymphocytes, where infection is predominantly latent and has the potential to induce growth-transformation of infected cells and (ii) epithelial cells, where infection is predominantly replicative. Whilst the exact mode of primary and persistent EBV infection and the relative contributions of B-cells and epithelial cells are uncertain, recent data point to the B-cell compartment as the main mediator of primary as well as persistent infection. Following primary infection of B lymphocytes, a chronic virus carrier state is established in which the outgrowth of EBV growth-transformed B-cells is controlled by an EBV-specific cytotoxic T lymphocyte (CTL) response reactivated from a pool of virus-specific memory T cells. At certain sites, presumably in the oropharynx, latently infected B-cells may become permissive for lytic EBV infection. Infectious virus released from these cells may be shed directly into the saliva or may infect epithelial cells and other B cells. In this way a virus-carrier state is established which is characterised by persistent, latent infection in circulating B cells and occasional EBV replication in B cells and epithelial cells.

potential interactions between epithelial and lymphoid compartments in a normal healthy virus carrier are illustrated diagrammatically in Figure 1.

EBV-associated tumors

Since the original observation of EBV infection in BL biopsy cells, the presence of EBV has been detected in a range of lymphoid malignancies and in certain carcinomas (Rickinson and Kieff, 1996). The development of more sensitive in situ hybridisation techniques and of monoclonal antibodies to specific EBV proteins has resulted in an ever-increasing number of different malignancies in which virus infection can be de-

Table 1. EBV-associated tumours

Tumour	Subtype	EBV genome positive
Burkitts lymphoma	Endemic	100%
	Sporadic	10-20%
	AIDS	30-40%
Nasopharngeal carcinoma	Undiff.	100%
Gastric carcinoma	Adenocarcinoma	6-16% ?
	UNCT	
Hodgkin's disease	Mixed cellularity	> 80%
	Nodular sclerosing	30%
	Lymphocyte predominant	< 10%
T cell lymphoma	Nasal	100%
	Others	10-20%
Immunoblastic lymphoma	Transplant	100%
	AIDS	> 90%

tected. However, this section will only consider those tumors for which an association with EBV infection is well-characterised. The tumors associated with EBV infection are summarised in Table 1.

Burkitt's lymphoma

The endemic form of BL which is found in areas of equatorial Africa and New Guinea represents the most common childhood cancer (peak age 7-9 years) in these regions with an incidence of up to 10 cases per 100,000 people per year. This high incidence of BL is associated with holoendemic malaria accounting for the climatic variation in tumor incidence first recognised by Dennis Burkitt who discovered the tumor in 1958 (Burkitt, 1962). More than 95% of these endemic BL tumors are EBV-positive compared with 20% of the low incidence, sporadic form of BL which occurs world-wide. In areas of intermediate BL incidence, such as Algeria and Malaysia, the increased number of cases correlates with an increased proportion of EBV-positive tumors. BL is also observed as a consequence of HIV infection frequently occurring before the development of full blown AIDS. Only 30-40% of these cases of AIDS-BL are associated with EBV infection (Rickinson and Kieff, 1996). A consistent feature of all BL tumors, irrespective of geographical location or AIDS association, are chromosomal translocations involving the long arm of chromosome 8 (8q24) in the region of c-*myc* proto-oncogene and either chromosome 14 in the region of the immunoglobulin heavy-chain gene or, less frequently, chromosomes 2 or 22 in the region of the immunoglobulin light-chain genes (Magrath and Bhatia, 1997). Seroepidemiological studies have demonstrated elevated antibody titres to EBV capsid antigen (VCA) and early antigens (EA) in BL patients compared to children without the tumor (Henle, and Henle. 1979). These elevated antibody titres have been found to precede the development of BL and can therefore be used to screen 'at risk' individuals.

The precise role of EBV in the pathogenesis of BL remains obscure. Monoclonal EBV episomes have been detected in virus-positive BL biopsies suggesting that EBV infection preceded proliferation of the precursor B cells (Neri et al., 1991). The apparent germinal centre origin of BL is based on phenotypic studies (see below) and is supported by the ability of BL risk factors such as holoendemic malaria and chronic HIV infection to stimulate germinal centre cell proliferation (Rickinson and Kieff, 1996; Magrath and Bhatia, 1997). These cells are also programmed to undergo somatic mutation of immunoglobulin genes and this event, in conjunction with the stimulation of germinal centre proliferation and EBV infection, may be responsible for the generation and selection of B cells carrying the c-myc translocation.

Nasopharyngeal carcinoma (NPC) and gastric carcinoma

The tumor showing the most consistent worldwide association with EBV is undifferentiated NPC, a carcinoma that is particularly common in areas of China and South-East Asia (Niedobitek et al., 1996; Rickinson and Kieff, 1996). This association was originally identified by serological analysis and later confirmed by the demonstration of EBV DNA in NPC biopsy material (Wolf et al., 1973; zur Hausen et al., 1970). NPC is particularly common in areas of China and South-East Asia reaching a peak incidence of around 20-30 per 100,000. Incidence rates are high in individuals of Chinese descent, irrespective of where they live, and particularly in Cantonese males. In addition to this genetic pre-disposition, environmental co-factors such as dietary components (i.e. salted fish) are thought to be important in the aetiology of NPC (Yu et al., 1986). Extensive serological screening has identified elevated EBV-specific antibody titres in high incidence areas, in particular IgA antibodies to EBV capsid antigen (VCA) and early antigens (EA), and these have proved useful in diagnosis and in monitoring the effectiveness of therapy (Zeng et al., 1985).

The revised WHO classification recognises two main histological types of NPC, squamous cell carcinoma (SCC) and non-keratinising carcinoma. This latter group can be subdivided into differentiated non-keratinising and undifferentiated carcinomas and the association of these tumors with EBV has been confirmed for many different racial groups whether these exhibit a high, intermediate or low incidence of the tumor (Niedobitek et al., 1996). These tumors are commonly associated with a prominent lymphoid stroma and similar tumors, referred to as undifferentiated carcinomas of nasopharyngeal type (UCNT), arising in the stomach, the salivary glands, the thymus and the lungs have been shown to be EBV positive (Niedobitek et al., 1996). Recent studies indicate that EBV can also be detected in the relatively rare SCCs arising in the nasopharynx although this association appears to be more geographically variable than that for the non-keratinising tumors (Pathmanathan et al., 1995a; Nicholls et al. 1997).

A proportion of typical gastric adenocarcinomas lacking a lymphoid stroma have been shown to harbour EBV and these, combined with the rarer UCNT type gastric tumors, have led to estimates that around 6-16% of gastric carcinomas are EBV-positive (Osato and Imai, 1996). Taking into account the incidence of gastric cancer in both developed and developing countries, this would amount to a worldwide figure of around 50,000 new cases of EBV-postive gastric cancer per year.

The exact contribution of EBV to the development of NPC and other carcinomas is unclear as is the stage in the oncogenic process at which EBV infection of epithelial cells occurs. In both NPC and EBV-positive gastric carcinoma the tumor cells carry monoclonal viral genomes indicating that EBV infection must have occurred prior to expansion of the malignant cell clone (Niedobitek et al., 1996; Osato and Imai, 1996) . Whilst EBV infection of normal nasopharyngeal mucosa has not been observed, EBER-positive dysplastic and carcinoma *in situ* lesions have been detected (Niedobitek et al., 1996). In one study these pre-invasive lesions were shown to harbor clonal EBV genomes and to express the oncogenic LMP1 protein (Pathmanathan et al., 1995b). These observations together with our data in epithelial cells expressing a transfected EBV receptor (CR2) demonstrating that stable EBV infection requires an undifferentiated phenotype (Knox et al., 1996) support the possibility that epithelial cells may become susceptible to EBV infection as a result of exposure to environmental carcinogens such as those dietary factors previously implicated in the aetiology of NPC. Thus, it appears that EBV infection of pre-neoplastic mucosa may be a rare but essential event in the development of NPC and other virus-associated carcinomas.

LYMPHOMAS IN PATIENTS WITH IMMUNODEFICIENCY
Patients with primary immunodeficiency diseases such as X-linked lymphoproliferative syndrome (XLP) and Wiscott-Aldrich syndrome are at increased risk of developing EBV-associated B cell lymphomas (Rickinson and Kieff, 1996; Niedobitek and Young, 1997). Because these tumors are extremely rare little is known of their association with EBV infection. Mortality from XLP is high with around 50% of patients developing fatal IM after primary infection with EBV and an additional 30% of patients developing malignant lymphoma. The XLP gene has recently been identified and found to encode a small T cell-specific protein (SAP) which inhibits signalling via SLAM (signalling lymphocyte-activation molecule), a membrane protein expressed on B and T cells which through homotypic interaction is involved in the regulation of lymphocyte growth and differentiation (Sayos et al., 1998). The mutation of SAP in XLP patients removes this control and impairs T cell responses to EBV thereby resulting in unchecked EBV-induced B cell proliferation.

Allograft recipients receiving immunosuppressive therapy and patients with AIDS are also at increased risk for development of EBV-associated lymphoproliferative disease and immunoblastic lymphomas (Rickinson and Kieff, 1996; Niedobitek and Young, 1997). The incidence of B cell lymphomas in allograft recipients varies with the type of organ transplanted and with the type of immunosuppressive regimen used. Allogeneic bone marrow transplantation into EBV seronegative children is a particular risk factor for the development of virus-associated B cell lymphomas. The incidence of non-Hodgkin lymphoma in AIDS patients is increased approximately 60-fold compared to the normal population. Around 60% of these tumors are large-cell lymphomas like those found in allograft recipients, 20% are primary brain lymphomas and 20% are of the BL type. Recent studies have demonstrated that 50% of AIDS lymphomas are EBV-positive and that this association varies with the histological tumor type (Hamilton-

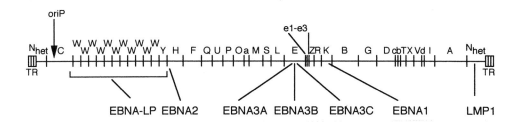

Figure 2. Location of open reading frames for the EBV latent proteins on the BamHI restriction map of the prototype B95.8 EBV genome. The BamHI fragments are named according to size with A being the largest. Note that the LMP2 proteins are produced from mRNAs that splice across the terminal repeats (TR) in the circularised EBV genome.

Dutoit et al., 1991). Thus, only 38% of the BL tumors are EBV-positive compared with 65% of the large-cell lymphomas.

T CELL LYMPHOMAS

Recent studies have demonstrated EBV infection in a considerable proportion of T cell non-Hodgkin's lymphomas (Meijer et al., 1996, Niedobitek and Young, 1997). Nasal T cell lymphomas, a tumor which is more common in the Far East, is invariably EBV-positive whereas around 20% of T cell lymphomas arising at other sites (gastro-intestinal, lung, lymph nodes) are associated with EBV. A rare form of virus-associated haemophagocytic syndrome (VAHS) involves the proliferation of EBV-infected T cells resulting in polyclonal lymphocytosis which can lead to monoclonal lymphoma (Kawa-guchi et al., 1993). An intriguing aspect of EBV-positive T cell lymphomas is the frequent detection of the virus in only a fraction (5-50%) of the tumor cells implying that EBV infection may have occurred subsequent to tumor development (Niedobitek and Young, 1997). The documented increase in the proportion of EBV-positive tumor cells with T cell lymphoma progression or recurrence suggests that the virus may provide an additional growth/survival advantage to the transformed T cells.

HODGKIN'S DISEASE

Epidemiological studies originally suggested a possible role for EBV in the aetiology of Hodgkin's disease (HD). Thus, elevated antibody titres to EBV antigens have been detected in patients with HD and these increased antibody levels are present before the diagnosis of disease (Herbst, 1996). Furthermore, there is an increased risk of HD following IM. EBV has been demonstrated in around 50% of HD cases with both viral nucleic acid (DNA/RNA) and virus latent antigens localised to the malignant compo-

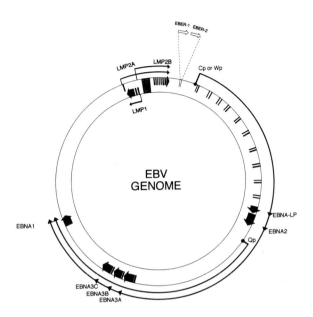

Figure 3. Location and transcription of the EBV latent genes on the double-stranded viral DNA episome. The large solid arrows represent coding exons for each of the latent proteins and the direction in which they are transcribed. EBNA-LP is transcribed from variable numbers of repetitive exons in the BamHI W fragments. LMP2 is composed of multiple exons located either side of the terminal repeat (TR) region which is formed during the circularization of the linear DNA to produce the viral episome. The open arrows represent the highly transcribed non-polyadenylated RNAs, EBER1 and EBER2, which are a consistent feature latent EBV infection. The outer long arrowed line represents EBV transcription in Lat III where all the EBNAs are transcribed from either the Cp or Wp promoter; the different EBNAs are encoded by individual mRNAs generated by differential splicing of the same long primary transcript. The inner shorter arrowed line represents the EBNA1 transcript originating from the Qp promoter located in the BamIII Q region, this is transcribed in latency types I and II.

nent of HD, the Reed-Sternberg cells and their variants (Weiss et al., 1989). The association of HD with EBV is age-related; paediatric and older adult cases are usually EBV-associated whereas HD in young adults is less frequently virus-positive (Jarrett, 1998). The proportion of EBV-positive HD in developing countries is high consistent with a greater incidence of HD in children and more frequent prevalence of the mixed cellularity histiotype. Although the incidence of HD is relatively low (1-3/100,000 per year) this tumor is not geographically restricted, making its association with EBV significant in world health terms.

EBV Latency In Vitro and In Vivo

The best characterised *in vitro* model of latency is provided by LCLs generated by infecting primary, resting B cells with EBV. Every cell in an LCL carries multiple copies of the viral episome and constitutively expresses a limited set of viral gene products, the so-called latent proteins, consisting of six nuclear antigens (EBNAs 1, 2, 3A, 3B, 3C and -LP) and three latent membrane proteins (LMPs 1, 2A and 2B) (Kieff, 1996). Transcripts from the BamHI A region of the viral genome, first identified in NPC cells, are also detected in LCLs although the ability of these mRNAs to encode proteins remains controversial (Brooks et al., 1993; Fries et al., 1997). In addition to the latent proteins, LCLs also show abundant expression of the small non-polyadenylated (and therefore non-coding) RNAs, EBERs 1 and 2; the function of these transcripts is not clear but they are consistently expressed in all forms of latent EBV infection (Kieff, 1996; Rickinson and Kieff, 1996).The relative positions and orientations of these viral genes are illustrated in Figure 2 under a linearised BamHI restriction map of the viral genome. The different EBNAs are encoded by individual mRNAs generated by differential splicing of the same long 'rightward' primary transcript expressed from one of two promotors (Cp and Wp) located close together in the BamHI C and W region of the genome (Speck and Strominger, 1989). These are illustrated in Figure 3 on the large (172 kilobase), covalently-closed EBV episome. The LMP transcripts are expressed from separate promoters in the BamHI N region of the EBV genome, with the leftward LMP1 and rightward LMP2B mRNAs apparently controlled by the same bidirectional promoter sequence (Figure 3; Speck and Strominger, 1989; Kieff, 1996). This pattern of latent EBV gene expression is referred to as the "latency III" (Lat III) form of EBV infection (Figure 4).

The consistent pattern of EBV latent protein expression in LCLs is matched by an equally consistent and characteristic cellular phenotype with high level expression of the B cell activation markers CD23, CD30, CD39 and CD70 and of the cellular adhesion molecules LFA1 (CD11a/18), LFA3 (CD58) and ICAM1 (CD54) (Rowe et al., 1987; Gregory et al., 1988). That these markers are either absent or expressed at low levels on resting B cells, but are transiently induced to high levels when these cells are activated into short-term growth by antigenic or mitogenic stimulation, suggests that EBV-induced immortalisation may be elicited through the constitutive activation of the same cellular pathways that drive physiological B cell proliferation. The ability of EBNA2, EBNA3C and LMP1 to induce LCL-like phenotypic changes when expressed individually in human B cell lines implicates these viral proteins as key effectors of the immortalisation process (Wang et al., 1987; Wang et al., 1990).

The cell surface phenotype of immunoblastic lymphomas that develop in solid organ or bone marrow transplant recipients resembles that of LCLs, with high level expression of the activation antigen CD23 and of the adhesion molecules, LFA1, LFA3

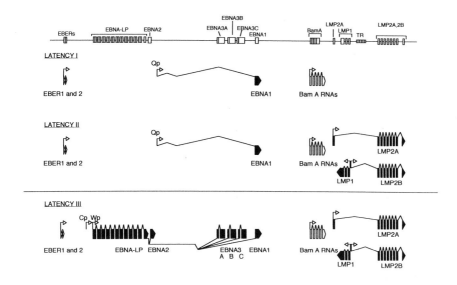

Figure 4. EBV gene transcription in the three forms of latency. The top panel shows the position of the exons on a linear map of the genome. The lower panels show the direction of transcription from each promoter (arrows), and the splicing structure between the exons. Coding exons are shown in black and non-coding exons in white.

and

ICAM1 (Young et al., 1989; Thomas et al., 1990; Rickinson and Kieff, 1996; Niedobitek and Young, 1997). This cellular phenotype is accompanied by a Lat III pattern of EBV latent protein expression as assessed by immunohistological analysis using monoclonal antibodies to EBNA2 and LMP1 and by immunoblotting analysis with polyvalent human sera (Young et al., 1989; Rickinson and Kieff, 1996; Niedobitek and Young, 1997). Thus, these lymphomas appear to represent the *in vivo* counterparts of *in vitro* immortalised LCLs and, by implication, are likely to be primarily driven by EBV. The LCL-like nature of the immunoblastic B cell lymphomas and their growth in immunosuppressed patients suggests that these tumors are sensitive to EBV-specific CTL control. Indeed, regression of lymphomas has been reported following relaxation of immunosuppressive therapy in transplant recipients and recent studies have demonstrated the clinical benefit of adoptive therapy using EBV-specific CTL even in patients with overt lymphoma (Rooney et al., 1995; Rickinson and Kieff, 1996). Whilst a role for secondary genetic events in the pathogenesis of these tumors has been proposed to account for the documented progression of immunoblastic B cell lymphomas from oligoclonality to monoclonality, there is in fact no evidence of consistent genetic or cytogenetic changes in the monoclonal lesions. The likelihood that EBV remains solely responsible for lymphoma growth even after progression to monoclonality is consistent with a phenomenon regularly observed *in vitro* , where EBV-immortalisation of resting B cells gives rise to an LCL which is initially polyclonal but which on serial passage becomes dominated by the fastest growing clone. Further support for this view comes from studies of EBV-induced B cell lymphomas in animal model systems. Thus, the lymphomas induced in cotton-top tamarins within a few weeks of experimental EBV infection (Cleary et al., 1985), and in SCID mice by inoculation of peripheral blood lymphocytes from healthy EBV-carrying individuals (Rowe et al., 1991) can be oligo-clonal or monoclonal, yet they all resemble LCLs in their Lat III pattern of EBV latent gene expression and in their cell surface phenotype. The remarkable efficiency of tumor development in both models is strong circumstantial evidence that the develop-ment of immunoblastic lymphomas in an immunosuppressed setting in man need only require EBV-induced B cell transformation with no necessity for secondary genetic change. This clearly sets these particular lesions apart from all other EBV-positive malignancies where viral infection is but one event in a complex multi-step oncogenic process.

A second form of EBV infection in B cells, referred to as "latency I" (Lat I), has been identified in BL tumor biopsy cells and in early passage BL cell lines where abun-dant EBER transcription is found and EBNA1 is selectively expressed in the absence of the other EBNA and LMP proteins (Figure 4; Rowe et al., 1987; Gregory et al., 1990). The selective expression of EBNA1 involves a different mRNA expressed from a novel EBNA1 promoter (Qp) in the BamHI Q region of the viral genome which is independ-ent of Cp or Wp promoter (Figure 4; Sample et al., 1991; Nonkwelo et al., 1996). In culture BL cells grow as a carpet of dispersed cells, in contrast to the multicellular aggregates that are observed in LCL cultures (Rickinson and Kieff, 1996). Furthermore, BL cells display a distinct cell surface marker phenotype characterised by expression of CD10 (CALLA) and CD77 (BLA) but little or no expression of the cellular activation antigens and adhesion molecules that are regularly expressed at high levels in LCLs (Gregory et al., 1990). The Lat I form of latency observed in BL cell lines is not always stably maintained *in vitro*, and on serial passage a drift to a Lat III pattern of gene expression can be observed concomitant with a change in the cellular phenotype to-wards that seen in LCLs (Gregory et al., 1990). A similar effect may occur *in vivo* as recent work has demonstrated that EBNA2 and LMP1 can occasionally be detected in a small proportion of BL cells in biopsy material (Niedobitek et al., 1995). This also highlights that the operational definitions of EBV latencies derived from cell lines *in vitro* may not readily apply to tumors *in vivo*.

Another form of EBV latency, Lat II, is characterised by selective expression of the Qp-driven EBNA1 mRNA, of the LMP 1, 2A and 2B transcripts, and of the EBERs (Figure 4; Brooks et al., 1992; Deacon et al., 1993). This form of infection was first identified at the protein level in NPC biopsies (Fahraeus et al., 1988; Young et al., 1988) but is clearly not restricted to epithelial cells since it is also observed in EBV-positive cases of Hodgkin's disease and in certain EBV-positive T cell lymphomas (Pallesen et al., 1991; Meijer et al., 1996; Rickinson and Kieff, 1996). All three forms

Table 2. Different patterns of EBV gene expression in EBV associated tumors

Tumour	Latent gene expression	Pattern of latency
BL, endemic	EBNA1	I
BL, sporadic/AIDS	EBNA1	I
Undiff. NPC	EBNA1; LMPs1, 2	II
Hodgkin's disease	EBNA1; LMPs1, 2	II
T lymphomas	EBNA1; LMPs1, 2	II
Immunoblastic lymphomas	EBNAs1-6;	III
	LMPs1, 2	III

Note that all EBV-positive tumours express the EBER RNAs and the BamHIA transcripts. Preliminary work suggests that another form of latency exists with expression of EBNA1 and LMP2 only and this is often observed in NPC and gastric adenocarcinomas.

of EBV latency can be interconverted in somatic cell hybrids between LCLs and either BL cells or certain non-lymphoid lines (Kerr et al., 1992). These transitions are influenced by the cell phenotype of the resultant hybrids, thus emphasising the complex interplay between cellular factors and the resident pattern of EBV latent gene expression. The intricate interaction between the host cell environment and the virus is elegantly depicted in a study in which deregulated c-myc expression introduced into an LCL with regulatable EBNA2 expression resulted in cells with a BL phenotype (growth as single cells, down-regulation of activation antigens, up-regulation of CD10) and a Lat I form of EBV latency (Polack et al., 1996). The different patterns of EBV gene expression in EBV associated tumors are summarised in Table 2.

EBV strain variation and virus-associated tumors

There are two major types of EBV isolate, originally referred to as A and B and now called types 1 and 2, which appear to be identical over the bulk of the EBV genome but show allelic polymorphism (with 50-80% sequence homology depending on the locus) in a subset of latent genes, namely those encoding EBNA-LP, EBNA2, EBNA3A, EBNA3B and EBNA3C (Dambaugh et al., 1989; Rowe et al., 1989; Sample et al., 1990). A combination of virus isolation and sero-epidemiological studies suggest that type 1 virus isolates are predominant (but not exclusively so) in many Western countries, whereas both types are widespread in equatorial Africa, New Guinea and perhaps certain other regions (Zimber et al., 1986; Young et al., 1987; Sixbey et al., 1989; Yao et al. 1991). *In vitro* studies suggest that type 1 isolates are more potent than type 2 in achieving B cell transformation *in vitro*; the type 2 virus-transformed LCLs characteristically show much slower growth especially in early passage (Rickinson et al., 1987). In addition to this broad distinction between EBV types 1 and 2, there is also minor heterogeneity within each virus type which is most easily detected as variation in the size of the EBNA proteins (Rickinson and Kieff, 1996). These differences have been used to trace virus transmission within families and from transplant donors to recipients. The balance of evidence to date suggests that healthy individuals are only infected with one virus type, although this changes in immunologically compromised patients where multiple EBV types including type 1 and type 2 strains can be detected in the same individual (Rickinson and Kieff, 1996).

As to the preferential association of EBV strains with virus-associated tumors, a number of studies have shown that the presence of a particular virus strain in the tumor reflects the prevalence of this strain in the same geographical location. For instance, original work demonstrated that around 20% of BL tumors from the endemic areas of Kenya and New Guinea were infected with a type 2 virus and that this reflected the 20% incidence of type 2 virus infection in normal, healthy individuals from these regions (Young et al., 1987). More recent work focussing on genetic variation in LMP1 (particularly a 30 bp deletion referred to as delLMP1) has produced confusing data suggesting an association of these alterations with more aggressive disease. However, more extensive analysis in relation to the normal population revealed that the EBV gene polymorphisms (including delLMP1) in virus-associated tumors occurred with similar frequency in EBV isolates from healthy virus carriers from the same geographical location (Khanim et al. 1996). Nevertheless, the increased incidence of EBV isolates carrying delLMP1 in the normal Chinese population may be a factor in the increased incidence of NPC and various T cell tumors in this region.

Function of the EBV latent proteins in cell transformation

The recent use of recombinant EBVs lacking individual latent genes has confirmed the absolute requirement for EBNA2 and LMP1 in the *in vitro* transformation of B cells and highlighted a role for EBNA-LP, EBNA3A, EBNA3C and LMP2A in this process (Kieff, 1996). These studies confirm that the transformation of B cells by EBV involves the co-ordinated action of several latent gene functions. With the demonstration of more restricted patterns of EBV gene expression involving LMP1 and LMP2 in NPC, HD and various T cell lymphomas, the function of these membrane proteins has been a focus of much interest.

EBNA1

EBNA1 is a DNA binding nuclear phosphoprotein which has a central role in the maintenance of latent EBV infection (Kieff, 1996). It is required for the replication and maintenance of the episomal EBV genome which is achieved through the binding of EBNA1 to the plasmid origin of viral replication, oriP (Kieff, 1996). EBNA1 can also interact with two sites immediately downstream of Qp, the promoter used to drive EBNA1 expression in Lat I and Lat II, thereby negatively regulating its own expression (Nonkwelo et al., 1996). Furthermore, EBNA1 can act as a transcriptional transactivator and has been shown to up-regulate Cp and the LMP1 promoter (Kieff, 1996). The EBNA1 protein is separated into amino and carboxy terminal domains by a glycine-glycine-alanine (gly-ala) repeat sequence which varies in size in different EBV isolates (Kieff, 1996; Rickinson and Kieff, 1996). This gly-ala repeat domain is a *cis*-acting inhibitor of MHC class I-restricted presentation and appears to function by inhibiting antigen processing via the ubiquitin/ proteosome pathway (Levitskaya et al., 1995; Levitskaya et al., 1997). This effect is also likely to be responsible for the long half-life of the EBNA1 protein (Levitskaya et al., 1997). Directing EBNA1 expression to B cells in transgenic mice results in B cell lymphomas suggesting that EBNA1 may have a direct role in oncogenesis (Wilson et al., 1996). Previous work has shown that stable EBNA1 expression in epithelial cells requires an undifferentiated cellular environment (Knox et al., 1996) and that EBNA1 expression can be toxic in certain cell lines (Smith, Dawson and Young, manuscript in preparation). This suggests that EBNA1 may have additional effects beyond its oriP maintenance function possibly by affecting the origins of replication of cellular genes.

The other EBNAs

The inability of an EBV strain, P3HR-1, carrying a deletion of the EBNA2 gene and the last two exons of EBNA-LP to transform B cells *in vitro* was the first indication of the crucial role of the EBNA2 protein in the transformation process (Kieff, 1996). Restoration of the EBNA2 gene into P3HR-1 by homologous recombination has unequivocally confirmed the importance of EBNA2 in B cell transformation and has allowed the functionally relevant domains of the EBNA2 protein to be identified (Hammerschmidt and Sugden, 1989; Cohen et al., 1989). EBNA2 is an acidic phosphoprotein which localizes in large nuclear granules. An amino terminal polyproline repeat is responsible for the variation in the size of EBNA2 protein in different EBV isolates. EBNA2 is a transcriptional activator of both cellular and viral genes up-regulating the expression of certain B cell antigens, CD21 and CD23, as well as LMP1 and LMP2 (Wang et al., 1987; Wang et al., 1990; Kieff, 1996). EBNA2 also transactivates the viral C promoter (Cp) thereby inducing the switch from Wp to Cp observed early in B cell infection. These EBNA2-responsive promoters have been extensively analysed and have been found to possess a common core sequence (GTGGGAA) which does not directly bind EBNA2. Thus EBNA2 interacts with a ubiquitous DNA binding protein, RBP-Jκ, and this is partly responsible for targeting EBNA2 to promoters which contain the RBP-Jκ sequence (Grossman et al., 1994; Henkel et al., 1994; Waltzer et al.,, 1994; Hsieh and Hayward, 1995). Interestingly, the RBP-Jκ homologue in Drosophila is involved in signal transduction via the Notch receptor, a pathway which is important in cell fate determination in the fruit fly and has been implicated in the development of T cell tumors in man (Artavanis-Tsakonas et al., 1995). Recent work demonstrates that EBNA2 can functionally replace the intracellular region of Notch (Sakai et al., 1998). The transactivation of genes by EBNA2 also involves PU.1, a transcription factor involved in B cell-specific gene transcription thereby accounting for ability of EBNA2 to induce LMP1 expression only in B cells.

The EBNA3A, 3B and 3C genes appear to have a common origin and encode hydrophilic nuclear proteins which contain heptad repeats of leucine, isoleucine or valine that may act as dimerisation domains (Kieff, 1996). Studies with EBV recombinants have demonstrated that EBNA3A and EBNA3C are essential for B cell transformation in vitro whereas EBNA3B is dispensable (Roberstson, 1997). Several lines of evidence suggest that the EBNA3 family are transcriptional regulators. Thus, EBNA3C can induce the up-regulation of both cellular (CD21) and viral (LMP1) gene expression (Wang et al., 1990; Allday and Farrell, 1994), repress the Cp promoter (Radkov et al., 1997) and may interact with pRb to promote transformation (Parker et al., 1996). Whilst not essential for transformation, EBNA3B has been shown to induce expression of vimentin and CD40 (Silins and Sculley, 1994). The EBNA3 proteins associate with the RBP-Jκ transcription factor and disrupt its binding to the cognate Jκ sequence and to EBNA2 thus repressing EBNA2-mediated transactivation (Robertson, 1997). Thus EBNA2 and the EBNA3 proteins work together to precisely control RBP-Jκ activity thereby regulating the expression of cellular and viral promoters containing Jκ cognate sequence.

EBNA-LP is encoded by the leader of each of the EBNA mRNAs and encodes a protein of variable size depending on the number of BamHIW repeats (see Figures 2 and 3) contained by a particular EBV isolate (Kieff, 1996). Molecular genetic analysis indicates that whilst not absolutely required for B cell transformation *in vitro*, EBNA-LP is required for the efficient outgrowth of LCLs (Allan et al., 1992). Transient trans-fection of EBNA-LP and EBNA2 into primary B cells induces G0 to G1 transition as measured by the up-regulation of cyclin D2 expression (Sinclair et al., 1994). EBNA-LP has been shown to co-localise with pRb in LCLs and *in vitro* biochemical studies have demonstrated an interaction of EBNA-LP with both pRb and p53 (Jiang et al., 1991; Szekely et al., 1993). However, this interaction has not been verified in LCLs and, unlike the situation with the HPV-encoded E6/E7 and adenovirus E1 proteins, EBNA-LP expression appears to have no effect on the regulation of the pRb and p53 pathways.

LMP1

The expression of LMP1 in a number of EBV-associated tumors including immunoblas-tic lymphoma, HD and NPC is consistent with its ability to transform rodent fibroblasts, to induce the up-regulation of CD40, CD54 and Bcl-2 family members, and to inhibit epithelial differentiation (Kieff, 1996; Rickinson and Kieff, 1996; Dawson et al., 1990). LMP1 comprises a short 23 amino acid amino terminal cytoplasmic domain, 6 putative membrane-spanning domains which are important for confering plasma membrane aggregation and a large 200 amino acid carboxy terminal cytoplasmic domain (Kieff, 1996). Mutational analysis has identified the cytoplasmic C-terminal domain of LMP1 as being important for cell growth transformation and induction of phenotypic changes (Kieff, 1996). Similarities between the effects of CD40, a member of the TNF receptor family, and LMP1 signalling suggest that common biochemical pathways may be acti-vated by these molecules. Both CD40 ligation and transient LMP1 expression are asso-ciated with activation of the transcription factor NF-κB, up-regulation of CD54, secre-tion of IL-6, induction of the anti-apoptotic A20 protein and growth inhibition (Kieff, 1996; Eliopoulos et al., 1996; Eliopoulos et al., 1997; Young et al., 1998). Thus, it is not surprising that LMP1 has recently been shown to function as a constitutively acti-vated CD40 by interacting with a common family of TNF receptor-associated factors

(TRAFs) (Mosialos et al., 1995). The six transmembrane spanning domains of LMP1 serve to promote aggregation of the protein in the plasma membrane thereby mimicking the receptor cross-linking effect induced by the interaction of trimeric CD40 ligand with its receptor (Gires et al., 1997; Floettmann and Rowe, 1997). The resultant clustering of the LMP1 cytoplasmic domain stimulates TRAF-mediated NF-κB activation as does clustering of the CD40 cytoplasmic tail induced by ligand binding (Rothe et al., 1995). A TRAF binding motif, PxQxT, is present in a region of LMP1 proximal to the plasma membrane (so-called C-terminal activating region 1 or CTAR1, residues 194-232) and is responsible for mediating TRAF2-dependent activation of NF-κB (Huen et al., 1995; Kaye et al., 1996; Devergne et al., 1996; Eliopoulos et al., 1997). TRAF1, 2, 3 and 5 directly associate with LMP1 through this PxQxT domain (TRAF binding domain), whilst TRAF6 does not bind to LMP1 (Devergne et al., 1996; Sandberg et al., 1997; Ishida et al., 1996a; Ishida et al., 1996b; Devergne *et al.*, 1998). A more distal region of the LMP1 cytoplasmic tail (CTAR2, residues 351-386) is the dominant NF-κB activating domain of LMP1 and this effect appears to be mediated indirectly via TRAF2; that is TRAF2 is unable to bind to CTAR2 but dominant negative (RING finger-deleted) TRAF2 blocks NF-κB activation from this region (Eliopoulos et al., 1997; Huen et al., 1995; Kaye et al., 1996; Devergne et al., 1996). It has recently been shown that TRADD (TNF receptor associated death domain), a death domain protein that interacts with TNF receptor I (TNFRI), directly associates with CTAR2 and probably recruits TRAF2 resulting in NF-κB activation (Izumi and Kieff, 1997). The precise mechanism responsible for TRAF-induced NF-κB activation is unknown but appears to involve a MAP kinase kinase kinase, NIK, which may function in the phosphorylation of I-κB leading to translocation of active NF-κB to the nucleus (Malinin et al., 1997; Sylla et al., 1998; Eliopoulos et al., 1999). A number of proteins exert a negative regulatory effect on NF-κB activation by either competing for the TRAF-binding domain (i.e. TRAF3) or by interacting with and inhibiting TRAF2 function (TANK/I-TRAF, A20) (Eliopoulos et al., 1997; Rothe et al., 1995; Devergne et al., 1996; Song et al., 1996). TRAF-mediated NF-κB activation in response to either LMP1 expression or CD40 ligation has been shown to result in induction of A20 expression and IL-6 secretion and TRAF3 has been implicated in LMP1 and CD40-induced epithelial cell growth inhibition (Eliopoulos et al., 1996; Eliopoulos et al., 1997; Cheng et al., 1995; Sarma et al., 1995). CD40 ligation also results in the activation of c-Jun N-terminal kinase (JNK, also known as the stress-activated protein kinase, SAPK) leading to activation of the AP-1 transcription factor family (Sutherland et al., 1996; Eliopoulos and Young, 1998). Recent work has demonstrated that LMP1 can also activate JNK and that this effect in mediated by CTAR2 and involves both TRADD and TRAF2 (Kieser et al., 1997; Eliopoulos et al., 1998; Eliopoulos et al., 1999a). The p38 stress-activated kinase is also activated by LMP1 predominantly through CTAR2 and this pathway via activation of the AP-1 and ATF2 transcription factors mediates LMP1-induced up-regulation of IL-8 synthesis and secretion (Eliopoulos et al., 1999b). Thus, LMP1 expression results in activation of both the NF-κB and AP-1/ATF2 transcription factors although the precise cell signalling pathways responsible for eliciting these effects remains unknown. The ability of the NF-κB pathway to mediate the transcription of anti-apoptotic genes (Baichwal and Baeuerle,

1997) and the role of the JNK/p38 pathway in both apoptosis and oncogenic transformation (Ip and Davis, 1998) suggests that these effects are responsible for the pleiotropic consequences of LMP1 expression.

The cloning and sequencing of the LMP1 gene from EBV isolates derived from either a Chinese or a Taiwanese NPC has identified several mutations as compared with the prototype B95.8 strain, including a point mutation leading to loss of an XhoI restriction site in the first exon, a 30bp deletion in the carboxy terminus immediately upstream of CTAR2 and multiple point mutations (Hu et al., 1991; Chen et al., 1992). These so-called delLMP1 variants (typified by Cao-LMP1) display increased tumorigenicity in rodent fibroblasts and epithelial cells (Chen et al., 1992; Hu et al., 1993; Zheng et al., 1994). Whilst initial studies using PCR suggested that EBV isolates carrying delLMP1 are more frequently detected in lymphoproliferative disorders, a more thorough analysis has shown that the incidence of delLMP1 in EBV-associated tumors reflects the frequency with which this isolate in detected in healthy virus carriers from the same geographical region (Khanim et al., 1996). However, given that delLMP1 is the predominant form of LMP1 in Chinese populations it remains possible that this variant contributes to the development of NPC. A recently published functional analysis has revealed that Cao-LMP1 is impaired in its ability to up-regulate CD40 and CD54 relative to B95.8-LMP1 eventhough Cao-LMP1 can induce greater activation of NF-κB than B95.8-LMP1 (Johnson et al., 1998). These studies concluded that the 30bp deletion was not responsible for these differences and that sequences outside CTAR2 were involved. Similar studies using a delLMP1 isolated from a different NPC (C15) have shown that this LMP1 isolate is also more efficient at activating NF-κB than B95.8-LMP1 with resultant enhanced induction of the EGF receptor in the C33A carcinoma cell line; these effects of C15-LMP1 were not due to the 30bp deletion (Miller et al., 1998). We have demonstrated that transient expression of Cao-LMP1 results in JNK activation (Eliopoulos and Young, 1998) but our recent studies suggest that Cao-LMP1 is impaired in its ability to induce various phenotypic changes in the SCC12F epithelial cell line (Dawson et al., 2000). Thus, continued study of delLMP1 may help to further dissect the LMP1 signalling pathway and to assess the contribution of LMP1 sequence variation to the pathogenesis of EBV-associated tumors such as HD and NPC.

LMP2

LMP2 is a hydrophobic membrane protein which is transcribed from two different promoters resulting in the expression of either LMP2A or LMP2B which differ only in the first exon (Kieff, 1996; Fruehling et al., 1997a). The first exon of LMP2A encodes a 119 amino acid amino terminal cytoplasmic domain while the first exon of LMP2B in non-coding. Both proteins contain 12 identical hydrophobic transmembrane domains and a 27 amino acid cytoplasmic carboxy domain and are expressed as small patches in the plasma membrane of LCLs. Neither LMP2A or LMP2B are essential for B cell transformation (Kieff, 1996; Fruehling et al., 1997a).. The LMP2A amino terminal domain contains 8 tyrosine residues, 2 of which (Y74 and Y85) form an immunoreceptor tyrosine-based activation motif (TAM) (Fruehling et al., 1997a; Fruehling et al.,

1997b) . When phosphorylated the TAM present in the B cell receptor (BCR) plays a central role in mediating lymphocyte proliferation and differentiation by the recruitment and activation of the *src* family of protein tyrosine kinases (PTKs) and the Syk PTK (Cambier et al., 1994) . LMP2A can also interact with these PTKs through its phosphorylated TAM and this association appears to negatively regulate PTK activity (Fruehling et al., 1997a; Fruehling et al., 1997b). Thus, the LMP2A TAM has been shown to be responsible for blocking BCR-stimulated calcium mobilisation, tyrosine phosphorylation and activation of the EBV lytic cycle in B cells (Miller et al., 1995; Fruehling et al., 1997a; Fruehling et al., 1997b). More recent work indicates that another tyrosine residue in the LMP2A amino terminal domain (Y112) is also required for efficient binding of src family PTKs (Fruehling et al., 1998). LMP2A is also phosphorylated on serine and threonine residues and two specific serine residues (S15 and S102) are phosphorylated by mitogen-activated protein (MAP) kinase *in vitro* (Panousis and Rowe, 1997). Interestingly, the Erk1 form of MAPK was found to directly interact with LMP2A but the functional significance of this effect remains unknown (Panousis and Rowe, 1997). Expression of LMP2A in the B cells of transgenic mice abrogates normal B cell development allowing immunoglobulin-negative cells to colonise peripheral lymphoid organs suggesting that LMP2A can drive the proliferation and survival of B cells in the absence of signalling through the B cell receptor (BCR) (Caldwell et al., 1998). Taken together these data support a role for LMP2 in modifying the normal B cell development programme to favour the maintenance of EBV latency in the bone marrow and to prevent inappropriate activation of the EBV lytic cycle. A modulatory role for LMP2B in regulating LMP2A function has been suggested (Fruehling et al., 1997a). The consistent expression of LMP2A in HD and NPC suggests an important function for this protein in oncogenesis but this remains to be shown.

Conclusions

Compelling evidence implicates EBV in the pathogenesis of tumors arising in both lymphoid and epithelial tissues. The virus appears to adopt different forms of latent infection in different tumor types reflecting the complex interplay between EBV and the host cell environment. Another important factor influencing EBV gene expression is the immune response such that those viral latent proteins to which immunodominant CTL responses are directed, namely the EBNA3 family of proteins, are down-regulated in virus-associated tumors arising in overtly immunocompetent individuals. EBNA1, an essential protein for the maintenance of EBV infection which is expressed in all currently known forms of EBV latency, has evolved to evade immunosurveillance by developing a strategy which prevents the protein being processed through the MHC class I pathway. Studies of the function of individual EBV latent genes have highlighted the ability of these proteins to target specific cell signalling pathways. Thus, as clearly evidenced by work with proteins encoded by other viruses, an understanding of the functions of EBV latent proteins will not only be relevant to the role of the virus in transformation but will also help to elucidate the mechanisms regulating cell growth, survival and differentiation. It is hoped that this work will also provide novel approaches to therapy. Adoptive transfer of EBV-specific CTLs has already proved useful in the treatment of immunoblastic B cell lymphomas and this approach as well as other vaccine strategies are currently being evaluated in patients with HD or NPC. The possibility of more direct therapeutic intervention targeting the function of essential EBV latent genes such as EBNA1 and LMP1 is also a possibility. Thus, drugs which prevent the ability of EBNA1 to bind to oriP or of the TRAFs to interact with LMP1 are likely to be developed. Finally, gene therapy strategies which exploit either the transcriptional regulation of the EBV genome or target the functional effects of EBV latent genes have been described (Franken et al., 1996; Piche et al., 1998).

Acknowledgements

Work in the author's laboratory is supported by the Cancer Research Campaign, U.K. and the Medical Research Council. Dr R. Tierney is thanked for help with the figures.

References

Allan, G.J., Inman, G.J., Parker, B.D., Rowe, D.T., Farrell, P.J. (1992). Cell growth effects of Epstein-Barr virus leader protein. J.Gen.Virol. 73, 1547-1551.

Allday, M.J. and Farell, P.J. (1994). Epstein-Barr virus nuclear antigen EBNA3C/6 expression maintains the level of latent membrane protein 1 in G1-arrested cells. J.Virol. 68, 3491-3498.

Artavanis-Tsakonas, S., Matsuno, K. and Fortini, M.E. (1995). Notch signaling. Science 268, 225-232.

Baichwal, V.R. and Baeuerle, P.A. (1997). Apoptosis: Activate NF-κB or die? Current Biol. 7, R94-R96.

Birkenbach, M., Tong, X., Bradbury, L.E., Tedder, T., and Kieff, E.(1992). Characterisation of an Epstein-Barr virus receptor on human epithelial cells. J. Exp. Med. 176, 1405-1414.

Brooks, L., Yao, Q.Y., Rickinson, A.B., and Young, L.S. (1992). Epstein-Barr virus latent gene transcription in nasopharyngeal carcinoma cells: coexpression of EBNA1, LMP1, and LMP2 transcripts. J.Virol. 66, 2689-2697.

Brooks, L.A., Lear, A.L., Young, L.S. and Rickinson, A.B. (1993). Transcripts from the Epstein-Barr virus BamHI A fragment are detectable in all three forms of virus latency. J. Virol. 67, 3182-3190.

Burkitt, D. (1962). A children's cancer dependent upon climatic factors. Nature, 194, 232-234.

Caldwell, R.G., Wilson, J. B., Anderson, S.J. and Longnecker, R. (1998) Epstein-Barr virus LMP2A drives B cell development and survival in the absence of normal B cell receptor signals. Immunity 9, 405-411.

Cambier, J.C., Pleiman, C.M. and Clark, M.R. (1994). Signal-transduction by the B-cell Antigen Receptor and its Coreceptors. Ann. Rev. Immunol. 12, 457-486.

Chen, M.L., Tsai, C.N.,, Liang, C.L., Shu, C.H., Huang, C.R., Sulitzeanu, D., Liu, S.T. and Chang, Y.S. (1992). Cloning and characterization of the latent membrane protein (LMP) of a specific Epstein-Barr virus variant derived from the nasopharyngeal carcinoma in the Taiwanese population. Oncogene, 7, 2131-2140

Cheng, G., Cleary, A.M., Ye, Z., Hong, D.I., Lederman, S. and Baltimore, D. (1995). Involvement of CRAF1, a Relative of TRAF, in CD40 Signaling. Science, 267, 1494-1498.

Cleary, M.L., Epstein, M.A., and Finerty, S. (1985). Individual tumors of multifocal Epstein-Barr virus-induced malignant lymphomas in Tamarins arise from different B-cell clones. Science, 228, 722-724.

Cohen, J. Wang, F. Mannick, J. and Kieff, E. (1989). Epstein-Barr cirus nuclear protein 2 is a key determinant of lymphocyte transformation. Proc.Natl.Acad.Sci. USA, 86, 9558-9562.

Dambaugh, T., Hennessy, K., Chamnankit, L., and Kieff, E. (1984). U2 region of Epstein-Barr virus DNA may encode Epstein-Barr nuclear antigen 2. Proc, Natl, Acad, Sci., USA, 81, 7632-7636.

Dawson, C.W., Rickinson, A.B. and Young, L.S. (1990). Epstein-Barr virus latent membrane protein inhibits human epithelial cell differentiation. Nature, 344, 777-780.

Dawson, C.W., Eliopoulos, A.G., Blake, S.M., Banker, R., and Young, L.S. (2000). Identification of functional differences between prototype Epstein-Barr virus-encoded LMP1 and a nasopharyngeal carcinoma-derived LMP1 in human epithelical cells. Virology 272, 204-217.

Deacon, E.M., Pallesen, G., Niedobitek, G., Crocker, J., Brooks, L., Rickinson, A.B., and Young, L.S. (1993). Epstein-Barr virus and Hodgkin's disease: transcriptional analysis of virus latency in the malignant cells. J, Exp, Med, 177, 339.

Deacon, E.M., Pallesen, G., Niedobitek, G. Crocker, J., Brooks, L., Rickinson, A.B., and Young, L.S. (1993). Epstein-Barr virus and Hodgkin's disease: Transcriptional analysis of virus latency in the malignant cells. J. Exp. Med. 177, 339-349.

Devergne, O., Hatzivassiliou, E., Izumi, K.M., Kaye, M.F., Kleijnen, E., Kieff, and Mosialos, G. (1996). Association of TRAF1, TRAF2, and TRAF3 with an Epstein-Barr virus LMP1 domain important for B-lymphocyte transformation: role in NF-κB activation. Mol. Cell. Biol. 16, 7098-7108.

Devergne, O., McFarland, E.C., Mosialos, G., Izumi, K.M., Ware, C.F. and Kieff, E. (1998) Role of TRAF binding site and NF-kB activation in Epstein-Barr virus latent membrane protein 1-induced cell gene expression. J. Virol. 72, 7900-7908.

Eliopoulos, A.G., Dawson, C.W., Mosialos, G. Floettmann, J.E., Rowe, M., Armitage, R.J., Dawson, J., Kerr, D.J., Wakelam, M.J.O., Reed, J.C., Kieff, E., and Young, L.S. (1996). CD40-induced growth inhibition in epithelial cells is mimicked by Epstein-Barr virus-encoded LMP1: involvement of TRAF3 as a common mediator. Oncogene 13, 2243-2254.

Eliopoulos, A.G., Stack, M., Dawson, C.W., Kaye, K.M., Hodgkin, L., Sihota, S., Rowe, M. and Young, L.S. (1997). Epstein-Barr virus-encoded LMP1 and CD40 mediate IL6 production in epithelial cells via and NF-κB pathway involving TNF receptor-associated factors. Oncogene 14, 2899-2916.

Eliopoulos, A.G. and Young, L.S. (1998). Activation of the cJun N-terminal kinase (JNK) pathway by the Epstein-Barr virus-encoded latent membrane protein 1 (LMP1). Oncogene 16, 1731-1742.

Eliopoulos, A.G., Blake, S.M.S., Floettmann, J.E., Rowe, M. and Young, L.S. (1999a). Epstein-Barr virus-encoded latent membrane protein 1 activates the JNK pathway through its extreme C-terminus via a mechanism involving TRADD and TRAF2. J. Virol. 73, 1023-1035.

Eliopoulos, A.G., Gallagher, N.J., Blake, S.M.S., Dawson, C.W. and Young, L.S. (1999b) Activation of the p38 MAPK pathway by Epstein-Barr virus-encoded latent membrane protein 1 (LMP1) co-regulates interleukin-6 and interleukin-8 production. J. Biol. Chem. 274, 16085-16096.

Fahraeus, R., Li-Fu, H., and Ernberg, I. (1988). Expression of Epstein-Barr virus-encoded proteins in nasopharyngeal carcinoma. Int. J. Cancer, 42, 329-338.

Floettmann, J.E. and Rowe, M. (1997). Epstein-Barr virus latent membrane protein-1 (LMP1) C-terminus activation region-2 (CTAR-2) maps to the far C-terminus and requires oligomerisation for NF-κB activation. Oncogene 15, 1851-1858.

Franken, M., Estabrooks, A., Cavacini, L., Sherburne, B., Wang, F. and Scadden, D.T. (1996) Epstein-Barr virus-driven gene therapy for EBV-related lymphomas. Nat. Med. 2, 1379-1382.

Fries, K.L., Sculley, T.B., Webster-Cyriaque, J., Rajadurai, P., Sadler, R.H., and Raabltraub, N. (1997). Identification of a novel protein encoded by the BamHI A region of the Epstein-Barr virus. J. Virol. 71, 2765-2771.

Fruehling, S., Caldwell, R. and Longnecker, R. (1997a). LMP2 Function in EBV latency. Epstein-Barr Virus Report 4, 151-159.

Fruehling, S and Longnecker, R (1997b) The immunoreceptor tyrosine based activation motif of Epstein Barr virus LMPA2 is essential for blocking BCR-mediated signal transduction. J. Virol., 235, 241-251.

Freuhling, S., Stuart, R., Dolwick, K.M., Kremmer, E. and Longnecker, R. (1998). Tyrosine 112 of latent membrane protein 2A is essential for a protein kinase loading and regulation of Epstein-Barr virus latency. J.Virol., 72, 7796-7806.

Gerber, P., Nonoyama, M., Lucas, S., Perlin, E., and Goldstein, L.I. (1972). Oral excretion of Epstein-Barr virus by healthy subjects and patients with infectious mononucleosis. Lancet ii, 988-989.

Gilligan, K., Sato, H., and Rajadurai, P. (1990). Novel transcription from the Epstein-Barr virus terminal EcoRI fragment, DIJhet, in a nasopharyngeal carcinoma. J. Virol 64, 4948-4956.

Gires, O., Zimber-Strobl, U., Gonnella, R., Ueffing, M., Marshall, G., Zeider, R., Pich, D. and Hammershcmidt, W. (1997). Latent membrane protein 1 of Epstein-Barr virus mimics a constituitively active receptor molecule. EMBO J. 16, 6131-6140.

Gregory, C.D., Murray, R.J., Edwards, C.F., and Rickinson, A.B. (1988). Downregulation of cell adhesion molecules LFA-3 and ICAM-1 in Epstein-Barr virus-positive Burkitt's lymphoma underlies tumor cell escape from virus-specific T cell surveillance. J,Exp. Med. 167, 1811-1824.

Gregory, C.D., Rowe, M., and Rickinson, A.B. (1990). Different Epstein-Barr virus (EBV)-B cell interactions in phenotypically distinct clones of a Burkitt lymphoma cell line. J,Gen, Virol, 71, 1481-1495.

Greenspan, J.S., Greenspan, D. Lennette, E.T., Abrams, D.I., Conant, M.A., Petersen, V., and Freese, U.K. (1985). Replication of Epstein-Barr virus within the epithelial cells of oral "hairy" leukoplakia, an AIDS-associated lesion. New Engl. J. Med. 313, 1564-1571.

Grossman, S.R., Johannsen, E., Tong, R., Yalamanchili, R. and Kieff, E. (1994). The Epstein-Barr virus nuclear antigen 2 transactivator is directed to response elements by the J☐ recombination signal binding protein. Proc. Natl. Acad. Sci. USA 91, 7568-7572.

Hamilton-Dutoit, S.J., Pallesen, G., Franzmann, M.B., Karkov, J., Black, F., Skinhoj, P., and Pedersen, C. (1991). AIDS-related lymphoma: histopathology, immunophenotype and association with Epstein-Barr virus as demonstrated by *in situ* nucleic acid hybridisation. Am.J.Pathol., 138, 149-163.

Hammerschmidt, W., and Sugden, B. (1989). Genetic analysis of immortalizing functions of Epstein-Barr virus in human B lymphocytes. Nature 340, 393-397.

Henkel, T.P., Ling, P.D., Hayward, S.D. and Peterson, M.G. (1994). Mediation of Epstein-Barr virus EBNA2 transactivation by recombination signal-binding protein J☐. Science, 265, 92-95.

Henle, W., and Henle, G., (1979). Seroepidemiology of the virus. The Epstein-Barr Virus, Berlin: Springer-Verlag, 61-78.

Herbst, H. (1996). Epstein-Barr virus in Hodgkin's disease. Seminars in Cancer Biology 7, 183-189.

Hsieh, J.J. and Hayward, S.D. (1995). Masking of the CBF1/RBPJk transcriptional repression domain by Epstein-Barr virus EBNA2. Science 268, 560-563.

Hu, L.F., Zabarovsky, E.R., and Chen, F. (1991). Isolation and sequencing of the Epstein-Barr virus BNLF-1 (LMP1) from a Chinese nasopharyngeal carcinoma. J. Gen. Virol. 72, 2399-2409.

Hu, L.F., Chen, F., and Zheng, X., Ernberg, I., Cao, S.L., Christensson, B., Klein, and G., Winberg, G. (1993). Clonability and tumorgenicity of human epithelial cells expressing the EBV encoded membrane protein LMP1. Oncogene 8, 1575-1583.

Huen, D.S., Henderson, S.A., Croom-Carter, D. and Rowe, M. (1995). The Epstein-Barr-virus latent membrane protein-1 (LMP1) mediates activation of the NF-B and cell surface phenotype via 2 effector regions in its carboxy-terminal cytoplasmic domain. Oncogene 10, 549-560.

Imai, S., Nishikawa, J. and Takada, K. (1998). Cell-to Cell Contact as an Efficient Mode of Epstein-Barr Virus Infection of Diverse Human Epithelial Cells. J. Virol. 72, 4371-4378.

Ip, Y.T. and Davis, R.J. (1998). Signal transduction by the c-Jun N-terminal kinase (JNK) – from inflammation to development. Curr. Op. Cell Biol. 10, 205-219.

Ishida, T., Tojo, T., Aoki, T. Kobayashi, N., Ohishi, T., Watanabe, T., Yamamoto, T., Inoue, J.I. (1996a). TRAF5, a novel tumor necrosis factor receptor-associated factor family protein, mediates CD40 signaling. Proc. Natl. Acad. Sci. *U.S.A.* 93, 9437-9442.

Ishida, T., Mizushima, S., Azuma, S., Kobayashi, N., Tojo, T., Suzuki, K., Aizawa, S., Watanabe, T., Mosialos, G., Kieff, E., Yamamoto, T., and Inoue, J. (1996b). Identification of TRAF6, a novel tumor necrosis factor receptor-associated factor protein that mediates signaling from an amino-terminal domain of the CD40 cytoplasmic region. J. Biol. Chem. 271, 28745-28748.

Izumi, K.M. and Kieff, E. (1997). The Epstein-Barr virus oncogene product latent membrane protein 1 engages the tumor necrosis factor receptor-associated death domain protein to mediate B lymphocyte growth transformation and activate NF-κB Proc. Natl. Acad. Sci. U.S.A. 94, 12592-12597.

Jarrett, R. (1998). Epstein-Barr virus and Hodgkin's disease. Epstein-Barr Virus Report, 5, 77-85.

Jiang, W.Q., Szekely, L., Wendel-Hansen, V., Ringertz, N. Klein, G., Rosen, A. (1991). Co-localization of the retinoblastoma protein and the Epstein-Barr virus-encoded nuclear antigen EBNA-5. Exp.Cell Res. 197, 314-318.

Johnson, R.J., Stack, M., Hazlewood, S.A., Jones, M., Blackmore, C.G., Hu, L.F., and Rowe, M. (1998). The 30-Base-Pair Deletion in Chinese Variants of the Epstein-Barr Virus LMP1 Gene Is Not the Major Effector of Functional Differences between Variant LMP1 Genes in Human Lymphocytes. J. Virol. 72, 4038-4048.

Kawaguchi, H., Miyashita, T., and Herbst, H. (1993). Epstein-Barr virus-infected T lymphocytes in Epstein-Barr virus-associated haemophagocytic syndrome. J. Clin.Invest., 92, 1444-1450.

Kaye, K.M., Devergne, O. Harada, J.N., Izumi, K.M., Yalamanchili, R., Kieff, E., and Mosialos, G. (1996). Tumor necrosis factor receptor associated factor 2 is a mediator of NF-κB activation by latent infection membrane protein 1, the Epstein-Barr virus transforming protein. Proc. Natl. Acad.Sci. U.S.A. 93, 11085-11090.

Kerr, B.M., Lear, A.L., Rowe, M., Croom-Carter, D., Young, L.S., Rookes, S.M., Gallimore, P.H., and Rickinson, A.B. (1992). Three transcriptionally distinct forms of Epstein-Barr virus latency in somatic cell hybrids: cell phenotype dependence of virus promoter usage. Virology 187, 189.

Khanim, F., Yao, Q-Y., Niedobitek, G., Sihota, S., Rickinson, A.B. and Young, L.S. (1996) Analysis of Epstein-Barr virus gene polymorphisms in normal donors and in virus-associated tumors from different geographical locations. Blood 88, 3491-3501.

Kieff, E. Epstein-Barr virus and its replication . In: Fields, B.N., Knipe, D.M., Howley, P.M. eds. Fields Virology. 3rd ed. Philadelphia: Lipincott-Raven Publishers, (1996), 2343-2396.

Kieser, A., Kilger, E., Gires, O., Ueffing, M., Kolch, W., and Hammerschmidt, W. (1997). Epstein-Barr virus latent membrane protein-1 triggers AP-1 activity via the c-Jun N-terminal kinase cascade. EMBO Journal, 16, 3478-6485.

Knox, P.G., Li, Q.X., Rickinson, A.B. and Young, L.S. (1996). In vitro production of stable Epstein-Barr virus-positive epithelial cell clones which resemble the virus: cell interaction observed in nasopharyngeal carcinoma Virology 215, 40-50.

Levitskaya, J., Coram, M., Levitsky, V., Imreh, S., Steigerwald-Mullen, P.M., Klein, G., Kurilla, M.G., and Masucci, M.G. (1995). Inhibition of antigen processing by the internal repeat region of the Epstein-Barr virus nuclear antigen-1. Nature 375, 685-688.

Levitskaya, J., Shapiro, A., Leonchiks, A., Ciechanover, A. and Masucci, M.G. (1997). Inhibition of ubiquitin/proteasome-dependent protein degradation by the Gly-Ala repeat domain of the Epstein-Barr virus nuclear antigen 1. Proc. Natl. Acad.Sci. U.S.A. 94, 12616-12621.

Magrath, I.T. and Bhatia, K. (1997). Exploitation of genetic abnormalities in the development of novel treatment strategies for hematological malignancies. The Non-Hodgkin's Lymphomas, 2nd ed. London: Arnold, 1065-1088.

Malinin, N.L., Boldin, M.P., Kovalenko, A.V. and Wallach, D. (1997) MAP3K-related kinase involved in NF-□B induction by TNF, CD95 and IL-1. Nature 385, 540-544.

Meijer, C.J.L.M., Meijer, N.M., Jiwa, D.F., Dukers, J.J., Oudejans, P.C., de Bruin, J.M.M. Walboomers and van den Brule, A.J.C. (1996). Epstein-Barr virus and human T-cell lymphomas. Seminars in Cancer Biology, 7, 191-196.

Miller, W.E., Cheshire, J.L., Baldwin, A.S., Raab-Traub, N. (1998). The NPC derived C15 LMP1 protein confers enhanced activation of NF-κB and induction of the EGFR in epithelial cells. Oncogene, 16, 1869-1877.

Miller, C.L., Burkhardt, A.L., and Lee, J.H. (1995). Integral membrane protein 2 (LMP2) of Epstein-Barr virus regulates reactivation from latency through dominant negative effects on protein tyrosine kinases. Immunity, 2, 155-166.

Mosialos, G., Birkenbach, M., VanArsdale, T., Ware, C., Yalamanchili, R., Kieff, E. (1995). The Epstein-Barr virus transforming protein LMP1 engages signaling proteins for the tumor necrosis factor receptor family. Cell 80, 389-399.

Neri, A., Barriga, F., and Ighirami, G. (1991). Epstein-Barr virus infection precedes clonal expansion in Burkitt's and acquired immunodeficiency syndrome-associated lymphoma. Blood, 11, 1092-1095.

Nicholls, J.M., Agathanggelou, A., Fung, K., Zeng, X.G., and Niedobitek, G. (1997). The association of squamous cell carcinomas of the nasopharynx with Epstein-Barr virus shows geographical variation reminiscent of Burkitt's lymphoma. J. Pathol. 183, 164-168.

Niedobitek, G. and Young, L.S. (1994). Epstein-Barr virus persistence and virus-associated tumors. Lancet, 343, 333-335.

Niedobitek, G., Agathanggelou, A., Rowe, M., Jones, E.L., Turyaguma, P., Oryema, J., Wright, D.H., and Young, L.S. (1995). Heterogeneous expression of Epstein-Barr virus latent proteins in endemic Burkitt's lymphoma. Blood, 86, 659-665.

Niedobitek, G., Agathanggelou, A. and Nicholls, J.M. (1996). Epstein-Barr virus infection and the pathogenesis of nasopharyngeal carcinoma: viral gene expression, tumor cell phenotype, and the role of the lymphoid stroma. Sem.Cancer Biol. 7, 165-174.

Niedobitek, G. and Young, L.S. (1997). Epstein-Barr virus and non-Hodgkin's lymphomas. The Non-Hodgkin's Lymphomas, 2nd ed., London: Arnold, 309-329.

Nonkwelo, C., Skinner, J., Bell, A., Rickinson, A., and Sample, J. (1996). Transcription start sites downstream of the Epstein-Barr virus (EBV) Fp promoter in early-passage Burkitt lymphoma cells define a fourth promoter for expression of the EBV EBNA-1 protein. J. Virol. 70, 623-627.

Osato, T. and Imai, S. (1996). Epstein-Barr virus and gastric carcinoma. Sem. Cancer Biol. 7, 175-182.

Pallesen, G., Hamilton-Dutoit, S.J., Rowe, M.,and Young, L.S.. (1991). Expression of Epstein-Barr virus latent gene products in tumor cells of Hodgkin's disease. Lancet 337, 320.

Panousis, C.G. and Rowe, D.T. (1997). Epstein-Barr virus latent membrane protein 2 associates with and is a substrate for mitogen-activated protein kinase. J. Virol. 71, 4752-4760.

Parker, G.A., Crook, T., Bain, M., Sara, E.A., Farrell, P.J., and Allday, M.J. (1996). Epstein-Barr virus nuclear antigen EBNA 3C is an immortalizing oncoprotein with similar properties to adenovirus E1A and papllomavirus E7. Oncogene, 13, 2541-9.

Pathmanathan, R., Prasad, U., Chandrika, G., Sadler, R. Flynn, K. and Raatraub, N. (1995). Undifferentiated, Nonkeratinizing, and Squamour-cell Carcinoma of the Naspharynx – Variants of Epstein-Barr Virus-infected Neoplasia. Am. J. Pathol. 146, 1355-1367.

Pathmanathan, R., Prasad, U., Sadler, R., Flynn, K., and Raabtraub, N. (1995). Clonal Proliferations of Cells Infected with Epstein-Barr-Virus in Preinvasive Lesions Related to Nasopharyngeal Carcinoma. New Engl. J. Med. 333, 693-698.

Piche, A., Kasono, K., Johanning, F., Curiel, T.J. and Curiel, D.T. (1998) Phenotypic knock-out of the latent membrane protein 1 of Epstein-Barr virus by an intracellular single-chain antibody. Gene Therapy 5, 1171-1179.

Polack, A., Hortnagel, K., Pajic, A., Christoph, B., Baier, B., Falk, M., Mautner, J., Geltinger, C., Bornkamm, G.W. and Kempkes, B. (1996). C-myc activation renders proliferation of Epstein-Barr virus (EBV)-transformed cells independent of EBV nuclear antigen 2 and latent membrane protein 1. Proc. Natl. Acad. Sci. USA 93, 10411-10416.

Radkov, S.A., Bain, M., Farrell, P.J., West, M., Rowe, M., Allday, M.J. (1997). Epstein-Barr virus EBNA3C represses Cp, the major promoter for EBNA expression, but has no effect on the promoter of the cell gene CD21. J.Virol. 71, 8552-8562.

Rickinson, A.B., Rowe, M., Hart, I.J., Yao, Q.Y., Henderson, L.E., Rabin, and H., Epstein, M.A. (1984). T-cell-mediated regression of "spontaneous" and of Epstein-Barr virus-induced B cell transformation in vitro: Studies with cyclosporin A. Cell Immunol. 87, 646-658.

Rickinson, A.B., Young, L.S., and Rowe, M. (1987). Influence of the Epstein-Barr virus nuclear antigen EBNA 2 on the growth phenotype of virus-transformed B cells. J. Virol. 61, 1310-1317.

Rickinson, A.B. and Kieff, E. Epstein-Barr virus. In: Fields, B.N., Knipe, D.M., Howley, P.M. eds. Fields Virology. 3rd ed. Philadelphia: Lipincott-Raven Publishers, (1996), 2397-2446.

Robertson, E.S (1997). The Epstein-Barr virus EBNA3 protein family as regulators of transcription. Epstein-Barr Virus Report 4, 143-150.

Rooney, C.M., Smith, C.A., Brenner, M.K., and Heslop, H.E., (1995). Prophylaxis and treatment of Epstein-Barr virus lymphoproliferative disease using genetically modified cytotoxic T lymphocytes. Lancet, 345, 9-13.

Rothe, M. Sarma, V. Dixit, V.M. and Goeddel, D.V. (1995). TRAF2-Mediated Activation of NF-κB by TNF Receptor 2 and CD40. Science 269, 1424-1427.

Rowe, M., Rowe, D.T., Gregory, C.D., Young, L.S., Farrell, P.J., Rupani, H., and Rickinson, A.B. (1987). Differences in B cell growth phenotype reflect novel patterns of Epstein-Barr virus latent gene expression in Burkitt's lymphoma cells. EMBO J 6, 2743-2751.

Rowe, M., Young, L.S., Cadwallader, K., Petti, L., Kieff, E., and Rickinson, A.B. (1989). Distinction between Epstein-Barr virus type A (EBNA 2A) and type B (EBNA 2B) isolates extends to the EBNA 3 family of nuclear proteins. J. Virol .63. 1031-1039.

Rowe, M., Young, L.S., Crocker, J., Stokes, H., Henderson, S., and Rickinson, A.B. (1991). Epstein-Barr virus (EBV)-associated lymphoproliferative disease in the SCID mouse model: implications for the pathogenesis of EBV-positive lymphomas in man. J.Exp.Med., 173, 147-158.

Sakai, T., Taniguchi, Y., Tamura, K., Minoguchi, S., Fukuhara, T., Strobl, L.J., Zimber-Strobl, U., Bornk-amm, G.W. and Honjo, T. (1998). Functional replacement of the intracellular region of the Notch 1 recep-tor by Epstein-Barr virus nuclear antigen 2. J. Virol. 72, 6034-6039.

Sample, J., Young, L., Martin, B., Chatman, T., Kieff, E., Rickinson, A., and Kieff, E. (1990). Epstein-Barr virus types 1 and 2 differ in their EBNA-3A, EBNA-3B, and EBNA-3C genes. J. Virol. 64, 4084.

Sample, J., Brooks, L., Sample, C., Young, L.S., Rowe, M., Rickinson, A., and Kieff, E. (1991). Restricted Epstein-Barr virus protein expression in Burkitt lymphoma is reflected in a novel EBNA-1 mRNA and transcriptional initiation site. Proc. Natl. Acad. Sci.. USA, 88, 6343.

Sandberg, M., Hammerschmidt, W. and Sugden, B. (1997). Characterization of LMP-1's Association with TRAF1, TRAF2, and TRAF3. J. Virol. 71, 4649-4656.

Sarma, V., Lin, Z., Clark, L., Rust, B.M., Tewari, M., Noelle, R.J., and Dixit, V.M. (1995). Activation of the B-cell Surface Receptor CD40 Induces A20, a Novel Zinc Finger Protein That Inhibits Apoptosis. J.Biol.Chem., 270, 12343-12346.

Sayos, J., Wu, C., Morra, M., Wang, N., Zhang, X., Allen, D., Van Schaik, S., Notarangelo, L., Geha, R., Roncarolo, M.G., Oettgen, H., De Vries, J.E., Aversa, G. and Terhorst, C. (1998) The X-linked lym-phoproliferative-disease gene product SAP regulates signals induced through the co-receptor SLAM. Na-ture 395, 462-469.

Silins, S.L. and Sculley, T.B (1994). Modulation of vimentin, the CD40 activation antigen and Burkitts lymphoma antigen (CD77) by the Epstein-Barr virus nuclear antigen EBNA 4. Virology 202, 16-24.

Sinclair, A.J., Palmero, I., Peters, G, and Farrell, P.J. (1994). EBNA-2 and EBNA-LP cooperate to cause G0 to G1 transition during immortalization of resting human B lymphocytes by Epstein-Barr virus. EMBO J. 13, 3321-3328.

Sixbey, J.W., Nedrud, J.G., Raab-Traub, N., Hanes, R.A., and Pagano, J.S. (1984). Epstein-Barr virus replication in oropharyngeal cells N. Engl. J. Med. 310, 1225-1230.

Sixbey, J.W., Shirley, P., Chesney, P.J., Buntin, D.M., and Resnick, L. (1989). Detection of a second wide-spread strain of Epstein-Barr virus. Lancet II, 761-765.

Song, H.Y., Rothe, M. and Goeddel, D.V. (1996). The tumor necrosis factor-inducible zinc finger protein A20 interacts with TRAF1/TRAF2 and inhibits NF-□B activation. Proc.Natl.Acad.Sci.U.S.A. 93, 6721-6725.

Speck, S.H., and Strominger, J.L. (1989). Transcription of Epstein-Barr virus in latently infected, growth-transformed lymphocytes. Adv. Viral. Oncol. 8, 133-150.

Strauch, B., Andrews, L.-L., Siegel, N., and Miller, G. (1974). Oropharyngeal excretion of Epstein-Barr virus by renal transplant recipients and other patients with immunosuppressive drugs. Lancet I, 234-237.

Sugiura, M., Imai, S., Tokunaga, M., Koizumi, S., Uchizawa, M., Okamoto, K. and Osato, T. (1996). Transcriptional analysis of Epstein-Barr virus gene expression in EBV-positive gastric carcinoma: unique viral latency in the tumor cells. Brit. J. Cancer, 74, 625-631.

Sutherland, C.L., Heath, A.W., Pelech, S.L., Young, P.R., and Gold, M.R. (1996). Differential Activation of the ERK, JNK, and p38 Mitogen-Activated Protein Kinases by CD40 and the B Cell Antigen Receptor. J.Immunol. 157, 3381-3390.

Sylla, B.S., Hung, S.C., Davidson, D.M., Hatzivassiliou, E., Malinin, N.L., Wallach, D., Gilmore, T.D., Kieff, E. and Mosialos, G. Epstein-Barr virus-transforming protein latent infection membrane protein 1 activates transcription factor NF-κB through a pathway that includes the NF-κB-inducing kinase and the IκB kinases IKKα and IKKβ. Proc. Natl. Acad. Sci. USA 95, 10106-10111.

Szekely, L. Selivanova, G., Magnusson, K.P., Klein, G., and Wiman, K.G. (1993). EBNA-5, an Epstein-Barr virus-coded nuclear antigen, binds to the retinoblastoma and p53 proteins. Proc.Natl.Acad.Sci.USA 90, 5455-9.

Thomas, J.A., Hotchin, N.A., Allday, M.J., Amlot, P., Rose, M., Yacoub, M., and Crawford, D.H. (1990). Immunohistology of Epstein-Barr virus-associated antigens in B cell disorders from immunocompromised individuals. Transplantation. 49, 944-953.

Waltzer, L., Logeat, F., Brou, C., Israel, A., Sergeant, A. and Manet, E. (1994). The human Jk recombination signal sequence binding protein (RBP-Jk) targets the Epstein-Barr virus EBNA2 protein to its DNA responsive elements. EMBO. J. 13, 5633-5638.

Wang, F., Gregory, C.D., Rowe, M., Rickinson, A.B., Wang, D., Birkenbach, M., Kikutani, H., Kishimoti, and T., Kieff, E. (1987). Epstein-Barr virus nuclear antigen 2 specifically induces expression of the B-cell activation antigen CD23. Proc. Natl. Acad. Sci. 84, 3452-3457.

Wang, F., Gregory, C., Sample, C., Rowe, M., Liebowitz, D., Murray, R., Rickinson, A., and Kieff, E. (1990). Epstein-Barr virus latent membrane protein (LMP1) and nuclear proteins 2 and 3c are effectors of phenotypic changes in B lymphocytes: EBNA-2 and LMP1 cooperatively induce CD23. J. Virol.. 64, 2309-2318.

Weiss, L.M., Movahed, L.A., Warnke, R.A. and Sklar, J. (1989). Detection of Epstein-Barr viral genomes in Reed-Sternberg cells of Hodgkin's disease. New Engl. J. Med. 320, 502-506.

Wilson, J.B., Bell, J.L. and Levine, A.J. (1996). Expression of Epstein-Barr virus nuclear antigen-1 induces B cell neoplasia in transgenic mice. EMBO J. 15, 3117-3126.

Wolf , H. zur Hausen, H., and Becker, V. (1973). EB viral genome in epithelial nasopharyngeal carcinoma cells. Nature New Biology, 244, 245-247.

Yao, Q.Y., Rickinson, A.B., and Epstein, M.A. (1985). A re-examination of the Epstein-Barr virus carrier state in healthy seropositive individuals. Int. J. Cancer, 35, 35-42.

Yao, Q.Y., Rowe, M., Martin, B., Young, and L.S., Rickinson, A.B. (1991). The Epstein-Barr virus carrier state: Dominance of a single growth-transforming isolate in the blood and in the oropharynx of healthy virus carriers. J. Gen,.Virol. 72, 1579-1590.

Young, L.S., Yao, Q.Y., Rooney, C.M., Sculley, T.B., Moss, D.J., Rupani, H., Laux, G., Bornkamm, G.W., and Rickinson, A.B. (1987). New type B isolates of Epstein-Barr virus from Burkitt's lymphoma and from normal individuals in endemic areas. J. Gen. Virol. 68, 2853-2862.

Young, L.S., Dawson, C., Clark, D. Rupani, H., Busson, P., Tursz, T., Johnson, A., and Rickinson, A.B. (1988). Epstein-Barr virus gene expression in nasopharyngeal carcinoma. J. Gen. Virol. 69, 1051-1065.

Young, L., Alfieri, C., Hennessy, K., Evans, H., O'Hara, C., Anderson, K.C., Ritz, J., Shapiro, R.S., Rickinson, A., Kieff, E., and Cohen, J.I. (1989). Expression of Epstein-Barr virus transformation-associated genes in tissues of patients with EBV lymphoproliferative disease. N. Engl. J. Med. 321, 1080-1085.

Young, L.S., Eliopoulos, A.G., Gallagher, N. and Dawson, C.W. (1998) CD40 and epithelial cells: across the great divide. Immunol. Today 19, 502-506.

Yu, M.C., Ho, J.H.C., Lai, S.H., Henderson, B.E. (1986). Cantonese-style salted fish as cause of nasopharyngeal carcinoma: report of a case-control study in Hong Kong. Cancer Res. 46, 956-961.

Zeng, Y. (1985). Seroepidemiological studies on nasopharyngeal carcinoma in China. Adv.Cancer Res. 44, 121-138.

Zheng, N., Yuan, F., Hu, L., Chen, F., Klein, G., and Christensson, B. (1994). Effect of B-lymphocyte- and NPC-derived EBV-LMP1 Gene Expression on In Vitro Growth and Differentiation of Human Epithelial Cells. Int. J. Cancer, 57, 747-753.

Zimber, U., Adldinger, H.K., Lenoir, G.M., Vuillaume, M., Knebel-Doeberitz, M., Laux, G., Desgranges, C., Wittmann, P., Freese, U.K., Schneider, U., and Bornkamm, G.W. (1986). Geographical prevalence of two types of Epstein-Barr virus. Virology 154, 56-.

Zur Hausen, H., Schulte-Holthauzen , and H., Klein, G. et al (1970). EBV DNA in biopsies of Burkitt tumors and anaplastic carcinomas of the nasopharynx. Nature, 228. 1956-1958.

HUMAN HERPESVIRUS-8

Ruth F. Jarrett

LRF Virus Centre, University of Glasgow

ABSTRACT

Since the discovery of human herpesvirus-8 (HHV-8) 4 years ago, a remarkable amount of data has accumulated on the biology and disease-associations of this virus. There is compelling evidence that HHV-8 is the long sought after agent which causes Kaposi's sarcoma. Unlike other human herpesviruses, HHV-8 infection does not appear to be ubiquitous and the distribution of HHV-8 appears similar to that of Kaposi's sarcoma. There is good evidence that the virus can be sexually transmitted and behaviours associated with acquisition of HHV-8 infection are the same as those associated with risk of developing Kaposi's sarcoma. Other routes of transmission are suggested by epidemiological studies in areas with a high incidence of Kaposi's sarcoma prior to the AIDS epidemic. The virus is also consistently and specifically associated with primary effusion lymphoma and multicentric Castleman's disease; both diseases are independently associated with Kaposi's sarcoma and interleukin-6 is implicated in the pathogenesis of both. The HHV-8 genome has been completely sequenced allowing the identification of potential viral oncogenes and facilitating functional studies. *In vitro* studies provide support for a causal role for the virus in Kaposi's sarcoma, and the available evidence suggests that HHV-8 is a new DNA tumour virus.

Introduction

Human herpesvirus 8 (HHV-8) genomic sequences were first identified in Kaposi's sarcoma (KS) tissue in 1994 by Chang et al using representational difference analysis. Two small fragments of DNA with homology to both herpesvirus saimiri (HVS) and Epstein-Barr virus (EBV) were identified and characterisation of the rest of the genome soon followed (Moore et al., 1996a; Russo et al., 1996; Neipel et al., 1997a). The virus was first referred to as Kaposi's sarcoma associated herpesvirus (KSHV) and, although HHV-8 is used in the remainder of this review, the terms HHV-8 and KSHV are both in current usage. A very frank account of the discovery of the virus has been written by Moore and Chang (1998).

The identification of nucleic acid sequences, which were unique to the virus, enabled polymerase chain reaction (PCR) primers to be designed and it was therefore possible to search for evidence of viral infection in a wide range of tissue samples. The presence of HHV-8 sequences in all forms of KS was soon established and there is now good evidence for a causal association between virus and disease. HHV-8 sequences were also found at high copy number in a sample from a body cavity-based lymphoma (Chang et al., 1994), and it became clear that the virus was also associated with this rare entity, now described as primary effusion lymphoma (PEL) (Nador et al., 1996).

The discovery that PELs were associated with HHV-8 was a major advance as PEL cell lines harbouring the viral genome and expressing viral antigens could be maintained in culture. The first such cell lines were co-infected with EBV but lines singly infected with HHV-8 were soon established (Cesarman et al., 1995a; Gaidano et al., 1996; Renne et al., 1996a; Boshoff et al., 1998). These lines have proved invaluable as a source of virus for both viral characterisation and serological studies. Viral particles were first definitively visualised in PEL cultures in 1996 (Renne et al., 1996a; Said et al., 1996a) and shortly afterwards in KS biopsy material (Orenstein et al., 1997; Said et al., 1997a). Thus, HHV-8 joins a growing list of viruses for which genomic sequences were identified prior to the visualisation of viral particles.

Overview of Genome Organisation

The family *Herpesviridae* is divided into three subfamilies, alpha, beta and gamma, on the basis of biological properties *in vivo* and *in vitro*. Some herpesviruses have been further classified into genera based on DNA sequence homology, similarities in genome arrangement and relatedness of viral proteins (Roizman, 1996). The genome of HHV-8 shares greatest sequence homology with HVS and is classified in the gamma-herpesvirus subfamily, genus *Rhadinovirus*. The most closely related human virus is the gamma-herpesvirus EBV, which is placed in the *Lymphocryptovirus* genus. Like other rhadino-viruses, the HHV-8 genome consists of a unique L-DNA which is flanked at each end by a tandemly repeated sequence with a high G+C content (Russo et al., 1996; Lagunoff & Ganem, 1997). Pulsed field gel electrophoresis showed that the viral genome is 160-170kb in size, consistent with other gamma-herpesviruses (Renne et al., 1996b). Genomes derived from PEL cell lines and KS lesions have essentially the same genome organisation and sequence, indicating that the same virus is associated with both conditions (Moore et al., 1996a; Russo et al., 1996; Nicholas et al., 1997a; Neipel et al., 1997a). The HHV-8 genome is maintained in latently infected B-cells in a monomeric, circular form and lytic infection is associated with the accumulation of linear genomes (Renne et al., 1996b).

The sequence of the unique coding region (minus a small region at the extreme right hand end) was published at the end of 1996, an amazing fete considering the first viral sequences were identified only two years earlier (Russo et al., 1996). Sequence analysis revealed 81 open reading frames (ORFs), consistent with other rhadinoviruses which encode 72-85 proteins. This number is certainly an underestimate as ORFs were assigned on a conservative basis and additional proteins, encoded by spliced transcripts, have already been identified (K8.1 and the latency-associated membrane protein [LAMP]) (Raab et al., 1998; Glenn et al., 1998).

Herpesvirus genomes contain many genes conserved throughout the virus family and also genes specific to each subfamily or individual virus. Genomes within the same subfamily show a greater degree of sequence conservation among homologous genes, and the homologous genes display similar genomic organisation. Despite this co-linearity among related herpesviruses, there are localised regions of appreciable genetic

Table 1: HHV-8 genes with homology to cellular genes

HHV-8 ORF	Cellular homologue	γ-herpesvirus with counterpart
ORF4	Complement binding protein	HVS, HVA
K2	IL-6	
ORF2	Dihydrofolate reductase	HVS
K3	Zinc finger motif	BHV-4
ORF70	Thymidylate synthase	HVS, HVA, EHV-2
K4	MIP-1 (CC chemokine)	
K4.1	CC chemokine	
K5	Zinc finger motif	BHV-4
K6	MIP-1 (CC chemokine)	
ORF16	bcl-2	HVS, HVA, BHV-4, EBV
K9	IRF	
ORF72	cyclin D	HVS, HVA
K14	ox-2 (N-CAM)	
ORF74	G-protein coupled receptor, IL-8 receptor	HVS, HVA, EHV-2

HVS, herpesvirus saimiri; HVA, herpesvirus ateles; BHV-4, bovine herpesvirus 4; MIP, macrophage inflammatory protein; EBV, Epstein-Barr virus; IRF, interferon regulatory factor.

divergence. These tend to occur at the genomic termini but also occur in clusters between blocks of conserved genes.

The HHV-8 genome contains seven blocks of conserved herpesvirus genes and eight non-conserved interblock (IB) regions, also referred to as divergent loci (Russo et al., 1996; Nicholas et al., 1997a, b) [Figure 1]. Divergent loci contain genes that are likely to confer biologically important properties to the virus. These include genes which are homologues of cellular genes (Table 1). A striking feature of the HHV-8 genome is the number of cellular genes which appear to have been pirated; the identification of these genes has enabled speculation as to likely features of the biology of the virus. The second divergent locus in HHV-8 encodes several cellular homologues including: an interleukin (IL)-6 homologue (vIL-6); two chemokines with weak homology to the macrophage inflammatory protein MIP-1 (vMIP-1A and vMIP-1B; ORFs K6 and K4 respectively) and a third with homology to MIP-1β; a bcl-2 family member (ORF16); and two genes which encode zinc finger proteins (named IE1-A and IE1-B by analogy with homologous genes in bovine herpesvirus 4). Another large non-conserved block (IBg) contains ORFs encoding proteins with weak but significant homology to members of the interferon regulatory factors (IRFs), of which K9 is the best studied to date. The divergent locus at the right end of the genome (IBh) contains: a G-protein coupled receptor protein with homology to the IL-8 receptor (ORF74); a cyclin D homologue (ORF72); and an ORF with homology to ox-2 membrane antigens. Functional studies relating to some of these proteins are discussed below. HHV-8 does not encode proteins with sequence homology to the EBV latent antigens or to the transforming protein of HVS.

The first sequences of HHV-8 which were identified by representational difference analysis are now known to be located within ORF26 and ORF75. ORF26 is a minor capsid antigen with homology to ORF26 of HVS and BDLF1 of EBV, while ORF75 encodes a putative tegument protein.

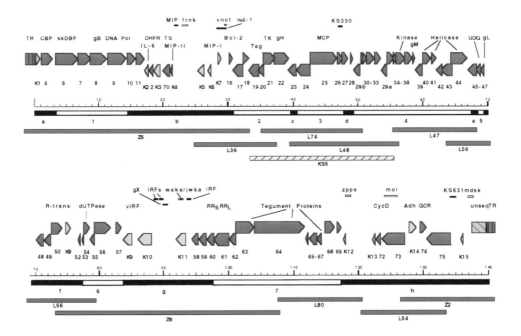

Figure 1: The HHV-8 genome. *Reproduced from Russo et al (1996) with kind permission from Patrick Moore. The open reading frames (ORFs) are numbered according to homology with the respective ORFs of HVS, even if positional homology is not maintained. HHV-8 ORFs not homologous to HVS genes are given the prefix K and numbered from left to right in consecutive order. The orientation of the reading frames is denoted by the direction of the arrows. Seven blocks (numbered) of conserved herpesvirus genes with nonconserved inter-block regions (lettered) are marked below the kilobase marker. The overlapping cosmid (Z prefix) and lambda (L prefix) clones used to map the HHV-8 genome are compared with the KS5 lambda phage clone from a KS lesion and shown below. Putative coding regions and features not specifically designated are shown above the ORF map. Repeat regions are shown as white lines (frnk, vnct, waka/jwka, zppa, moi, mdsk*

Viral Gene Expression

As with other herpesviruses, replication of HHV-8 can be latent or lytic. In latent infection the viral genome is episomal and replicates alongside host cell DNA. In lytic infection, transcription of viral genes occurs in a sequential fashion and results in release of progeny virions. Because of difficulties in passaging the virus *in vitro*, it has not been possible to classify HHV-8 genes as latent, immediate-early and late replication cycle genes.

Gene expression has largely been studied in PEL lines and at present RNAs are divided into 3 classes as follows: type I are constitutively expressed under standard growth conditions and are not induced by TPA; type II transcripts are detected at varying levels in unstimulated cells but are induced to higher levels by TPA; type III RNAs are only detectable after RNA induction (Sarid et al., 1998). Type I RNAs include 2 polycistronic messages which encode ORF73, ORFK13 (vFLIP), and ORF72 (v-cyc). A large transcript of ~ 6.6kb encodes all three proteins whereas the smaller 2.2kb spliced form encodes only ORFK13 and ORF72 (Rainbow et al., 1997). A third latent transcript LT3 originates from the extreme right end of the genome but has not been completely characterised to date (Sarid et al., 1998).

The class II transcripts include the very abundant T1.1 RNA (also called nut-1) and the T0.7 transcript (ORFK12) which encodes a membrane protein referred to as kaposin. These RNAs were originally identified as being highly expressed in non-stimulated cells from the BCBL-1 cell line (Zhong et al., 1996). This class also includes transcripts from non-conserved parts of the genome which encode signal transduction and regulatory protein homologues, including vIL-6 (ORFK2), vMIP-II (ORFK4), and vIRF (ORFK9). It is possible that transcription patterns differ in different cell types, for instance vIL-6 is expressed in latently-infected haematopoietic cells but is expressed in only rare KS spindle cells (Moore et al., 1996b). Class III transcripts encode viral enzymes and structural proteins such as ORF25 (major capsid protein) and the DNA polymerase (ORF21).

Prevalence and tropism

Serological assays

Antibody tests have been widely used to detect asymptomatic infection by many viruses, including herpesviruses, and to study viral prevalence. Since the identification of HHV-8 sequences there has therefore been an intense effort to develop serological assays for this virus. Cell lines derived from PELs have provided a useful source of HHV-8 antigens for these assays. A major deficiency of the cell lines used initially was that they were co-infected by EBV and therefore strategies had to be devised to eliminate detection of EBV antigens. Immunoblotting studies using the BC-1 cell line revealed a doublet of nuclear antigens, migrating with a relative molecular mass of 226/234 kilo Daltons, which was detected by serum from KS patients and was not related to any known EBV proteins (Gao et al., 1996a). The antigen detected in this assay is now known to be the latency nuclear antigen-1 (LNA-1), encoded by ORF73 (Rainbow et al., 1997; Kellam et al., 1997; Kedes et al., 1997). A second assay exploited the observation that BC-1 cells could be selectively induced into HHV-8 lytic replication by treatment with sodium butyrate (Miller et al., 1996). Induction of lytic cycle was accompanied by the appearance of several antigenic peptides which were recognised by sera from KS patients and were not present in EBV-producer cell lines. The presence of one antigen in particular (p40) appeared to represent specific expression of HHV-8 in the induced cells and reactivity with this antigen was taken as indicative of a positive serological result. Using these assays it was shown that the majority of individuals with KS were HHV-8 seropositive and that individuals at risk of KS, for example, HIV-infected homosexual men, had a lower seroprevalence (Gao et al., 1996a; Miller et al., 1996)[Table 2]. Seropositivity was not detected in the general population (Gao et al., 1996a), providing the first evidence that HHV-8 infection is not widely prevalent in the general population.

Other more specific serological assays followed quickly, many making use of the EBV-negative PEL cell lines BCBL-1 and BCP-1 (Renne et al., 1996a; Boshoff et al., 1998). Reactivity with an antigen or antigenic complex expressed during latent infection was found to produce a distinctive, punctate, nuclear staining pattern (Kedes et al., 1996). This complex is referred to as the latency-associated nuclear antigen (LANA) and includes the LNA-1 protein discussed above. The LANA immunofluorescence assay (IFA), using slightly different methodologies and serum dilutions, is in widespread use in various laboratories and is generally regarded as a very specific test for HHV-8 infection (Gao et al., 1996b; Simpson et al., 1996). Non-specific cytoplasmic fluorescence is frequently observed at low serum dilutions and this can be overcome by dilution of serum samples or by using isolated nuclei as the source of antigen (Kedes et al., 1996).

Lennette et al (1996) developed a mouse monoclonal antibody-enhanced IFA which utilises TPA-stimulated BCBL-1 cells and can detect antibodies to both lytic and latent antigens. Higher seroprevalence rates have been reported using this assay system, as compared to other assays, raising suspicion that it may be detecting cross-reactive antibodies. However cross-reactivity with EBV and detection of autoantibodies were excluded in the assay optimisation.

In order to circumvent problems associated with cross-reactivity to EBV antigens many tests using recombinant antigens have been developed. Of these the best results have been obtained with recombinant ORF65 proteins (Simpson et al., 1996), and with a recombinant protein derived from the recently recognised ORFK8.1, identified by virtue of its robust reactivity with HHV-8-positive sera (Raab et al., 1998). An ELISA utilising purified virus from the producer line KS-1, derived from a PEL, has also given promising results (Chatlynne et al., 1998).

Table 2. Representative results from serological studies using a range of assays to investigate the prevalence of antibodies to HHV-8 in Kaposi's sarcoma patients, risk groups and control populations. Dilution, serum dilution at which assay scored; IB, immunoblot; AIDS, acquired immunodeficiency syndrome; KS, Kaposi's sarcoma; EBV, Epstein-Barr virus; LANA, latency-associated nuclear antigen; IFA, immunofluorescence assay, HIV, human immunodeficiency virus; STD; sexually transmitted disease; MIFA, mouse monoclonal antibody-enhanced immunofluorescence assay. #, mixed ethnicity; *, isolated nuclei used as source of antigen; [r], reactivity to latent and lytic antigens scored separately but only results of latter reported here; [s], reported as positive if either assay positive.

Table 2: Serological studies of HHV-8 infection

Reference	Assay	Dilution	Subject group	Country	Positive/total	%Positive
Gao et al., 1996a	BC-1 IB	1:100	AIDS-KS homosexual	US	32/40	80
			AIDS non-KS homosexual	US	7/40	18
			Haemophiliacs	US	0/20	0
			Blood donors	US	0/122	0
			Individuals with high EBV titres	US	0/22	0
Gao et al., 1996b	BCP-1 IFA	1:160	HIV-negative KS	Italy	11/11	100
			HIV-negative KS	Uganda	1/1	100
			AIDS-KS	N. America	35/40	88
			AIDS-KS	Italy	10/14	71
			AIDS-KS	Uganda	14/18	78
			AIDS non-KS homosexual	N. America	12/40	30
			HIV-positive non-KS	Uganda	18/35	51
			HIV-positive haemophiliacs	N. America	0/20	0
			Blood donors	N. America	0/122	0
			Blood donors	Italy	4/107	4
			HIV-negative non-KS	Uganda	24/47	51
			EBV-positive individuals	N. America	0/69	0
Kedes et al., 1996	BCBL-1 IFA*	1:40	HIV-positive blood donors	US	41/138	30
			HIV-positive transfusion recipients	US	2/44	5
			HIV-positive haemophiliacs	US	9/300	3
			STD clinic attendees	US	23/176	13
			Blood donors	US	2/141	1
Lennette et al., 1996	BCBL-1 MIFA	1:10	KS	Africa	28/28	100
			KS	US	87/91	96
			HIV-positive homosexual asymptomatic	US	23/23	100
			HIV-positive heterosexual IVDA		3/13	23
			HIV-positive women	US	7/33	21
			Blood donors	US	9/44	20
			Adults non-specified	US	33/174	19
			Women	US	15/54	28
			Not specified	Zimbabwe	12/37	32
			Not specified	Nigeria	29/52	56
			Not specified	Zaire	13/16	82
			Not specified	Uganda	63/82	77
			Not specified	The Gambia	38/45	84
			Not specified	Ivory Coast	7/7	100
			Not specified	Haiti	15/52	29
			Not specified	Dominican Republic	5/40	12
			Not specified	Guatemala	2/20	10
Miller et al., 1996	BC-1 p40 IB	1:100	AIDS-KS	US#	32/48	67
			HIV-positive non KS various risk groups	US#	7/54	13
Simpson et al., 1996	ORF65 ELISA	1:100	AIDS-KS	UK/US	46/57	81
			AIDS-KS	Uganda	14/17	82
			Classical KS	Greece	17/18	94
			HIV-positive homosexual non KS	UK	5/16	31
			HIV-positive hemophiliacs	UK	0/28	0
			HIV-negative hemophiliacs	UK	1/56	1.8
			HIV-positive IVDA	UK	2/38	5.2
			HIV-negative IVDA	UK	0/25	0
			Blood donors	UK	3/174	1.7
			Blood donors	US	6/117	5
			Controls for Greek KS patients	Greece	3/26	12
			HIV-positive non-KS	Uganda	16/34	47
			HIV-negative non-KS	Uganda	6/17	35
Simpson et al., 1996	BCP-1 IFA	1:150	AIDS-KS	UK/US	84/103	81.5
			Classical KS	Greece	17/18	94
			HIV-positive homosexual non-KS	UK	10/33	30
			Female STD clinic attendees	UK	3/15	20
			HIV-positive haemophiliacs	UK	0/26	0
			HIV-positive IVDA	UK	0/38	0
			HIV-negative IVDA	UK	0/25	0
			HIV-negative homosexual male STD clinic attendees	UK	8/65	12
			HIV-negative heterosexual male STD clinic attendees	UK	4/75	5
			HIV-negative heterosexual female STD clinic attendees	UK	2/26	8
			Children with rash and fever	UK	0/24	0
			Blood donors	UK	4/150	3
			Blood donors	US	0/117	0
			Controls for Greek KS patients	Greece	3/26	12
			HIV-positive non-KS	Uganda	18/34	53
			HIV-negative non-KS	Uganda	9/17	53
Raab et al., 1998	K8.1 IB	1:50	Classic KS	Germany	2/2	100
			AIDS-KS	Germany	17/19	89
			Blood donors	Germany	2/50	4
			EBV primary infection	Germany	0/10	0
			Nasopharyngeal carcinoma	Germany	0/9	0
Chatlynne et al., 1998	Whole virus ELISA	1:80	Classic KS		67/72	93
			AIDS-KS	US	57/62	92
			Pre-KS	US	26/31	84
	n		HIV-positive homosexual non-KS	US	7/14	50
			HIV-negative homosexual non-KS	US	2/14	14
			HIV-negative heterosexual non-KS	US	1/19	5
			Blood donors	US	10/91	11
			HIV-negative heterosexual non-KS	US	1/19	5
Calabro et al., 1998	BCP-1 IFA & ORF65 ELISA		Blood donors	Italy	188/779	24

A blinded comparison of seven immunofluorescence and ELISA tests was recently performed (Rabkin et al., 1998). With the exception of an ELISA based on ORF26 which performed poorly, the tests detected reactivity in most classic KS patients (80-100%) and AIDS-KS patients (67-91%), in an intermediate number of HIV-positive non-KS patients (27-60%) and a small proportion of healthy blood donors (0-29%). However, on individual samples the results frequently differed, particularly for blood donor samples. Furthermore, latent and lytic tests did not appear to identify distinct sets of positive samples. It was concluded that while the assays are clearly able to detect a specific and sensitive association between HHV-8 infection and KS, and are useful for epidemiological studies, they could not be used to determine the absolute prevalence of HHV-8 infection. Despite this important caveat, serological studies have provided much useful data regarding HHV-8 prevalence, transmission routes and disease associations.

Results from Serological Studies

Results from a representative selection of serological surveys are shown in Table 2. Several clear patterns emerge from these studies. First, the vast majority of patients with KS are HHV-8 seropositive. Irrespective of the assays used most have reported seropositivity rates in excess of 80%, and several have reported 100% seropositivity for HIV-negative KS (Gao et al., 1996b; Lennette et al., 1996; Raab et al., 1998). Secondly, unlike other human herpesviruses, with the exception of Herpes simplex-2, HHV-8 does not appear to be ubiquitous. Thirdly, there appears to be significant geographical variation in prevalence. Although the exact rates remain to be determined, prevalence among healthy blood donors in the UK and US is low (0-20%) (Gao et al., 1996a, b; Simpson et al., 1996; Lennette et al., 1996). In contrast, prevalence in Africa is high with reports of seropositivity rates of 66-100% in West Africa and 33-53% in Uganda (Whitby, 1999; Simpson et al., 1996; Lennette et al., 1996). Mediterranean countries such as Greece and Italy have intermediate seroprevalence rates, 12 and 24% respectively (Simpson et al., 1996; Calabro et al., 1998). Lastly, seroprevalence is higher in persons at risk of KS, for example HIV-positive homosexual men, than in the general population. Seroprevalence in HIV-positive individuals who have acquired their infection parenterally and are at low risk of KS, for example haemophiliacs, have a seroprevalence rate similar to that of the general population.

PCR studies

PCR has been used to study the prevalence of HHV-8 infection, disease associations and possible routes of transmission; studies relating to particular diseases and transmission are considered in the relevant sections below. Unfortunately PCR studies have been complicated by two issues. First, contamination leading to false positive results, or high detection rates leading to the suspicion of PCR contamination, appear to have been a feature of these studies. This issue has been discussed in a somewhat humorous, although serious, fashion by Moore (1998) in a letter to the Lancet. A second concern relates to sampling error when dealing with latent herpesvirus infection. In the case of EBV only a very small proportion of peripheral blood B-cells is latently infected by the virus, ~1-50 per 10^6 B-cells (Khan et al., 1996). Therefore, in order to detect reliably the virus in peripheral blood, the sample should contain in excess of 10^6 B-cells or 10^7 peripheral blood mononuclear cells (PBMCs). The prevalence of latent infection would therefore be underestimated, at least for EBV, if samples containing only 1μg of DNA or 1.5 x 10^5 PBMCs were analysed.

Most PCR studies have used primers which amplify a 233 base pair fragment derived from the ORF26 fragment identified in the original study by Chang at al (1994). Such studies have generally detected a low prevalence of HHV-8 in PBMCs from healthy persons. No positive samples were reported from three separate studies assaying samples from a total of 431 healthy HIV-negative individuals (Marchioli et al., 1996; Whitby et al., 1995; De Milito et al., 1997). Two studies examining healthy HIV-negative individuals from Italy have reported higher positivity rates, 9% and 11% respectively (Bigoni et al., 1996; Viviano et al., 1997), consistent with the higher seroprevalence rate in this locale. Kikuta reported positive PBMC samples from 12/15 healthy adults from Japan and suggested that infection was widespread in Japan (Kikuta et al., 1997). Further studies from this area are clearly needed to confirm or refute this association.

In a study examining multiple aliquots of PBMCs, Decker et al (1996) found evidence of infection in 3/5 healthy individuals and 4/5 allograft recipients from the US. In the latter study at least 10 replicates of 1 x 10^6 cells were analysed for each individual, and a maximum of 2 out of 10 replicates were positive. This study raises the possibility that the use of small samples may have led to an underestimate of HHV-8 prevalence in previous studies. However, given the very large number of samples which have been examined with negative results other explanations must be considered.

Cell fractionation studies suggest that infected cells within the peripheral blood are mainly CD19-positive B-cells, although less frequent infection of T-cells has also been reported (Ambroziak et al., 1995; Harrington et al., 1996; Sirianni et al., 1997)

Saliva and semen samples have been extensively studied in attempts to define both viral prevalence and potential routes of transmission. HHV-8 is detectable in the saliva of KS patients, as discussed below, but has not been detected in the saliva of healthy HIV-negative individuals (Lucht et al., 1998). Studies of semen and prostate have led to more controversial findings. The original report that HHV-8 sequences could be detected in 23% of artificial insemination donors was subsequently retracted (Lin et al., 1998). However, Monini et al (1996) reported an even higher prevalence (30/33) following PCR analysis of semen samples from the Po valley in Italy. This study also found evidence of infection in samples from the urinary tract (2/20), female genital tract (3/16), glans or foreskin (4/18), and prostate (7/16). They concluded that HHV-8 infection was present in a large proportion of healthy adults from this area. This study provoked much comment from other workers who failed to detect HHV-8 sequences in samples of prostate and urogenital cancers from other areas of Italy and elsewhere (Corbellino et al., 1996; Tasaka et al., 1996; Diamond et al., 1997; Lebbe et al., 1997; Howard et al., 1997).

Overall, both serological and molecular studies suggest that HHV-8 is not a ubiquitous virus and that there is significant geographical variation in prevalence. However, PCR studies have given rise to some conflicting results, and current serological tests show a lack of concordance in the analysis of samples from presumed low seroprevalence groups. Refinements in serological assays should resolve this important issue in the near future.

Disease Associations

There is very good evidence that certain diseases are closely associated with HHV-8 infection including KS, PEL and MCD. For other diseases notably multiple myeloma (MM) the association with HHV-8 is much more controversial. The virus has been detected less frequently in other conditions including primary cerebral lymphomas and reactive lymphadenopathies.

Kaposi's sarcoma

EPIDEMIOLOGY

KS occurs in four forms: classic; African endemic; iatrogenic; and acquired immunodeficiency syndrome-associated (AIDS-KS). Classic KS is typically described as a rare, indolent disease affecting elderly men of Eastern European or Mediterranean descent. The original description of this disease included patients with widespread lesions and visceral involvement (Kaposi, 1872) and it is possible that a more aggressive sub-type of classic KS exists (Lospalluti et al., 1995). In the 1960s interest was aroused by reports from Africa suggesting that KS was prevalent in equatorial Africa, and represented 10% of all cases of malignancy in Uganda (Oettle, 1962). The African endemic form of the disease largely affects children and young adults, is generally more aggressive and may occur in a lymphadenopathic form resembling lymphoma. The next decade saw the advent of iatrogenic KS in patients receiving immunosuppressive therapy; this form of the disease may regress following withdrawal of immunosuppressive treatment, underscoring the importance of immunosuppression in KS pathogenesis (Myers et al., 1974; Farge, 1993).

An aggressive form of KS, frequently involving viscera, became apparent in young men in the US around 1980 (Friedman-Kien et al., 1982). This epidemic form of the disease is usually associated with HIV infection and presaged the onset of the AIDS (acquired immunodeficiency syndrome) epidemic.

Prior to the identification of HHV-8, epidemiological studies strongly suggested involvement of an infectious agent in KS (Beral et al., 1990; Peterman et al., 1993). The sudden and dramatic increase in the incidence of KS in the US in the 1980s alone, suggested the likely importance of environmental factors. Data relating to AIDS-KS further predicted that the infectious agent was predominantly sexually transmitted. In the US, KS in persons with AIDS was at least 20,000 times more common than in the general population, and 300 times more common than in other immunosuppressed groups. It was commoner in individuals who acquired HIV through sexual contact than parenterally - 21% of homosexual or bisexual men compared to 1% of haemophiliacs. Women were more likely to have KS if their husbands were bisexual rather than if they were intravenous drug abusers. A variety of sexual behaviours was also associated with increased risk of disease (Jacobson et al., 1990). These data were consistent with the presence of a sexually transmitted agent which was transmitted in blood less efficiently than HIV. Geographical variation in KS incidence within the US was also evident with the highest incidence in New York and the San Francisco area, suggesting introduction of an infectious agent to these areas at around the same time as HIV (Beral et al., 1990). Although the evidence pointed to immunosuppression as an important factor in KS pathogenesis, the documentation of KS occurring in HIV-negative homosexual men suggested involvement of an infectious agent distinct from HIV.

CLINICO-PATHOLOGIC FEATURES OF KAPOSI'S SARCOMA

Clinically KS represents a spectrum of lesions from plaque to patch to nodular stages. Early lesions are characterised by jagged, thin-walled dilated vascular spaces surrounded by inflammatory cells and extravasated blood. Later nodular lesions consist of plump, spindle-shaped stromal cells containing irregular, angulated slit-like spaces lined by endothelium and filled with red cells. Angiomatous and spindle cell elements blend together almost imperceptibly. The lineage of the spindle cells remains unresolved; immunophenotyping studies have suggested an origin from both lymphatic and vascular endothelium, and also cells with both monocyte and endothelial cell markers (Jussila et al., 1998; Jones et al., 1986; Rutgers et al., 1986; Uccini et al., 1994). An expansion of KS-like spindle cells, or their progenitors, is present in the peripheral blood of patients with all forms of KS (Browning et al., 1994).

There is continuing debate about whether KS is a truly malignant condition or whether it is a reactive process. Studies by Rabkin and co-workers (1997) suggest that the lesions are clonal on the basis of unbalanced methylation patterns of X-linked genes. Other studies using similar techniques have not confirmed these findings, both with regard to the clonality of individual lesions and the relationship between multiple lesions in an individual patient (Delabesse et al., 1997; Gill et al., 1998). Inflammatory cytokines, such as basic fibroblast growth factor, γ-interferon, tumor necrosis factor and IL-6, secreted by infiltrating cells and the KS spindle cells clearly play an important role in KS pathogenesis (Fiorelli et al., 1998). Soluble HIV Tat protein also increases the KS-like forming activity of endothelial spindle cells and it is suggested that this protein plays a role in disease progression (Ensoli et al., 1994). On the basis of the latter findings, it has been proposed that KS, at least in the early stages, is not a true cancer but rather a hyperplastic-proliferative disease (reviewed in Fiorelli et al., 1998).

DETECTION OF HHV-8 IN KAPOSI'S SARCOMA LESIONS BY PCR AND SOUTHERN BLOTTING

HHV-8 sequences were first identified in KS tissue and were subsequently shown, by PCR and Southern blotting, to be present in samples from most patients with AIDS-KS (Chang et al., 1994). A large number of studies followed showing that HHV-8 genomic sequences could be detected in all forms of KS from a wide variety of geographical

Table 3. *All studies used the PCR KS330$_{233}$ assay utilising primers derived from the 330 base pair fragment, originally described by Chang et al., (1994), which amplify a fragment of 233 base pairs. Boshoff et al., (1995) used a nested assay which incorporated these primers as the inner primer set. AIDS, acquired immunodeficiency syndrome; KS, Kaposi's sarcoma.*

Table 3: Detection of HHV-8 in lesions of Kaposi's sarcoma

Reference	Patient Group	Positive/Total	% Positive
Chang et al., 1994	AIDS-KS	25/27	93
Su et al., 1995	AIDS-KS	4/4	100
	Non-AIDS KS	2/3	66
Dupin et al., 1995	AIDS-KS	4/4	100
	Classic KS	5/5	100
Huang et al., 1995	AIDS-KS	12/12	100
	Classic KS	7/8	87.5
	African KS	7/10	70
Boshoff et al., 1995a	AIDS-KS	14/14	100
	Classic KS	16/17	94
	Transplant-associated KS	8/8	
	HIV-negative homosexual male with KS	1/1	
Lebbe et al., 1995	AIDS-KS	2/2	100
	Classic KS	10/10	
	African KS	3/3	
	Iatrogenic KS	1/1	
Ambroziak et al., 1995	AIDS-KS, homosexual males	12/12	100
	HIV-negative homosexual male with KS	1/1	
Moore & Chang, 1995	AIDS-KS	10/11	91
	Classic KS	6/6	
	HIV-negative homosexual males with KS	4/4	
Schalling et al., 1995	AIDS-KS	25/25	100
	Classic KS	3/3	
	African KS	18/18	100

locations (Su et al., 1995; Dupin et al., 1995; Huang et al., 1995; Boshoff et al., 1995a; Lebbe et al., 1995; Ambroziak et al., 1995; Moore and Chang, 1995; Schalling et al., 1995). Viral sequences were detected in all stages of disease, from patch to nodular, although detection rates were higher in nodular compared to patch-stage lesions (Noel et al., 1996). Multiple tissue types including skin, lymph node, gut and oral mucosa were also found to harbour viral sequences. Representative results of these studies are summarised in Table 3. Examination of paraffin-embedded tissues necessitated the use of nested PCR in many studies and failure to detect viral sequences may relate to quality of archival material. It is therefore plausible that viral genomes are present in all KS lesions.

Viral sequences have been detected less frequently in unaffected skin from KS patients, usually, but not always, in skin adjacent to lesions. In contrast, viral sequences are almost never detected in skin lesions and other vascular tumours from patients without KS (Chang et al., 1994; Boshoff et al., 1995a; Buonaguro et al., 1996; Cathomas et al., 1996; Jin et al., 1996; Dictor et al., 1996). Rady et al (1995) detected HHV-8 sequences in the majority of skin lesions from patients who were iatrogenically immunosuppressed following organ transplantation, but these findings have not been supported by other studies (Dupin et al., 1997; Foreman et al., 1997a; Kohler et al., 1997).

Southern blotting using a probe from the TR of the genome has been used to assess the clonality of virally-infected cells. By analogy with EBV, the presence of a single band in this analysis indicates the presence of a clonal, episomal genome whereas a ladder of bands indicates lytic replication. Analysis of DNA from a KS lesion revealed a single band, consistent with latent infection and suggestive of clonality (Russo et al., 1996). However it remains to be determined whether this is a reliable marker of clonality in the case of HHV-8 infection.

IN SITU AND GENE EXPRESSION STUDIES

HHV-8 DNA has been localised to lesional spindle cells and endothelial cells using PCR *in situ* hybridisation, DNA and RNA *in situ* hybridisation, and immunohistochemistry (Boshoff et al., 1995b; Li et al., 1996; Foreman et al., 1997b; Rainbow et al., 1997; Staskus et al., 1997; Sturzl et al., 1997; Reed et al., 1998). Using the T0.7 probe, Sturzl et al (1997) showed viral gene expression in 50-70% of cells within nodular lesions but in only 1-3% of the cells in patch stage lesions. In this study, the surrounding cells were all found to be negative. Using a similar approach, Staskus et al (1997) also found expression of the T0.7 mRNA in at least 85% of cells in advanced lesions. Viral sequences are clearly detectable in lesions at all stages, but in early lesions a much smaller percentage of cells is positive (Foreman et al., 1997b). HHV-8 has also been detected in keratinocytes, eccrine cells, and infiltrating mononuclear cells (Foreman et al., 1997b; Reed et al., 1998; Orenstein et al., 1997).

In situ hybridisation studies have detected the expression of T0.7 (K12), K13 (vFLIP), ORF72 (v-cyc) mRNAs in most spindle cells; in addition expression of ORF73 (LNA-1) has been demonstrated at the protein level (Sturzl et al., 1997; Staskus et al., 1997; Davis et al., 1997; Reed et al., 1998; Rainbow et al., 1997). Expression of T1.1 and ORF26 transcripts has been detected within 10% of cells in advanced lesions

(Staskus et al., 1997), consistent with the presence of a subpopulation of cells undergoing productive HHV-8 replication. RT-PCR (reverse transcriptase-PCR) has been used to demonstrate expression of ORF74 (vGCR) but it is not clear whether expression is limited to cells undergoing lytic replication (Cesarman et al., 1996a). Human IL-6 is expressed within KS lesions but the viral homologue appears to be poorly expressed, in contrast to the situation in PELs and MCD (Moore & Chang, 1995).

TEMPORAL ASSOCIATIONS

Serological and molecular studies show a strong association between KS and HHV-8 positivity, and cross-sectional studies suggest that seroprevalence correlates with risk of developing KS. Few longitudinal studies have been performed to date but these support the idea that infection precedes disease development, and suggest that seropositivity and the ability to detect viral sequences in PBMCs are associated with risk of KS development (Whitby et al., 1995; Gao et al., 1996a, b; Lefrere et al., 1996). Whitby et al (1996) detected HHV-8 sequences in the peripheral blood of approximately 50% of KS patients and in 11/143 homosexual men with HIV infection. During a follow-up period of 30 months, 6 of the 11 men (54%) with detectable viral sequences developed KS compared to 12/132 men (9%) with negative results (odds ratio 7.0, 95% CI, 2.8-1.3). These findings suggest that 50% of HIV-infected patients progress to KS within 3.5 years of HHV-8 being detected in peripheral blood. Gao et al (1996a) performed a serological study on 40 patients who developed AIDS-KS over a period of 13-103 months. Eleven patients were HHV-8 seropositive at all time points whereas 21 seroconverted 6-75 months before the diagnosis of KS. The median duration of seropositivity before diagnosis was 33 months and antibody titres remained constant from seroconversion to KS diagnosis. A recent study of HHV-8 seroprevalence in the 'Amsterdam Cohort Studies of HIV infection and AIDS' shows that individuals who are infected with HHV-8 after HIV are at greater risk of developing KS than those who are infected with HHV-8 prior to HIV (Renwick et al., 1998). The median time from seroconversion to development of KS in the former group was around 5 years.

HHV-8 sequences are detected more frequently in body fluids, such as saliva and semen, from KS patients and HHV-8-infected individuals as compared to HIV-infected individuals without KS or healthy individuals; HIV-infected individuals without KS are also more likely to harbour viral sequences than healthy individuals (Boldogh et al., 1996; Diamond et al., 1997; Blackbourn et al., 1998; Lucht et al., 1998; Whitby, 1999). Detection of HHV-8 sequences in broncheolar lavage specimens appears to predict the presence or subsequent development of pulmonary KS (Howard et al., 1995).

CORRELATION BETWEEN KS INCIDENCE AND HHV-8 SEROPREVALENCE

Serological studies suggest that HHV-8 is not ubiquitous and that there is geographical variation in prevalence. There is a good correlation between the incidence of KS and HHV-8 seroprevalence. In Italy and Greece, countries in which classic KS is found, HHV-8 seroprevalence in the general population is higher than in countries, such as the UK and US, with low KS incidence (Table 2). Within Italy, regional differences in HHV-8 seroprevalence, sometimes over quite small distances, have been described and

Table 4: Detection of HHV-8 in lymphomas

Histology	Number positive/tested
AIDS-related	
Burkitt's lymphoma	0/28
Diffuse large B-cell lymphoma	2*/41
Plasmacytoma/myeloma	0/3
Primary effusion lymphoma	44/44
Peripheral T-cell lymphoma	0/2
Anaplastic large cell lymphoma	0/2
Hodgkin's disease	0/11
Non-AIDS-related	
Precursor B-cell lymphoblastic lymphoma/leukaemia	0/42
B-cell chronic lymphocytic leukaemia/prolymphocytic leukaemia/small lymphocytic lymphoma	0/90
Lymphoplasmacytoid lymphoma	0/3
Mantle cell lymphoma	0/14
Follicular center lymphoma	0/60
Marginal zone lymphoma (extra-nodal and nodal) and MALT lymphoma	0/21
Hairy cell leukaemia	0/18
Splenic lymphoma with villous lymphocytes	0/9
Plasmacytoma and myeloma	0/28
Diffuse large cell lymphoma	0/107
Burkitt's lymphoma	0/40
Post-transplant lymphoproliferative disease	0/23
Primary effusion lymphoma	8/8
T-cell chronic lymphocytic leukaemia/prolymphocytic leukaemia	0/43
Large granular lymphocytic leukaemia	0/46
Mycosis fungoides/Sezary syndrome	0/57
Peripheral T-cell lymphoma	0/24
Angioimmunoblastic T-cell lymphoma	3#/24
Adult T-cell lymphoma/leukaemia	0/15
Anaplastic large cell lymphoma	0/13
Hodgkin's disease	0/75

For the purpose of this table, lymphomas have been classified as far as possible according to the REAL classification (Harris et al., 1994). *Positive samples were a gingival mass from a patient with Kaposi's sarcoma (low level positivity) (Otsuki et al., 1996) and a large cell immunoblastic lymphoma from a case with cutaneous Kaposi's sarcoma (Gessain et al., 1997). #The 3 positive samples were from the study by Luppi et al., (1996a). Data are derived from (Chang et al., 1994; Pastore et al., 1995; Cesarman et al., 1995b; Karcher et al., 1995; Nador et al., 1995; Ansari et al., 1996; Arvanitakis et al., 1996; Luppi et al., 1996; Nador et al., 1996; Otsuki et al., 1996; Said et al., 1996b; Strauchen et al., 1996; Pawson et al., 1996; Gessain et al., 1997; Karcher & Alkan, 1997; Armstrong et al., 1998; Jones et al., 1998) these again correlate with KS incidence in the pre-AIDS era. Generally, KS incidence and HHV-8 seroprevalence are higher in Southern Italy (21.9-24.6%) than in Northern Italy (7.3%) (Calabro et al., 1998; Whitby et al., 1998). In Sicily, Sardinia and the Po valley, areas with a relatively high incidence of classic KS, HHV-8 seroprevalence is greater (35%, 32% and 27.4% respectively) than in regions with a lower KS incidence (13.3% in Conegliano, 3.8% in Lombardi) (Calabro et al., 1998; Whitby et al., 1998).

In countries, such as Uganda, with endemic KS the seroprevalence of HHV-8 is high with rates in excess of 50% reported (Simpson et al., 1996; Lennette et al., 1996). The situation seems rather different in West Africa where the HHV-8 seroprevalence is similarly high but the incidence of KS is much lower (Ariyoshi et al., 1998). In general, geometric mean titres of HHV-8 antibodies are greater in areas with a high seroprevalence, for instance Italy and Uganda, however this is not the case in the Gambia where the reported geometric mean titres are low. It is possible that the low incidence of KS is related to low antibody titres among infected individuals, plus the fact that, until recently, HIV-2 infection was the predominant cause of AIDS in this region.

Lymphoproliferative disease

Early reports indicated that HHV-8 DNA was detectable in an unusual lymphoma previously called body cavity-based lymphoma and now referred to as PEL. This finding, coupled with the tropism of HHV-8 for B and T-cells, led to many studies investigating the distribution of HHV-8 sequences in both benign and malignant lymphoproliferative disease. Representative studies are summarised in Table 4. A striking and consistent feature of these studies is that HHV-8 is associated with PELs but not with other types of leukaemia and lymphoma. Similarly among benign lymphoproliferative lesions HHV-8 is significantly associated with Castleman's disease but is found infrequently in other conditions (Chadburn et al., 1997).

PRIMARY EFFUSION LYMPHOMA
Prior to the discovery of HHV-8, cases of non-Hodgkin's lymphoma presenting in body cavities in the absence of clinically identifiable tumour masses were referred to as body cavity-based lymphomas. However, the existence of a distinct biological entity which is associated with HHV-8 is now evident. It is recommended that this disease is referred to as primary effusion lymphoma in order to avoid confusion with other, albeit rare, lymphomas which occur in body cavities (Nador et al., 1995; Nador et al., 1996; Cesarman et al., 1996b). PELs usually arise in HIV-positive homosexual men and are frequently associated with KS, but are also found less frequently in HIV-negative individuals usually in older age groups (Cesarman et al., 1995b; Nador et al., 1996; Karcher & Alkan, 1997). The precise incidence of this tumour remains to be established but PELs account for ~3% of AIDS-related lymphomas (Carbone & Gaidano, 1997).

PELs display a confined spreading along serous membranes without invasive or destructive features. Simultaneous involvement of multiple cavities without dissemination to other sites is sometimes observed. Tumour cells are described as having a morphology bridging large cell immunoblastic and anaplastic large cell lymphoma

(Nador et al., 1996). They rarely express pan-B markers and lack surface immuno-globulin, but are usually CD45-positive and have clonal immunoglobulin gene rear-rangements consistent with a B-cell origin (Nador et al., 1995; Nador et al., 1996). In addition they usually express EMA, HLA-DR, CD38 and CD71 and about half are CD30-positive. Most express late stage B-cell markers including CD138 suggesting that PEL cells represent a pre-terminal stage of B-cell differentiation (Gaidano et al., 1997a).

In addition to HHV-8, clonal EBV genomes are detected in AIDS-related PELs, but are only rarely found in tumour cells from HIV-negative cases (Cesarman et al., 1995b; Ansari et al., 1996; Nador et al., 1996; Said et al., 1996b; Nador et al., 1996; Komanduri et al., 1996). PELs are generally devoid of alteration of Bcl-2, Bcl-6 and p53 genes and, in contrast to Burkitt's or Burkitt-like lymphoma which sometimes occur in body cavi-ties, they do not have c-myc rearrangements (Nador et al., 1996).

Consistent with the association between PELs and HHV-8, PELs occurring both with and without HIV infection are strongly associated with KS (Nador et al., 1995; Said et al., 1996b; Strauchen et al., 1996). PELs contain a greater number of HHV-8 genomes per cell compared to KS lesions (40-80 copies in contrast to $\sim$ 1 copy) and retain the virus when established in culture (Cesarman et al., 1995a, b). Growth of PEL cell lines appears dependent on the availability of IL-6; both human IL-6 and the IL-6 receptor are expressed by these lines and it has been suggested that the stimulatory signal is trans-mitted via an intracellular interaction between IL-6 and its receptor (Asou et al., 1998). Viral IL-6 is also expressed by PELs (Moore et al., 1996b) but the role of this cytokine in promoting tumour growth is not clear at present. Expression of other viral genes in PEL is summarised in an earlier section.

Despite intensive searching, HHV-8 genomes have been detected only rarely in other lymphomas (Table 4). Corboy et al., (1998) detected viral sequences in 15/27 primary CNS B-cell lymphomas examined by nested PCR; detection rates were similar in tu-mours from HIV-positive and negative individuals. The cellular localisation of the viral sequences was not examined and it was suggested that infiltrating cells adjacent to the tumour could be infected and contributing to lymphomagenesis by a paracrine mecha-nism. HHV-8 detection rates are lower using single round PCR with positivity rates of 4/65 and 4/23 for AIDS and non-AIDS-related primary B-cell lymphoma respectively (Luppi et al., 1996a; Luppi et al., 1996b; Morgello et al., 1997; Gaidano et al., 1997b; Corboy et al., 1998; Luppi et al., 1998). The collective data therefore indicate that it is highly unlikely that primary CNS lymphomas represent clonal expansions of HHV-8-infected cells.

Multicentric Castleman's disease

Castleman's disease is a rare atypical lymphoproliferative disorder which is clinically and morphologically heterogeneous. It is associated with an increased risk of developing malignant disease. KS is the most commonly associated malignancy, but non-Hodgkin's lymphoma, Hodgkin's disease and plasmacytomas all occur at increased frequency (Peterson & Frizzera, 1993). Castleman's disease occurs in localised and multicentric forms. Multicentric Castleman's disease (MCD) occurs in older patients, is frequently associated with systemic symptoms and usually runs an aggressive course with a poor prognosis. In contrast, the localised form occurs mainly in young people and exists as a solitary mass. HIV infection is associated with the multicentric form of this disease. Two histological types of Castleman's disease are described: the more common hyaline-vascular type is associated with small hyalinized and hypervascular germinal centres whereas the plasma cell type is characterised by plasma cell accumulations. MCD is almost exclusively of the plasma cell type.

Soulier et al (1995) examined a series of 31 cases of MCD including 14 HIV-positive cases, 9 of which also had KS, for the presence of HHV-8. All of the lesions from HIV-positive individuals were HHV-8-positive as were 7/17 of the remaining cases. The strong association between HHV-8 and MCD has been confirmed by many subsequent studies although some have found a lower proportion of non-HIV-associated cases to be positive (Corbellino et al., 1996; Gessain et al., 1996; Luppi et al., 1996a; Smir et al., 1996; Parravicini et al., 1997a; Chadburn et al., 1997). Differences between series probably relate to sample selection; HHV-8-positive cases appear more likely to be elderly, and have multicentric disease and plasma cell histology.

HHV-8-positive MCD lesions contain a high viral load and viral sequences have been detected in the peripheral blood of these cases. Grandadam et al (1997) showed that the viral load in PBMCs was related to exacerbation of symptoms in the 3 HIV-positive cases studied.

Prior to the identification of HHV-8, IL-6 was known to be associated with the pathogenesis of Castleman's disease. Using immunohistochemistry and in situ hybridi-sation, IL-6 expression had been demonstrated in germinal centres and in cells in inter-follicular areas of lesions (Yoshizaki et al., 1989; Leger-Ravet et al., 1991; Ishiyama et al., 1994). Elevated levels of IL-6 had also been described in serum and in cell suspensions from lesions (Yoshizaki et al., 1989). Animal models support a central role for IL-6 secretion in disease pathogenesis (Brandt et al., 1990), and temporary clinical improvement has been achieved following treatment with monoclonal antibodies to IL-6 (Beck et al., 1994). Parravicini et al (1997a) detected vIL-6 expression in 6/6 cases of HHV-8-positive Castleman's disease providing evidence to support the idea that vIL-6 is likely to contribute to the pathogenesis in HHV-8-associated cases.

Several additional associations between HHV-8 and benign lymphoproliferative disease are worthy of mention. A significant minority of cases of HIV-associated lymph-adenopathy, including 3/12 cases in the original study by Chang et al (1994), are HHV-8 positive (Su et al., 1995; Luppi et al., 1996a; Gessain et al., 1996). Luppi et al (1996a) described 5 benign lymphoproliferations with florid germinal centre hyperplasia and increased vascularity and 4 of these were HHV-8 positive. An HHV-8-positive lesion with similar histology was reported by Soulier et al (1995) and was the only positive sample out of 34 reactive nodes examined.

Controversial associations

There is controversy regarding the reported association between HHV-8 and two rather different conditions - MM and sarcoidosis. Di Alberti et al (1997) detected HHV-8 sequences by nested PCR in 8/8 lung and 26/27 lymph node samples from 17 patients with sarcoidosis. Other workers have not confirmed this association (Regamey et al., 1998a; Belec et al., 1998) which is not considered further in this review. The association between HHV-8 and MM has attracted a great deal of interest but the controversy continues.

MULTIPLE MYELOMA

The cytokine IL-6 is known to be a growth factor for MM. The association between HHV-8 and both PEL and Castleman's disease, two diseases in which IL-6 is also thought to play a role in pathogenesis, coupled with the presence of a functional IL-6 homologue in the genome of HHV-8, prompted Rettig et al (1997) to look for evidence of HHV-8 infection in MM. HHV-8 DNA sequences were detected in 15/15 bone marrow stromal cell cultures from MM patients and also in 2/8 patients with monoclonal gammopathy of uncertain significance, a precursor to MM. Control samples were negative. HHV-8 was not detected by PCR in bone marrow mononuclear cell fractions from 23 patients indicating that the virus was not present in the tumour cells. vIL-6 expression was detected in 3/3 bone marrow stromal cell samples suggesting the virus may support growth of myeloma cells by a paracrine mechanism. In a follow-up study, *in situ* hybridisation and PCR were used to confirm the presence of HHV-8 in bone marrow dendritic cells in 17/20 patients with myeloma (Said et al., 1997b).

Many studies investigating the association between HHV-8 and MM quickly followed the original report, largely with negative results. Serological studies have generally found that myeloma patients, as a group, have a similar HHV-8 seroprevalence to controls from the same geographical region (MacKenzie et al., 1997; Marcelin et al., 1997; Parravicini et al., 1997b; Masood et al., 1997; Whitby et al., 1997; Cathomas et al., 1998; Santarelli et al., 1998; Bouscary et al., 1998). An exception to this is a study from Gao et al (1998) who found 81% of MM patients were HHV-8 seropositive compared to 22% of controls. The authors suggested that failure to detect a higher HHV-8 seroprevalence in MM patients in other studies may have been due to the high cut-off used in ELISA assays. However, in the study by MacKenzie et al (1997) sera from MM patients actually had slightly lower optical density readings in the ORF65 ELISA than the control group (unpublished results). Failure to detect HHV-8 antibodies in MM does not appear to relate to decreased humoral immunity since antibodies to other viruses are detectable in these patients.

Similarly, PCR studies have generally failed to find evidence of increased HHV-8 infection rates in MM patients.A diverse range of samples has been investigated including: PBMCs; dendritic cells enriched from leukapheresis samples; bone marrow mononuclear cells; bone marrow stromal cells; bone marrow stromal cell cultures; long-term bone marrow cultures; and bone marrow biopsies (Parravicini et al., 1997b; Masood et al., 1997; Tarte et al., 1998; Tarte et al., 1998; Cathomas et al., 1998; Mitterer et al., 1998; Cull et al., 1998; Bouscary et al., 1998; Yi et al., 1998). In contrast to these negative findings, Brousset et al (1997) and Agbalika et al (1998) detected HHV-8 in bone marrow biopsies from 18/20 and 5/10 MM patients respectively. In the latter study 2/3 long-term bone marrow cultures were also positive however there was no increase in seroprevalence in this group of patients.

Epidemiological studies do not favour the association between MM and HHV-8. MM and HHV-8 do not share a similar geographical variation in incidence (based on current serological assays) and there is no evidence that MM incidence is increased in KS patients (Cottoni & Uccini, 1997; Hjalgrim et al., 1998). However, the incidence rate of MM is increased 4.5-fold in patients with AIDS, consistent with the idea that a virus is involved in MM pathogenesis (Goedert et al., 1998).

Further studies are clearly needed to confirm or refute this association. Different results do not appear to be due to different patients groups or different geographical locales; most negative PCR studies have demonstrated good assay sensitivity and most serological studies have demonstrated antibodies to other common viruses in MM sera. Careful attention needs to be paid to sample collection and preparation (in order to preserve sufficient bone marrow dendritic cells) and to absence of contamination in PCR assays.

Transmission

As described above, the epidemiology of AIDS-KS implicated a sexually transmissible agent long before the discovery of HHV-8 and, in general, the risk of HHV-8 infection conforms to that of a sexually transmitted pathogen. Homosexual men are at higher risk of infection than heterosexuals and behaviours associated with increased risk of KS appear to be the same as those associated with HHV-8 infection (Jacobson et al., 1990; Jacobson et al., 1998). In a cohort of Danish homosexual men studied from 1981 to 1996, seropositivity at enrolment was associated with number of receptive anal intercourses and with sex with US men (Melbye et al., 1998). Seroconversion was highest between 1981 and 1982 and, during the study period, was associated with having visited homosexual communities in the US and with current HIV status. In a study of unmarried San Francisco men, the prevalence of HHV-8 infection was highest in homosexual men and correlated with the number of homosexual partners in the preceding 2 years (Martin et al., 1998). Exclusively homosexual men had a seroprevalence of 39.6% compared to 0% in exclusively heterosexual men. In this study there was also an association between HHV-8 and HIV infection suggesting that some specific sexual practice may be associated with the acquisition of both infections.

HHV-8 infection is not exclusively associated with homosexual or bisexual behaviour. Among HIV-infected women, HHV-8 infection is more common in those whose partners are bisexual than in those whose partners are intravenous drug abusers. In a study investigating seroprevalence in Honduras, seropositivity was found to be 4 times higher in HIV-positive commercial sex workers (36%) than in HIV-negative non-commercial sex workers suggesting that commercial sex work is a risk factor for HHV-8 infection (Sosa et al., 1998).

Although most of the data point to a sexual route of transmission, it is clear from studies of children and studies of geographical differences in prevalence that other routes of infection must exist. In the US and UK there is a very low seroprevalence in childhood (Lennette et al., 1996; Blauvelt et al., 1997a), but in Italy and in Africa much higher rates have been reported. Calabro et al (1998) reported a seroprevalence of 15% among 13 year old children from Sardinia, an area with a high incidence of classic KS, consistent with a non-sexual mode of transmission. Similarly, in a cross-sectional study of Ugandan children, Mayama et al (1998) found that HHV-8 seroprevalence increased during childhood and reached a plateau before the age of puberty. HHV-8 infection was strongly associated with hepatitis B, but not A or C, virus infection suggesting that the virus is not spread by the faecal oral route. Bourboulia et al (1998) found a strong correlation between seropositivity in mothers and their children in South Africa - 8/19 children with seropositive mothers were also seropositive. Although this suggests mother to child transmission, the age at which infection occurred could not be established and therefore the route of infection is not clear.

Laboratory studies suggest the potential for transmission of the virus in semen and saliva. Among KS patients HHV-8 has been detected in semen from 4/31 (Marchioli et al., 1996), 1/3 (Diamond et al., 1997), 3/12 (Huang et al., 1997), 3/15 (Howard et al., 1997), thus viral sequences are consistently detected in semen samples from a minority of infected individuals. HHV-8 has been detected in cervical brushings, consistent with a sexual mode of transmission, but overall the rate of detection in the genital tract is low compared with other herpesviruses (Whitby, 1999; Tasaka et al., 1997; Viviano et al., 1997).

A range of detection rates has been reported from studies analysing saliva from KS patients - 16/23 individuals with active KS (Koelle et al., 1997); 4/8 patients with KS (Blackbourn et al., 1998); 4/42 patients with AIDS-KS (Whitby, 1999). Differences between studies are probably attributable to case selection and different methods of sample preparation, and it would appear likely that viral sequences are present in saliva from a significant number of infected individuals. Vieira et al (1997) have detected infectious virus in the saliva of subjects with KS confirming that saliva is a potential vehicle for transmission of this virus. Viral sequences have also been detected in nasal secretions, throat swabs, sputum, plasma, and serum from KS patients (Whitby et al., 1995; Blackbourn et al., 1998). An investigation of stool specimens failed to find evidence of viral particles (Whitby et al., 1995) and there is currently no direct evidence to support transmission in faeces.

Blood donor studies and the low level of HHV-8 infection amongst haemophiliacs argue against a major role for parenteral transmission (Lennette et al., 1996). Blackbourn et al (1997) rescued infectious virus from stimulated CD19-positive B-cells from a blood donor sample indicating that this mode of infection is theoretically possible. Despite this, AIDS-KS is rare in people infected with HIV following blood transfusion and risk of KS is not increased in recipients of blood transfusions (Lefrere et al., 1997). Operskalski et al (1997) studied blood donor-recipient pairs; from 14 donors who were co-infected with HIV and HHV-8, 10 recipients became infected with HIV but HHV-8 seroconversion was not observed during a period of 19 months.

Another potential route of transmission is through organ transplantation. Parravicini et al (1997c) studied 18 Italian transplant patients, 11 of whom developed KS following transplantation. Serum samples collected prior to transplantation were positive in 10/11 KS patients as compared to 2/17 controls. Following this case series, the authors studied a transplant patient who received an organ from a seropositive donor, subsequently seroconverted and developed KS and Castleman's disease. This report provided evidence that HHV-8 can be transmitted by organ transplantation but suggested that KS occurring following transplantation wss usually related to pre-existing HHV-8 infection. In contrast, a more recent study from Switzerland (a low prevalence area) described an increase in seroprevalence from 6.4 to 17.7% one year after transplantation (Regamey et al., 1998b). In 5 of 6 patients who seroconverted, donor samples tested positive for HHV-8 antibodies. Thus, transmission of HHV-8 by renal transplantation is a risk factor for transplantation-associated KS, particularly in non-endemic regions.

Strain variation

Nucleotide sequence analysis of 5 loci of the HHV-8 genome reveals 4 different viral subgroups, A to D, which show 15-30% variation in the ORFK1 coding region (Zong et al., 1998). A and C subgroup viruses are found in Europe, B in Africa and D in southern Asia and Pacific Islands. The variation observed in ORFK1 is 10-20 fold greater than that observed at the other loci examined and ~85% of the nucleotide changes result in amino acid changes. Evaluation of the patterns of ORFK1 variation suggest there are 11 clades of the virus that have close associations with the ethnic and geographic background of the individuals. The patterns appear to reflect the known major migrationary events in modern human populations. Variation is also observed at the extreme right end of the genome where two unrelated sequences referred to as Prototype and Minor are found and vary essentially independently of the K1 genotypes. It is suggested, on the basis of these results, that the major HHV-8 subtypes arose in human populations in paleoloithic times. Studies of viral variation are consistent with the idea that a) transmission of the virus is generally by close contact and b) only a small number of distinct exogenous isolates have been transmitted within the AIDS epidemic.

In Vitro Cell Culture Studies

Cell lines established from PEL lesions retain viral genomes and express viral antigens and have therefore been extremely useful for serological studies and the characterisation of the viral genome. In contrast, cultures established from KS lesions do not contain HHV-8 and primary KS cultures lose the virus after a few passages in culture (Flamand et al., 1996; Ambroziak et al., 1995; Lebbe et al., 1995).

Difficulties encountered in the serial passage of the virus in culture have limited *in vitro* studies on the temporal regulation of viral gene expression and on viral gene function. Infection of a range of cell lines has been reported by several laboratories but infection is inefficient; of the cell lines tested the human kidney cell line 293 appears to be the most readily infectable. Foreman et al (1997c) reported serial passage of virus from KS skin biopsies for 20 passages in 293 cells. This observation has been questioned by others who used electronmicroscopy or RT-PCR to monitor viral infection and were unable to demonstrate serial propagation, although they could infect 293 cells (Blauvelt et al., 1997b; Renne et al., 1998; Denise Whitby, personal communication). There is currently an urgent need for a continuous cell line which can be readily infected and in which the virus can be serially passaged.

Primary endothelial cell cultures can be infected with HHV-8 (Panyutich et al., 1998; Flore et al., 1998). Flore et al (1998) infected early-passage bone marrow endothelial cells and subsequently human umbilical vein endothelial cells and maintained the cultures in the presence of VEGF. HHV-8 induced transformation as evidenced by extended survival, acquisition of telomerase activity and anchorage-independent growth. The mechanism of transformation, however, was different from that observed with other transforming viruses in that only a small proportion, ~5%, of the cultured cells were HHV-8 infected. Proliferation of the remaining cells appeared to be due to the up-regulation of KDR (kinase domain receptor/Flk-1/VEGF receptor 2) enabling these cells to respond to VEGF. In contrast to the requirements for long-term survival only HHV-8 infected cells were able to grow in soft agar. The results of this study are consistent with a transforming role for HHV-8 in the pathogenesis of KS, but suggest that paracrine effects may also be involved.

Potential viral oncogenes

The cloning and sequencing of the HHV-8 genome have facilitated the initiation of functional studies of individual HHV-8 genes, and many studies investigating the transforming potential of this virus are now under way. Attention has focused on viral homologues of cellular genes with potential transforming activity, and on HHV-8 genes which share features with EBV latent genes or the HVS STP (saimiri transforming protein). HHV-8 does not encode genes with sequence homology to the EBV latent genes, but does encode several viral genes whose cellular homologues are up-regulated by EBV infection, suggesting that these two viruses may share some common mechanisms. Similarly, HHV-8 does not encode a homologue of the HVS transforming protein STP, however the positional homologue of STP in HHV-8 (K1) can substitute for STP in the transformation of T-cells, as discussed below. By analogy with EBV, it is likely that proteins associated with transformation are expressed during latency, and therefore will be encoded by type I and perhaps, type II transcripts.

Proteins encoded by type I transcripts

ORF73 encodes a protein which is expressed in the nuclei of infected cells with a distribution similar to that of the EBV latent proteins EBNA-2 and LP. It is a hydrophilic, proline-rich protein with an extensive repetitive region and a leucine zipper motif. The latter features suggest its activity may be modulated by protein-protein interactions. Yeast two hybrid experiments reveal interaction between LNA-1 and ubiquitin conjugating enzyme 9 and histone H1 (Wiezorek et al., 1998). EBNA-2 interacts with histone

H1 further suggesting that there may be some functional similarity between LNA-1 and EBNA-2.

ORF71 (also called ORFK13) encodes a vFLIP (viral FLICE inhibitory protein), a member of a recently identified family of proteins which contain two domains with homology to cellular death effector domains (Bertin et al., 1997; Thome et al., 1997). Interaction between vFLIPs and the adapter protein FADD inhibits recruitment and activation of the FLICE protease by CD95/Fas. Cells expressing vFLIPs are therefore protected from apoptosis induced by Fas/CD95 or related death receptors. Other members of this family include the HVS lytic cycle protein ORF71, equine herpesvirus 2 ORFE8 and the MC159 protein of Molluscum contagiosum.

ORF72 encodes a viral cyclin (v-cyc) which has 31-32% sequence identity and 53-54% similarity to mammalian cyclin D2 (Li et al., 1997). During the G1 phase of the cell cycle, D-type cyclins associate with cyclin-dependent kinases (CDKs) resulting in the phosphorylation and inactivation of pRB and entry into S phase. HHV-8 v-cyc can form active kinase complexes with CDK6, the catalytic sub-unit for type D cyclins which appears to predominate in lymphoid cells (Li et al., 1997; Godden-Kent et al., 1997). HVS also encodes a cyclin homologue (Jung et al., 1994) which has been shown to phosphorylate pRB through activation of CDK6. Both viral cyclins show profound resistance to the CDK inhibitor proteins p21, p27 and p16 (Swanton et al., 1997). Ectopic expression of v-cycs prevents G1 arrest imposed by each of these inhibitors and stimulates cell cycle progression in quiescent fibroblasts (Swanton et al., 1997).

Proteins encoded by type II transcripts

The abundantly expressed transcript T0.7 contains 3 small ORFs, one of which (ORFK12) encodes a hydrophobic protein of 66 amino acids, referred to as kaposin. Constructs expressing kaposin induce morphological transformation of Rat-3 cells and, on injection into nude mice, these cells form high grade, highly vascular, undifferentiated sarcomas (Muralidhar et al., 1998). Expression of T0.7 is readily detectable in KS spindle cells using *in situ* hybridisation (Staskus et al., 1997; Sturzl et al., 1997) and expression of kaposin has been demonstrated in PEL cell lines (Muralidhar et al., 1998).

ORFK2 is the first example of an IL-6 homologue in a viral genome (Neipel et al., 1997b). The overlap between diseases associated with IL-6 dysregulation and HHV-8 suggests the likely importance of this gene in the pathogenesis of HHV-8-associated diseases. The predicted protein has 25% identity and 50% similarity to IL-6 and homology is most pronounced within a region known to be involved in binding to the IL-6 receptor. vIL-6 is a secreted cytokine which has been shown to prevent apoptosis of the IL-6-dependent murine hybridoma line B9 (Moore et al., 1996b; Neipel et al., 1997b) and the IL-6-dependent myeloma cell line INA-6 (Burger et al., 1998). Like human IL-6, vIL-6 has been shown to activate the JAK/STAT signalling pathway in HepG2 cells (Molden et al., 1997); however, human IL-6 requires to bind to both the α and β sub-units of the receptor, whereas the viral protein can induce signalling by binding to the gp130 (IL-6 receptor β) alone (Molden et al., 1997). vIL-6 is expressed by PEL cells and in MCD but is poorly expressed in KS lesions (Moore & Chang, 1995; Parravicini et al., 1997a).

HHV-8 includes 3 proteins with homology to CC chemokines and 2 of these, vMIP-I and vMIP-II, show 30-40% amino acid identity to human MIP-1α. Unlike their human homologues, both vMIP-I and vMIP-II have been shown to induce angiogenesis in chick chorioallantoic membranes suggesting that they may play a role in KS pathogenesis (Boshoff et al., 1997).

The vIRF was the first HHV-8 protein shown to have transforming activity *in vitro.* The IRF family of transcription factors are cellular DNA binding proteins that act as activators or repressors of promoters containing variations of the IRF binding sequence; IRF-1 is a transcriptional activator while IRF-2 is a negative regulator of interferon-stimulated genes. Transfection of IRF-2 can transform NIH 3T3 cells and this can be reversed by co-transfection with IRF-1 (Taniguchi et al., 1995). vIRF inhibits interferon-induced signal transduction and suppresses genes regulated by interferon (Gao et al., 1997; Zimring et al., 1998). In addition, transfection of vIRF expression constructs into NIH 3T3 cells leads to transformation, and the transformed cells cause tumours in nude mice (Gao et al., 1997; Li et al., 1998).

RT-PCR and cDNA cloning experiments suggest the presence of a gene with multiple exons situated between ORF75 and the terminal repeat, referred to as LAMP (Glenn et al., 1998). In non-induced PEL cells, the LAMP transcript is predicted to encode a membrane-spanning protein with 12 transmembrane domains followed by a hydrophilic, presumably cytoplasmic, carboxy-terminus. The presence of a YxxI/L motif in the presumed cytoplasmic tail and the 12 transmembrane domains suggest similarities to the EBV LMP-2 protein. In TPA induced cells alternative splicing produces a family of transcripts predicted to encode proteins with the same C-terminus but with fewer transmembrane domains, features more reminiscent of LMP-1.

Proteins encoded by type III transcripts

Transformation by HVS *in vitro* is associated with the protein encoded by ORF1, or STP. The K1 gene of HHV-8 occupies an equivalent position in the HHV-8 genome but has no sequence homology to STP. However K1 has been shown to transform rodent fibroblasts, and a recombinant HVS containing the K1 gene in place of STP was found to immortalise primary T-cells and induce lymphomas in common marmosets (Lee et al., 1998). The K1 protein is a 289 amino acid, transmembrane glycoprotein with a distinctive immunoreceptor tyrosine-based activation signalling motif (ITAM) in its cytoplasmic domain (Lagunoff & Ganem, 1997; Lee et al., 1998). As discussed above, K1 is the most variable gene in the HHV-8 genome and may differ by up to 30% between isolates; however most variation is present in the central region of the protein and the amino and carboxy-terminal regions are conserved.

Many viruses encode Bcl-2 homologues which are thought to prolong the life of the cell during lytic viral infection in order to allow effective viral replication (Shen & Shenk, 1995). The Bcl-2 protein family is characterised by the ability to modulate cell death; members of this family share two highly conserved domains, called Bcl-2 homology 1 and 2, which have been shown to be critical for the death-repressor activity of Bcl-2 and Bcl-x$_L$. The overall homology between ORFK16 (vBcl-2) and other Bcl-2 homologues is low, although within the range for most family members, but is concentrated within the Bcl-2 homology 1 and 2 domains. Over-expression of vBcl-2 blocks apoptosis. There is contradictory evidence, however, as to whether vBcl-2 can hetero-dimerise with human Bcl-2 (Sarid et al., 1997), or whether it escapes negative regulatory mechanisms by failing to homo- or heterodimerise with other members of the Bcl-2 family (Li et al., 1997). Although it is attractive to suggest that vBcl-2 may play some role in viral transformation, expression of this protein is only detected in PEL cells following TPA treatment (Li et al., 1997).

ORF74 encodes a G-protein coupled receptor (GCR) with significant homology to the IL-8 receptor (Cesarman et al., 1996a). GCR homologues are also found in HVS, equine herpesvirus 2, MHV-68, herpesvirus ateles and HHV-6 and, although EBV does not encode a GCR, infection by EBV results in up-regulation of the GCR EBI1 (Birkenbach et al., 1993). Transient expression studies show that the HHV-8 GCR is constitutively active although it is also able to bind chemokines of the CXC and CC families. Transfection of vGCR expression constructs into rat kidney fibroblasts results in increased proliferation, suggesting that this gene may be involved in tumour formation (Arvanitakis et al., 1997). NIH 3T3 cells are transformed by vGCR and, in addition, the transfected cells release angiogenic growth factors (Bais et al., 1998). It is therefore possible that vGCR expression contributes to KS development by both direct and indirect mechanisms. vGCR is not expressed in latently infected B-cells and further studies are required to determine its role in KS.

HHV-8: A New DNA Tumour Virus?

There is very good evidence for a causal association between HHV-8 and both KS and PEL. Viral genomes are consistently found in all, or almost all, lesions and only rarely detected in other conditions. Patients with KS usually have antibodies to HHV-8 and seropositivity precedes the development of disease. Epidemiologically, the distribution of HHV-8 antibodies reflects the geographical distribution of KS. HHV-8 sequences are frequently detectable in the peripheral blood of KS patients, and HIV-positive individuals with HHV-8 genomes in the peripheral blood are more likely to develop KS than those in whom the virus is not detectable.

In the case of PEL, the evidence that HHV-8 is involved in transformation is compelling. The lesions are clonal and viral genomes are present within all tumour cells. A group of HHV-8 genes is expressed in PEL cells including ORFK1 which is transforming *in vitro*, a cyclin homologue ORF72, a FLICE gene encoding an anti-apoptotic function and two genes, ORF73 and the gene encoding LAMP, which share features with EBV latent genes. In addition, IL-6 is known to be an important growth factor in PEL and the viral homologue, vIL-6, is expressed by tumour cells. It is therefore not difficult to envisage a role for the virus in the pathogenesis of this condition. For KS, the situation is more complex since there is ongoing debate as to whether KS is a true malignancy or a reactive process. In nodular lesions the virus is present in a latent form in the vast majority of spindle cells, and viral genes with potential transforming activity are expressed. These features are consistent with a transforming role for the virus. In early lesions it remains possible that paracrine effects are important and factors secreted by HHV-8-infected infiltrating cells and lytically-infected cells may contribute to the pathology.

Immunosuppression most probably plays a role in HHV-8-associated diseases since both PEL and KS are found at increased frequency in immunocompromised individuals. The very high incidence of KS in HIV-positive male homosexuals suggests that HHV-8 infection, coupled with immunosuppression, is sufficient for disease development, and other genetic events need not be implicated. In the absence of HIV infection, PEL and KS usually affect elderly patients, consistent with the age-related decline in immune function. It remains to be determined whether additional genetic events are required for tumourigenesis in the latter group of patients.

It is extremely difficult to determine unequivocally that a virus is playing a causal role in the development of a human cancer; however, the available evidence suggests that HHV-8 should be added to the list of human tumour viruses.

Acknowledgements

I would like to thank Bill Jarrett, David Blackbourn and Thomas Schulz for critical reading of the manuscript, and Denise Whitby for making her Ph.D. thesis available to me.

References

Agbalika, F., Mariette, X., Marolleau, J.P., Fermand, J.P., & Brouet, J.C. 1998 Detection of human herpesvirus-8 DNA in bone marrow biopsies from patients with multiple myeloma and Waldenstrom's macroglobulinemia. Blood 91:4393-4394.

Ambroziak, J.A., Blackbourn, D.J., Herndier, B.G., Glogau, R.G., Gullett, J.H., McDonald, A.R., Lennette, E.T., & Levy, J.A. 1995 Herpes-like sequences in HIV-infected and uninfected Kaposi's sarcoma patients. Science 268:582-583.

Ansari, M.Q., Dawson, D.B., Nador, R., Rutherford, C., Schneider, N.R., Latimer, M.J., Picker, L., Knowles, D.M., & McKenna, R.W. 1996 Primary body cavity-based AIDS-related lymphomas. Am J Clin Pathol 105:221-229.

Ariyoshi, K., Schim van der Loeff, M., Cook, P., Whitby, D., Corrah, T., Jaffar, S., Cham, F., Sabally, S., O'Donovan, D., Weiss, R.A., Schulz, T.F., & Whittle, H. 1998 Kaposi's sarcoma in the Gambia, West Africa is less frequent in human immunodeficiency virus type 2 than in human immunodeficiency type 1 infection despite a high prevalence of human herpesvirus 8. Journal of Human Virology 1:193-199

Armstrong, A.A., Shield, L., Gallagher, A., & Jarrett, R.F. 1998 Lack of involvement of known oncogenic DNA viruses in Epstein-Barr virus-negative Hodgkin's disease. Br J Cancer 77:1045-1047.

Arvanitakis, L., Geras-Raaka, E., Varma, A., Gershengorn, M.C., & Cesarman, E. 1997 Human herpesvirus KSHV encodes a constitutively active G-protein- coupled receptor linked to cell proliferation. Nature 385:347-350.

Arvanitakis, L., Mesri, E.A., Nador, R.G., Said, J.W., Asch, A.S., Knowles, D.M., & Cesarman, E. 1996 Establishment and characterization of a primary effusion (body cavity- based) lymphoma cell line (BC-3) harboring Kaposi's sarcoma- associated herpesvirus (KSHV/HHV-8) in the absence of Epstein-Barr virus. Blood 88:2648-2654.

Asou, H., Said, J.W., Yang, R., Munker, R., Park, D.J., Kamada, N., & Koeffler, H.P. 1998 Mechanisms of growth control of Kaposi's sarcoma-associated herpes virus-associated primary effusion lymphoma cells. Blood 91:2475-2481.

Bais, C., Santomasso, B., Coso, O., Arvanitakis, L., Raaka, E.G., Gutkind, J.S., Asch, A.S., Cesarman, E., Gershengorn, M.C., Mesri, E.A., & Gerhengorn, M.C. 1998 G-protein-coupled receptor of Kaposi's sarcoma-associated herpesvirus is a viral oncogene and angiogenesis activator. Nature 391:86-89.

Beck, J.T., Hsu, S.M., Wijdenes, J., Bataille, R., Klein, B., Vesole, D., Hayden, K., Jagannath, S., & Barlogie, B. 1994 Brief report: alleviation of systemic manifestations of Castleman's disease by monoclonal anti-interleukin-6 antibody. N Engl J Med 330:602-605.

Belec, L., Mohamed, A.S., Lechapt-Zalcman, E., Authier, F.J., Lange, F., & Gherardi, R.K. 1998 Lack of HHV-8 DNA sequences in sarcoid tissues of French patients. Chest 114:948-949.

Belec, L., Tevi-Benissan, C., Mohamed, A.S., Carbonel, N., Matta, M., & Gresenguet, G. 1998 Enhanced detection of human herpesvirus-8 and cytomegalovirus in semen of HIV-seropositive asymptomatic heterosexual men living in Central Africa. AIDS 12:674-676.

Beral, V., Peterman, T.A., Berkelman, R.L., & Jaffe, H.W. 1990 Kaposi's sarcoma among persons with AIDS: a sexually transmitted infection? Lancet 335:123-128.

Bertin, J., Armstrong, R.C., Ottilie, S., Martin, D.A., Wang, Y., Banks, S., Wang, G.H., Senkevich, T.G., Alnemri, E.S., Moss, B., Lenardo, M.J., Tomaselli, K.J., & Cohen, J.I. 1997 Death effector domain-containing herpesvirus and poxvirus proteins inhibit both Fas- and TNFR1-induced apoptosis. Proc Natl Acad Sci U S A 94:1172-1176.

Bigoni, B., Dolcetti, R., de Lellis, L., Carbone, A., Boiocchi, M., Cassai, E., & Di Luca, D. 1996 Human herpesvirus 8 is present in the lymphoid system of healthy persons and can reactivate in the course of AIDS. J Infect Dis 173:542-549.

Birkenbach, M., Josefsen, K., Yalamanchili, R., Lenoir, G., & Kieff, E. 1993 Epstein-Barr virus-induced genes: first lymphocyte-specific G protein-coupled peptide receptors. J Virol 67:2209-2220.

Blackbourn, D.J., Ambroziak, J., Lennette, E., Adams, M., Ramachandran, B., & Levy, J.A. 1997 Infectious human herpesvirus 8 in a healthy North American blood donor. Lancet 349:609-611.

Blackbourn, D.J., Lennette, E.T., Ambroziak, J., Mourich, D.V., & Levy, J.A. 1998 Human herpesvirus 8 detection in nasal secretions and saliva. J Infect Dis 177:213-216.

Blauvelt, A., Sei, S., Cook, P.M., Schulz, T.F., & Jeang, K.T. 1997a Human herpesvirus 8 infection occurs following adolescence in the United States. J Infect Dis 176:771-774.

Blauvelt, A., Herndier, B.G., & Orenstein, J.M. 1997b Propagation of a human herpesvirus from AIDS-associated Kaposi's sarcoma. N Engl J Med 336:1837-1839.

Boldogh, I., Szaniszlo, P., Bresnahan, W.A., Flaitz, C.M., Nichols, M.C., & Albrecht, T. 1996 Kaposi's sarcoma herpesvirus-like DNA sequences in the saliva of individuals infected with human immunodeficiency virus. Clin Infect Dis 23:406-407.

Boshoff, C., Whitby, D., Hatziioannou, T., Fisher, C., van der Walt, J., Hatzakis, A., Weiss, R., & Schulz, T. 1995a Kaposi's-sarcoma-associated herpesvirus in HIV-negative Kaposi's sarcoma. Lancet 345:1043-1044.

Boshoff, C., Schulz, T.F., Kennedy, M.M., Graham, A.K., Fisher, C., Thomas, A., McGee, J.O., Weiss, R.A., & O'Leary, J.J. 1995b Kaposi's sarcoma-associated herpesvirus infects endothelial and spindle cells. Nat Med 1:1274-1278.

Boshoff, C., Endo, Y., Collins, P.D., Takeuchi, Y., Reeves, J.D., Schweickart, V.L., Siani, M.A., Sasaki, T., Williams, T.J., Gray, P.W., Moore, P.S., Chang, Y., & Weiss, R.A. 1997 Angiogenic and HIV-inhibitory functions of KSHV-encoded chemokines. Science 278:290-294.

Boshoff, C., Gao, S.J., Healy, L.E., Matthews, S., Thomas, A.J., Coignet, L., Warnke, R.A., Strauchen, J.A., Matutes, E., Kamel, O.W., Moore, P.S., Weiss, R.A., & Chang, Y. 1998 Establishing a KSHV+ cell line (BCP-1) from peripheral blood and characterizing its growth in Nod/SCID mice. Blood 91:1671-1679.

Bourboulia, D., Whitby, D., Boshoff, C., Newton, R., Beral, V., Carrara, H., Lane, A., & Sitas, F. 1998 Serologic evidence for mother-to-child transmission of Kaposi sarcoma- associated herpesvirus infection. JAMA 280:31-32.

Bouscary, D., Dupin, N., Fichelson, S., Grandadam, M., Fontenay-Roupie, M., Marcelin, A.G., Blanche, P., Picard, F., Freyssinier, J.M., Ravaud, P., Dreyfus, F., & Calvez, V. 1998 Lack of evidence of an association between HHV-8 and multiple myeloma. Leukemia 12:1840-1841.

Brandt, S.J., Bodine, D.M., Dunbar, C.E., & Nienhuis, A.W. 1990 Retroviral-mediated transfer of interleukin-6 into hematopoietic cells of mice results in a syndrome resembling Castleman's disease. Curr Top Microbiol Immunol 166:37-41.

Brousset, P., Meggetto, F., Attal, M., & Delsol, G. 1997 Kaposi's sarcoma-associated herpesvirus infection and multiple myeloma. Science 278:1972-1973.

Browning, P.J., Sechler, J.M., Kaplan, M., Washington, R.H., Gendelman, R., Yarchoan, R., Ensoli, B., & Gallo, R.C. 1994 Identification and culture of Kaposi's sarcoma-like spindle cells from the peripheral blood of human immunodeficiency virus-1-infected individuals and normal controls. Blood 84:2711-2720.

Buonaguro, F.M., Tornesello, M.L., Beth-Giraldo, E., Hatzakis, A., Mueller, N., Downing, R., Biryamwaho, B., Sempala, S.D., & Giraldo, G. 1996 Herpesvirus-like DNA sequences detected in endemic, classic, iatrogenic and epidemic Kaposi's sarcoma (KS) biopsies. Int J Cancer 65:25-28.

Burger, R., Neipel, F., Fleckenstein, B., Savino, R., Ciliberto, G., Kalden, J.R., & Gramatzki, M. 1998 Human herpesvirus type 8 interleukin-6 homologue is functionally active on human myeloma cells. Blood 91:1858-1863.

Calabro, M.L., Sheldon, J., Favero, A., Simpson, G.R., Fiore, R., Gomes, E., Angarano, G., Chieco-Bianchi, L., & Schulz, T.F. 1998 Seroprevalence of Kaposi's sarcoma-associated herpesvirus/human herpesvirus 8 in several regions of Italy. Journal of Human Virology 1:207-213.

Carbone, A. and Gaidano, G. 1997 HHV-8-positive body-cavity-based lymphoma: a novel lymphoma entity. Br J Haematol 97:515-522.

Cathomas, G., McGandy, C.E., Terracciano, L.M., Itin, P.H., De Rosa, G., & Gudat, F. 1996 Detection of herpesvirus-like DNA by nested PCR on archival skin biopsy specimens of various forms of Kaposi sarcoma. J Clin Pathol 49:631-633.

Cathomas, G., Stalder, A., Kurrer, M.O., Regamey, N., Erb, P., & Joller-Jemelka, H.I. 1998 Multiple myeloma and HHV8 infection. Blood 91:4391-4393.

Cesarman, E., Moore, P.S., Rao, P.H., Inghirami, G., Knowles, D.M., & Chang, Y. 1995a In vitro establishment and characterization of two acquired immunodeficiency syndrome-related lymphoma cell lines (BC-1 and BC-2) containing Kaposi's sarcoma-associated herpesvirus-like (KSHV) DNA sequences. Blood 86:2708-2714.

Cesarman, E., Chang, Y., Moore, P.S., Said, J.W., & Knowles, D.M. 1995b Kaposi's sarcoma-associated herpesvirus-like DNA sequences in AIDS- related body-cavity-based lymphomas. N Engl J Med 332:1186-1191.

Cesarman, E., Nador, R.G., Bai, F., Bohenzky, R.A., Russo, J.J., Moore, P.S., Chang, Y., & Knowles, D.M. 1996a Kaposi's sarcoma-associated herpesvirus contains G protein-coupled receptor and cyclin D homologs which are expressed in Kaposi's sarcoma and malignant lymphoma. J Virol 70:8218-8223.

Cesarman, E., Nador, R.G., Aozasa, K., Delsol, G., Said, J.W., & Knowles, D.M. 1996b Kaposi's sarcoma-associated herpesvirus in non-AIDS-related lymphomas occurring in body cavities. Am J Pathol 149:53-57.

Chadburn, A., Cesarman, E., Nador, R.G., Liu, Y.F., & Knowles, D.M. 1997 Kaposi's sarcoma-associated herpesvirus sequences in benign lymphoid proliferations not associated with human immunodeficiency virus. Cancer 80:788-797.

Chang, Y., Cesarman, E., Pessin, M.S., Lee, F., Culpepper, J., Knowles, D.M., & Moore, P.S. 1994 Identification of herpesvirus-like DNA sequences in AIDS- associated Kaposi's sarcoma. Science 266:1865-1869.

Chatlynne, L.G., Lapps, W., Handy, M., Huang, Y.Q., Masood, R., Hamilton, A.S., Said, J.W., Koeffler, H.P., Kaplan, M.H., Friedman-Kien, A., Gill, P.S., Whitman, J.E., & Ablashi, D.V. 1998 Detection and titration of human herpesvirus-8-specific antibodies in sera from blood donors, acquired immunodeficiency syndrome patients, and Kaposi's sarcoma patients using a whole virus enzyme-linked immunosorbent assay. Blood 92:53-58.

Corbellino, M., Bestetti, G., Galli, M., & Parravicini, C. 1996 Absence of HHV-8 in prostate and semen. N Engl J Med 335:1237-1239.

Corbellino, M., Poirel, L., Aubin, J.T., Paulli, M., Magrini, U., Bestetti, G., Galli, M., & Parravicini, C. 1996 The role of human herpesvirus 8 and Epstein-Barr virus in the pathogenesis of giant lymph node hyperplasia (Castleman's disease). Clin Infect Dis 22:1120-1121.

Corboy, J.R., Garl, P.J., & Kleinschmidt-DeMasters, B.K. 1998 Human herpesvirus 8 DNA in CNS lymphomas from patients with and without AIDS. Neurology 50:335-340.

Cottoni, F. and Uccini, S. 1997 Kaposi's sarcoma-associated herpesvirus infection and multiple myeloma. Science 278:1972-1973.

Cull, G.M., Timms, J.M., Haynes, A.P., Russell, N.H., Irving, W.L., Ball, J.K., & Thomson, B.J. 1998 Dendritic cells cultured from mononuclear cells and CD34 cells in myeloma do not harbour human herpesvirus 8. Br J Haematol 100:793-796.

Davis, M.A., Sturzl, M.A., Blasig, C., Schreier, A., Guo, H.G., Reitz, M., Opalenik, S.R., & Browning, P.J. 1997 Expression of human herpesvirus 8-encoded cyclin D in Kaposi's sarcoma spindle cells. J Natl Cancer Inst 89:1868-1874.

De Milito, A., Venturi, G., Catucci, M., Romano, L., Bianchi, B.M., & Zazzi, M. 1997 Lack of evidence of HHV-8 DNA in blood cells from heart transplant recipients. Blood 89:1837b-1838.

Decker, L.L., Shankar, P., Khan, G., Freeman, R.B., Dezube, B.J., Lieberman, J., & Thorley-Lawson, D.A. 1996 The Kaposi sarcoma-associated herpesvirus (KSHV) is present as an intact latent genome in KS tissue but replicates in the peripheral blood mononuclear cells of KS patients. J Exp Med 184:283-288.

Delabesse, E., Oksenhendler, E., Lebbe, C., Verola, O., Varet, B., & Turhan, A.G. 1997 Molecular analysis of clonality in Kaposi's sarcoma. J Clin Pathol 50:664-668.

Di Alberti, L., Piattelli, A., Artese, L., Favia, G., Patel, S., Saunders, N., Porter, S.R., Scully, C.M., Ngui, S.L., & Teo, C.G. 1997 Human herpesvirus 8 variants in sarcoid tissues. Lancet 350:1655-1661.

Diamond, C., Huang, M.L., Kedes, D.H., Speck, C., Rankin, G.W.J., Ganem, D., Coombs, R.W., Rose, T.M., Krieger, J.N., & Corey, L. 1997 Absence of detectable human herpesvirus 8 in the semen of human immunodeficiency virus-infected men without Kaposi's sarcoma. J Infect Dis 176:775-777.

Dictor, M., Rambech, E., Way, D., Witte, M., & Bendsoe, N. 1996 Human herpesvirus 8 (Kaposi's sarcoma-associated herpesvirus) DNA in Kaposi's sarcoma lesions, AIDS Kaposi's sarcoma cell lines, endothelial Kaposi's sarcoma simulators, and the skin of immunosuppressed patients. Am J Pathol 148:2009-2016.

Dupin, N., Gorin, I., Escande, J.P., Calvez, V., Grandadam, M., Huraux, J.M., & Agut, H. 1997 Lack of evidence of any association between human herpesvirus 8 and various skin tumors from both immunocompetent and immunosuppressed patients. Arch Dermatol 133:537.

Dupin, N., Grandadam, M., Calvez, V., Gorin, I., Aubin, J.T., Havard, S., Lamy, F., Leibowitch, M., Huraux, J.M., & Escande, J.P. 1995 Herpesvirus-like DNA sequences in patients with Mediterranean Kaposi's sarcoma. Lancet 345:761-762.

Ensoli, B., Gendelman, R., Markham, P., Fiorelli, V., Colombini, S., Raffeld, M., Cafaro, A., Chang, H.K., Brady, J.N., & Gallo, R.C. 1994 Synergy between basic fibroblast growth factor and HIV-1 Tat protein in induction of Kaposi's sarcoma. Nature 371:674-680.

Farge, D. 1993 Kaposi's sarcoma in organ transplant recipients. The Collaborative Transplantation Research Group of Ile de France. Eur J Med 2:339-343.

Fiorelli, V., Gendelman, R., Sirianni, M.C., Chang, H.K., Colombini, S., Markham, P.D., Monini, P., Sonnabend, J., Pintus, A., Gallo, R.C., & Ensoli, B. 1998 gamma-Interferon produced by CD8+ T cells infiltrating Kaposi's sarcoma induces spindle cells with angiogenic phenotype and synergy with human immunodeficiency virus-1 Tat protein: an immune response to human herpesvirus-8 infection? Blood 91:956-967.

Flamand, L., Zeman, R.A., Bryant, J.L., Lunardi-Iskandar, Y., & Gallo, R.C. 1996 Absence of human herpesvirus 8 DNA sequences in neoplastic Kaposi's sarcoma cell lines. J Acquir Immune Defic Syndr Hum Retrovirol 13:194-197.

Flore, O., Rafii, S., Ely, S., O'Leary, J.J., Hyjek, E.M., & Cesarman, E. 1998 Transformation of primary human endothelial cells by Kaposi's sarcoma-associated herpesvirus. Nature 394:588-592.

Foreman, K., Bonish, B., & Nickoloff, B. 1997a Absence of human herpesvirus 8 DNA sequences in patients with immunosuppression-associated dermatofibromas. Arch Dermatol 133:108-109.

Foreman, K.E., Bacon, P.E., Hsi, E.D., & Nickoloff, B.J. 1997b In situ polymerase chain reaction-based localization studies support role of human herpesvirus-8 as the cause of two AIDS-related neoplasms: Kaposi's sarcoma and body cavity lymphoma. J Clin Invest 99:2971-2978.

Foreman, K.E., Friborg, J.J., Kong, W.P., Woffendin, C., Polverini, P.J., Nickoloff, B.J., & Nabel, G.J. 1997c Propagation of a human herpesvirus from AIDS-associated Kaposi's sarcoma. N Engl J Med 336:163-171.

Friedman-Kien, A.E., Laubenstein, L.J., Rubinstein, P., Buimovici-Klein, E., Marmor, M., Stahl, R., Spigland, I., Kim, K.S., & Zolla-Pazner, S. 1982 Disseminated Kaposi's sarcoma in homosexual men. Ann Intern Med 96:693-700.

Gaidano, G., Cechova, K., Chang, Y., Moore, P.S., Knowles, D.M., & Dalla-Favera, R. 1996 Establishment of AIDS-related lymphoma cell lines from lymphomatous effusions. Leukemia 10:1237-1240.

Gaidano, G., Gloghini, A., Gattei, V., Rossi, M.F., Cilia, A.M., Godeas, C., Degan, M., Perin, T., Canzonieri, V., Aldinucci, D., Saglio, G., Carbone, A., & Pinto, A. 1997a Association of Kaposi's sarcoma-associated herpesvirus-positive primary effusion lymphoma with expression of the CD138/syndecan-1 antigen. Blood 90:4894-4900.

Gaidano, G., Capello, D., Pastore, C., Antinori, A., Gloghini, A., Carbone, A., Larocca, L.M., & Saglio, G. 1997b Analysis of human herpesvirus type 8 infection in AIDS-related and AIDS- unrelated primary central nervous system lymphoma. J Infect Dis 175:1193-1197.

Gao, S.J., Kingsley, L., Hoover, D.R., Spira, T.J., Rinaldo, C.R., Saah, A., Phair, J., Detels, R., Parry, P., Chang, Y., & Moore, P.S. 1996a Seroconversion to antibodies against Kaposi's sarcoma-associated herpesvirus-related latent nuclear antigens before the development of Kaposi's sarcoma. N Engl J Med 335:233-241.

Gao, S.J., Kingsley, L., Li, M., Zheng, W., Parravicini, C., Ziegler, J., Newton, R., Rinaldo, C.R., Saah, A., Phair, J., Detels, R., Chang, Y., & Moore, P.S. 1996b KSHV antibodies among Americans, Italians and Ugandans with and without Kaposi's sarcoma. Nat Med 2:925-928.

Gao, S.J., Boshoff, C., Jayachandra, S., Weiss, R.A., Chang, Y., & Moore, P.S. 1997 KSHV ORF K9 (vIRF) is an oncogene which inhibits the interferon signaling pathway. Oncogene 15:1979-1985.

Gao, S.J., Alsina, M., Deng, J.H., Harrison, C.R., Montalvo, E.A., Leach, C.T., Roodman, G.D., & Jenson, H.B. 1998 Antibodies to Kaposi's sarcoma-associated herpesvirus (human herpesvirus 8) in patients with multiple myeloma. J Infect Dis 178:846-849.

Gessain, A., Sudaka, A., Briere, J., Fouchard, N., Nicola, M.A., Rio, B., Arborio, M., Troussard, X., Audouin, J., & Diebold, J. 1996 Kaposi sarcoma-associated herpes-like virus (human herpesvirus type 8) DNA sequences in multicentric Castleman's disease: is there any relevant association in non-human immunodeficiency virus-infected patients? Blood 87:414-416.

Gessain, A., Briere, J., Angelin-Duclos, C., Valensi, F., Beral, H.M., Davi, F., Nicola, M.A., Sudaka, A., Fouchard, N., Gabarre, J., Troussard, X., Dulmet, E., Audouin, J., Diebold, J., & de The, G. 1997 Human herpes virus 8 (Kaposi's sarcoma herpes virus) and malignant lymphoproliferations in France: a molecular study of 250 cases including two AIDS-associated body cavity based lymphomas. Leukemia 11:266-272.

Gill, P.S., Tsai, Y.C., Rao, A.P., Spruck, C.H., Zheng, T., Harrington, W.A.J., Cheung, T., Nathwani, B., & Jones, P.A. 1998 Evidence for multiclonality in multicentric Kaposi's sarcoma. Proc Natl Acad Sci U S A 95:8257-8261.

Glenn, M.A., L. Rainbow, A.J. Davison, and T.F. Schulz 1998 Identification of a spliced KSHV/HHV 8 gene predicted to encode a latency associated membrane protein (LAMP). The first annual meeting on Kaposi's sarcoma associated herpesvirus (KSHV) and related agents, University of California, Santa Cruz.

Godden-Kent, D., Talbot, S.J., Boshoff, C., Chang, Y., Moore, P., Weiss, R.A., & Mittnacht, S. 1997 The cyclin encoded by Kaposi's sarcoma-associated herpesvirus stimulates cdk6 to phosphorylate the retinoblastoma protein and histone H1. J Virol 71:4193-4198.

Goedert, J.J., Cote, T.R., Virgo, P., Scoppa, S.M., Kingma, D.W., Gail, M.H., Jaffe, E.S., & Biggar, R.J. 1998 Spectrum of AIDS-associated malignant disorders. Lancet 351:1833-1839.

Grandadam, M., Dupin, N., Calvez, V., Gorin, I., Blum, L., Kernbaum, S., Sicard, D., Buisson, Y., Agut, H., Escande, J.P., & Huraux, J.M. 1997 Exacerbations of clinical symptoms in human immunodeficiency virus type 1-infected patients with multicentric Castleman's disease are associated with a high increase in Kaposi's sarcoma herpesvirus DNA load in peripheral blood mononuclear cells. J Infect Dis 175:1198-1201.

Harrington, W.J.J., Bagasra, O., Sosa, C.E., Bobroski, L.E., Baum, M., Wen, X.L., Cabral, L., Byrne, G.E., Pomerantz, R.J., & Wood, C. 1996 Human herpesvirus type 8 DNA sequences in cell-free plasma and mononuclear cells of Kaposi's sarcoma patients. J Infect Dis 174:1101-1105.

Harris, N.L., Jaffe, E.S., Stein, H., Banks, P.M., Chan, J.K.C., Cleary, M.L., Delsol, G., de Wolf-Peeters, C., Falini, B., Gatter, K.C., Grogan, T.M., Isaacson, P.G., Knowles, D.M., Mason, D.Y., Muller-Hermelink, H.-K., Pileri, S.A., Piris, M.A., Ralfkiaer, E., & Warnke, R.A. 1994 A revised European-American classification of lymphoid neoplasms: a proposal from the International Lymphoma Study Group. Blood 84:1361-1392.

Hjalgrim, H., Frisch, M., & Melbye, M. 1998 Incidence rates of classical Kaposi's sarcoma and multiple myeloma do not correlate. Br J Cancer 78:419-420.

Howard, M., Brink, N., Miller, R., & Tedder, R. 1995 Association of human herpes virus with pulmonary Kaposi's sarcoma. Lancet 346:712.

Howard, M.R., Whitby, D., Bahadur, G., Suggett, F., Boshoff, C., Tenant-Flowers, M., Schulz, T.F., Kirk, S., Matthews, S., Weller, I.V., Tedder, R.S., & Weiss, R.A. 1997 Detection of human herpesvirus 8 DNA in semen from HIV-infected individuals but not healthy semen donors. AIDS 11:F15-F19.

Huang, Y.Q., Li, J.J., Kaplan, M.H., Poiesz, B., Katabira, E., Zhang, W.C., Feiner, D., & Friedman-Kien, A.E. 1995 Human herpesvirus-like nucleic acid in various forms of Kaposi's sarcoma. Lancet 345:759-761.

Huang, Y.Q., Li, J.J., Poiesz, B.J., Kaplan, M.H., & Friedman-Kien, A.E. 1997 Detection of the herpesvirus-like DNA sequences in matched specimens of semen and blood from patients with AIDS-related Kaposi's sarcoma by polymerase chain reaction in situ hybridization. Am J Pathol 150:147-153.

Ishiyama, T., Nakamura, S., Akimoto, Y., Koike, M., Tomoyasu, S., Tsuruoka, N., Murata, Y., Sato, T., Wakabayashi, Y., & Chiba, S. 1994 Immunodeficiency and IL-6 production by peripheral blood monocytes in multicentric Castleman's disease. Br J Haematol 86:483-489.

Jacobson, L.P., F. Jenkins, G. Springer, A. Munoz, K. Shah, and H. Armenian 1998 Behaviors associated with HHV-8 infection: Results from the multicenter AIDS cohort study (MACS). The first annual meeting on Kaposi's sarcoma associated herpesvirus (KSHV) and related agents, University of California, Santa Cruz.

Jacobson, L.P., Munoz, A., Fox, R., Phair, J.P., Dudley, J., Obrams, G.I., Kingsley, L.A., & Polk, B.F. 1990 Incidence of Kaposi's sarcoma in a cohort of homosexual men infected with the human immunodeficiency virus type 1. The Multicenter AIDS Cohort Study Group. J Acquir Immune Defic Syndr 3 Suppl 1:S24-S31.

Jin, Y.T., Tsai, S.T., Yan, J.J., Hsiao, J.H., Lee, Y.Y., & Su, I.J. 1996 Detection of Kaposi's sarcoma-associated herpesvirus-like DNA sequence in vascular lesions. A reliable diagnostic marker for Kaposi's sarcoma. Am J Clin Pathol 105:360-363.

Jones, D., Ballestas, M.E., Kaye, K.M., Gulizia, J.M., Winters, G.L., Fletcher, J., Scadden, D.T., & Aster, J.C. 1998 Primary-effusion lymphoma and Kaposi's sarcoma in a cardiac-transplant recipient. N Engl J Med 339:444-449.

Jones, R.R., Spaull, J., Spry, C., & Jones, E.W. 1986 Histogenesis of Kaposi's sarcoma in patients with and without acquired immune deficiency syndrome (AIDS). J Clin Pathol 39:742-749.

Jung, J.U., Stager, M., & Desrosiers, R.C. 1994 Virus-encoded cyclin. Mol Cell Biol 14:7235-7244.

Jussila, L., Valtola, R., Partanen, T.A., Salven, P., Heikkila, P., Matikainen, M.T., Renkonen, R., Kaipainen, A., Detmar, M., Tschachler, E., Alitalo, R., & Alitalo, K. 1998 Lymphatic endothelium and Kaposi's sarcoma spindle cells detected by antibodies against the vascular endothelial growth factor receptor-3. Cancer Res 58:1599-1604.

Kaposi, M. 1872 Idiopathisches multiples pigmentsarcom der haut. Archives Dermatol und Syphillis 4:265-273.

Karcher, D.S., Alkan, S., Dupin, N., Gorin, I., Deleuze, J., Agut, H., Huraux J, M., Escande, J.P., Moore, P.S., Chang, Y., Cesarman, E., & Knowles, D.M. 1995 Herpes-like DNA sequences, AIDS-related tumors, and Castleman's disease. N Engl J Med 333:797-799.

Karcher, D.S. and Alkan, S. 1997 Human herpesvirus-8-associated body cavity-based lymphoma in human immunodeficiency virus-infected patients: a unique B-cell neoplasm. Hum Pathol 28:801-808.

Kedes, D.H., Lagunoff, M., Renne, R., & Ganem, D. 1997 Identification of the gene encoding the major latency-associated nuclear antigen of the Kaposi's sarcoma-associated herpesvirus. J Clin Invest 100:2606-2610.

Kedes, D.H., Operskalski, E., Busch, M., Kohn, R., Flood, J., & Ganem, D. 1996 The seroepidemiology of human herpesvirus 8 (Kaposi's sarcoma- associated herpesvirus): distribution of infection in KS risk groups and evidence for sexual transmission. Nat Med 2:918-924.

Kellam, P., Boshoff, C., Whitby, D., Matthews, S., Weiss, R.A., & Talbot, S. 1997 Identification of a major latent nuclear antigen, LNA-1, in the human herpesvirus 8 genome. Journal of Human Virology 1:19-29.

Khan, G., Miyashita, E.M., Yang, B., Babcock, G.J., & Thorley-Lawson, D.A. 1996 Is EBV persistence in vivo a model for B cell homeostasis? Immunity 5:173-179.

Kikuta, H., Itakura, O., Ariga, T., & Kobayashi, K. 1997 Detection of human herpesvirus 8 DNA sequences in peripheral blood mononuclear cells of children. J Med Virol 53:81-84.

Koelle, D.M., Huang, M.L., Chandran, B., Vieira, J., Piepkorn, M., & Corey, L. 1997 Frequent detection of Kaposi's sarcoma-associated herpesvirus (human herpesvirus 8) DNA in saliva of human immunodeficiency virus-infected men: clinical and immunologic correlates. J Infect Dis 176:94-102.

Kohler, S., Kamel, O.W., Chang, P.P., & Smoller, B.R. 1997 Absence of human herpesvirus 8 and Epstein-Barr virus genome sequences in cutaneous epithelial neoplasms arising in immunosuppressed organ-transplant patients. J Cutan Pathol 24:559-563.

Komanduri, K.V., Luce, J.A., McGrath, M.S., Herndier, B.G., & Ng, V.L. 1996 The natural history and molecular heterogeneity of HIV-associated primary malignant lymphomatous effusions. J Acquir Immune Defic Syndr Hum Retrovirol 13:215-226.

Lagunoff, M. and Ganem, D. 1997 The structure and coding organization of the genomic termini of Kaposi's sarcoma-associated herpesvirus. Virology 236:147-154.

Lebbe, C., de Cremoux, P., Rybojad, M., Costa, d.C., Morel, P., & Calvo, F. 1995 Kaposi's sarcoma and new herpesvirus. Lancet 345:1180.

Lebbe, C., Pellet, C., Tatoud, R., Agbalika, F., Dosquet, P., Desgrez, J.P., Morel, P., & Calvo, F. 1997 Absence of human herpesvirus 8 sequences in prostate specimens. AIDS 11:270.

Lee, H., Veazey, R., Williams, K., Li, M., Guo, J., Neipel, F., Fleckenstein, B., Lackner, A., Desrosiers, R.C., & Jung, J.U. 1998 Deregulation of cell growth by the K1 gene of Kaposi's sarcoma- associated herpesvirus. Nat Med 4:435-440.

Lefrere, J.J., Mariotti, M., Girot, R., Loiseau, P., & Herve, P. 1997 Transfusional risk of HHV-8 infection. Lancet 350:217.

Lefrere, J.J., Meyohas, M.C., Mariotti, M., Meynard, J.L., Thauvin, M., & Frottier, J. 1996 Detection of human herpesvirus 8 DNA sequences before the appearance of Kaposi's sarcoma in human immunodeficiency virus (HIV)-positive subjects with a known date of HIV seroconversion. J Infect Dis 174:283-287.

Leger-Ravet, M.B., Peuchmaur, M., Devergne, O., Audouin, J., Raphael, M., Van Damme, J., Galanaud, P., Diebold, J., & Emilie, D. 1991 Interleukin-6 gene expression in Castleman's disease. Blood 78:2923-2930.

Lennette, E.T., Blackbourn, D.J., & Levy, J.A. 1996 Antibodies to human herpesvirus type 8 in the general population and in Kaposi's sarcoma patients. Lancet 348:858-861.

Li, J.J., Huang, Y.Q., Cockerell, C.J., & Friedman-Kien, A.E. 1996 Localization of human herpes-like virus type 8 in vascular endothelial cells and perivascular spindle-shaped cells of Kaposi's sarcoma lesions by in situ hybridization. Am J Pathol 148:1741-1748.

Li, M., Lee, H., Guo, J., Neipel, F., Fleckenstein, B., Ozato, K., & Jung, J.U. 1998 Kaposi's sarcoma-associated herpesvirus viral interferon regulatory factor. J Virol 72:5433-5440.

Lin, J.C., Lin, S.C., Mar, E.C., Pellett, P.E., Stamey, F.R., Stewart, J.A., & Spira, T.J. 1998 Retraction: Is Kaposi's sarcoma-associated herpesvirus in semen of HIV- infected homosexual men? [retraction of Lin JC, Lin SC, Mar EC, Pellett PE, Stamey FR, Stewart JA, Spira TJ. In: Lancet 1995 Dec 16;346(8990):1601-2]. Lancet 351:1365.

Lospalluti, M., Mastrolonardo, M., Loconsole, F., Conte, A., & Rantuccio, F. 1995 Classical Kaposi's sarcoma: a survey of 163 cases observed in Bari, south Italy. Dermatology 191:104-108.

Lucht, E., Brytting, M., Bjerregaard, L., Julander, I., & Linde, A. 1998 Shedding of cytomegalovirus and herpesviruses 6, 7, and 8 in saliva of human immunodeficiency virus type 1-infected patients and healthy controls. Clin Infect Dis 27:137-141.

Luppi, M., Barozzi, P., Maiorana, A., Artusi, T., Trovato, R., Marasca, R., Savarino, M., Ceccherini-Nelli, L., & Torelli, G. 1996a Human herpesvirus-8 DNA sequences in human immunodeficiency virus- negative angioimmunoblastic lymphadenopathy and benign lymphadenopathy with giant germinal center hyperplasia and increased vascularity. Blood 87:3903-3909.

Luppi, M., Barozzi, P., Marasca, R., Savarino, M., & Torelli, G. 1996b HHV-8-associated primary cerebral B-cell lymphoma in HIV-negative patient after long-term steroids. Lancet 347:980.

Luppi, M., Barozzi, P., Marasca, R., Savarino, M., & Torelli, G. 1998 Polymerase chain reaction detection of human herpesvirus 8 sequences in primary central nervous system lymphomas. J Infect Dis 177:520-521.

MacKenzie, J., Sheldon, J., Morgan, G., Cook, G., Schulz.T.F., & Jarrett, R.F. 1997 HHV-8 and multiple myeloma in the UK. Lancet 350:1144-1145.

Marcelin, A.G., Dupin, N., Bouscary, D., Bossi, P., Cacoub, P., Ravaud, P., & Calvez, V. 1997 HHV-8 and multiple myeloma in France. Lancet 350:1144.

Marchioli, C.C., Love, J.L., Abbott, L.Z., Huang, Y.Q., Remick, S.C., Surtento-Reodica, N., Hutchison, R.E., Mildvan, D., Friedman-Kien, A.E., & Poiesz, B.J. 1996 Prevalence of human herpesvirus 8 DNA sequences in several patient populations. J Clin Microbiol 34:2635-2638.

Martin, J.N., Ganem, D.E., Osmond, D.H., Page-Shafer, K.A., Macrae, D., & Kedes, D.H. 1998 Sexual transmission and the natural history of human herpesvirus 8 infection. N Engl J Med 338:948-954.

Masood, R., Zheng, T., Tupule, A., Arora, N., Chatlynne, L., Handy, M., & Whitman, J.J. 1997 Kaposi's sarcoma-associated herpesvirus infection and multiple myeloma. Science 278:1970-1971.

Mayama, S., Cuevas, L.E., Sheldon, J., Omar, O.H., Smith, D.H., Okong, P., Silvel, B., Hart, C.A., & Schulz, T.F. 1998 Prevalence and transmission of Kaposi's sarcoma-associated herpesvirus (human herpesvirus 8) in Ugandan children and adolescents. Int J Cancer 77:817-820.

Melbye, M., Cook, P.M., Hjalgrim, H., Begtrup, K., Simpson, G.R., Biggar, R.J., Ebbesen, P., & Schulz, T.F. 1998 Risk factors for Kaposi's-sarcoma-associated herpesvirus (KSHV/HHV-8) seropositivity in a cohort of homosexual men, 1981-1996. Int J Cancer 77:543-548.

Miller, G., Rigsby, M.O., Heston, L., Grogan, E., Sun, R., Metroka, C., Levy, J.A., Gao, S.J., Chang, Y., & Moore, P. 1996 Antibodies to butyrate-inducible antigens of Kaposi's sarcoma- associated herpesvirus in patients with HIV-1 infection. N Engl J Med 334:1292-1297.

Mitterer, M., Mair, W., Gatti, D., Sheldon, J., Vachula, M., Coser, P., & Schultz, T.F. 1998 Dendritic cells derived from bone marrow and CD34+ selected blood progenitor cells of myeloma patients, cultured in serum-free media, do not contain the Kaposi sarcoma herpesvirus genome. Br J Haematol 102:1338-1340.

Molden, J., Chang, Y., You, Y., Moore, P.S., & Goldsmith, M.A. 1997 A Kaposi's sarcoma-associated herpesvirus-encoded cytokine homolog (vIL- 6) activates signaling through the shared gp130 receptor subunit. J Biol Chem 272:19625-19631.

Monini, P., de Lellis, L., Fabris, M., Rigolin, F., & Cassai, E. 1996 Kaposi's sarcoma-associated herpesvirus DNA sequences in prostate tissue and human semen. N Engl J Med 334:1168-1172.

Moore, P.S. and Chang, Y. 1995 Detection of herpesvirus-like DNA sequences in Kaposi's sarcoma in patients with and without HIV infection. N Engl J Med 332:1181-1185.

Moore, P.S., Gao, S.J., Dominguez, G., Cesarman, E., Lungu, O., Knowles, D.M., Garber, R., Pellett, P.E., McGeoch, D.J., & Chang, Y. 1996a Primary characterization of a herpesvirus agent associated with Kaposi's sarcoma. J Virol 70:549-558.

Moore, P.S., Boshoff, C., Weiss, R.A., & Chang, Y. 1996b Molecular mimicry of human cytokine and cytokine response pathway genes by KSHV. Science 274:1739-1744.

Moore, P.S. and Chang, Y. 1998a The discovery of KSHV (HHV 8). Epstein Barr Virus Report 5:1-2.

Moore, P.S. 1998b Human herpesvirus 8 variants. Lancet 351:679-680.

Morgello, S., Tagliati, M., & Ewart, M.R. 1997 HHV-8 and AIDS-related CNS lymphoma. Neurology 48:1333-1335.

Muralidhar, S., Pumfery, A.M., Hassani, M., Sadaie, M.R., Azumi, N., Kishishita, M., Brady, J.N., Doniger, J., Medveczky, P., & Rosenthal, L.J. 1998 Identification of kaposin (open reading frame K12) as a human herpesvirus 8 (Kaposi's sarcoma-associated herpesvirus) transforming gene. J Virol 72:4980-4988.

Myers, B.D., Kessler, E., Levi, J., Pick, A., Rosenfeld, J.B., & Tivkah, P. 1974 Kaposi sarcoma in kidney transplant recipients. Arch Intern Med 133:307-311.

Nador, R.G., Cesarman, E., Chadburn, A., Dawson, D.B., Ansari, M.Q., Said, J., & Knowles, D.M. 1996 Primary effusion lymphoma: A distinct clinicopathologic entity associated with the Kaposi's sarcoma-associated herpes virus. Blood 88:645-656.

Nador, R.G., Cesarman, E., Knowles, D.M., & Said, J.W. 1995 Herpes-like DNA sequences in a body-cavity-based lymphoma in an HIV- negative patient. N Engl J Med 333:943.

Neipel, F., Albrecht, J.C., & Fleckenstein, B. 1997a Cell-homologous genes in the Kaposi's sarcoma-associated rhadinovirus human herpesvirus 8: determinants of its pathogenicity? J Virol 71:4187-4192.

Neipel, F., Albrecht, J.C., Ensser, A., Huang, Y.Q., Li, J.J., Friedman-Kien, A.E., Fleckenstein, B. 1997b Human herpesvirus 8 encodes a homolog of interleukin-6. J Virol 71:839-842.

Nicholas, J., Ruvolo, V., Zong, J., Ciufo, D., Guo, H.G., Reitz, M.S., & Hayward, G.S. 1997a A single 13-kilobase divergent locus in the Kaposi sarcoma-associated herpesvirus (human herpesvirus 8) genome contains nine open reading frames that are homologous to or related to cellular proteins. J Virol 71:1963-1974.

Nicholas, J., Ruvolo, V.R., Burns, W.H., Sandford, G., Wan, X., Ciufo, D., Hendrickson, S.B., Guo, H.G., Hayward, G.S., & Reitz, M.S. 1997b Kaposi's sarcoma-associated human herpesvirus-8 encodes homologues of macrophage inflammatory protein-1 and interleukin-6. Nat Med 3:287-292.

Noel, J.C., Hermans, P., Andre, J., Fayt, I., Simonart, T., Verhest, A., Haot, J., & Burny, A. 1996 Herpesvirus-like DNA sequences and Kaposi's sarcoma: relationship with epidemiology, clinical spectrum, and histologic features. Cancer 77:2132-2136.

Oettle, A.G. 1962 Geographic and racial differences in the frequency of Kaposi's sarcoma as evidence of environmental or genetic causes. In: Symposium on Kaposi's sarcoma. L.V. Ackerman and Murray, J.F., eds. Karger, Basel.

Operskalski, E.A., Busch, M.P., Mosley, J.W., & Kedes, D.H. 1997 Blood donations and viruses. Lancet 349:1327.

Orenstein, J.M., Alkan, S., Blauvelt, A., Jeang, K.T., Weinstein, M.D., Ganem, D., & Herndier, B. 1997 Visualization of human herpesvirus type 8 in Kaposi's sarcoma by light and transmission electron microscopy. AIDS 11:F35-F45.

Otsuki, T., Kumar, S., Ensoli, B., Kingma, D.W., Yano, T., Stetler-Stevenson, M., Jaffe, E.S., & Raffeld, M. 1996 Detection of HHV-8/KSHV DNA sequences in AIDS-associated extranodal lymphoid malignancies. Leukemia 10:1358-1362.

Panyutich, E.A., Said, J.W., & Miles, S.A. 1998 Infection of primary dermal microvascular endothelial cells by Kaposi's sarcoma-associated herpesvirus. AIDS 12:467-472.

Parravicini, C., Corbellino, M., Paulli, M., Magrini, U., Lazzarino, M., Moore, P.S., & Chang, Y. 1997a Expression of a virus-derived cytokine, KSHV vIL-6, in HIV-seronegative Castleman's disease. Am J Pathol 151:1517-1522.

Parravicini, C., Lauri, E., Baldini, L., Neri, A., Poli, F., Sirchia, G., Moroni, M., Galli, M., & Corbellino, M. 1997b Kaposi's sarcoma-associated herpesvirus infection and multiple myeloma. Science 278:1969-1970.

Parravicini, C., Olsen, S.J., Capra, M., Poli, F., Sirchia, G., Gao, S.J., Berti, E., Nocera, A., Rossi, E., Bestetti, G., Pizzuto, M., Galli, M., Moroni, M., Moore, P.S., & Corbellino, M. 1997c Risk of Kaposi's sarcoma-associated herpes virus transmission from donor allografts among Italian posttransplant Kaposi's sarcoma patients. Blood 90:2826-2829.

Pastore, C., Gloghini, A., Volpe, G., Nomdedeu, J., Leonardo, E., Mazza, U., Saglio, G., Carbone, A., & Gaidano, G. 1995 Distribution of Kaposi's sarcoma herpesvirus sequences among lymphoid malignancies in Italy and Spain. Br J Haematol 91:918-920.

Pawson, R., Catovsky, D., & Schulz, T.F. 1996 Lack of evidence of HHV-8 in mature T-cell lymphoproliferative disorders. Lancet 348:1450-1451.

Peterman, T.A., Jaffe, H.W., & Beral, V. 1993 Epidemiologic clues to the etiology of Kaposi's sarcoma. AIDS 7:605-611.

Peterson, B.A. and Frizzera, G. 1993 Multicentric Castleman's disease. Semin Oncol 20:636-647.

Raab, M.S., Albrecht, J.C., Birkmann, A., Yaguboglu, S., Lang, D., Fleckenstein, B., & Neipel, F. 1998 The immunogenic glycoprotein gp35-37 of human herpesvirus 8 is encoded by open reading frame K8.1. J Virol 72:6725-6731.

Rabkin, C.S., Janz, S., Lash, A., Coleman, A.E., Musaba, E., Liotta, L., Biggar, R.J., & Zhuang, Z. 1997 Monoclonal origin of multicentric Kaposi's sarcoma lesions. N Engl J Med 336:988-993.

Rabkin, C.S., Schulz, T.F., Whitby, D., Lennette, E.T., Magpantay, L.I., Chatlynne, L., & Biggar, R.J. 1998 Interassay correlation of human herpesvirus 8 serologic tests. HHV-8 Interlaboratory Collaborative Group. J Infect Dis 178:304-309.

Rady, P.L., Yen, A., Rollefson, J.L., Orengo, I., Bruce, S., Hughes, T.K., & Tyring, S.K. 1995 Herpesvirus-like DNA sequences in non-Kaposi's sarcoma skin lesions of transplant patients. Lancet 345:1339-1340.

Rainbow, L., Platt, G.M., Simpson, G.R., Sarid, R., Gao, S.J., Stoiber, H., Herrington, C.S., Moore, P.S., & Schulz, T.F. 1997 The 222- to 234-kilodalton latent nuclear protein (LNA) of Kaposi's sarcoma-associated herpesvirus (human herpesvirus 8) is encoded by orf73 and is a component of the latency-associated nuclear antigen. J Virol 71:5915-5921.

Reed, J.A., Nador, R.G., Spaulding, D., Tani, Y., Cesarman, E., & Knowles, D.M. 1998 Demonstration of Kaposi's sarcoma-associated herpes virus cyclin D homolog in cutaneous Kaposi's sarcoma by colorimetric in situ hybridization using a catalyzed signal amplification system. Blood 91:3825-3832.

Regamey, N., Erb, P., Tamm, M., & Cathomas, G. 1998a Human herpesvirus 8 variants. Lancet 351:680.

Regamey, N., Tamm, M., Wernli, M., Witschi, A., Thiel, G., Cathomas, G., Erb, P. 1998b Transmission of human herpesvirus 8 infection from renal-transplant donors to recipients. N Engl J Med 339:1358-1363.

Renne, R., Zhong, W., Herndier, B., McGrath, M., Abbey, N., Kedes, D., & Ganem, D. 1996a Lytic growth of Kaposi's sarcoma-associated herpesvirus (human herpesvirus 8) in culture. Nat Med 2:342-346.

Renne, R., Lagunoff, M., Zhong, W., & Ganem, D. 1996b The size and conformation of Kaposi's sarcoma-associated herpesvirus (human herpesvirus 8) DNA in infected cells and virions. J Virol 70:8151-8154.

Renne, R., Blackbourn, D., Whitby, D., Levy, J., & Ganem, D. 1998 Limited transmission of Kaposi's sarcoma-associated herpesvirus in cultured cells. J Virol 72:5182-5188.

Renwick, N., Halaby, T., Weverling, G.J., Dukers, N.H., Simpson, G.R., Coutinho, R.A., Lange, J.M., Schulz, T.F., & Goudsmit, J. 1998 Seroconversion for human herpesvirus 8 during HIV infection is highly predictive of Kaposi's sarcoma. AIDS 12:2481-2488.

Rettig, M.B., Ma, H.J., Vescio, R.A., Pold, M., Schiller, G., Belson, D., Savage, A., Nishikubo, C., Wu, C., Fraser, J., Said, J.W., & Berenson, J.R. 1997 Kaposi's sarcoma-associated herpesvirus infection of bone marrow dendritic cells from multiple myeloma patients. Science 276:1851-1854.

Roizman, B. 1996 Herpesviridae. In: Fields Virology. B.N. Fields, D.M. Knipe and P.M. Howley, eds. Lippincott-Raven, Philadelphia, pp. 2221-2230.

Russo, J.J., Bohenzky, R.A., Chien, M.C., Chen, J., Yan, M., Maddalena, D., Parry, J.P., Peruzzi, D., Edelman, I.S., Chang, Y., & Moore, P.S. 1996 Nucleotide sequence of the Kaposi sarcoma-associated herpesvirus (HHV8). Proc Natl Acad Sci U S A 93:14862-14867.

Rutgers, J.L., Wieczorek, R., Bonetti, F., Kaplan, K.L., Posnett, D.N., Friedman-Kien, A.E., & Knowles, D.M. 1986 The expression of endothelial cell surface antigens by AIDS-associated Kaposi's sarcoma. Evidence for a vascular endothelial cell origin. Am J Pathol 122:493-499.

Said, W., Chien, K., Takeuchi, S., Tasaka, T., Asou, H., Cho, S.K., de Vos, S., Cesarman, E., Knowles, D.M., & Koeffler, H.P. 1996a Kaposi's sarcoma-associated herpesvirus (KSHV or HHV8) in primary effusion lymphoma: ultrastructural demonstration of herpesvirus in lymphoma cells. Blood 87:4937-4943.

Said, J.W., Tasaka, T., Takeuchi, S., Asou, H., de Vos, S., Cesarman, E., Knowles, D.M., & Koeffler, H.P. 1996b Primary effusion lymphoma in women: report of two cases of Kaposi's sarcoma herpes virus-associated effusion-based lymphoma in human immunodeficiency virus-negative women. Blood 88:3124-3128.

Said, J.W., Chien, K., Tasaka, T., & Koeffler, H.P. 1997a Ultrastructural characterization of human herpesvirus 8 (Kaposi's sarcoma-associated herpesvirus) in Kaposi's sarcoma lesions: electron microscopy permits distinction from cytomegalovirus (CMV). J Pathol 182:273-281.

Said, J.W., Rettig, M.R., Heppner, K., Vescio, R.A., Schiller, G., Ma, H.J., Belson, D., Savage, A., Shintaku, I.P., Koeffler, H.P., Asou, H., Pinkus, G., Pinkus, J., Schrage, M., Green, E., & Berenson, J.R. 1997b Localization of Kaposi's sarcoma-associated herpesvirus in bone marrow biopsy samples from patients with multiple myeloma. Blood 90:4278-4282.

Santarelli, R., Angeloni, A., Farina, A., Gonnella, R., Gentile, G., Martino, P., Petrucci, M.T., Mandelli, F., Frati, L., & Faggioni, A. 1998 Lack of serologic association between human herpesvirus-8 infection and multiple myeloma and monoclonal gammopathies of undetermined significance. J Natl Cancer Inst 90:781-782.

Sarid, R., Sato, T., Bohenzky, R.A., Russo, J.J., & Chang, Y. 1997 Kaposi's sarcoma-associated herpesvirus encodes a functional bcl-2 homologue. Nat Med 3:293-298.

Sarid, R., Flore, O., Bohenzky, R.A., Chang, Y., & Moore, P.S. 1998 Transcription mapping of the Kaposi's sarcoma-associated herpesvirus (human herpesvirus 8) genome in a body cavity-based lymphoma cell line (BC-1). J Virol 72:1005-1012.

Schalling, M., Ekman, M., Kaaya, E.E., Linde, A., & Biberfeld, P. 1995 A role for a new herpes virus (KSHV) in different forms of Kaposi's sarcoma. Nat Med 1:707-708.

Shen, Y. and Shenk, T.E. 1995 Viruses and apoptosis. Curr Opin Genet Dev 5:105-111.

Simpson, G.R., Schulz, T.F., Whitby, D., Cook, P.M., Boshoff, C., Rainbow, L., Howard, M.R., Gao, S.J., Bohenzky, R.A., Simmonds, P., Lee, C., de Ruiter, A., Hatzakis, A., Tedder, R.S., Weller, I.V., Weiss, R.A., & Moore, P.S. 1996 Prevalence of Kaposi's sarcoma associated herpesvirus infection measured by antibodies to recombinant capsid protein and latent immunofluorescence antigen. Lancet 348:1133-1138.

Sirianni, M.C., Vincenzi, L., Topino, S., Scala, E., Angeloni, A., Gonnella, R., Uccini, S., & Faggioni, A. 1997 Human herpesvirus 8 DNA sequences in CD8+ T cells. J Infect Dis 176:541.

Smir, B.N., Greiner, T.C., & Weisenburger, D.D. 1996 Multicentric angiofollicular lymph node hyperplasia in children: a clinicopathologic study of eight patients. Mod Pathol 9:1135-1142.

Sosa, C., Klaskala, W., Chandran, B., Soto, R., Sieczkowski, L., Wu, M.H., Baum, M., & Wood, C. 1998 Human herpesvirus 8 as a potential sexually transmitted agent in Honduras. J Infect Dis 178:547-551.

Soulier, J., Grollet, L., Oksenhendler, E., Cacoub, P., Cazals-Hatem, D., Babinet, P., d'Agay, M.F., Clauvel, J.P., Raphael, M., & Degos, L. 1995 Kaposi's sarcoma-associated herpesvirus-like DNA sequences in multicentric Castleman's disease. Blood 86:1276-1280.

Staskus, K.A., Zhong, W., Gebhard, K., Herndier, B., Wang, H., Renne, R., Beneke, J., Pudney, J., Anderson, D.J., Ganem, D., & Haase, A.T. 1997 Kaposi's sarcoma-associated herpesvirus gene expression in endothelial (spindle) tumor cells. J Virol 71:715-719.

Strauchen, J.A., Hauser, A.D., Burstein, D., Jimenez, R., Moore, P.S., & Chang, Y. 1996 Body cavity-based malignant lymphoma containing Kaposi sarcoma- associated herpesvirus in an HIV-negative man with previous Kaposi sarcoma. Ann Intern Med 125:822-825.

Sturzl, M., Blasig, C., Schreier, A., Neipel, F., Hohenadl, C., Cornali, E., Ascherl, G., Esser, S., Brockmeyer, N.H., Ekman, M., Kaaya, E.E., Tschachler, E., & Biberfeld, P. 1997 Expression of HHV-8 latency-associated T0.7 RNA in spindle cells and endothelial cells of AIDS-associated, classical and African Kaposi's sarcoma. Int J Cancer 72:68-71.

Su, I.J., Hsu, Y.S., Chang, Y.C., & Wang, I.W. 1995 Herpesvirus-like DNA sequence in Kaposi's sarcoma from AIDS and non- AIDS patients in Taiwan. Lancet 345:722-723.

Swanton, C., Mann, D.J., Fleckenstein, B., Neipel, F., Peters, G., & Jones, N. 1997 Herpes viral cyclin/Cdk6 complexes evade inhibition by CDK inhibitor proteins. Nature 390:184-187.

Taniguchi, T., Harada, H., & Lamphier, M. 1995 Regulation of the interferon system and cell growth by the IRF transcription factors. J Cancer Res Clin Oncol 121:516-520.

Tarte, K., Olsen, S.J., Rossi, J.F., Legouffe, E., Lu, Z.Y., Jourdan, M., Chang, Y., & Klein, B. 1998 Kaposi's sarcoma-associated herpesvirus is not detected with immunosuppression in multiple myeloma. Blood 92:2186-2188.

Tarte, K., Olsen, S.J., Yang, L.Z., Legouffe, E., Rossi, J.F., Chang, Y., & Klein, B. 1998 Clinical-grade functional dendritic cells from patients with multiple myeloma are not infected with Kaposi's sarcoma-associated herpesvirus. Blood 91:1852-1857.

Tasaka, T., Said, J.W., & Koeffler, H.P. 1996 Absence of HHV-8 in prostate and semen. N Engl J Med 335:1237-1238.

Tasaka, T., Said, J.W., Morosetti, R., Park, D., Verbeek, W., Nagai, M., Takahara, J., & Koeffler, H.P. 1997 Is Kaposi's sarcoma—associated herpesvirus ubiquitous in urogenital and prostate tissues? Blood 89:1686-1689.

Thome, M., Schneider, P., Hofmann, K., Fickenscher, H., Meinl, E., Neipel, F., Mattmann, C., Burns, K., Bodmer, J.L., Schroter, M., Scaffidi, C., Krammer, P.H., Peter, M.E., & Tschopp, J. 1997 Viral FLICE-inhibitory proteins (FLIPs) prevent apoptosis induced by death receptors. Nature 386:517-521.

Uccini, S., Ruco, L.P., Monardo, F., Stoppacciaro, A., Dejana, E., La, P., I, Cerimele, D., & Baroni, C.D. 1994 Co-expression of endothelial cell and macrophage antigens in Kaposi's sarcoma cells. J Pathol 173:23-31.

Vieira, J., Huang, M.L., Koelle, D.M., & Corey, L. 1997 Transmissible Kaposi's sarcoma-associated herpesvirus (human herpesvirus 8) in saliva of men with a history of Kaposi's sarcoma. J Virol 71:7083-7087.

Viviano, E., Vitale, F., Ajello, F., Perna, A.M., Villafrate, M.R., Bonura, F., Arico, M., Mazzola, G., & Romano, N. 1997 Human herpesvirus type 8 DNA sequences in biological samples of HIV- positive and negative individuals in Sicily. AIDS 11:607-612.

Whitby, D., Howard, M.R., Tenant-Flowers, M., Brink, N.S., Copas, A., Boshoff, C., Hatzioannou, T., Suggett, F.E., Aldam, D.M., & Denton, A.S. 1995 Detection of Kaposi sarcoma associated herpesvirus in peripheral blood of HIV-infected individuals and progression to Kaposi's sarcoma. Lancet 346:799-802.

Whitby, D., Boshoff, C., Luppi, M., & Torelli, G. 1997 Kaposi's sarcoma-associated herpesvirus infection and multiple myeloma. Science 278:1971-1972.

Whitby, D., Luppi, M., Barozzi, P., Boshoff, C., Weiss, R.A., & Torelli, G. 1998 Human herpesvirus 8 seroprevalence in blood donors and lymphoma patients from different regions of Italy. J Natl Cancer Inst 90:395-397.

Whitby, D. Humaherpesvirus 8 (HHV-8) and Kaposi's sarcoma. 1999. University of London Ph.D. thesis.

Wiezorek, J.S., R. Sarid, S. Bhattacharyya, K. Low, Y. Chang, and P.S. Moore 1998 KSHV encoded latency associated nuclear antigen binds to ubiquitin conjugating enzyme 9 and histone H1. The first annual meeting on Kaposi's sarcoma associated herpesvirus (KSHV) and related agents, University of California, Santa Cruz.

Yi, Q., Ekman, M., Anton, D., Bergenbrant, S., Osterborg, A., Georgii-Hemming, P., Holm, G., Nilsson, K., & Biberfeld, P. 1998 Blood dendritic cells from myeloma patients are not infected with Kaposi's sarcoma-associated herpesvirus (KSHV/HHV-8). Blood 92:402-404.

Yoshizaki, K., Matsuda, T., Nishimoto, N., Kuritani, T., Taeho, L., Aozasa, K., Nakahata, T., Kawai, H., Tagoh, H., & Komori, T. 1989 Pathogenic significance of interleukin-6 (IL-6/BSF-2) in Castleman's disease. Blood 74:1360-1367.

Zhong, W., Wang, H., Herndier, B., & Ganem, D. 1996 Restricted expression of Kaposi sarcoma-associated herpesvirus (human herpesvirus 8) genes in Kaposi sarcoma. Proc Natl Acad Sci U S A 93:6641-6646.

Zimring, J.C., Goodbourn, S., & Offermann, M.K. 1998 Human herpesvirus 8 encodes an interferon regulatory factor (IRF) homolog that represses IRF-1-mediated transcription. J Virol 72:701-707.

Zong, J.C., D.M. Cuifo, I.J. Su, K. Forman, S. Alkan, B. Nickoloff, C. Rabkin, M. Melbye, M. Croxson, J. Orenstein, J. Schaeffer-Cannon, R. Ambinder, P. Rady, P. Browning, and G.S. Hayward 1998 Complex patterns of sequence variability at multiple loci across the KSHV/HHV8 genome reveal both global cladal features and evidence for subtype recombination in some lineages. The first annual meeting on Kaposi's sarcoma associated herpesvirus (KSHV) and related agents, University of California, Santa Cruz.

HUMAN HERPESVIRUS-8:

DYSREGULATION OF CELL GROWTH AND APOPTOSIS

Frank Neipel and Edgar Meinl

Institut für Klinische und Molekulare Virologie,
Friedrich-Alexander-Universität Erlangen-Nürnberg, Germany

Introduction: Diseases Associated with Human Herpesvirus -8

A. *Kaposi's sarcoma*

Kaposi's sarcoma (KS) was first described by Moritz Kaposi as "multiple idiopathic pigmented sarcoma of the skin" in 1872. It is a multifocal, proliferative lesion of spindle-shaped cells with slit-like vascular spaces in skin and mucous membranes of the oral cavity, gastrointestinal tract, and pleura. The tumor cells, termed KS spindle cells, are thought to be of endothelial origin. These tumor cells are certainly not monoclonal in the early stages of KS (Delabesse et al., 1997; Diaz-Cano et al., 1997). However, nodular KS may eventually progress to true sarcoma as indicated by monoclonality of the lesions (Rabkin et al., 1997; Gill et al., 1998). The "classic" form of Kaposi's sarcoma is a rare and slowly progressing tumor of elderly males, generally of Mediterranean or Jewish descent. Usually, the skin lesions of classic KS arise multifocally on the lower limbs and develop from patches to plaques and then nodules over several years. More aggressive, disseminated forms of KS have been described in Africa in the 1950s, and later in immunosuppressed organ transplant recipients. The etiology of this peculiar semi-malignant neoplasia has always been an enigma, the favored hypothesis being a model where proliferation and transformation of endothelial cells are triggered in a paraendocrine manner by a host of proinflammatory cytokines and growth factors (Nakamura et al., 1988; Ensoli et al., 1989). Although this model is consistent with some of the clinical features of this uncommon malignancy, it does not answer the question of what initiates the abnormal release of cytokines. An early hypothesis linked Kaposi's sarcoma to infectious agents. The epidemiology of Kaposi's sarcoma (KS) amongst patients with AIDS clearly indicated that an infectious agent other than the human immunodeficiency virus must be involved in its pathogenesis. Kaposi's sarcoma has been found to be at least 20,000 times more common in AIDS patients than expected (Beral et al., 1990). Most notably, whereas up to 21% of homosexual AIDS patients suffered from KS during the first decade of the AIDS epidemic, the tumor was observed in only 1% of age and sex matched AIDS patients with hemophilia. Representational difference analysis (RDA), a PCR based technique targeted at the identification of relatively small differences in complex genomes, was developed in 1993 (Lisitsyn et al., 1993). Application of this technique to biopsy specimens from AIDS-associated KS resulted in the discovery of a novel human herpesvirus, now termed human herpesvirus 8 (HHV-8) or Kaposi's sarcoma-associated herpesvirus (KSHV). Numerous studies revealed soon that HHV-8 DNA is invariably found in all types of Kaposi's sarcoma (Albini et al., 1996; Corbellino et al., 1996) where the majority of KS spindle cells is positive for HHV-8 DNA and transcripts (Boshoff et al., 1995; Davis et al., 1997; Stürzl et al., 1997). Searches in normal and diseased tissues other than KS showed that, at least in Northern Europe and the United States, HHV-8 DNA is infrequently detected in Caucasians not belonging to one of the groups at increased risk of KS.

B. *Lymphoproliferative diseases*

It is well established that HHV-8 is consistently found in a rare B cell lymphoma, called primary effusion lymphoma (PEL) or Body cavity based B cell lymphoma (BCBL) and also in lymphoproliferative syndromes such as Castleman's disease and possibly angio-immunoblastic lymphadenopathy (Cesarman et al., 1995; Nador et al., 1996; Cesarman et al., 1996; Luppi et al., 1996; Soulier et al., 1995). A number of permanent B cell lines could be established from PEL. These PEL-derived cell lines invariably harbor the HHV-8 genome at approximately 20 - 50 copies per cell. Some PEL-derived cell lines also contain EBV. HHV-8 is in a latent state in the vast majority of PEL cells. However, stimulation of the tumor cell line BCBL-1 by phorbolester induces the lytic replication of HHV-8 and the production of infectious virus (Renne et al., 1996; Lagunoff et al., 1997). An association with a third B-lymphoproliferative disorder, multiple Myeloma (MM), was first noted by R. Rettig and colleagues (Rettig et al., 1997), although numerous groups have not been able to confirm this association (Cathomas et al., 1998; Cottoni et al., 1997; Parravicini et al., 1997; Masood et al., 1997; MacKenzie et al., 1997; Marcelin et al., 1997; Cull et al., 1998; Yi et al., 1998). In particular, serological methods have not been able to confirm a link between MM and HHV-8. However, it is too early to judge whether HHV-8 may be involved in MM pathogenesis as there have been a few exceptions confirming the initial work by R. Renne and colleagues (Agbalika et al., 1998; Brousset et al., 1997; Chauhan et al., 1999; Gao et al., 1998).

Modulators of Cytokines and Cytokine Reaction

A. *Structure of the HHV-8 genome*

HHV-8 is the first human member of the genus *rhadinoviridae* or γ_2-herpesviruses. It has the characteristic genome structure of rhadinoviruses: a central low-GC (53.3% G+C) coding fragment is flanked by numerous tandem repeats high in GC-content (84.5% GC, H-DNA). The central L-DNA comprises approximately 140kbp (Russo et al., 1996b; Neipel et al., 1997b) and contains at least 80 open reading frames, most of which have homologs in other herpesviruses, most notably the closely related tumor virus *Herpesvirus saimiri* (*H. saimiri*). Like other rhadinoviruses, HHV-8 has numerous open reading frames with striking homology to known cellular genes. All known rhadinoviruses have non-spliced genes that seem to be captured from the host cell during viral evolution. Typically, they code for proteins which interfere with the immune system, for enzymes of the nucleotide metabolism, and for putative regulators of cell growth (Tables 1 and 2). Although the cell-homologous rhadinoviral genes are usually located at equivalent genomic regions between conserved gene blocks, some viruses have a distinct pattern. Several of the HHV-8 cell homologies are not shared by other rhadinoviruses; examples are the viral genes for an interleukin-6 (vIL-6), three CC-chemokines, at least one interferon response factor, and the N-CAM family transmembrane protein ox-2. Two reading frames of HHV-8, for which equivalents are found in *H. saimiri,* are related to cellular genes cyclin-D2 and *bcl-2.*

B. *Cytokine, chemokine, and chemokine-receptor genes encoded by HHV-8*

The amino acid sequence of the HHV-8 interleukin-6 homolog (vIL-6) is 24.7 % identical to human interleukin-6 (hIL-6) (Neipel et al., 1997a). This is intriguing, as hIL-6 has been suspected for some time to be involved in KS pathogenesis. The highest conservation is in the IL-6 domain known to be involved in receptor binding. Several groups were able to show that the cytokine encoded by vIL-6 is functional and supports the growth of both murine (Moore et al., 1996; Nicholas et al., 1997; Molden et al., 1997) and human (Burger et al., 1998a) IL-6 dependent cells. The interleukin-6 receptor consists of two chains. The β-chain, also termed gp130, is shared by several receptors such as interleukin-6, interleukin-11, ciliary neurotrophic factor, cardiotrophin-1, oncostatin M, and leukemia inhibitory factor (LIF). It is this almost ubiquitously expressed β-chain which is responsible for signal transduction. The affinity of hIL-6 to the β-chain alone is not sufficient for binding. hIL-6 needs to bind to IL6Rα first. This complex then associates with a homodimer of two gp130 molecules before signal transduction occurs. Stimulation of human cells expressing both chains of the interleukin-6 receptor by vIL-6 can be reduced by antibodies against IL6Rα, the IL-6 specific chain of the IL6-receptor (Burger et al., 1998a). This indicates that vIL-6 is able to bind IL6Rα, albeit with reduced affinity. However, there is compelling evidence that IL6Rα is not required for binding of vIL-6 to the signal transducer gp130 ((Molden et al., 1997 and R. Burger et al., unpublished). This may be particularly important as data on the expression of the IL6Rα chain in KS spindle cells both in situ and in cell culture are controversial. Similarly, cultured KS cells did not invariably respond to human IL-6. The ability of viral IL-6, however, to bind to the signal transducing gp130 component of the IL-6 receptor would make the gp80 chain dispensable and could greatly increase the spectrum of cells susceptible to growth stimulation by vIL-6 (Table 1).

Three genes with homology to the family of macrophage inflammatory protein (MIP) have been identified in a non-conserved region of the HHV-8 genome (Neipel et al., 1997b). Two of them, also termed vMIP-I and vMIP-II, are most closely related to human macrophage inflammatory protein-α (table 1). A third HHV-8 reading frame is related to the CC-chemokine family, but sequence data did not allow an assignment discriminating between MIP-1β and the macrophage chemoattractant factor MCP; it may also be derived from another member of the CC-chemokine family. At present, functional data are available for vMIP-I and the closely related vMIP-II. Both have been shown to encode functional cytokines (Boshoff et al., 1997). They attract and activate eosinophils via CCR3. In contrast

Table 1: HHV-8 encoded cytokines and modulators of cytokine reaction

ORF	gene product	experimental evidence	putative function in infection and viral persistence	possible function in HHV-8 associated malignancy (KS, BCBL, MCD)
K2	vIL-6	proliferation of human B-cells (Burger et al., 1998b), binding to IL6Rα not required (Molden et al., 1997)	controlled para/autocrine amplification of host cells	para/autocrine growth stimulation of KS spindle cells, B-cells
K4	vMIP-II (vMIP-1α)	chemoattraction via CCR3, angiogenic in chorioallantoic assay (Boshoff et al., 1997)	chemotaxis of hematopoietic cells	chemoattraction of persistently infected cells, induction of angiogenesis
K4.1	vMIP-III	*none*	chemotaxis of hematopoietic cells	
K6	vMIP-I	angiogenic in chick embryo (Boshoff et al., 1997)	chemotaxis of hematopoietic cells	chemoattraction of persistently infected cells, induction of angiogenesis
K9	vIRF	inhibits signal trans duction by interferon-α, -β, -γ (Li et al., 1998; Gao et al., 1997; Zimring et al., 1998)	counteract interferon-mediated virus suppression	interfering with the antiproliferative action of IRF
ORF74	vIL8R	constitutively active, induces VEGF secretion (Arvanitakis et al., 1997; Bais et al., 1998)	amplification of the natural habitat	angiogenesis

to its cellular homologue, the macrophage inflammatory protein 1α, vMIP-II does also bind to the CXC-type chemokine receptor CXCR4. Thus, as with vIL-6, the HHV-8 encoded chemokine codes for a functional protein with an increased spectrum of target cells. In addition, both vMIP-I and vMIP-II have also gained a function which may be of particular importance for the pathogenesis of the highly vascularized Kaposi's sarcoma: in contrast to cellular chemokines they were able to efficiently induce angiogenesis in the chorioallantoic assay (Table 1).

Angiogenesis is also one of the prominent, albeit indirect, effects of the interleukin-8 receptor homologue (vIL8R) encoded by HHV-8 (Table 1). The interleukin-8 receptor

Table 2: Putatively transforming genes of HHV-8

ORF	gene product	experimental evidence	putative function in infection and viral persistence	possible function in KS, BCBL, MCD
K1	transmembrane glycoprotein	transformation of Rat1 cells, lymphoma induction (Lee et al., 1998)	?	positional and (possibly) functional analog to other rhadinoviral oncoproteins
K9	vIRF	transformation of 3T3 cells (Zimring et al., 1998; Li et al., 1998; Gao et al., 1997)	counteracting IFN-mediated virus suppression	interfering with the antiproliferative action of IFN
K12	kaposin ?	transformation of Rat-2 cells (Muralidhar et al., 1998)	?	cell growth transformation
ORF72	k-Cyclin	activates cdk6, not inhibited by CDK-inhibitors, destabilization of p27 (Swanton et al., 1997; Mann et al., 1999; Ellis et al., 1999)	revokes cell cycle arrest in and thus guarantees efficient virus replication	dysregulated cell cycle progression
ORF74	vIL-8R	rodent fibroblast transformation, angiogenesis (Bais et al., 1998)	amplification of the natural habitat	cell growth transformation, angiogenesis
K15	integral membrane protein reminiscent of EBV LMP-2	none		

belongs to the family of 7-transmembrane G-protein coupled receptor (GPR) genes frequently found in herpesviral genomes. In contrast to other viral and cellular GPR proteins, however, the protein encoded by vIL8R exhibited constitutive activity (Arvanitakis et al., 1997). Thus, even without binding of a suitable chemokine, vIL8R induced signal transduction via the JNK/SAPK and p38-MAPK protein kinase pathways which are characteristic of inflammatory cytokines (Bais et al., 1998). Most interestingly, this was associated with an increased secretion of vascular endothelial growth factor (VEGF). NIH3T3 cells transfected with an vIL8R expression construct were able to induce angiogenic responses both in cell culture and in nude mice.

This effect could be blocked by antibodies against VEGF. Receptors for VEGF are not only expressed on vascular endothelium, but also on KS-spindle cells (Jussila et al., 1998).

VEGF has always been regarded as one of the key players in paraendocrine models of KS-pathogenesis (reviewed in (Ensoli et al., 1998).

In summary, the HHV-8 genome contains an unusually large number of genes with homology to cytokines, chemokines, and cytokine-receptors involved in inflammatory reactions. Whenever examined, these genes were found to encode not only functional proteins, but proteins with additional functions acting on a broadened spectrum of target cells (Table 1). It likely that these viral gene products are of relevance for the pathogenesis of KS, an unusual malignancy which more often resembles a hyperplastic, inflammatory reaction than true sarcoma.

Putative Transforming Genes

Genes with transforming potential usually map towards the ends of the non-repetitive central DNA portion of γ-herpesvirus genomes. Examples are the oncoproteins STP (**s**aimiri **t**ransforming **p**rotein) of the prototypic *H. saimiri*, Tio (**t**wo-**i**n-**o**ne-protein) of *Herpesvirus ateles (H. ateles)*, and LMP-1 (**l**atent **m**embrane **p**rotein) of the more distantly related Epstein-Barr Virus. None of these transformation related genes is conserved in HHV-8. However, several HHV-8 genes have been found to be transforming, at least in *in-vitro* assays using rodent fibroblasts (Table 2).

A. *K1*

K1 is the left-most reading frame of HHV-8 and thus analogous in position to STP of *H. saimiri*. Due to the lack of an HHV-8 cell culture system suitable for the generation of recombinant viruses, *H. saimiri* has been used as a model system. K1 recombinants were generated using *H. saimiri* group C strain 488. This revealed that K1 could complement the transforming function of STP-C both in cell culture and in an animal model (table 2). K1 was able to induce lymphoma in common marmosets when expressed in the context of the *H. saimiri* genome (Lee et al., 1998). Although functional data obtained in this heterologous system and the positional analogy to known transforming genes of other γ-herpesviruses are intriguing, the relevance of these findings remains controversial as it is not clear whether K1 is expressed in cells transformed by HHV-8. Data available to date indicate that this may not be the case, as it appears that K1 is expressed only during the lytic, productive phase of HHV-8 infection, but not in latently infected malignant cells (Lagunoff et al., 1997).

B. *Transformation of rodent fibroblasts: vIRF, K12, and vIL8R*

Several other genes of HHV-8 have been shown to be able to transform rodent fibroblasts (Table 2). Open reading frame K9 of HHV-8 encodes a gene with homology to interferon-regulatory factors (IRF), a family of transcription factors. Expression of recombinant vIRF induced transformation of NIH 3T3 cells, resulting in changes in morphology, focus formation, and growth in reduced-serum conditions (Li et al., 1998). Similar data were obtained when reading frame K12, also termed *kaposin*, was expressed either from its endogenous promoter or from a heterologous promoter. It induced focal transformation upon transfection into Rat-3 cells, and these cells gave rise to highly undifferentiated sarcomas following injection into athymic nude mice (Muralidhar et al., 1998).

Another gene with the potential to transform rodent fibroblasts in cell culture is the constitutively active viral interleukin-8 receptor homologue encoded by reading frame 74. It has been shown to induce the protein kinase C (PKC) pathway in transfected cells, which is associated with stimulated cell proliferation and growth transformation of rodent fibroblasts (Arvanitakis et al., 1997).

C. k-cyclin

In contrast to other rhadinoviruses, where transformation-related genes encoded at the left end of the genome are expressed in malignant cells, the HHV-8 genes expressed in both KS spindle cells and also the majority of cultured PEL cells, are clustered at the right end of the genome. One group of bi- or tri-cistronic latent transcripts has the potential to encode the viral cyclin (k-cyclin), viral FLICE inhibitory-protein homolog (vFLIP) (Thome et al., 1997), and open reading frame 73. Open reading frame 73 encodes a nuclear protein which is part of the antigen detected by the LNA-IFA (Rainbow et al., 1997). The function of ORF73 is unknown, as is the function of the homologous reading frames found in other rhadinoviruses. The function of k-cyclin is better understood. The protein is functional as a cyclin D (Li et al., 1997) that associates primarily with cyclin-dependent-kinase 6 (cdk6). Interestingly, the k-cyclin/cdk6 complex evades inhibition by cdk-inhibitors, resulting in a constitutive kinase activity in cells expressing cdk6 (Swanton et al., 1997). The k-cyclin/cdk6 holoenzyme is not only resistant to inhibition by cdk-inhibitors like $p27^{Kip}$, it is also able to phosphorylate a broad spectrum of substrates including histone (Li et al., 1997), $p27^{Kip}$, and a subset of proteins usually phosphorylated by activated cdk2. Phosphorlyation of $p27^{Kip}$ results in the proteolytic degradation of this regulatory protein (Ellis et al., 1999; Mann et al., 1999). This is likely to be of relevance for cell cycle dysregulation by HHV-8, as $p27^{Kip}$ normally inhibits the activity of both cyclinD/cdk6 and cyclinE/cdk2 complexes. Thus, the cyclin D homolog encoded by HHV-8 may also be considered a candidate oncogene (table 2).

HHV-8 Encoded Inhibitors of Apoptosis

A. General considerations

Apoptosis, also called programmed cell death, is used amongst other functions as a defence mechanism of the host to combat harmful infectious agents and oncogenesis. It is beneficial for the organism to eliminate infected cells rather than to try to preserve them with the drawback that the virus may spread. On the other hand, it is advantageous for the virus to prolong the life of infected cells in order to sustain ongoing viral replication. Different viruses have developed a variety of strategies to interfere with host cell apoptosis (Meinl et al., 1998).

B. *FLIP*

Rhadinoviruses such as HHV-8 and *H. saimiri* code for two different anti-apoptotic proteins with homology to cellular regulators of apoptosis. One of them belongs to a class of cell death regulating proteins that interfere with apoptosis mediated by death receptors (Thome et al., 1997; Hu et al., 1997; Bertin et al., 1997; Wang et al., 1997) such as CD95, TNF-R1, TRAMP and two of the four identified receptors for the cytotoxic ligand TRAIL. These molecules share a cytoplasmic domain that is required for transmission of a pro-apoptotic signal and is therefore called a death domain (DD). Apoptotic signaling of CD95 has been most extensively studied, but there is evidence that the other death receptors use similar death signaling pathways. Binding of CD95 to its ligand leads to the recruitment of a death-inducing signaling complex (Kischkel et al., 1995). This complex consists of adaptor proteins that contain protein-protein interaction motifs. The adaptor molecule FADD is recruited to CD95 by interactions of their respective death domains. FADD then recruits FLICE (caspase 8, MACH, Mch-5) via interactions of their death effector domains (DED), leading to FLICE activation by autocleavage. Activated FLICE subsequently cleaves caspase 3 and initiates a proteolytic cascade that result in apoptosis (Figure 1). TNF-R1 and TRAMP use an additional adaptor molecule, named TRADD, to recruit FADD and then FLICE.

The knowledge of the adaptor molecules involved in programmed cell death provided the basis for identifying a novel class of viral anti-apoptotic effectors (Thome et al., 1997; Hu et al., 1997; Bertin et al., 1997). Searches for homology to death effector domains using multiple alignment analysis yielded viral proteins with two DEDs (Table 3). These viral anti-apoptotic molecules block the acitvity of FLICE (caspase 8) and were therefore named FLIPs (FLICE inhibitory proteins) (Thome et al., 1997). Shortly thereafter, cellular FLIPs (Irmler et al., 1997) were discovered by other groups (reviewed by Wallach, 1997).

The homology between viral FLIPs and their cellular counterpart is restricted to key amino acids of the DEDs. In addition, there is a splice variant of cellular FLIP that contains a C-terminal caspase-like domain which, however, lacks the active site cysteine and is therefore inactive (Irmler et al., 1997). The identified viral proteins have two DEDs and bind to cellular proteins with a DED like FADD and FLICE (Thome et al., 1997; Hu et al., 1997; Bertin et al., 1997), and thereby block the formation of the death inducing signaling complex (Thome et al., 1997). Viral FLIPs block cell death mediated by the death receptors Fas, TNF-R1, TRAMP, and induced by TRAIL (Thome et al., 1997; Hu et al., 1997; Bertin et al., 1997; Wang et al., 1997). Up to now, no functional data concerning the FLIP of HHV-8 have been reported. However, based on sequence homology it is very likely that it exhibits a similar function to that described for the v-FLIP encoded by EHV-2, *H.saimiri*, BHV-4 and MCV (Thome et al., 1997; Wang et al., 1997; Hu et al., 1997; Bertin et al., 1997). Very recently it was also reported that a rhesus macaque rhadinovirus with similarity to HHV-8 codes for a FLIP homolog (Searles et al., 1999).

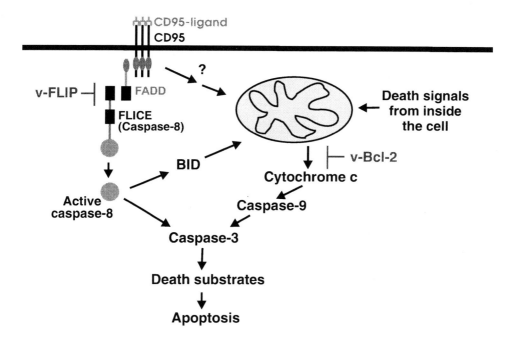

Figure 1. Mode of action of herpesvirus-encoded FLIP and Bcl-2 homologs. Viral FLIPs specifically inhibit apoptosis mediated through death receptors such as CD95 (Thome et al., 1997). Herpesviral Bcl-2 stabilizes mitochondria and thereby protects cells from apoptosis induced by a variety of stimuli (Derfuss et al., 1998). In some cell types CD95-mediated apoptosis is signaled through mitochondria (Scaffidi et al., 1998) and in such cells v-Bcl-2 also inhibits CD95-mediated apoptosis (Derfuss et al., 1998).

C. Bcl-2

Different viruses, most of them lymphotropic herpesviruses, code for a homolog to the cellular anti-apoptotic protein Bcl-2. Cellular Bcl-2 was discovered as an oncogenic protein involved in the development of follicular B cell lymphoma. The number of cellular bcl-2 family members is still growing, with more than ten family members having already been described (Reed, 1997; Kroemer, 1997). Cellular Bcl-2 family members can be divided in two groups, either promoting or inhibiting apoptosis. The ratio of inhibitors to activators of apoptosis determines life or death. The best studied anti-apoptotic cellular Bcl-2 family members are Bcl-2 itself and Bcl-x_L, while Bax and Bak promote apoptosis.

Table 3. Cellular and viral proteins with a death effector domain

	Death effector domain (DED)	Caspase domain
Cellular proteins		
FADD	1 DED	
FLICE/Caspase-8	2 DED	Caspase
Mch4/Caspase-10	2 DED	Caspase
FLIP-L	2 DED	I-caspase [a]
FLIP-S	2 DED	

Viral FLIPs

Virus	Gene	Death effector domain (DED)
HHV-8	K13 / Orf 71	2 DED
H.saimiri	Orf 71	2 DED
Rhesus rhadinovirus	Orf 71	2 DED
EHV-2	E8	2 DED
BHV-4	BORFE2	2 DED
MCV	Orf 159L	2 DED
MCV	Orf 160L	2 DED

[a] The caspase domain of FLIP-L is inactive.

HHV-8 encodes a member of the Bcl-2 family (Sarid et al., 1997a; Cheng et al., 1997) that is located at the same position in the genome as the *H. saimiri*-encoded Bcl-2 homolog (Albrecht et al., 1992; Russo et al., 1996a). A Bcl-2 homolog was found in virtually all lymphotropic γ-herpesviruses sequenced so far and is also encoded by the African swine fever virus. The adenovirus encoded E1B19K protein has similar functional properties to Bcl-2, but does not show strong structural homology. An important function of the anti-apoptotic herpesviral Bcl-2 homologs in the life cycle of these viruses is suggested by the finding that lymphotropic herpesviruses of distantly related species code for a Bcl-2 homolog (Ensser et al., 1997; Virgin et al., 1997; Derfuss et al., 1998; Searles et al., 1999). All viral Bcl-2 family members studied so far block the progress of apoptosis (Meinl et al., 1998).

Homology of Bcl-2 family members is restricted to distinct Bcl-2 homology regions, BH1, BH2, BH3, and BH4. Most of the cellular Bcl-2 members have a membrane anchor at their C-terminus and are localized at the outer mitochondrial, outer nuclear, and endoplasmic membranes.

The Bcl-2 homologs encoded by herpeviruses are shorter than cellular Bcl-2 or Bcl-x_L – they lack a strong homology to the BH3 and BH4 domain, but contain, like their cellular counterparts, a membrane anchor at the C-terminus (Meinl et al., 1998). The function of the different Bcl-2 homology domains can be identified to some extent. BH1 and BH2 domains are involved in Bcl-2 homodimer formation. The BH3 domain of death agonists like Bax or Bak is required for heterodimerization with Bcl-2 and Bcl-x_L and to promote apoptosis. The BH4 domain of Bcl-2 and Bcl-x_L is involved in binding to death-regulatory proteins like Raf-1, Bag-1, calcineurin and CED-4 (Kroemer, 1997; Reed, 1997; Huang et al., 1998). The anti-apoptotic cellular Bcl-2 can be converted to a death promotor upon cleavage by caspases (Cheng et al., 1997), and this death promoting activity is dependent on BH3. It was suggested that the lack of BH3 allows the herpesviral Bcl-2 homologs to evade regulation by caspases and conversion into a proapoptotic protein (Cheng et al., 1997).

Bcl-2 family members form homodimers or heterodimers. Since the function of Bcl-2 family members is regulated through binding to each other, potential binding partners of HHV-8 have been analysed. Cheng and coworkers performed coimmunoprecipitation assays of ^{35}S-labelled in cotranslated proteins. They reported that HHV-8 Bcl-2 forms homodimers but does not form heterodimers with Bcl-2, Bcl-x_L, Bax or Bak. The authors suggested that this allows HHV-8 Bcl-2 to escape any negative regulatory effects of Bax or Bak. It was reported in another study which addressed the binding properties of HHV-8 Bcl-2 in a yeast two hybrid system, however, that cellular Bcl-2 and HHV-8 Bcl-2 did bind to each other (Sarid et al., 1997b).

Cellular Bcl-2 is a multifunctional protein and different mechanisms have been implicated in the protection of cells from apoptotic stimuli. Prevention of the loss of mitochondrial membrane potential that is induced by a number of apoptotic stimuli (Marchetti et al., 1996; Susin et al., 1997), interaction with several proteins participating in cell death regulation such as the mammalian homolog of CED-4 (Apaf-1), Raf-1, BAG-1, calcineurin, p53BP-2, and other members of the Bcl-2 family are possible modes of action of cellular Bcl-2 (reviewed by Reed, 1997; Kroemer, 1997).

The HHV-8 encoded Bcl-2 was found to protect against apoptosis in different assay systems (Figure 1). One study reported that HHV-8 Bcl-2 inhibited Bax-induced cytotoxicity in yeast and in human GM701 fibroblasts (Sarid et al., 1997a). HHV-8 Bcl-2 also inhibited Sindbis virus induced apoptosis (Cheng et al., 1997). A detailed analysis of the anti-apoptotic spectrum and of the mode of action of the homologous viral Bcl-2 encoded by *H.saimiri* has been performed (Derfuss et al., 1998). The *H.saimiri* encoded Bcl-2 protected against apoptosis induced by irradiation, dexamethasone, and oxygen radicals. Inhibition of CD95-mediated cell death was cell type dependent. Analysis of the mode of action of *H.saimiri*-Bcl-2 revealed that it protected against this broad range of apoptotic stimuli by stabilizing mitochondria and by functioning upstream of the generation of caspase-3 like activity (Derfuss et al., 1998).

Taken together, the viral FLIP and the viral Bcl-2 are complementary in their anti-apoptotic activity. The FLIP protects against apoptosis from outside the cell mediated by death receptors, whereas the viral Bcl-2 protects against cell-autonomous apoptosis induced by intracellular stress. In addition, the viral Bcl-2 protects against apoptosis mediated by death receptors in certain cell types.

Table 4: Properties of human virus transformed lymphocytes

Properties	Transforming virus			
	HHV-8	*H.saimiri*	HTLV-I	EBV
Transformed cell type	B	T	T	B
Antigen receptor persistence	-	+	+ / -	+
Expression of lineage specific differentiation markers	-	+	+	+
Viral persistence	episomal	episomal	integrated	episomal
Release of virus	inducible	not seen	spontaneously	inducible
Oncogenic potential in SCID mice	+ (Boshoff et al., 1998; Picchio et al., 1997)	- (Huppes et al., 1994)	- / + (Feuer et al., 1993)	- (Ramqvist et al., 1991)

D. *Expression of HHV-8 encoded Bcl-2 and FLIP during latency or lytic replication*

Lymphotropic herpesviruses such as *H.saimiri*, EBV or KSHV can be found in two principally different conditions. The virus may replicates in infected lymphocytes or certain epithelial cells – this is associated with expression of all viral genes and eventually leads to destruction of the infected cell and release of progeny virus. Alternatively, the virus persists episomally in lymphocytes; in this case only few viral genes are expressed, and the infected lymphocytes may be transformed to stable growth (Table 4).

The HHV-8 encoded *flip* gene is transcribed during episomal persistence along with the viral cyclin (Sarid et al., 1998) as seen in a tumor cell line derived from a body cavity-based B cell lymphoma (Rainbow et al., 1997; Sarid et al., 1998). This is remarkable, since the homologous FLIP of *Herpesvirus .saimiri* is only expressed during lytic replication, but not during latency (Kraft et al., 1998).

Expression of HHV-8-encoded Bcl-2 homolog was detected in Kaposi´s sarcoma tissue and in HHV-8-containing B-cell (Sarid et al., 1997a). Another study did not detect constitutive expression of HHV-8 encoded Bcl-2 in the cell line BCBL-1(Cheng et al., 1997). Both groups, however, described a strong expression after activation of these B cell lines with phorbol ester acetate indicating that KSHV-Bcl-2 is mainly expressed during lytic replication. The detection of expression of HHV-8 Bcl-2 in Kaposi´s sarcoma is not surprising, since a proportion of HHV-8 infected cells in these tumors support lytic replication of HHV-8.

Conclusions

Induction of apoptosis, cell cycle arrest, and activation of cellular immunity are the typical responses of the host to viral infection. Different viruses appear to have developed different strategies to overcome these defense mechanisms. For example, whereas Epstein-Barr virus induces cellular Bcl-2 and codes for a Bcl-2 homolog, HHV-8 encodes two inhibitors of apoptosis. Block of apoptosis is required to ensure efficient production of progeny before lysis of the cell occurs. Similarly, expression of human IL-6 and the IL-8 receptor are induced by EBV (Tanner et al., 1996), whereas homologs to both genes can be found in the HHV-8 genome. The function of these genes may be to stimulate proliferation of target cells, thus both increasing the pool of cells that can be infected and enhancing the conditions for viral replication in stimulated cells, as herpesviruses, like most other viruses, are not able to replicate in resting cells. Similarly, to ensure efficient replication, viruses have a vital interest to overcome the typical cell cycle arrest in G_0/G_1. This may well be ensured by k-cyclin, a cyclin-D homologue resistant to inhibition by several cyclin-dependant-kinase-inhibitors. Deregulation of the G1/S checkpoint is a common feature not only of many oncogenic viruses but of several malignant tumors. The HHV-8-encoded cyclin makes it particularly obvious that anti-viral and tumor-suppressing pathways frequently converge at the same regulatory proteins. Thus, by ensuring persistent infection and efficient productive replication, viruses accidentally contribute to oncogenesis.

References

Agbalika, F., Mariette, X., Marolleau, J.P., Fermand, J.P. and Brouet, J.C. (1998). Detection of human herpesvirus-8 DNA in bone marrow biopsies from patients with multiple myeloma and Waldenstrom's macroglobulinemia. Blood 91, 4393-4394.

Albini, A., Aluigi, M.G., Benelli, R., Berti, E., Biberfeld, P., Blasig, C., Calabro, M.L., Calvo, F., Chieco-Bianchi, L., Corbellino, M., Del Mistro, A., Ekman, M., Favero, A., Hofschneider, P.H., Kaaya, E., Lebbe, C., Morel, P., Neipel, F., Noonan, D.M., Parravicini, C., Repetto, L., Schalling, M., Stürzl, M. and Tschachler, E. (1996). Oncogenesis in HIV-infection: KSHV and Kaposi's sarcoma. Int.J.Onc. 9, 5-8.

Albrecht, J.C., Nicholas, J., Biller, D., Cameron, K.R., Biesinger, B., Newman, C., Wittmann, S., Craxton, M.A., Coleman, H., Fleckenstein, B. and Honess, R.W. (1992). Primary structure of the herpesvirus saimiri genome. J.Virol. 66, 5047-5058.

Arvanitakis, L., Geras Raaka, E., Varma, A., Gershengorn, M.C. and Cesarman, E. (1997). Human herpesvirus KSHV encodes a constitutively active G-protein- coupled receptor linked to cell proliferation. Nature 385, 347-350.

Bais, C., Santomasso, B., Coso, O., Arvanitakis, L., Raaka, E.G., Gutkind, J.S., Asch, A.S., Cesarman, E., Gerhengorn, M.C. and Mesri, E.A. (1998). G-protein-coupled receptor of Kaposi's sarcoma-associated herpesvirus is a viral oncogene and angiogenesis activator. Nature 391, 86-89.

Beral, V., Peterman, T.A., Berkelman, R.L. and Jaffe, H.W. (1990). Kaposi's sarcoma among persons with AIDS: a sexually transmitted infectiony Lancet 335, 123-128

Bertin, J., Armstrong, R.C., Ottilie, S., Martin, D.A., Wang, Y., Banks, S., Wang, G.H., Senkevich, T.G., Alnemri, E.S., Moss, B., Lenardo, M.J., Tomaselli, K.J. and Cohen, J.I. (1997). Death effector domain-containing herpesvirus and poxvirus proteins inhibit both Fas- and TNFR1-induced apoptosis. Proc.Natl.Acad.Sci.U.S.A. 94, 1172-1176.

Boshoff, C., Endo, Y., Collins, P.D., Takeuchi, Y., Reeves, J.D., Schweickart, V.L., Siani, M.A., Sasaki, T., Williams, T.J., Gray, P.W., Moore, P.S., Chang, Y. and Weiss, R.A. (1997). Angiogenic and HIV-inhibitory functions of KSHV-encoded chemokines. Science. 278, 290-294.

Boshoff, C., Gao, S.J., Healy, L.E., Matthews, S., Thomas, A.J., Coignet, L., Warnke, R.A., Strauchen, J.A., Matutes, E., Kamel, O.W., Moore, P.S., Weiss, R.A. and Chang, Y. (1998). Establishing a KSHV+ cell line (BCP-1) from peripheral blood and characterizing its growth in Nod/SCID mice. Blood 91, 1671-1679.

Boshoff, C., Schulz, T.F., Kennedy, M.M., Graham, A.K., Fisher, C., Thomas, A., McGee, J.O., Weiss, R.A. and O'Leary, J.J. (1995). Kaposi's sarcoma-associated herpesvirus infects endothelial and spindle cells. Nat.Med. 1, 1274-1278.

Brousset, P., Meggetto, F., Attal, M. and Delsol, G. (1997). Kaposi's sarcoma-associated herpesvirus infection and multiple myeloma [letter]. Science. 278, 1972.

Burger, R., Neipel, F., Fleckenstein, B., Savino, R., Ciliberto, G., Kalden, J.R. and Gramatzki, M. (1998a). Human herpesvirus type 8 interleukin-6 homologue is functionally active on human myeloma cells. Blood 91, 1858-1863.

Burger, R., Neipel, F., Fleckenstein, B., Savino, R., Ciliberto, G., Kalden, J.R. and Gramatzki, M. (1998b). Human herpesvirus type 8 interleukin-6 homologue is functionally active on human myeloma cells. Blood 91, 1858-1863.

Cathomas, G., Stalder, A., Kurrer, M.O., Regamey, N., Erb, P. and Joller-Jemelka, H.I. (1998). Multiple myeloma and HHV8 infection. Blood 91, 4391-4393.

Cesarman, E., Moore, P.S., Rao, P.H., Inghirami, G., Knowles, D.M. and Chang, Y. (1995). In vitro establishment and characterization of two acquired immunodeficiency syndrome-related lymphoma cell lines (BC-1 and BC-2) containing Kaposi's sarcoma-associated herpesvirus-like (KSHV) DNA sequences. Blood 86, 2708-2714.

Cesarman, E., Nador, R.G., Bai, F., Bohenzky, R.A., Russo, J.J., Moore, P.S., Chang, Y. and Knowles, D.M. (1996). Kaposi's sarcoma-associated herpesvirus contains G protein- coupled receptor and cyclin D homologs which are expressed in Kaposi's sarcoma and malignant lymphoma. J.Virol. 70, 8218-8223.

Chauhan, D., Bharti, A., Raje, N., Gustafson, E., Pinkus, G.S., Pinkus, J.L., Teoh, G., Hideshima, T., Treon, S.P., Fingeroth, J.D. and Anderson, K.C. (1999). Detection of Kaposi's Sarcoma Herpesvirus DNA Sequences in Multiple Myeloma Bone Marrow Stromal Cells. Blood 93, 1482-1486.

Cheng, E.H.Y., Kirsch, D.G., Clem, R.J., Ravi, R., Kastan, M.B., Bedi, A., Ueno, K. and Hardwick, J.M. (1997). Conversion of Bcl-2 to a Bax-like death effector by caspases. Science 278, 1966-1968.

Cheng, E.H., Nicholas, J., Bellows, D.S., Hayward, G.S., Guo, H.G., Reitz, M.S. and Hardwick, J.M. (1997). A Bcl-2 homolog encoded by Kaposi sarcoma-associated virus, human herpesvirus 8, inhibits apoptosis but does not heterodimerize with Bax or Bak. Proc.Natl.Acad.Sci.U.S.A. 94, 690-694.

Corbellino, M., Poirel, L., Bestetti, G., Pizzuto, M., Aubin, J.T., Capra, M., Bifulco, C., Berti, E., Agut, H., Rizzardini, G., Galli, M. and Parravicini, C. (1996). Restricted tissue distribution of extralesional Kaposi's sarcoma- associated herpesvirus-like DNA sequences in AIDS patients with Kaposi's sarcoma. AIDS Res.Hum.Retroviruses 12, 651-657.

Cottoni, F. and Uccini, S. (1997). Kaposi's sarcoma-associated herpesvirus infection and multiple myeloma [letter]. Science. 278, 1972.

Cull, G.M., Timms, J.M., Haynes, A.P., Russell, N.H., Irving, W.L., Ball, J.K. and Thomson, B.J. (1998). Dendritic cells cultured from mononuclear cells and CD34 cells in myeloma do not harbour human herpesvirus 8. Br.J.Haematol. 100, 793-796.

Davis, M.A., Stürzl, M., Blasig, C., Schreier, A., Guo, H.G., Reitz, M., Opalenik, S.R. and Browning, P.J. (1997). Expression of human herpesvirus 8-encoded cyclin D in Kaposi's sarcoma spindle cells. J.Natl.Cancer Inst. 89, 1868-1874.

Delabesse, E., Oksenhendler, E., Lebbe, C., Verola, O., Varet, B. and Turhan, A.G. (1997). Molecular analysis of clonality in Kaposi's sarcoma. J.Clin.Pathol. 50, 664-668.

Derfuss, T., Fickenscher, H., Kraft, M.S., Henning, G., Lengenfelder, D., Fleckenstein, B. and Meinl, E. (1998). Antiapoptotic Activity of the Herpesvirus Saimiri-Encoded Bcl-2 Homolog: Stabilization of Mitochondria and Inhibition of Caspase-3-Like Activity. J.Virol. 72, 5897-5904.

Diaz-Cano, S.J. and Wolfe, H.J. (1997). Clonality in Kaposi's sarcoma [letter; comment]. N.Engl.J.Med. 337, 571-572.

Ellis, M., Chew, Y.P., Fallis, L., Freddersdorf, S., Boshoff, C., Weiss, R.A., Lu, X. and Mittnacht, S. (1999). Degradation of p27(Kip) cdk inhibitor triggered by Kaposi's sarcoma virus cyclin-cdk6 complex. EMBO J. 18, 644-653.

Ensoli, B., Nakamura, S., Salahuddin, S.Z., Biberfeld, P., Larsson, L., Beaver, B., Wong-Staal, F. and Gallo, R.C. (1989). AIDS-Kaposi's sarcoma-derived cells express cytokines with autocrine and paracrine growth effects. Science. 243, 223-226.

Ensoli, B. and Stürzl, M. (1998). Kaposi's sarcoma: a result of the interplay among inflammatory cytokines, angiogenic factors and viral agents. Cytokine.Growth Factor.Rev. 9, 63-83.

Ensser, A., Pflanz, R. and Fleckenstein, B. (1997). Primary structure of the alcelaphine herpesvirus 1 genome. J.Virol. 71, 6517-6525.

Feuer, G., Zack, J.A., Harrington, W.J., Jr., Valderama, R., Rosenblatt, J.D., Wachsman, W., Baird, S.M. and Chen, I.S. (1993). Establishment of human T-cell leukemia virus type I T-cell lymphomas in severe combined immunodeficient mice. Blood 82, 722-731.

Gao, S.J., Alsina, M., Deng, J.H., Harrison, C.R., Montalvo, E.A., Leach, C.T., Roodman, G.D. and Jenson, H.B. (1998). Antibodies to Kaposi's sarcoma-associated herpesvirus (human herpesvirus 8) in patients with multiple myeloma. J.Infect.Dis. 178, 846-849.

Gao, S.J., Boshoff, C., Jayachandra, S., Weiss, R.A., Chang, Y. and Moore, P.S. (1997). KSHV ORF K9 (vIRF) is an oncogene which inhibits the interferon signaling pathway. Oncogene 15, 1979-1985.

Gill, P.S., Tsai, Y.C., Rao, A.P., Spruck, C.H., Zheng, T., Harrington, W.A.J., Cheung, T., Nathwani, B. and Jones, P.A. (1998). Evidence for multiclonality in multicentric Kaposi's sarcoma. Proc.Natl.Acad.Sci.U.S.A. 95, 8257-8261.

Hu, S., Vincenz, C., Buller, M. and Dixit, V.M. (1997). A novel family of viral death effector domain-containing molecules that inhibit both CD-95- and tumor necrosis factor-1-induced apoptosis. J.Biol.Chem. 272, 9621-9624.

Huang, D.C.S., Adams, J.M. and Cory, S. (1998). The conserved N-terminal BH4 domain of Bcl-2 homologues is essential for inhibition of apoptosis and interaction with CED-4. EMBO J. 17, 1029-1039.

Huppes, W., Fickenscher, H., 'tHart, B.A. and Fleckenstein, B. (1994). Cytokine dependence of human to mouse graft-versus-host disease. Scand.J.Immunol. 40, 26-36.

Irmler, M., Thome, M., Hahne, M., Schneider, P., Hofmann, K., Steiner, V., Bodmer, J.-L., Schröter, M., Burns, K., Mattmann, C., Rimoldi, D., French, L.E. and Tschopp, J. (1997). Identification of death receptor signals by cellular FLIP. Nature 388, 190-195.

Jussila, L., Valtola, R., Partanen, T.A., Salven, P., Heikkila, P., Matikainen, M.T., Renkonen, R., Kaipainen, A., Detmar, M., Tschachler, E., Alitalo, R. and Alitalo, K. (1998). Lymphatic endothelium and Kaposi's sarcoma spindle cells detected by antibodies against the vascular endothelial growth factor receptor-3. Cancer Res. 58, 1599-1604.

Kischkel, F.C., Hellbardt, S., Behrmann, I., Germer, M., Pawlita, M., Krammer, P.H. and Peter, M.E. (1995). Cytotoxicity-dependent APO-1 (Fas/CD95)-associated proteins form a death-inducing signaling complex (DISC) with the receptor. EMBO J. 14, 5579-5588.

Kraft, M.S., Henning, G., Fickenscher, H., Lengenfelder, D., Tschopp, J., Fleckenstein, B. and Meinl, E. (1998). Herpesvirus saimiri transforms human T cells to stable growth without inducing resistance to apoptosis. J.Virol. 72, 3138-3145.

Kroemer, G. (1997). The proto-oncogene Bcl-2 and its role in regulating apoptosis. Nat.Med. 3, 614-620.

Lagunoff, M. and Ganem, D. (1997). The structure and coding organization of the genomic termini of Kaposi's sarcoma-associated herpesvirus. Virology 236, 147-154.

Lee, H., Veazey, R., Williams, K., Li, M., Guo, J., Neipel, F., Fleckenstein, B., Lackner, A., Desrosiers, R.C. and Jung, J.U. (1998). Deregulation of cell growth by the K1 gene of Kaposi's sarcoma- associated herpesvirus. Nat.Med. 4, 435-440.

Li, M., Lee, H., Guo, J., Neipel, F., Fleckenstein, B., Ozato, K. and Jung, J.U. (1998). Kaposi's sarcoma-associated herpesvirus viral interferon regulatory factor. J.Virol. 72, 5433-5440.

Li, M., Lee, H., Yoon, D. W., Albrecht, J.C., Fleckenstein, B., Neipel, F. and Jung, J.U. (1997). Kaposi's sarcoma associated herpesvirus encodes a functional cyclin. J.Virol. 71, 1984-1991.

Lisitsyn, N.A., Lisitsyn, N.M. and Wigler, M. (1993). Cloning the differences between to complex genomes. Science. 259, 946-951.

Luppi, M., Barozzi, P., Maiorana, A., Artusi, T., Trovato, R., Marasca, R., Savarino, M., Ceccherini Nelli, L. and Torelli, G. (1996). Human herpesvirus-8 DNA sequences in human immunodeficiency virus-negative angioimmunoblastic lymphadenopathy and benign lymphadenopathy with giant germinal center hyperplasia and increased vascularity. Blood 87, 3903-3909.

MacKenzie, J., Sheldon, J., Morgan, G., Cook, G., Schulz, T.F. and Jarrett, R.F. (1997). HHV-8 and multiple myeloma in the UK [letter]. Lancet 350, 1144-1145.

Mann, D.J., Child, E.S., Swanton, C., Laman, H. and Jones, N. (1999). Modulation of p27(Kip1) levels by the cyclin encoded by Kaposi's sarcoma-associated herpesvirus. EMBO J. 18, 654-663.

Marcelin, A.G., Dupin, N., Bouscary, D., Bossi, P., Cacoub, P., Ravaud, P. and Calvez, V. (1997). HHV-8 and multiple myeloma in France [letter]. Lancet 350, 1144.

Marchetti, P., Castedo, M., Susin, S.A., Zamzami, N., Hirsch, T., Macho, A., Haeffner, A., Hirsch, F., Geuskens, M. and Kroemer, G. (1996). Mitochondrial permeability transition is a central coordinating event of apoptosis. J.Exp.Med. 184, 1155-1160.

Masood, R., Zheng, T., Tupule, A., Arora, N., Chatlynne, L., Handy, M. and Whitman, J., Jr. (1997). Kaposi's sarcoma-associated herpesvirus infection and multiple myeloma [letter]. Science. 278, 1970-1971.

Meinl, E., Fickenscher, H., Thome, M., Tschopp, J. and Fleckenstein, B. (1998). Anti-apoptotic strategies of lymphotropic viruses. Immunol.Today 19, 474-479.

Molden, J., Chang, Y., You, Y., Moore, P.S. and Goldsmith, M.A. (1997). A Kaposi's sarcoma-associated herpesvirus-encoded cytokine homolog (vIL-6) activates signaling through the shared gp130 receptor subunit. J.Biol.Chem. 272, 19625-19631.

Moore, P.S., Boshoff, C., Weiss, R.A. and Chang, Y. (1996). Molecular mimicry of human cytokine and cytokine response pathway genes by KSHV. Science. 274, 1739-1744.

Muralidhar, S., Pumfery, A.M., Hassani, M., Sadaie, M.R., Azumi, N., Kishishita, M., Brady, J.N., Doniger, J., Medveczky, P. and Rosenthal, L.J. (1998). Identification of kaposin (open reading frame K12) as a human herpesvirus 8 (Kaposi's sarcoma-associated herpesvirus) transforming gene. J.Virol. 72, 4980-4988.

Nador, R.G., Cesarman, E., Chadburn, A., Dawson, D.B., Ansari, M.Q., Sald, J. and Knowles, D.M. (1996). Primary effusion lymphoma: a distinct clinicopathologic entity associated with the Kaposi's sarcoma-associated herpes virus. Blood 88, 645-656.

Nakamura, S., Salahuddin, S.Z., Biberfeld, P., Ensoli, B., Markham, P.D., Wong-Staal, F. and Gallo, R.C. (1988). Kaposi's sarcoma cells: long-term culture with growth factor from retrovirus-infected CD4+ T cells. Science. 242, 426-430.

Neipel, F., Albrecht, J.C., Ensser, A., Huang, Y.Q., Li, J.J., Friedman-Kien, A.E. and Fleckenstein, B. (1997a). Human herpesvirus 8 encodes a homolog of interleukin-6. J.Virol. 71, 839-842.

Neipel, F., Albrecht, J.C. and Fleckenstein, B. (1997b). Cell-homologous genes in the Kaposi's sarcoma-associated rhadinovirus human herpesvirus 8: determinants of its pathogenicityγ J.Virol. 71, 4187-4182.

Nicholas, J., Ruvolo, V.R., Burns, W.H., Sandford, G., Wan, X., Ciufo, D., Hendrickson, S.B., Guo, H.G., Hayward, G.S. and Reitz, M.S. (1997). Kaposi's sarcoma-associated human herpesvirus-8 encodes homologues of macrophage inflammatory protein-1 and interleukin-6. Nat.Med. 3, 287-292.

Parravicini, C., Lauri, E., Baldini, L., Neri, A., Poli, F., Sirchia, G., Moroni, M., Galli, M. and Corbellino, M. (1997). Kaposi's sarcoma-associated herpesvirus infection and multiple myeloma [letter]. Science. 278, 1969-1970.

Picchio, G.R., Sabbe, R.E., Gulizia, R.J., McGrath, M., Herndier, B.G. and Mosier, D.E. (1997). The KSHV/HHV8-infected BCBL-1 lymphoma line causes tumors in SCID mice but fails to transmit virus to a human peripheral blood mononuclear cell graft. Virology 238, 22-29.

Rabkin, C.S., Janz, S., Lash, A., Coleman, A.E., Musaba, E., Liotta, L., Biggar, R.J. and Zhuang, Z. (1997). Monoclonal origin of multicentric Kaposi's sarcoma lesions. N.Engl.J.Med. 336, 988-993.

Rainbow, L., Platt, G.M., Simpson, G.R., Sarid, R., Gao, S.J., Stoiber, H., Herrington, C.S., Moore, P.S. and Schulz, T.F. (1997). The 222- to 234-kilodalton latent nuclear protein (LNA) of Kaposi's sarcoma-associated herpesvirus (human herpesvirus 8) is encoded by orf73 and is a component of the latency-associated nuclear antigen. J.Virol. 71, 5915-5921.

Ramqvist, T., Noren, L., Iwarsson, K. and Klein, G. (1991). Tumorigenicity of EBV-carrying lymphoblastoid cell lines (LCLs): distinctive grading in SCID mice. Int.J.Cancer 49, 587-591.

Reed, J.C. (1997). Double identity for proteins of the Bcl-2 family. Nature 387, 773-776.

Renne, R., Zhong, W., Herndier, B., McGrath, M.S., Abbey, N., Kedes, D.H. and Ganem, D.E. (1996). Lytic growth of Kaposi's sarcoma-associated herpesvirus (human herpesvirus 8) in culture. Nature Medicine 2, 342-346.

Rettig, M.B., Ma, H.J., Vescio, R.A., Pold, M., Schiller, G., Belson, D., Savage, A., Nishikubo, C., Wu, C., Fraser, J., Said, J.W. and Berenson, J.R. (1997). Kaposi's sarcoma-associated herpesvirus infection of bone marrow dendritic cells from multiple myeloma patients. Science. 276, 1851-1854.

Russo, J.J., Bohenzky, R.A., Chen, M.C., Chen, J., Yan, M., Maddalena, D., Parry, J.P., Peruzzi, D., Edelman, I.S., Chang, Y. and Moore, P.S. (1996a). Nucleotide sequence of the Kaposi's sarcoma-accociated herpesvirus (HHV8). Proc.Natl.Acad.Sci.U.S.A. 93, 14862-14867.

Russo, J.J., Bohenzky, R.A., Chien, M.C., Chen, J., Yan, M., Maddalena, D., Parry, J.P., Peruzzi, D., Edelman, I.S., Chang, Y. and Moore, P.S. (1996b). Nucleotide sequence of the Kaposi sarcoma-associated herpesvirus (HHV8). Proc.Natl.Acad.Sci.U.S.A. 93, 14862-14867.

Sarid, R., Flore, O., Bohenzky, R.A., Chang, Y. and Moore, P.S. (1998). Transcription mapping of the Kaposi's sarcoma-associated herpesvirus (human herpesvirus 8) genome in a body cavity-based lymphoma cell line (BC-1). J.Virol. 72, 1005-1012.

Sarid, R., Sato, T., Bohenzky, R.A., Russo, J.J. and Chang, Y. (1997a). Kaposi's sarcoma-associated herpesvirus encodes a functional bcl- 2 homologue. Nat.Med. 3, 293-298.

Sarid, R., Sato, T., Bohenzky, R.A., Russo, J.J. and Chang, Y. (1997b). Kaposi's sarcoma-associated herpesvirus encodes a functional bcl- 2 homologue. Nat.Med. 3, 293-298.

Scaffidi, C., Fulda, S., Srinivasan, A., Friesen, C., Li, F., Tomaselli, K.J., Debatin, K.M., Krammer, P.H. and Peter, M.E. (1998). Two CD95 (Apo-1/Fas) signaling pathways. EMBO J. 17, 1675-1687.

Searles, R.P., Bergquam, E.P., Axthelm, M.K. and Wong, S.W. (1999). Sequence and genomic analysis of a rhesus macaque rhadinovirus with similarity to Kaposi's sarcoma-associated Herpesvirus/Human herpesvirus 8. J.Virol. 73, 3040-3053.

Soulier, J., Grollet, L., Oksenhendler, E., Cacoub, P., Cazals Hatem, D., Babinet, P., d'Agay, M.F., Clauvel, J.P., Raphael, M., Degos, L. and Sigaux, F. (1995). Kaposi's sarcoma-associated herpesvirus-like DNA sequences in multicentric Castleman's disease. Blood 86, 1276-1280.

Stürzl, M., Blasig, C., Schreier, A., Neipel, F., Hohenadl, C., Cornali, E., Ascherl, G., Esser, S., Brockmeyer, N.H., Ekman, M., Kaaya, E.E., Tschachler, E. and Biberfeld, P. (1997). Expression of HHV-8 latency-associated T0.7 RNA in spindle cells and endothelial cells of AIDS-associated, classical and African Kaposi's sarcoma. Int.J.Cancer 72, 68-71.

Susin, S.A., Zamzami, N., Castedo, M., Daugas, E., Wang, H.G., Geley, S., Fassy, F., Reed, J.C. and Kroemer, G. (1997). The central executioner of apoptosis: multiple connections between protease activation and mitochondria in Fas/APO-1/CD95- and ceramide-induced apoptosis. J.Exp.Med. 186, 25-37.

Swanton, C., Mann, D.J., Fleckenstein, B., Neipel, F., Peters, G. and Jones, N. (1997). Herpes viral cyclin/cdk6 complexes evade inhibition by cdk inhibitor proteins. Nature 390, 184-187.

Tanner, J.E., Alfieri, C., Chatila, T.A. and Diaz Mitoma, F. (1996). Induction of interleukin-6 after stimulation of human B-cell CD21 by Epstein-Barr virus glycoproteins gp350 and gp220. J.Virol. 70, 570-575.

Thome, M., Schneider, P., Hofmann, K., Fickenscher, H., Meinl, E., Neipel, F., Mattmann, C., Burns, K., Bodmer, J.-L., Schröter, M., Scaffidi, C., Krammer, P.H., Peter, M.E. and Tschopp, J. (1997). Viral FLICE-inhibitory proteins (FLIPs) prevent apoptosis induced by death receptors. Nature 386, 517-521.

Virgin IV, H.W., Latreille, P., Wamsley, P., Hallsworth, K., Weck, K., Dal Canto, A.J.D. and Speck, S.H. (1997). Complete sequence and genomic analysis of murine gammaherpesvirus 68. J.Virol. 71, 5894-5904.

Wallach, D. (1997). Placing death under control. Nature 388, 123-126.

Wang, G.H., Bertin, J., Wang, Y., Martin, D.A., Wang, J., Tomaselli, K.J., Armstrong, R.C. and Cohen, J.I. (1997). Bovine herpesvirus 4 BORFE2 protein inhibits Fas- and tumor necrosis factor receptor 1-induced apoptosis and contains death effector domains shared with other gamma-2 herpesviruses. J.Virol. 71, 8928-8932.

Yi, Q., Ekman, M., Anton, D., Bergenbrant, S., Osterborg, A., Georgii-Hemming, P., Holm, G., Nilsson, K. and Biberfeld, P. (1998). Blood dendritic cells from myeloma patients are not infected with Kaposi's sarcoma-associated herpesvirus (KSHV/HHV 8). Blood 92, 402-404.

Zimring, J.C., Goodbourn, S. and Offermann, M.K. (1998). Human herpesvirus 8 encodes an interferon regulatory factor (IRF) homolog that represses IRF-1-mediated transcription. J.Virol. 72, 701-707.

HUMAN T-CELL LEUKEMIA VIRUS TYPE I ONCOPROTEIN, TAX :
CELL CYCLE DYSREGULATION AND CELLULAR TRANSFORMATION

Kenneth G. Low[1] and Kuan-Teh Jeang[2]

[1]Lead Discovery Screening, Bristol-Myers Squibb, Wallingford, CT
[2]Laboratory of Molecular Microbiology, National Institutes of Allergy
and Infectious Diseases, Bethesda, MD

1. Introduction

Human tumor viruses induce cellular transformation through various mechanisms. Commonly, viruses encode oncoproteins which target critical cellular processes such as transcription/gene expression, signal transduction, cell cycle progression and apoptosis (Fields, 1990). Some human tumor viruses such as Kaposi's sarcoma herpesvirus (KSHV)/human herpesvirus-8 (HHV8) have evolved multiple viral oncoproteins, each capable of targeting a unique cellular process (Beck et al., 1998; Nead and McCance, 1998; Schulz et al., 1998). On the other hand, several other tumor viruses such as adenoviruses, papillomaviruses, polyomaviruses and hepatitis viruses express multifunctional viral oncoproteins each capable of targeting multiple cellular processes (Cann and Chen, 1995). The human T-cell leukemia viruse type 1 (HTLV-1) Tax oncoprotein is a prototypic example of such a multifunctional oncoprotein with well-documented effects on cellular transcription and gene expression (Gitlin et al., 1993; Franklin and Nyborg, 1995).

Many studies on cellular transformation have focused on the contributory interactions of HTLV-1 Tax and cellular transcription factors. In this regard, Tax has been shown to be capable of direct modulation of gene expression through interactions with both coactivators and the basal transcriptional complex. However, it remains clear that Tax-dependent alterations in the expression of cellular genes cannot wholly explain its transforming potential. The recent identification of novel cellular targets of HTLV-1 Tax suggests that other cellular processes which serve critical and pivotal roles in regulating normal cell cycle progression, signal transduction pathways and apoptosis are likely also to be targeted by HTLV-I in its transformation of T-cells leading to the development of adult T-cell leukemia (ATL). This chapter will review some of these studies and discuss the relative contribution of various molecular events towards cellular transfomation.

2. Tax transforms cells *in vitro* and induces tumors *in vivo*

The transforming potential of HTLV-1 Tax has been explored in several independent studies. Tax has been demonstrated not only to initiate the immortalization and transformation of human thymocytes, cord blood lymphocytes and murine fibroblast cells in vitro (Grassmann et al., 1989; Tanaka et al., 1990; Grassmann et al., 1992) but also to maintain the transformed phenotype (Yamaoka et al., 1992). Tax-transformed fibroblast and lymphoid cells induce tumor formation in vivo when injected into nude mice (Tanaka et al., 1990; Yamaoka et al., 1992; Oka et al., 1992). Overexpression of HTLV-1 Tax in transgenic mice can result in the formation of mesenchymal tumors (Nerenberg et al., 1987), salivary and lacrimal gland exocrinopathy (Green et al., 1989), lympadenopathy or splenomegaly (Peebles et al., 1995) and lymphoma or leukemia (Grossman et al., 1995). Additionally, when Tax is deleted from a replication competent HTLV-I proviral genome, the resulting molecular entity shows a loss of transforming potential (Ross et al., 1996).

The descriptive observations that Tax transforms cells *in vitro* and induces tumor formation *in vivo* are clear. Less clear are the molecular mechanisms that lead to the phenotypic changes in cellular proliferation. Initial hypotheses suggest that the transforming capacities of Tax are linked to its transcriptional function(s). Indeed, there have been several compelling studies which delineated the transcriptional activation of genes involved in regulating cell cycle progression by Tax (Uittenbogaard et al., 1995; Akagi et al., 1996; Ressler et al., 1997). However, later it was shown that mutations which abrogate the transcriptional activities of Tax did not result in a concomitant loss of transforming potential (Willems et al., 1992) suggesting that transcriptional activity cannot wholly account for transformation. Indeed, several findings are consistent with non-transcriptional roles for Tax in modulating intracellular signal transduction pathways. Thus, Tax acts synergistically with Ras to immortalize and transform rat fibroblasts in vitro; these cells form tumors when they are injected into nude mice (Pozatti et al., 1990). Recent results further verified that Tax has another role in a separate signal transducing pathway which leads to the activation of Jun-kinase (Jin et al., 1997). Additionally, there is also evidence that direct protein-protein interaction between Tax and cell cycle regulatory proteins results in profound alterations in cell cycle progression (Suzuki et al., 1996; Low et al., 1997; Neuveut et al., 1998; Jin et al., 1998).

3. Dysregulation of normal cell cycle progression by HTLV-1 Tax

A common mechanism employed by from oncoproteins encoded by tumor viruses is the abrogation of cellular tumor suppressor functions (e.g. pRb and p53; McCance, Human Tumor Viruses). Hence, simian virus 40 (SV40) large T antigen, adenovirus E1A and human papillomavirus type 16 (HPV-16) E6 and E7 inactivate tumor suppressor pathways by interacting directly with pRb and p53 (Lane and Crawford, 1979; Linzer and Levine, 1979; Sarnow et al., 1982; Werness et al., 1990; DeCaprio et al., 1988; Whyte et al., 1988; Whyte et al., 1989; Dyson et al., 1989). Consistent with this idea, it has been noted recently that HTLV-1 Tax can similarly target p53 and/or pRb. In these latter instances, Tax binds neither pRb nor p53 directly. Instead, Tax can activate the transcription of the gene for p53 (Uittenbogaard et al., 1995), extend the half-life of the p53 protein (Reid et al., 1993; Akagi et al., 1997; Pise-Masison et al., 1998a), and inhibit p53-dependent gene transcription (Pise-Masison et al., 1998a; 1998b; Mulloy et al.,

1998). Furthermore, Tax can also affect events "upstream" of tumor suppressor functions by directly interacting with critical cellular factors independently involved in two different checkpoints: G1/S transition (Suzuki et al., 1996; Mori, 1997; Low et al., 1997; Neuveut et al. 1998; Lemasson et al., 1998), and the mitotic (M) checkpoint (Jin et al., 1998). Finally, Tax can also alter the expression of genes involved in normal cell cycle control (Akagi et al., 1996; Ressler et al., 1997) or act synergistically with the proteins expressed by these genes (Parker et al., 1996).

4. HTLV-1 Tax binds several cell cycle regulatory proteins

The progression of cells through various checkpoints in the cell cycle is regulated by the activities of distinct cyclin-dependent kinases (cdks) which are activated by phosphorylation and complex formation with specific cyclin partners (Hunter and Pines, 1994; Morgan, 1995; Peter and Herskowitz, 1994; Sherr, 1994; Sherr and Roberts, 1995). The activities of different cdk/cyclin complexes are also regulated by specific cdk inhibitors which act either by binding complexes of cdks/cyclins or displacing cyclins from the cdk/cyclin complex (Hunter and Pine, 1994; Morgan, 1995; Peter and Herskowitz, 1994; Sherr, 1994; Sherr and Roberts, 1995). The primary substrates of activated cdks/cyclins are tumor suppressors such as pRb which when hyperphosphorylated release transcription factors such as E2Fs which activate the transcription and expression of genes involved with S phase progression (Nevins, 1992).

While many tumor viruses perturb cell cycle progression through a direct protein-protein interaction between viral oncoproteins and the cellular tumor suppressors, p53 and pRB , HTLV-1 Tax has been shown to bind neither p53 nor pRb. Instead, Tax binds at least three classes of proteins involved in regulating progression through the cell cycle (Suzuki et al., 1996; Low et al., 1997; Neuveut et al., 1998; Jin et al., 1998). In binding to and inactivating cdk inhibitor, p16INK4a, Tax describes a novel mechanism for cell cycle dysregulation (Suzuki et al., 1996; Low et al., 1997). p16INK4a is a member of a family of cdk inhibitors which include p15INK4b, p18INK4c and p19INK4d that inhibit cdk4 and cdk6 kinases by displacing D-type cyclins from the cdk/cyclin complex (Sherr, 1995). Although all the cdk inhibitors of this family share amino acid homology, Tax interacts specifically with p16INK4a and not with p18INK4c nor with p19INK4d (Low et al., 1997, Neuveut et al., 1998). Through this interaction , Tax inactivates p16INK4a function leading to a net increase in phosphorylation of pRb by cdk4/cyclin D complexes (Suzuki et al., 1996; Low et al., 1997). Thus, Tax releases a p16INK4a-induced cell cycle arrest at the G1/S transition (Low et al., 1997).

There is a p16INK4a-independent mechanism through which Tax dysregulates normal cell cycle control (Neuveut et al., 1998). In this separate route, Tax stimulates the progression of p16INK4a-null cells through the G1/S restriction by means of direct protein-protein interaction with D-type cyclins (Neuveut et al., 1998). In the absence of p16INK4a, this binding between Tax and cyclin Ds leads to increased cdk4 and cdk6 kinase activities, without changing the ambient protein levels of cdk4, cdk6 or D-type cyclins, resulting in hyperphosphorylation of pRb (Neuveut et al., 1998). Hence, Tax might independently stimulate pRb hyperphosphorylation by stabilizing complexes of cdk4/cdk6 with D-type cyclins possibly through a mechanism involving the phosphorylation of D-type cyclins (Neuveut et al., 1998). Hyperphosphorylated pRb poorly sequesters E2F. Thus, indirectly, Tax is envisioned to increase the level of E2F-dependent transcription (although a direct interaction between E2Fs and Tax remains to be formally excluded) (Mori, 1997; Neuveut et al., 1998; Lemasson et al., 1998).

A third class of cell-cycle regulatory proteins targeted by Tax is the human mitotic spindle assembly checkpoint protein, MAD1 (Jin et al., 1998). The mitotic spindle assembly checkpoint serves to guard against aneuploidogenic chromosomal damages. HTLV-1 Tax was shown to interfere with the MAD checkpoint; this interference plausibly leads to the formation of multinucleated and karyotypically abnormal cells (Jin et al., 1998). The recently reported ex vivo tissue culture results are fully consistent with established findings that a significant burden of damaged DNA exist in adult T-cell leukemic (ATL) cells in vivo. Interestingly, in an independent screen of 7, 202 cellular transcripts, human MAD1 was found to be one of thirteen genes which are transcriptionally induced 10 fold or more by p53 (Polyak et al., 1997). Conceivably, then, human MAD1 is a downstream effector of p53 in M phase of the cell cycle (comparable to the p53-induced role served by p21Cip1 in G1/S), and that the identification of hsMAD1 and its perturbation by Tax molecularly explains the previously postulated p53 function in the mitotic phase of the cell cycle.

5. Transcriptional effects of Tax on cellular genes relevant to cell cycle progression

As an activator that can directly activate transcription from a minimal RNA pol II TATAA box (Semmes and Jeang, 1995), it is likely that Tax can directly influence the expression of many cellular genes relevant for cell cycle progression. Indeed, one study reported differences between uninfected and HTLV-1 infected cells for the expression of genes such as cyclins, cdks and cdk inhibitors which are involved in cell cycle progression (Akagi et al., 1996). However, since other studies have failed to detect significant differences in D-type cyclins and cdk4 or cdk6 mRNA or protein levels after singular induction of Tax expression in stable cells lines (Suzuki et al., 1996; Neuveut et al., 1997), it is unclear whether these differences in gene expression are a direct effect of HTLV-1 Tax as opposed to other events that occurred as a consequence of infection by HTLV.

Recently it has become increasingly clear that HTLV-1 Tax can target transcriptionally the p53 tumor suppressor pathway at multiple points. Tax can act downstream of p53 by transactivating genes synergistically with p21Cip1 through kB enhancer elements (Parker et al., 1996). Tax can also act upstream of p53 by repressing basal p53 gene transcription through an E-box enhancer element located in the promoter of the p53 gene (Uittenbogaard et al., 1995). E-box enhancer elements mediate transcriptional activation of the basic helix-loop-helix (bHLH) family of transcription factors including c-Myc, Max and Mad which can regulate cell cycle progression and apoptosis (Fracchini and Penn, 1998; Grandori and Eisenman, 1997). Thus, Tax represses c-Myc transcriptional activation of p53 gene expression and adenoviral major late promoter transcription through the E-box (Uittenbogaard et al., 1995; Semmes et al., 1996), and Tax also represses β-polymerase gene expression (a DNA repair enzyme) through E-box enhancer elements (Jeang et al., 1990). In these regards, the concomitant repression of p53 gene expression and the inactivation of the DNA repair enzyme β-polymerase by HTLV-1 Tax could contribute significantly towards early events in HTLV-1 tumorigenesis.

HTLV-1 Tax also been demonstrated to interact with basal transcription factors such as TATA-binding protein (TBP)(Caron et al., 1993), TFIIA (Clemens et al., 1996) and TAFII28 (Caron et al., 1997) and/or transcriptional coactivators such as the cyclic AMP-response element (CRE) binding protein (CREB) binding protein (CBP) and/or p300 (Kwok et al., 1996; Giebler et al., 1997; Lenzmeier et al., 1998; Bex et al., 1998; Yan et al., 1998; Harrod et al., 1990; Colgin and Nyborg, 1998). Recent studies have identified a requirement for CBP/p300 in mediating p53-dependent transcriptional activation (Somasundaram and El, 1997; Avantaggiati et al., 1997; Gu et al., 1997; Lill et al., 1997) through the acetylation of p53 and the subsequent enhancement of p53 DNA-binding (Gu and Roeder, 1997). Thus another possible mechanism explaining the effects of HTLV-1 Tax on p53-dependent gene transcription would be through an effect on the p53/histone acetylase activities of CBP/p300 (Gu et al., 1997; Ogryzko et al., 1996; Bannister and Kouzarides, 1996).

6. Tax and phosphorylation of proteins

Wild-type p53 protein levels appear to be stabilized in long-term HTLV-1 immortalized/transformed cell cultures (Reid et al., 1995; Akagi et al., 1997) in a Tax-dependent manner (Pise-Masison, et al., 1998). This increase in an HTLV-1 Tax-dependent manner of wild-type p53 was unexpected since this would appear to augment the p53 tumor suppressor pathway. However the wild-type p53 protein in HTLV-1 transformed cell lines was found to be functionally inactive; and it was shown that Tax overexpression inhibited p53-dependent transcriptional activation and p53-induced G1/S cell cycle arrest and apoptosis (Gartenhaus and Wang, 1995; Pise-Masison, et al., 1998; Mulloy et al., 1998). Tax does not bind p53 directly (Gartenhaus and Wang, 1995), nor affect p53 subcellular localization, nor p53 DNA binding (Pise-Masison et al., 1998; Mulloy et al., 1998). A suggested mechanism of p53-inactivation involves a change in the phosphorylation status of p53 by HTLV-1 Tax (Pise-Masison et al., 1998). Thus, it was proposed that changes in the phosphorylation of serines in the amino terminal domain of p53 by HTLV-1 Tax could alter p53 conformation and inhibit interactions between p53 and the basal transcription complex or transcriptional coactivators (Pise-Masison et al., 1998). Although the p53 protein kinase affected by HTLV-1 Tax has not yet been identified, HTLV-1 Tax has recently been found to interact with and alter the kinase activities of a number of different cellular protein kinases such as the protein kinase C isozymes (Lindholm et al., 1996), mitogen-activated protein/extracellular signal-regulated kinase

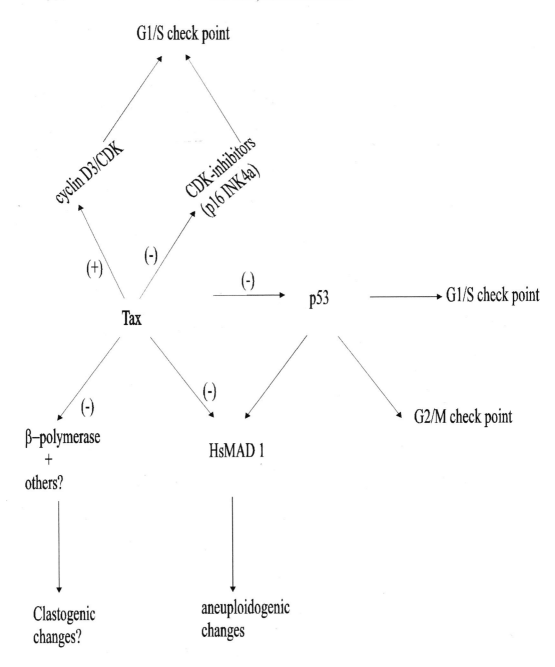

Fig. 1.   Multiple pathways that summarize the effects of Tax on cell-cycle progression and potentially account for Tax- induced clastogenic and/or aneuploidogenic changes. Tax affects cy-
clinD/cdks, cdk inhibitors, and p53. Tax can also directly interfere with chromosome repair or
fidelity of chromosome segregation through •-polymerase or Hsmad 1, respectively. Surveillence
of DNA-fidelity could also be indirectly engendered through suppression of p53 function. It has
been shown by Polyak et al. (1997) that HsMAD1 (Jin et al., 1998) is transcriptionally unregulated by p53.

kinase 1 (MEKK1), the IkB kinase (IKK) complex (Yin et al., 1998; Chu et al., 1998; Geleziunas et al., 1998), and Jun-kinase (Jin et al., 1997). More studies are needed to dissect the independent and inter-related effects of these phosphorylation networks.

7. Concluding remarks

The p53 and pRb tumor suppressor pathways are targeted by many viral oncoproteins. Some of these oncoproteins dysregulate a singular cellular process while others are multifunctional in their action and can dysregulate many cellular processes. HTLV-1 Tax is an excellent example of the latter in not only dysregulating normal cell cycle control by targeting the p53 and pRb tumor suppressor pathways, but also dysregulating cellular transcription as well as cellular signal transduction. Tax targets the p53 and pRb tumor suppressor pathways in a manner distinct from other viral oncoproteins. Whereas many viral oncoproteins target the p53 and pRb by direct binding, Tax appears not to bind directly with either p53 or pRb but acts at many points upstream or downstream of these tumor suppressors. It should be pointed out that while we have focused our discussion to Tax and p53 and pRb here, Tax likely targets additional tumor suppressors. Indeed, Tax was recently shown to also bind to the hDlg/SAP97 tumor suppressor protein (Lee et al., 1997). Relevance of this finding to transformation is supported by the observation that differences in the C-terminal sequences between the transforming Tax protein from HTLV-I versus the non-transforming Tax protein from HTLV-II (Semmes et al., 1996) specifies for association (lack of association) for the hDlg/SAP97 tumor suppressor.

Cellular transformation is thought to be a multiple-step process where single events are insufficient and where multiply linked events lead to tumorigenesis. Thus it is reasonable that there would be an evolutionary selection for multifunctional oncoproteins in tumor viruses. The pleiotropic functions of the Tax protein (see figure 1) would be fully consistent with this evolution. The many aspects of Tax function in adult T-cell leukemia present exciting and important challenges for HTLV researchers.

References

Akagi, T., Ono, H. and Shimotohno, K. 1996. Expression of cell-cycle regulatory genes in HTLV-I infected T-cell lines: possible involvement of Tax1 in the altered expression of cyclin D2, p18Ink4 and p21Waf1/Cip1/Sdi1. Oncogene 12:1645-1652.

Akagi, T., Ono, H., Tsuchida, N. and Shimotohno, K. 1997. Aberrant expression and function of p53 in T-cells immortalized by HTLV-1 Tax1. Febs Lett 406:263-266.

Avantaggiati, M. L., Ogryzko, V., Gardner, K., Giordano, A., Levine, A.S. and Kelly, K.. 1997. Recruitment of p300/CBP in p53-dependent signal pathways. Cell 89:1175-1184.

Bannister, A. J., and T. Kouzarides. 1996. The CBP co-activator is a histone acetyltransferase. Nature 384:641-643.

Beck Jr., G. R., B. R. Zerler, and E. Moran. 1998. Introduction to tumor viruses: adenovirus, simian virus 40 and polyomavirus, p. 51-86. In D. J. McCance (ed.), Human Tumor Viruses, Second ed. ASM Press, Washington DC.

Bex, F., M. J. Yin, A. Burny, and R. B. Gaynor. 1998. Differential transcriptional activation by human T-cell leukemia virus type 1 Tax mutants is mediated by distinct interactions with CREB binding protein and p300. Mol Cell Biol 18:2392-2405.

Cann, A. J., and I. S. Y. Chen. 1995. Human T-cell leukemia virus types I and II, p. 1849-1880. In B. N. Fields, D. M. Knipe, P. M. Howley, R. M. Chanock, J. L. Melnick, T. P. Monath, B. Roizman, and S. E. Straus (ed.), Virology, Second ed, vol. 2. Lippincott-Raven Publishers, Philadelphia.

Caron, C., G. Mengus, V. Dubrowskaya, A. Roisin, I. Davidson, and P. Jalinot. 1997. Human TAF(II)28 interacts with the human T cell leukemia virus type I Tax transactivator and promotes its transcriptional activity. Proc Natl Acad Sci U S A 94:3662-7.

Caron, C., R. Rousset, C. Beraud, V. Moncollin, J. M. Egly, and P. Jalinot. 1993. Functional and biochemical interaction of the HTLV-I Tax1 transactivator with TBP. Embo J 12:4269-78.

Chu, Z. L., J. A. DiDonato, J. Hawiger, and D. W. Ballard. 1998. The tax oncoprotein of human T-cell leukemia virus type 1 associates with and persistently activates IkappaB kinases containing IKKalpha and IKKbeta. J Biol Chem 273:15891-4.

Clemens, K. E., G. Piras, M. F. Radonovich, K. S. Choi, J. F. Duvall, J. DeJong, R. Roeder, and J. N. Brady. 1996. Interaction of the human T-cell lymphotropic virus type 1 tax transactivator with transcription factor IIA. Mol Cell Biol 16:4656-64.

Colgin, M. A., and J. K. Nyborg. 1998. The human T-cell leukemia virus type 1 oncoprotein Tax inhibits the transcriptional activity of c-Myb through competition for the CREB binding protein. J Virol 72:9396-9.

DeCaprio, J. A., J. W. Ludlow, J. Figge, J. Y. Shew, C. M. Huang, W. H. Lee, E. Marsilio, E. Paucha, and D. M. Livingston. 1988. SV40 large tumor antigen forms a specific complex with the product of the retinoblastoma susceptibility gene. Cell 54:275-83.

Dyson, N., P. M. Howley, K. Munger, and E. Harlow. 1989. The human papilloma virus-16 E7 oncoprotein is able to bind to the retinoblastoma gene product. Science 243:934-7.

Francchini, L. M., and L. Z. Penn. 1998. The molecular role of Myc in growth and transformation: recent discoveries lead to new insights. Faseb J 12:633-51.

Gartenhaus, R. B., and P. Wang. 1995. Functional inactivation of wild-type p53 protein correlates with loss of IL-2 dependence in HTLV-I transformed human T lymphocytes. Leukemia 9:2082-6.

Geleziunas, R., S. Ferrell, X. Lin, Y. Mu, E. J. Cunningham, M. Grant, M. A. Connelly, J. E. Hambor, K. B. Marcu, and W. C. Greene. 1998. Human T-cell leukemia virus type 1 Tax induction of NF-kappaB involves activation of the IkappaB kinase alpha (IKKalpha) and IKKbeta cellular kinases. Mol Cell Biol 18:5157-65.

Giebler, H. A., J. E. Loring, O. K. van, M. A. Colgin, J. E. Garrus, K. W. Escudero, A. Brauweiler, and J. K. Nyborg. 1997. Anchoring of CREB binding protein to the human T-cell leukemia virus type 1 promoter: a molecular mechanism of Tax transactivation. Mol Cell Biol 17:5156-64.

Franklin, A.A., and Nyborg, J.K. 1995. Mechanisms of Tax regulation of human T cell leukemia virus type I gene expression. J. Biomed. Sci. 2: 17-29.

Gitlin, S. D., J. Dittmer, R. L. Reid, and J. N. Brady. 1993. The molecular biology of human T-cell leukemia viruses, p. 159-192. In B. R. Cullen (ed.), Human Retroviruses. Oxford University Press, New York.

Grandori, C., and R. N. Eisenman. 1997. Myc target genes. Trends Biochem Sci 22:177-81.

Grassmann, R., S. Berchtold, I. Radant, M. Alt, B. Fleckenstein, J. G. Sodroski, W. A. Haseltine, and U. Ramstedt. 1992. Role of human T-cell leukemia virus type 1 X region proteins in immortalization of primary human lymphocytes in culture. J Virol 66:4570-5.

Grassmann, R., C. Dengler, F. I. Muller, B. Fleckenstein, K. McGuire, M. C. Dokhelar, J. G. Sodroski, and W. A. Haseltine. 1989. Transformation to continuous growth of primary human T lymphocytes by human T-cell leukemia virus type I X-region genes transduced by a Herpesvirus saimiri vector. Proc Natl Acad Sci U S A 86:3351-5.

Green, J. E., S. H. Hinrichs, J. Vogel, and G. Jay. 1989. Exocrinopathy resembling Sjogren's syndrome in HTLV-1 tax transgenic mice. Nature 341:72-4.

Grossman, W. J., J. T. Kimata, F. H. Wong, M. Zutter, T. J. Ley, and L. Ratner. 1995. Development of leukemia in mice transgenic for the tax gene of human T- cell leukemia virus type I. Proc Natl Acad Sci U S A 92:1057-61.

Gu, W., and R. G. Roeder. 1997. Activation of p53 sequence-specific DNA binding by acetylation of the p53 C-terminal domain. Cell 90:595-606.

Gu, W., X. L. Shi, and R. G. Roeder. 1997. Synergistic activation of transcription by CBP and p53. Nature 387:819-23.

Harrod, R., Y. Tang, C. Nicot, H. S. Lu, A. Vassilev, Y. Nakatani, and C. Z. Giam. 1998. An exposed KID-like domain in human T-cell lymphotropic virus type 1 Tax is responsible for the recruitment of coactivators CBP/p300. Mol Cell Biol 18:5052-61.

Hunter, T., and J. Pines. 1994. Cyclins and cancer. II: Cyclin D and CDK inhibitors come of age. Cell 79:573-82.

Jeang, K. T., S. G. Widen, O. J. Semmes, and S. H. Wilson. 1990. HTLV-I trans-activator protein, tax, is a trans-repressor of the human beta-polymerase gene. Science 247:1082-4.

Jin, D. Y., F. Spencer, and K. T. Jeang. 1998. Human T cell leukemia virus type 1 oncoprotein Tax targets the human mitotic checkpoint protein MAD1. Cell 93:81-91.

Jin, D.-Y., Teramoto, H., Giam, C. Z., Chun, R. F., Gutkind, J. S., and Jeang, K.- T. 1997. A human suppressor of c-Jun N-terminal kinase 1 (JNK1)-activation by tumor necrosis factor-alpha. *J. Biol. Chem.* 272, 25816-25823.

Kwok, R. P., M. E. Laurance, J. R. Lundblad, P. S. Goldman, H. Shih, L. M. Connor, S. J. Marriott, and R. H. Goodman. 1996. Control of cAMP-regulated enhancers by the viral transactivator Tax through CREB and the co-activator CBP. Nature 380:642-6.

Lane, D. P., and L. V. Crawford. 1979. T antigen is bound to a host protein in SV40-transformed cells. Nature 278:261-3.

Lee, S., Weiss, R.S., and Javier, R. T. 1997. Binding of hman virus oncoproteins to hDlg/SAP97, a mammalian homolog of the Drosophila discs large tumor suppressor protein. Proc. Natl. Acad. Sci. USA 94: 6670-6675

Lemasson, I., S. Thebault, C. Sardet, C. Devaux, and J. M. Mesnard. 1998. Activation of E2F-mediated transcription by human T-cell leukemia virus type I Tax protein in a p16(INK4A)-negative T-cell line. J Biol Chem 273:23598-604.

Lenzmeier, B. A., H. A. Giebler, and J. K. Nyborg. 1998. Human T-cell leukemia virus type 1 Tax requires direct access to DNA for recruitment of CREB binding protein to the viral promoter. Mol Cell Biol 18:721-31.

Lill, N. L., S. R. Grossman, D. Ginsberg, J. DeCaprio, and D. M. Livingston. 1997. Binding and modulation of p53 by p300/CBP coactivators. Nature 387:823-7.

Lindholm, P. F., M. Tamami, J. Makowski, and J. N. Brady. 1996. Human T-cell lymphotropic virus type 1 Tax1 activation of NF-kappa B: involvement of the protein kinase C pathway. J Virol 70:2525-32.

Linzer, D. I., and A. J. Levine. 1979. Characterization of a 54K dalton cellular SV40 tumor antigen present in SV40-transformed cells and uninfected embryonal carcinoma cells. Cell 17:43-52.

Low, K. G., L. F. Dorner, D. B. Fernando, J. Grossman, K. T. Jeang, and M. J. Comb. 1997. Human T-cell leukemia virus type 1 Tax releases cell cycle arrest induced by p16INK4a. J Virol 71:1956-62.

Morgan, D. O. 1995. Principles of CDK regulation. Nature 374:131-4.

Mori, N. 1997. High levels of the DNA-binding activity of E2F in adult T-cell leukemia and human T-cell leukemia virus type I-infected cells: possible enhancement of DNA-binding of E2F by the human T-cell leukemia virus I transactivating protein, Tax. Eur J Haematol 58:114-20.

Mulloy, J. C., T. Kislyakova, A. Cereseto, L. Casareto, A. LoMonico, J. Fullen, M. V. Lorenzi, A. Cara, C. Nicot, C. Giam, and G. Franchini. 1998. Human T-cell lymphotropic/leukemia virus type 1 Tax abrogates p53- induced cell cycle arrest and apoptosis through its CREB/ATF functional domain. J Virol 72:8852-60.

Nead, M. A., and D. J. McCance. 1998. Activities of the transforming proteins of human papillomaviruses, p. 223-250. *In* D. J. McCance (ed.), Human Tumor Viruses, Second ed. ASM Press, Washington DC.

Nerenberg, M., S. H. Hinrichs, R. K. Reynolds, G. Khoury, and G. Jay. 1987. The tat gene of human T-lymphotropic virus type 1 induces mesenchymal tumors in transgenic mice. Science 237:1324-9.

Neuveut, C., K. G. Low, F. Maldarelli, I. Schmitt, F. Majone, R. Grassmann, and K. T. Jeang. 1998. Human T-cell leukemia virus type 1 Tax and cell cycle progression: role of cyclin D-cdk and p110Rb. Mol Cell Biol 18:3620-32.

Nevins, J. R. 1992. E2F: a link between the Rb tumor suppressor protein and viral oncoproteins. Science 258:424-9.

Nevins, J. R., and P. K. Vogt. 1995. Cellular transformation by viruses, p. 301-344. *In* B. N. Fields, D. M. Knipe, P. M. Howley, R. M. Chanock, J. L. Melnick, T. P. Monath, B. Roizman, and S. E. Straus (ed.), Virology, Second ed, vol. 2. Lippincott-Raven Publishers, Philadelphia.

Ogryzko, V. V., R. L. Schiltz, V. Russanova, B. H. Howard, and Y. Nakatani. 1996. The transcriptional coactivators p300 and CBP are histone acetyltransferases. Cell 87:953-9.

Oka, T., H. Sonobe, J. Iwata, I. Kubonishi, H. Satoh, M. Takata, Y. Tanaka, M. Tateno, H. Tozawa, S. Mori, T. Yoshiki, and Y. Ohtsuki. 1992. Phenotypic progression of a rat lymphoid cell line immortalized by human T-lymphotropic virus type 1 to induce lymphoma/leukemia-like disease in rats. J Virol 66:6686-6694.

Parker, S. F., N. D. Perkins, S. D. Gitlin, and G. J. Nabel. 1996. A cooperative interaction of human T-cell leukemia virus type 1 Tax with the p21 cyclin-dependent kinase inhibitor activates the human immunodeficiency virus type 1 enhancer. J Virol 70:5731-4.

Peebles, R. S., C. R. Maliszewski, T. A. Sato, H. J. Hanley, I. G. Maroulakou, R. Hunziker, J. P. Schneck, and J. E. Green. 1995. Abnormal B-cell function in HTLV-I-tax transgenic mice. Oncogene 10:1045-51.

Peter, M., and I. Herskowitz. 1994. Joining the complex: cyclin-dependent kinase inhibitory proteins and the cell cycle. Cell 79:181-4.

Pise, M. C., K. S. Choi, M. Radonovich, J. Dittmer, S. J. Kim, and J. N. Brady. 1998a. Inhibition of p53 transactivation function by the human T-cell lymphotropic virus type 1 Tax protein. J Virol 72:1165-70.

Pise, M. C., M. Radonovich, K. Sakaguchi, E. Appella, and J. N. Brady. 1998b. Phosphorylation of p53: a novel pathway for p53 inactivation in human T- cell lymphotropic virus type 1-transformed cells. J Virol 72:6348-55.

Polyak, K., Y. Xia, J. L. Zweier, K. W. Kinzler, and B. Vogelstein. 1997. A model for p53-induced apoptosis . Nature 389:300-5.

Pozzatti, R., J. Vogel, and G. Jay. 1990. The human T-lymphotropic virus type I tax gene can cooperate with the ras oncogene to induce neoplastic transformation of cells. Mol Cell Biol 10:413-7.

Reid, R. L., P. F. Lindholm, A. Mireskandari, J. Dittmer, and J. N. Brady. 1993. Stabilization of wild-type p53 in human T-lymphocytes transformed by HTLV-I. Oncogene 8:3029-36.

Ressler, S., G. F. Morris, and S. J. Marriott. 1997. Human T-cell leukemia virus type 1 Tax transactivates the human proliferating cell nuclear antigen promoter. J Virol 71:1181-90.

Ross, T. M., S. M. Pettiford, and P. L. Green. 1996. The tax gene of human T-cell leukemia virus type 2 is essential for transformation of human T lymphocytes. J Virol 70:5194-202.

Sarnow, P., Y. S. Ho, J. Williams, and A. J. Levine. 1982. Adenovirus E1b-58kd tumor antigen and SV40 large tumor antigen are physically associated with the same 54 kd cellular protein in transformed cells. Cell 28:387-94.

Schulz, T. F., Y. Chang, and P. S. Moore. 1998. Kaposi's sarcoma-associated herpesvirus (human herpesvirus 8), p. 87-132. *In* D. J. McCance (ed.), Human Tumor Viruses, Second ed. ASM Press, Washington DC.

Semmes, O. J., J. F. Barret, C. V. Dang, and K. T. Jeang. 1996. Human T-cell leukemia virus type I tax masks c-Myc function through a cAMP-dependent pathway. J Biol Chem 271:9730-8.

Semmes, O. J., Majone. F., Cantemir, C., Turchetto, L., Hjelle, B. and Jeang, K-T. 1996. HTLV-I and HTLV-II Tax: differences in induction of micronuclei in cells and transcriptional activation of viral LTRs. *Virology,* 217: 373-379.

Semmes, OJ, and Jeang, K-T. 1995. Definition of a minimal activation domain in HTLV-I Tax. *J. Virol.,* 69: 1827-1833

Sherr, C. J. 1995. D-type cyclins. Trends Biochem Sci 20:187-90.

Sherr, C. J. 1994. G1 phase progression: cycling on cue. Cell 79:551-5.

Sherr, C. J., and J. M. Roberts. 1995. Inhibitors of mammalian G1 cyclin-dependent kinases. Genes Dev 9:1149-63.

Somasundaram, K., and D. W. El. 1997. Inhibition of p53-mediated transactivation and cell cycle arrest by E1A through its p300/CBP-interacting region. Oncogene 14:1047-57.

Suzuki, T., S. Kitao, H. Matsushime, and M. Yoshida. 1996. HTLV-1 Tax protein interacts with cyclin-dependent kinase inhibitor p16INK4A and counteracts its inhibitory activity towards CDK4. Embo J 15:1607-14.

Tanaka, A., C. Takahashi, S. Yamaoka, T. Nosaka, M. Maki, and M. Hatanaka. 1990. Oncogenic transformation by the tax gene of human T-cell leukemia virus type I in vitro. Proc Natl Acad Sci U S A 87:1071-5.

Uittenbogaard, M. N., H. A. Giebler, D. Reisman, and J. K. Nyborg. 1995. Transcriptional repression of p53 by human T-cell leukemia virus type I Tax protein. J Biol Chem 270:28503-6.

Werness, B. A., A. J. Levine, and P. M. Howley. 1990. Association of human papillomavirus types 16 and 18 E6 proteins with p53. Science 248:76-9.

Whyte, P., K. J. Buchkovich, J. M. Horowitz, S. H. Friend, M. Raybuck, R. A. Weinberg, and E. Harlow. 1988. Association between an oncogene and an anti-oncogene: the adenovirus E1A proteins bind to the retinoblastoma gene product. Nature 334:124-9.

Whyte, P., N. M. Williamson, and E. Harlow. 1989. Cellular targets for transformation by the adenovirus E1A proteins. Cell 56:67-75.

Willems, L., C. Grimonpont, H. Heremans, N. Rebeyrotte, G. Chen, D. Portetelle, A. Burny, and R. Kettmann. 1992. Mutations in the bovine leukemia virus Tax protein can abrogate the long terminal repeat-directed transactivating activity without concomitant loss of transforming potential. Proc Natl Acad Sci U S A 89:3957-61.

Yamaoka, S., T. Tobe, and M. Hatanaka. 1992. Tax protein of human T-cell leukemia virus type I is required for maintenance of the transformed phenotype. Oncogene 7:433-7.

Yan, J. P., J. E. Garrus, H. A. Giebler, L. A. Stargell, and J. K. Nyborg. 1998. Molecular interactions between the coactivator CBP and the human T-cell leukemia virus Tax protein. J Mol Biol 281:395-400.

Yin, M. J., L. B. Christerson, Y. Yamamoto, Y. T. Kwak, S. Xu, F. Mercurio, M. Barbosa, M. H. Cobb, and R. B. Gaynor. 1998. HTLV-I Tax protein binds to MEKK1 to stimulate IkappaB kinase activity and NF-kappaB activation. Cell 93:875-84.

PROVIRAL TAGGING: A STRATEGY USING RETROVIRUSES
TO IDENTIFY ONCOGENES

Tarik Möröy[1], Martin Zörnig[2] and Thorsten Schmidt[1]

[1]Institut für Zellbiologie, Universitätsklinikum Essen, Germany
[2]Biochemistry of the Cell Nucleus Laboratory, Imperial Cancer Research Fund, London

Introduction

Retrovirus infection can be the cause of a number of malignant diseases in animals with a few selected cases in humans. Retroviruses can elicit diseases in the course of a natural infection but also under experimental conditions in the laboratory. In contrast to many other viruses retroviral infections do not provoke the death of their host cells but rather establish a latent infection and assure viral multiplication through a chronic infection of susceptible host cells. The oncogenic activity of retroviruses and the potency by which they can malignantly transform cells depends on the presence of an oncogene in their genome. Viruses that do not contain oncogenes transform host cells slowly i.e. with a long latency period and are termed "non acute transforming retroviruses". In contrast, viruses with oncogenes are able to provoke tumor formation quickly in their hosts and can be designated "acute transforming retroviruses".

The ability of retroviruses to establish themselves persistently in a host cell and the fact that they can principally infect a wide range of host cells has made them an ideal tool for the manipulation of eukaryotic cells and even whole organisms. In addition retroviruses are readily amenable to experimental manipulation and have considerable tolerance to foreign genetic material incorporated into their genome. For these reasons retroviruses are now established as an experimental tool suitable for the investigation of the molecular processes that underlie oncogenesis and development. Retroviruses have also been used as vectors to introduce and express foreign genes in eukaryotic cells. Today a large number of different retroviral vectors are routinely used in molecular biology labs. Most of them are derived from defective strains that can only be produced with helper cells and infect the target cell once without producing new virus from the final target cell of interest. This strategy allowed the establishment of retroviral vectors as safe molecular tools to alter the genetic information of target cells. Recently, retroviral vectors have been at the center of attention for the design of vehicles for human gene therapy. Retroviruses have also been used to infect stem cells and even whole early murine embryos to be able to trace differentiation lineages. This review will focus on the use of retroviruses as insertional mutagens and in particular the use of the non acute transforming retrovirus MoMuLV for the induction of lymphoid malignancies in mice which has been shown to be a powerful method to identify new oncogenes and to gain more insight into the molecular wiring that underlies oncogene cooperation.

Table 1: Classification of retroviridae

Oncoviridae	Type B:	<u>murine:</u>
		Mouse mammary tumor viruses (MMTV)
	Type C:	<u>avian:</u>
		Rous sarcoma virus (RSV)
		Rous associated viruses (RAV)
		Leukosis viruses (ALV)
		Reticuloendotheliosis viruses
		Pheasant viruses
		<u>mammalian:</u>
		Murine sarcoma viruses (MSV)
		Murine leukemia viruses (MuLV, e.g. AKR type)
		Murine leukemia viruses (Moloney, Friend, Rauscher)
		Feline leukemia viruses (FeLV)
		Gippon ape leukemia virus (GALV)
		Simian sarcoma viruses (SSV)
		Baboon endogenous virus (BaEV)
		Human T-cell leukemia viruses (HTLV-I, -II)
		Bovine leukemia viruses (BLV)
		Ape T-lymphotrophic viruses (STLV-I)
		<u>reptilian:</u>
		Viper virus
	Type D	<u>mammalian:</u>
		Mason- Pfizer-Monkey virus (MPMV)
		Langur virus
		Squirrel Monkey virus
		Sheep pulmonary adenomatosis
Lentiviridae		<u>mammalian:</u>
		Visna virus of sheep
		Maedi virus
		Human immunodeficiency viruses (HIV)
		Simian immunodeficiency viruses (SIV)
Spumaviridae		<u>mammalian:</u>
		Simian foamy viruses (SFV)
		Human foamy viruses

Source: (Davis *et al.,*1980)

Retroviruses

Morphology

Retroviruses are viruses of eukaryotes that carry as a genome two identical, single (+) stranded RNA molecules that are connected to each other by hydrogen bonds at their 5'-ends. Both RNA strands carry a cellular t-RNA molecule that is attached to their primer binding sites (PBS). The length of the viral RNA genome varies between 2 and 10 kb (for a review see Varmus, 1988). Retroviruses are spherical with a diameter of about 80-130 nm and are made up of a complex of ribonucleoproteins, a nucleocapsid and an outer envelope (Davis et al., 1980; Fig. 1). The virus core contains the diploid RNA genome as well as the viral-encoded reverse transcriptase, which is a RNA-dependent DNA polymerase, and two other enzymes- an integrase and a protease. The outer envelope membrane is provided by the infected host cell during the budding process of the viral core. The host cell membrane also contains the viral Env glycoproteins that form the so called "spikes" on the outer side of the virion (Bolognesi et al., 1978, Fig. 1). All the virus proteins are encoded by its RNA genome. The three open reading frames *gag*, *pol*, *env* that can be found in all non defective retroviruses encode precursor proteins that are subsequently processed by a viral protease to give rise to the different envelope and core constituents (Fig. 1, for a detailed description see Davis et al., 1980 or Varmus, 1982; 1988).

Classification

Retroviruses are today grouped into 3 subfamilies (Table 1), oncoviridae, lentiviridae and spumaviridae. The biggest subgroup are the oncoviridae which are further subdivided in to types B, C, and D. The systematics of retroviridae is in general based on morphological criteria and on data obtained from electrophotomicrographs, on serology and on host range. One important difference among oncoviridae is their degree of oncogenicity. Those viruses which carry only their structural genes namely *gag*, *pol* and *env* (see below) are non acute oncogenic viruses and induce tumors in their host only after a considerable latency period. In contrast, acute transforming oncoviruses quickly induce tumors and have a different organization of their genome. They carry altered cellular sequences called "oncogenes" in their genome that account for their increased ability to provoke tumor outgrowth. Classical examples are the RSV that carries the v-*src* gene or the Abelson virus which is a derivative of the MoMuLV and carries the gene for the v-Abl kinase. In addition, the v-*myc* oncogene was discovered when a specific strain of ALV the myelocytomatosis virus MC29 was analyzed (for a review see Varmus, 1988). Experiments with retroviruses and their detailed analysis were the basis of the concept of proto-oncogenes and oncogene activation as we know it today.

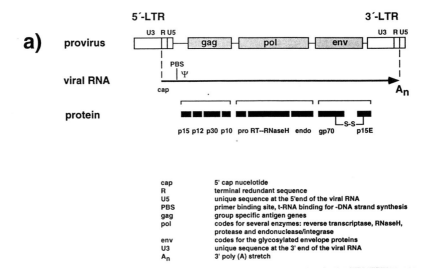

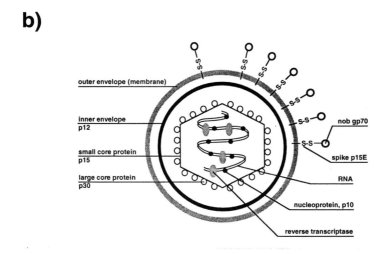

Figure 1. (a) Schematic representation of the retroviral genome and the three open reading frames gag, *pol and* env *representative of a murine leukemia virus (MuLV). All three reading frames can give rise to different proteins that are represented by black bars underneath (see also Davis et al., 1980). The viral RNA molecule is shown as a black arrow. It is transcribed from the integrated provirus. The 5' end is generated at the transcription initiation site (TATA box) within the 5' LTR at the boundary between U3 and R. Termination of this genomic viral RNA takes place at the polyadenylation site in the 3' LTR. The polyadenylation site in the 5' LTR that immediately follows the promotor in the R region is read through. (For details of the viral LTR see Fig. 4). (b) Assembly of the different part of a retrovirus (Davis et al., 1980).*

Structure of the Retroviral Genome

All retroviruses that are competent to replicate without any helper virus have an RNA genome that is similar in structure to that shown in Figure 1. The viral RNA has features of a eukaryotic mRNA molecule because it possesses a cap structure at its 5'-end, a poly (A) sequence at its 3'-end and methylated bases. After the virus has penetrated the membrane of its host cell (see Fig. 2) its genomic RNA is reverse transcribed by the viral encoded polymerase and gives rise to a double stranded complementary DNA molecule that is integrated as a "provirus" into the host genome (Fig. 2 and also below). Due to the specific replication mechanism of retroviruses (see below) the provirus has a particular structure: The U3, R and U5 sequences form two identical "long terminal repeats" (LTRs) which flank the proviral genome on both ends (Fig. 1). Transcription starts at the transition from the U3 region to the sequence in the 5' LTR (Fig. 1, 4). The R sequence is important for the reverse transcription and the viral replication cycle whereas the U3 region contains the transcriptional control elements (see below). The 5' non-coding part of proviral mRNA immediately upstream of the *gag* open reading frame is a leader sequence that also contains the primer binding site for the t-RNA molecule responsible for the initial step of the viral replication cycle. In addition, in this region a sequence called Ψ is localized that is essential for the packaging of viral RNA into viral particles. The regions designated *gag*, *pol* and *env* code for all viral proteins; the *gag* and Pol proteins are translated from the viral RNA and the Env protein from a subgenomic DNA that is generated by alternative splicing. A number of different proteins can be generated upon translation of the genetic information that is stored in the viral genomic mRNA. The three open reading frames *gag, pol* and *env* give rise to the proteins that are depicted in Fig.1. This is achieved by translating larger proteins from the open reading frames and subsequent proteolytic processing of these precursors into the different polypeptides that make up the envelope, the core and the different enzymes of the virus (for more detailed descriptions of this process see Davis, 1980; Varmus, 1988; Bolognesi, 1978).

The *pol* open reading frame encodes the viral reverse transcriptase which is a RNA dependent DNA polymerase and is responsible for the generation of a double stranded DNA molecule from the single stranded RNA template. Moreover this protein also contains a RNase H activity. This activity is necessary to degrade the RNA:DNA hybrids that are intermediate products in the generation of the double stranded viral genomic DNA molecule. The 3' part of the *pol* frame encodes an endonuclease/integrase (Fig. 1) that is necessary for the integration of the double stranded DNA molecule generated from the RNA genome into the host genomic DNA. (Schwartzberg et al., 1984; Donehower and Varmus, 1984; Panganiban and Temin, 1984).

The Retroviral Life Cycle

The life cycle of a retrovirus comprises the penetration of the virion into a host cell, the synthesis of a new proviral DNA and its integration into the genome using the activities

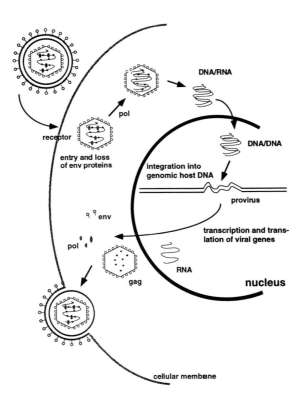

Figure 2.   The retroviral life cycle: The entry of the virus into the host cell is mediated by a receptor on the cellular membrane. Entry of the virus is accompanied with the loss of the Env proteins and is followed by the replication of the RNA genome by the viral enzyme reverse transcriptase. The DNA/RNA hybrid is converted into an DNA/DNA hybrid and imported into the nucleus where it integrates as a provirus. Transcription and expression of proviral DNA leads to new synthesis of viral proteins and the packaging of two copies of the genomic RNA into new virions that bud at the cell surface to give rise to new viruses.

encoded within the *pol* open reading frame (see above). Also part of the cycle is the expression of the viral genes i.e. transcription and translation of the viral genome using the integrated provirus as template. Finally, the subsequent modification of the viral proteins, their maturation and the budding of the new virion through the host cell membrane completes the cycle (Fig. 2).

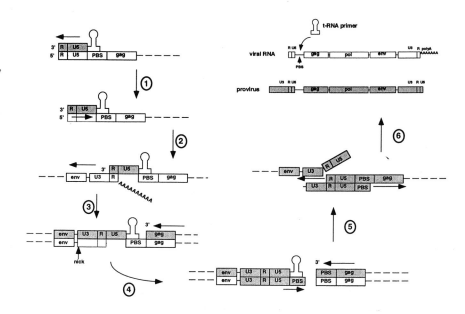

Figure 3. Schematic representation of the different steps during the replication cycle of the viral RNA genome (details see text).

Replication

After the penetration of the virion into host cells, its uncoating and partial lysis of nu-cleoproteins by cellular proteases, the RNA genome of the virus will be reverse tran-scribed into a double stranded DNA molecule. The enzyme reverse transcriptase that catalyses all the necessary steps needs a primer to initiate the DNA synthesis. This is provided by a cellular t-RNA molecule which is carried along by the virus from the previously infected cell. The t-RNA molecule remains attached to a short nucleotide sequence 5' of the *gag* sequences (primer binding site, PBS; see Fig. 1, 3). New DNA synthesis starts from here in the direction of the 5'-end of the genomic viral RNA mole-cule (see Fig. 3 and Davis et al., 1980 for a detailed description). To be able to elongate the (-) DNA strand further the RNA:DNA hybrid is degraded by the intrinsic RNase H activity of the reverse transcriptase molecule (Fig. 3-1). The R-region of the newly syn-thesized (-) DNA strand is now able to hybridize with the R-region at the 3'-end of the RNA molecule resulting in a cyclic intermediate (Fig. 3-2). The synthesis of the (-) DNA strand is continued from the 3'-end to the 5'-end of the RNA strand until the primer binding site is reached (Fig. 3-3). The RNase H activity now introduces a nick into the original RNA molecule at the 5'-end of the U3 region and is degraded towards the 3'-end. Using the residual RNA molecule as a primer the reverse transcriptase syn-

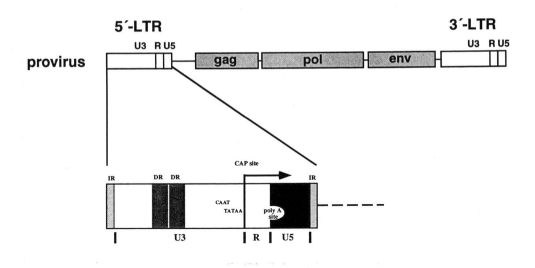

Figure 4. The LTR sequence of a MuLV: the different regions and transcriptional control sequences are described in the text; IR: inverted repeat, DR: direct repeat.

thesizes from the position of the nick the (+) DNA strand up to the primer binding site PBS; the residual RNA molecule and the t-RNA are degraded at the same time (see Fig. 3-5). Hybridization of the PBS sequence on the (+) DNA strand with the complementary sequence on the (-) DNA strand allows a complete synthesis of both DNA strands in 5' to 3' direction (Fig. 3-6).

Integration

After reverse transcription, linear and double stranded DNA will be transported into the nucleus and integrated into the host chromosomal DNA. This is either achieved directly as is described for MoMuLV, or via a circular intermediate depending on the particular viral strain (Fujiwara and Mizuuchi 1988; Panganiban and Temin 1984a,b). Once integrated, the proviral DNA behaves like a cellular gene and remains part of the chromosome thereby conferring on the host a status as a life long carrier of retroviral DNA. For the spleen necrosis virus (SNV) which integrates its proviral DNA by a circular intermediate the 12 terminal base pairs are of the U3 region and the 8 terminal base pairs of the U5 region are essential for the integration via a ring structure with the two LTRs present (Panganiban and Temin, 1984). In this case the double stranded DNA is circularized via the short inverted repeat (IR) sequences at the LTRs (see Fig. 4). Thus a palindromic sequence is generated that is recognized as a substrate by the p46 integrase which endonucleolytically cleaves the proviral DNA two bases before the ends of the repeats i.e. of the LTR sequence-4 bases will be lost upon integration. The integrase cleaves the chromosomal host DNA at random and during the integration of the proviral DNA 4-6 bases at the integration site will be duplicated (Temin, 1980). The integration does not require specific sites in the chromosomal host DNA; it is considered to be completely random. Although there is speculation that integration occurs preferentially at transcribed sequences or within or near DNase hypersensitive sites, but definite proof for this is still lacking.

Control of Retroviral Gene Expression

The expression of viral genes and the production of viral proteins depends on cellular enzymes but the transcriptional control elements that are located in the LTR sequences have a key role in this process. All the important transcriptional regulatory sequences are located in the U3 region of the LTRs (Fig. 4). Transcriptional initiation occurs at the transition between the U3 and R regions (Fig. 4, "Cap" site); a TATA box is situated 25-30 nucleotides upstream of this site whilst a CAAT box further 20-70 bp 5' constitutes a classical RNA polymerase II promotor (Fig. 4). Further upstream of this location and contained in the direct repeated sequences (DR) the enhancer elements are located (Fig. 4). These enhancers are 30-100 bp long tandem-like repeated nucleotide sequences which affect, independently, of their position or orientation, the efficiency of transcription. A number of eukaryotic expression vectors make use of these structures employing the whole LTR unit to drive expression of foreign genes in mammalian cells. The fact that these enhancers act in a position- and orientation-independent fashion can lead to the transcriptional activation of host genes that are located in the vicinity of the integrated provirus. This particular effect of retroviral integration can have dramatic consequences when a host gene whose product governs such essential cellular processes as growth, proliferation or cell death (see also below) is activated.

Another level of control that regulates the expression of retroviral genes occurs during RNA synthesis and translation and is achieved through terminal suppression of RNA translation or ribosomal frameshifting (Varmus, 1982). Thus, the Gag and Pol proteins are translated from a single genomic RNA, whereas the Env proteins are translated from a subgenomic RNA molecule. In the murine leukemia viruses the *gag* and *pol* genes are separated by a stop codon, in RSV and HIV they are encoded by different reading frames, in the MMTV and the HTLV subtypes both are separated by a third open reading frame that encodes a viral protease (Varmus, 1988).

Retroviruses in Malignant Transformation

Retroviruses can induce a wide variety of malignant diseases in their respective hosts as well as conditions of immundeficiency in humans and primates (HIV, SIV). A large number of retroviral strains are responsible for neoplasia in the hematopoietic system among them malignant T- and B- cell lymphoma, erythroleukemia or myeloid leukemias. Of critical importance for the course of the disease is the presence of an oncogene in the retroviral genome. Viruses that carry v-*onc* sequences induce diseases in their hosts that manifest after a short latency periods (usually days to weeks). Moreover retroviruses carrying oncogenes are able to malignantly transform cells *in vitro* which is not possible with non-acute transforming retroviruses that lack v-*onc* sequences (Weiss et al., 1982). The viral *onc* sequences are mutated versions of cellular proto-oncogenes that have gained some notoriety since their discovery in the late 70's and early 80's. The most studied representatives are Ras, Myc, Abl and Src (Hunter, 1991). The function of these oncoproteins as G-proteins, transcription factors and kinases, respectively have attracted a lot of attention and have been the target of intense investigation in many laboratories. The alterations of the cellular sequences have been recognized as critical for the transforming properties of the v-*onc* sequences. Point mutations, partial deletions of coding regions and in particular the fusion with the *gag* open reading frame have been identified as critical mechanisms for the activation of a cellular proto-*onc* sequence to a viral *onc* gene.

Viruses without v-*onc* sequences induce tumors with a long latency period (several months) and are unable to transform cells in culture. Thus, the infection per se represents only one of several steps in the process of tumorigenesis. Among the viruses that fall under the group of "non-acute transforming viruses" are, for instance, ALV which can induce bursal B-cell lymphomas in chicken as well as the Moloney and Friend substrains of the murine leukemia ·viruses (MoMuLV and FMuLV). Whereas MoMuLV induces T-cell lymphomas that are typically located in the thymus of affected animals the Friend viruses can cause splenic erythroleukemia. Interestingly, studies using "swap mutants" from both viruses have shown that differences in the LTR sequences of both strains are responsible for the tissue tropism of MoMuLv and FMuLV (Lowy, 1986). In this multistep process evidence for viral infection occurs well before the final stage tumors appear (Weiss et al., 1982). Here, the activation of cellular proto-oncogenes by viral insertion (see below) may be a relatively late event in leukemogenesis (O'Donnell et al., 1985, van der Putten et al., 1988). Clearly, the formation of mink cell focus forming virus (MCF) plays an important role in retroviral induced leukemia although its precise role in this process remains to be fully elucidated (Hartley et al., 1977). MCF viruses emerge during an infection with a MuLV as a chimeric virus between RNA genomes from the ecotropic MuLV and endogenous xenotropic viruses probably via co-packaging of both RNAs. They are able to superinfect cells which have been infected with MuLV and some of the MCF viruses are strong leukemogenic agents; they are most probably involved in accelerating the tumorigenic process initiated by infection with the original MuLV.

Mechanisms of Insertional Activation

The non acute transforming retroviruses contribute to the process of malignant transformation by activating cellular target genes. The ability of an integrated provirus to activate flanking DNA sequences always depends on the transcriptional control sequences in the viral LTR (see Fig. 4). These sequences are able to initiate, enhance or

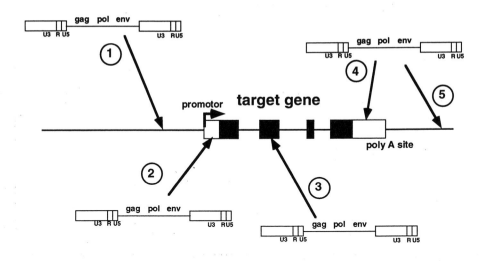

Figure 5. Different mechanisms of target gene activation by proviral insertion. Insertion in regions 5' and 3' outside of the gene result in enhanced transcription of the target gene (1, 5). Insertion in the 3' UTR results in replacement of the endogenous target gene promotor and transcriptional initiation from either the viral 3' or 5' LTR (2). Insertion of proviral DNA into the 5' UTR results in enhancement of transcription of the target due to the presence of the viral LTR enhancer elements as in (1) and (5) but also in the production of truncated transcripts and altered RNA stability (4). Integration within the coding part of the cellular target gene results in N-terminally or C-terminally truncated mRNA molecules and expression of altered target gene products (3).

terminate transcription of the cellular gene in the vicinity of the provirus depending of its orientation relative to the target sequence.

A direct insertion of the provirus in the 5' region outside the target gene coding region but within the 5' UTR results in a replacement of the target gene promotor by a promotor from the proviral 3' or 5' LTR. This requires the integration of the provirus in the same transcriptional orientation as the target gene (Fig. 5-2). Transcription can now initiate from the promotor in either LTR; use of the 3' promotor results in a mRNA with unaltered coding potential whilst use of the 5' promotor can produce different large fusion transcripts between viral and cellular sequences due to the frequent negligence of the poly (A) site in the 3' LTR and the splice sites present in the proviral sequences.

A second and very common activation mechanism is that of transcriptional enhancement. The high frequency is explained by the multiple mechanisms that can lead to transcriptional enhancement upon proviral insertion. The enhancer elements in the proviral LTRs can act over considerable distances (several 100 kb) and are orientation independent. Thus, the integration of a provirus can enhance transcription of a target gene after insertion in a region outside of the gene either in the 3' or 5' region. Transcription then initiates from the normal endogenous target gene promotor and the enhancer elements increase the efficiency of transcriptional initiation and act as typical cis-acting transcriptional control elements (Fig. 5-1,5).

If integration of the provirus takes place in the 3' untranslated region (Fig. 5-4) the affected gene could be activated in addition to transcriptional enhancement due to the loss of sequences involved in generating mRNA instability. The elimination of destabilizing mRNA motifs like "AUUUA" can contribute to a higher steady state level of the mRNA, resulting in a forced expression of the gene at the protein level (Meylink et al., 1985; Selten et al., 1986; Shaw and Kamen, 1986). Proviral integrations are also found within coding sequences of cellular genes (Fig. 5-3). In this case malignant transformation is mediated by protein fragments with altered function or activity expressed by truncated 5'-end and/or 3'-end mRNA transcripts (Habets et al., 1994; Patriotis et al., 1993).

Insertional Mutagenesis and "Proviral Tagging"

Comparing the transforming activity of both types of retroviruses and the deciphering of their target genes as well as the study of their *onc* sequences have provided a wealth of information about the molecular mechanisms underlying malignant transformation. In particular, this led to the clarification that tumorigenesis requires multiple distinct steps which a normal cell has to accumulate in order to become an aggressive metastasizing cancer cell. Today it is well accepted that these distinct steps are reflected by the accumulation of activated oncogenes or the loss of tumor suppressor genes. During the last 10-15 years, genetically manipulated animals, in particular transgenic and knock-out mice, have been invaluable in identifying the roles of oncogenes and tumor suppressor genes in malignant transformation. Using these genetically altered mice, it has been possible to dissect the different steps and their biological consequence, e.g. growth factor independence, cell cycle progression, lack of apoptosis and metastasis. In addition, it has been possible to demonstrate synergistic effects of the combined expression of more than one oncogene or the combined effect of the loss of a tumor suppressor gene in a deficient mouse mutant and the concomitant gain of an activated oncogene. These systems have also facilitated the study of the influence of neighboring cells or the immune system of a whole animal on the development of a tumor.

To be able to follow the development of a particular tumor and to identify the molecular steps involved, Berns and colleagues have designed a strategy called "retroviral tagging" (Berns, 1991, Jonkers and Berns, 1996). This technique, using non acute transforming retroviruses, made it possible to induce a particular tumor in animals and at the same time allowed the identification of the consecutive steps necessary for the development of a full-blown tumor. The virus used for this "retroviral tagging" strategy is MoMuLV which induces T-cell lymphomas after a mean latency period of several months in C57/BL/6 mice. It has to be kept in mind that the integration of proviral sequences into the host genome occurs at random. Within the infected T-cell population, a selection of cells that have acquired a specific insertion conferring a growth or survival advantage will allow the preferential outgrowth of such cells all now carrying the same proviral integration. If this insertion site is found in several independently generated tumors the site will be designated as a common proviral integration site. Other cells carrying an insertion that does not provide such an advantage will be selected against and be eliminated from the pool of infected cells in the animal. Due to the multistep character of tumor development other events have to occur, but if a gene activated at the insertion site contributes to the process it will be found in the DNA of the tumor tissue. The identification of such a gene and its molecular cloning is then made possible by the presence of the known proviral sequences used as a molecular probe. A considerable number of new oncogenes that act as dominant factors in tumorigenesis have been cloned using this approach (Berns et al., 1994, Berns and Jonkers, 1996).

An even more useful aspect of the proviral tagging method is achieved when transgenic mice are used that dominantly overexpress an oncogene and already are predisposed to a certain type of cancer. In addition genetically engineered mice that are deficient for a tumor suppressor gene or carry a natural mutation in a gene that is relevant to cancer have been used. By applying retroviral insertional mutagenesis to such animals one can identify genes that functionally collaborate with the present transgene or a given "loss of function" mutation. Interestingly, in the case of mice which are deficient for a particular gene it is possible to identify genes that act downstream or in parallel signal transduction pathways from the depleted gene product. Using wild type and transgenic mice Berns and colleagues, as well as other groups, have identified a large number of genes that contribute to tumorigenesis or synergize with other already known oncogenes (Berns et al., 1994, Jonkers and Berns 1996).

The oncogenes cloned by proviral tagging over the last 10-15 years fall in different categories. Among them are genes encoding transcription factors (e.g. Myc, Evi-5, Fli-1, p53 and Gfi-1), serine threonine kinases (Pim-1, Pim-2, Tpl-2, c-Mos, Lck), polycomb genes (*bmi-1*), genes for GTPases (Ras family), genes for growth factors and their receptors (e.g. IL-2, IL-6, CSF-1 and c-Fms, IL-6R, Erb-2), G1 cyclins (cyclin D1 and D2 resp., Vis-1 and Fin-1), GAPs (Evi-2), and GDS proteins (Tiam-1) as well as genes that encode proteins with as yet unknown functions (*frat-1*). Several of these genes have also been identified as oncogenes in an independent way or have been found as v-*onc* sequences in acute transforming retroviruses.

Targets in MuLV Induced T-Cell Lymphomas

Among the murine leukemia viruses the Moloney subtype MoMuLV induces T-cell lymphoma with a preferential location in the thymus and subsequently in other lymphoid organs such as spleen and lymph nodes. There are a large number of integration sites that have been isolated either from infected T-cell lines in culture or from tumors which have developed in infected animals. This review will focus on genes from the *myc* family, the *pim* family, the *gfi-1/pal-1* locus and on the insertion sites that affect G1 regulators of cell cycle progression (*vin-1* and *fis-2*).

PIM-1 AND *PIM*-2

PIM-1 AND *PIM*-2

The *pim*-1 gene encodes a cytoplasmic protein serine/threonine kinase (Saris et al., 1991) and was discovered as the first locus frequently activated by proviral insertion in Moloney murine leukemia virus (MoMuLV) induced T-cell lymphomas (Cuypers et al., 1984; Selten et al., 1985, 1986; Mucenski et al., 1987). Evidence that *pim*-1 is directly implicated in the tumorigenic process and therefore has oncogenic potential was provided by the analysis of Eμ *pim*-1 transgenic animals (van Lohuizen et al., 1989b). The Eμ *pim*-1 transgene was expressed at equal levels in both B- and T-cells, but the animals were clearly predisposed to the development of T-cell neoplasia with an incidence of 10% and a latency period of 7 months (van Lohuizen et al., 1989b). While the oncogenic activity of high levels of *pim*-1 is undisputed, the regular physiological function of this cytoplasmic kinase remains completely unknown. Mice carrying a homozygous deletion of *pim*-1 generated by gene targeting show a very subtle phenotype (Domen et al., 1993a,b; Laird et al., 1993). This was very surprising given the strong phenotypic changes in *pim*-1 transgenic animals. One possible explanation was that *pim*-1 is a member of several redundant signaling pathways and that other members could substitute for the lost *pim*-1. Infection of *pim*-1 deficient mice with MoMuLV showed indeed that a second gene *pim*-2 with a homology to *pim*-1 of 53% amino acid identity exists (van der Lugt et al., 1995). Pim-2 can replace *pim*-1 in lymphoma genesis when constitutively expressed in transgenic mice (Allen et al., 1997).

MYC FAMILY GENES

c-*myc* has been identified as the cellular counterpart of the viral *onc* sequence in substrains of ALV in particular MC29. In addition, and of interest here, the c-*myc* gene has been isolated as a frequent target gene for proviral insertions of MuLV in various lymphoma and leukemia of mice (Corcoran et al., 1984; Selten et al., 1984) but also of ALV in birds (Hayward et al., 1981) and of FeLV in cats (Neil et al., 1985). The closely related N-*myc* gene was found to be a target of MoMuLV proviral integration with insertion taking place in the 3' UTR of the gene (Dolcetti et al., 1989, van Lohuizen et al.,1989a).

The Myc nuclear phosphoproteins have been under intense investigation for the last 10-15 years (for a review see Henriksson and Lüscher, 1996). While c-*myc* is found in almost all proliferating cells, expression of N- and L-*myc* is more restricted to specific cell types (for a review see Henriksson and Lüscher, 1996, Meichle et al., 1992). All three Myc family members have key roles in normal cellular proliferation. The c-*myc* gene for instance is induced in serum-stimulated cells as a typical immediate early response gene. Microinjection of c-Myc protein directly into the nuclei of quiescent cells rapidly drives the cells through G1 into S-phase; a similar effect is seen after inducible activation of Myc through a conditional allele (reviewed in Meichle et al., 1992 and in Henriksson and Lüscher, 1996). Moreover, a block of Myc function can lead to arrest of cells in the G1 phase of the cell cycle. In a large number of human cancers *myc* family genes are transcriptionally activated either by gene amplification or specific chromosomal alterations (reviewed in Henriksson and Lüscher, 1996). In addition to its activation by proviral insertion in retroviral-induced lymphomagenesis Myc is able to malignantly transform cells in culture either alone or in cooperation with other activated oncogenes such as Ha-Ras (Land et al., 1983). Surprisingly, under growth factor deprivation constitutive Myc expression can drive cells into apoptosis (programmed cell death; Evan et al., 1992). It still remains controversial how the growth promoting and death promoting effects of *myc* can be reconciled.

One example for *myc* activation in human malignancies is the Burkitt type lymphoma that carries a reciprocal translocation between chromosomes 8 and 14. As a consequence of this rearrangement the *myc* gene that is normally located on chromosome 8 is placed in the region of immunoglobulin heavy chain genes on chromosome 14 in the direct vicinity of the strong transcriptional Eμ enhancer element. Transgenic mice carrying a DNA construct in their germline that contains sequences of the immunoglobulin enhancer Eμ and the *myc* gene downstream mimicking the situation found in the human Burkitt lymphoma cells quickly succumb with B-cell lymphoma (Adams et al., 1985). This particular B-lymphoma is very similar to the human malignancy demonstrating a causal role of constitutive Myc expression in the generation of this human malignancy (Adams and Cory, 1991). In addition, there are numerous other similar examples which emphasize the key role Myc proteins play in genesis and progression of tumors.

First hints of the molecular function of Myc proteins were provided by the finding that all Myc family members contain a transactivation domain at the amino termnus and a basic region directly followed by a helix loop helix-leucine zipper motif (b-HLH-LZip) at the carboxy terminus (Henriksson and Lüscher, 1996). The b-HLH-LZip domain is responsible for DNA binding and heterodimerization with specific partner proteins. One of the known proteins that interact with Myc family members through this domain is the Max protein that also has a b-HLH-LZip domain. The Myc/Max complex specifically binds to E-box sequences with a preference for the sequence CACGTG. Max can form homodimers but can also interact with two other proteins that contain b-HLH-LZip structures, namely Mad and Mxi-1. Both Mad and Mxi-1 can efficiently antagonize the effects of Myc by regulating the availability of Max and thereby the relative abundance of active Myc/Max complexes (Henriksson and Lüscher, 1996). A number of other proteins have been identified that bind to Myc or regulate its activity. While the biochemical details of Myc function have still to be completely elucidated its role as a transcriptional transactivator regulating G1 phase progression of the cell cycle appears to be established (Steiner et al., 1995, Haas et al., 1996).

GFI-1

The *gfi*-1 gene was discovered as a MoMuLV integration site in an infected rat T-cell line that was selected for IL-2 independence (Gilks et al., 1993). Other experiments with MoMuLV infected transgenic mice, that already carried *myc* and *pim*-1 transgenes, showed rapid tumor development and the presence of proviral insertions near *gfi*-1 in a high percentage of tumors indicating a synergistic function of Gfi-1, Myc and Pim-1 (Zörnig et al., 1996, Schmidt et al., 1996, Scheijen et al., 1997). Further studies demonstrated that Gfi-1 acts as a transcriptional repressor that mediates its activity by sequence specific DNA binding in a position independent manner (Grimes et al., 1996a,

Zweidler-McKay et al., 1996). Gfi-1 is normally expressed at high levels in thymus but only appears after antigenic stimulation in peripheral T-cells. Although the biological role of Gfi-1 remains to be clarified several *in vitro* studies indicated that a constitutive expression can relieve peripheral mature T-cells from a requirement of Il-2 to overcome a G1 arrest (Grimes et al., 1996) or in general could help to sustain cell proliferation of Il-2 dependent cells in the absence of the cytokine (Zörnig et al., 1996). Studies with transgenic mice have shown that overexpression of Gfi-1 weakly predisposes mice to the development of T-cell lymphoma indicating that the proviral activation in MoMuLV induced lymphomas is causally linked to the process of tumorigenesis. This experiment also established *gfi-1* as a bona fide proto-oncogene next to the previously identified MoMuLV targets *myc* and *pim*-1 (Schmidt et al., 1998).

FIS-1 AND *VIN*-1

Two integration sites that were found in retrovirally-induced T-cell lymphomas targeted positive G1 regulators are *fis*-1 and *vin*-1 which represent proviral insertions that activate the genes for cyclin D1 and cyclin D2 (Lammie et al., 1992, Tremblay et al., 1992). This is particularly intriguing as the gene encoding cyclin D1 was found to be amplified in human breast carcinoma, squaemous cell carcinoma and mouse skin carcinoma. Furthermore, the gene for cyclin D1 appeared to be rearranged in human parathyroid adenomas (reviewed in Hall and Peters, 1996). In addition, cyclin D1 represents the product of the *bcl-1* gene that is located in the vicinity of the breakpoint in the chromosomal translocation t(11:14) typical of low malignant human B-cell lymphoma affecting centrocytic B-cells and B-cells of intermediate differentiation (Tsujimoto et al., 1985; Meeker et al., 1989; Withers et al., 1991; Motokura and Arnold, 1993). This t(11:14) translocation juxtaposes the cyclin D1 gene to the locus encoding the immunoglobulin μ heavy chain. This is very similar to the well-characterized situation found in Burkitt lymphoma (see above) where the c-*myc* proto-oncogene is placed under the control of this transcriptional control element. Under this circumstance the retroviral insertions *vin*-1 and *fis*-1 provided additional strong evidence that the genes for cyclin D1 and D2 are both proto-oncogenes and their activation a prerequisite for the generation of lymphoid malignancies. First direct experimental evidence for a transforming activity of cyclin D1 came from cotransfection of primary rat embryonic fibroblasts with activated c-*myc* or Ha-*ras* genes. Together with an activated Ha-Ras protein, high levels of cyclin D1 and cyclin D2 were able to morphologically transform primary cells, to abrogate their anchorage dependence and to enable them to grow rapidly as fibrosarcomas in nude mice (Lovec et al., 1994a; Kerkhoff et al., 1995). In another experiment constitutive expression of cyclin D1 was shown to transform BRK cells in the presence of activated Ha-Ras and an altered E1A (Hinds et al., 1994). Studies with transgenic mice from different laboratories have shown directly the potential of cyclin D1 to malignantly transform lymphoid cells (Bodrug et al., 1994; Lovec et al., 1994b).

In a normal physiological situation D-type cyclins are regulators of cell cycle progression and act specifically during early G1. They form complexes cyclin dependent kinases (CDKs) which can phosphorylate pocket proteins. One of the most prominent representatives is the tumor suppresser protein Rb. Upon phosphorylation Rb can release bound transcription factors of the E2F family that transcriptionally regulate genes needed to progress to the next stage in the cell cycle. In addition, D-type cyclin/CDK complexes can be blocked in their activity to phosphorylate pocket proteins by specific cyclin dependent kinase inhibitors (CKIs) such as p21, p27, p57, or p16. The latter binds and blocks specifically CDK4 the partner of cyclin D1 and cyclin D2 (for a review see Bartek et al., 1996). This particular situation has also been interpreted as a p16/cyclin D/CDK4/Rb pathway that controls the restriction point in the G1 phase of the cell cycle. Intriguingly, each member of this pathway is involved in tumorigenesis either as a proto-oncogene or as a tumor suppresser gene (details see Bartek et al., 1996).

Targets in MuLV-Induced B-Cell Lymphomas

BMI-1

To identify potential partners that could collaborate with *myc* in lymphomagenesis, Eμ c-*myc* transgenic mice that are predisposed to develop pre B and B-cell tumors (Adams et al., 1985) have been subjected to a proviral tagging experiment (Haupt et al., 1991; van Lohuizen et al., 1991). MoMuLV infection led to accelerated development of B- and T-lymphoid tumors. Analysis of the proviral insertion sites revealed the anticipated *pim*-1 site and insertion at two new loci: *bmi*-1 and *pal*-1 (Haupt et al., 1991; van Lohuizen et al., 1991). A third to half of the B-cell tumors but none of the T-cell tumors harbored MoMuLV proviral insertions in the *bmi*-1 locus. The *bmi*-1 gene was activated in most cases by insertion of the provirus within the first exon of the *bmi*-1 gene leading to enhanced transcription driven from the 3' LTR promotor. As for the previously identified genes activated by proviral insertion the *bmi*-1 gene was used to construct transgenic mice overexpressing Bmi-1 in the T- and B- cell compartment. It could be shown that *bmi*-1 transgenics develop lymphomas in both lineages after a short latency period which demonstrated the oncogenic potential of Bmi-1 (Haupt et al., 1993). The *bmi*-1 gene encodes a protein highly conserved in evolution with zinc finger structures and a putative helix turn helix domain that belongs to the polycomb family (van Lohuizen et al.,1991). The Bmi-1 protein seems to be important in regulating the proliferation of a number of hematopoietic cells throughout pre- and postnatal life and for morphogenesis during embryonic development (van der Lugt et al., 1994).

EVI-5 AND THE *PAL*-1 LOCUS

Further analysis of proviral insertion sites in B-cell tumors that arose in MoMuLV infected Eμ *myc* transgenic mice led to the identification of another common integration site denoted *pal*-1 (van Lohuizen et al., 1991). This locus coincided in its chromosomal location with *gfi*-1 (see above) and two other integration sites *evi*-5 and *ico*-1 (Liao et al., 1995 , Scheijen et al., 1996). The *pal*-1 locus that stretches over 50 kb is very frequently rearranged in MoMuLV-induced lymphoid tumors and is in this respect comparable to the *pim*-1 and *myc* loci. Which of the insertion sites is the most relevant for tumorigenesis remains an open question. However, the *gfi*-1 gene seems the best candidate as it is highly expressed also in tumors that bear only integration at the *evi*-5 locus

(Schmidt et al., 1996; Scheijen et al., 1996). In addition, Gfi-1 has been shown to be tumorigenic when overexpressed in transgenic mice (Schmidt et al., 1998, A. Berns personal communication) and therefore seems to be causally involved in the malignant transformation of both T- and B-lymphoid cells. Interestingly, although both the *gfi-1* and *bmi-1* genes are proviral targets in MoMuLV induced B-lymphoid tumors an integration in both loci has never been observed in the same tumor or the same tumor cell. Thus the activation of both the *pal*-1 locus and *bmi*-1 appears to be mutually exclusive indicating that both act on redundant or parallel signaling pathways (Berns et al., 1994).

Evi-5 had also been isolated from tumors that appear in a set of inbred mouse strains, termed AKXD, that have a high incidence for T-cell lymphomas (Liao et al., 1995). AKXD mice stem from a cross between AKR mice and animals from the DBA strain. AKR mice are highly predisposed to develop T-cell lymphoma that arise in the thymus at 6-12 months of age. Later in life B-cell lymphomas arise in these mice in the peripheral lymphoid organs. The high predisposition of lymphomagenesis in AKR mice is mediated by the expression of endogenous ecotropic MuLV and also by recombinant MCFs (Jenkins et al., 1982). Detailed analysis of the *evi*-5 integration site within the *pal*-1 locus revealed a new gene that bears some resemblance to the *tre*-2 oncogene and other genes whose products had been implicated in cell cycle control (Liao et al., 1997). Although the integration site *evi*-5 now correlates with a gene, the question as to whether its activation by proviral insertion is really necessary for lymphomagenesis has still to be answered. This can only be solved by generating transgenic mouse models in analogy to all the other genes isolated as proviral insertion sites.

Targets in other MuLV-Induced Leukemias

EPOR, FLI-1 AND SPI-1

Viruses of the Friend subclass also called the Friend virus complex (FV) induce primarily erythroid leukemia. The FV complex comprises two different strains of viruses namely the Friend spleen focus-forming virus (SFFV) which is replication-defective and the Friend murine leukemia virus (FMuLV) an ecotropic helper virus. One particular interesting aspect of SFFV is that it behaves as an acute transforming retrovirus and does not need the replication-defective component to induce disease. It has been recognized that this effect of SFFV is due to a mutated Env gp55 glycoprotein that binds and activates the Epo receptor (EpoR) in cells infected by the virus (Hoatlin et al., 1990, Li et al., 1990). Further evidence that activation of the Epo receptor plays a causal role in the disease process of erythroid leukemias was provided by the finding that SFFV integrations can occur in the *epoR* gene in several erythroleukemia cell lines. In these cases the proviral FV integration led to an increased expression of the EpoR (Lacombe *et al.*, 1991, Chretien et al., 1994, Hino et al., 1991). However the majority of proviral integrations in FV infected erythroleukemia cells occur in the *spi-1* locus upstream of the transcriptional start site of *spi-1* (Moreau-Gachelin et al., 1988, 1990) which represents a gene that belongs to the *ets* family of transcription factors. Another integration site that appears to be specific for FmuLV-induced erythroid leukemia and is never found in FmuLV-induced lymphoid or myeloid tumors is the *fli-1* locus. This gene is hit by proviral integration in 75-90% of the tested cell lines (Sels et al., 1992, Ben David et al., 1990) and also encodes a transcription factor of the *ets* family. More recently, the human *fli-1* gene was found to be rearranged in a number of Ewing sarcomas that belong to a class of peripheral neuroectodermal tumors or round cell tumors and typically arise during early adulthood. This rearrangement manifests as a chromosomal translocation, t(11;22)(q24;q12), that juxtaposes the amino-terminal end of the *ews* gene to the carboxy-terminal end of the *fli-1* gene (Delattre et al., 1992) producing a chimeric fusion protein termed EWS-FLI-1. This fusion protein still functions as a transcription factor and is apparently able to transform cells in vitro (May et al., 1993, Ohno et al., 1993).

MYB, EVI-1 AND EVI-2

Mice that are infected with the Moloney type murine leukemia virus develop T- cell lymphoma as already described. However, when pristane treated Balb/c mice are infected with MoMuLV they develop promonocytic myeloid leukemia instead of T-cell lymphoma (Wolff et al., 1991, Shen-Ong and Wolff, 1987). The proviral insertions that are normally found associated with MoMuLV T-cell lymphoma are not found in the pristane/MoMuLV-induced myeloid tumors. Instead, proviral integration occurs almost exclusively in the *myb* proto-oncogene in a way that leads to the production of a truncated Myb protein (Shen -Ong and Wolff, 1987, Mukhopadhaya and Wolff, 1992, Nazarov and Wolff, 1995). The *myb* gene codes for a transcription factor that specifically binds DNA and exerts a key role in hematopoietic cell differentiation (reviewed in Lüscher and Eisenmann, 1990).

Among the recombinant inbred mouse strains of the AKXD series that were derived by crossing mice from two inbred strains with different incidences of lymphoma, namely AKR/J and DBA/2/ several are predisposed to develop myeloid malignancies (Mucenski et al., 1988). In tumors from those animals an ecotropic viral integration site was identified and termed *evi-1* . Integrations in *evi-1* occur about 90 kb upstream leaving the coding region of the gene intact but provoking an overexpression of the *evi-1* mRNA (Morishita et al., 1988, Bartholomew et al., 1989, Bartholomew and Ihle, 1991). The *evi-1* gene codes for a transcription factor with two separate zinc-finger domains: one N-terminal with 7 zinger repeats and the second with 3 repeats (Morishita et al., 1988, Matsugi et al., 1990). Both separated domains are able to bind DNA in a sequence specific manner. Overexpression of Evi-1 can interfere with G-CSF induced differentiation from precursors into granulocytes suggesting that this ability to block terminal differentiation of precursor is the biochemical function of Evi-1 that is responsible for malignant transformation (Morishita et al., 1992).

The *evi-2* gene locus was found in BXH-2 mice that develop myeloid malignancies upon infection with MuLV (Buchberg et al., 1988). Most proviral insertions, in cells that have survived selection and become a tumor cell upon retroviral infection, produce a "gain of function" mutation i.e. the insertion results in an inappropriately or overexpressed target gene product. The *evi-2* locus appears to be different. It has been shown that proviral integrations in the *evi-2* locus are on mouse chromosome 11 and occur within a large intron of the neurofibromatosis type I gene *Nf1* which encodes a GAP related tumor suppressor gene (Buchberg et al., 1990, Xu et al., 1990a, b). Several genes were identified in this region but none of them seemed to be affected by the proviral insertion. By contrast, proviral insertion in this locus led to the production of truncated Nf-1 transcripts and the absence of a normal full-length NF1 protein (Largaespada et al., 1990). Interestingly, the second Nf1 allele was inactivated, in some cases by the insertion of proviruses.

Targets Associated with Tumor Progression

The emergence of cancer is now recognized as the result of an accumulation of genetic lesions in a particular cell triggering a multistep process that drives the conversion of normal cells to fully malignant tumor cells (Vogelstein and Kinzler, 1993). We have described here that a number of genetic lesions can be provoked by insertion of proviral DNA into or near genes whose products regulate cellular biochemical processes that are critical for proliferation or survival. It is conceivable that proviral insertion can also activate genes that are associated with tumor progression i.e. progression of a transformed cell into a more malignant cell that has gained the ability to metastasize, leave blood vessels, break intracellular matrix restrictions or acquire growth factor independence. The observation that several independent proviral integrations in different sites can occur in a single tumor has led to a model in which different activated targets have to cooperate to produce a malignant tumor in a way that some of the targets assures proliferation of the cell and others activate their metastatic potential and hence assure tumor progression. *In vivo* and *in vitro* models have been used to isolate proviral insertions and targeted genes associated with tumor progression. Two of theses loci are described here in more detail.

TIAM-1

One strategy to clone genes that are associated with a higher invasive potential was applied on T-lymphoma cells from the hybridoma line BW5147. These already-transformed cells were infected with MoMuLV and selected for their ability to invade monolayers of hepatocytes or fibroblasts (Habets et al., 1994). Several subclones that had been derived from MuMoLV-infected cells with invasive behavior showed a common proviral integration that was designated *tiam-1* (Habets et al., 1994). The insertions of proviral DNA occurred in two clusters within the *tiam-1* locus. In both cases the *tiam-1* open reading frame was disrupted which led to the production of truncated transcripts and the expression of N- or C-terminal Tiam-1 polypeptide fragments. The sequence homologies found within the *tiam-1* open reading frame suggested that the *tiam-1* protein is a GDP/GTP exchanger for the *rho* family of GTPases (Habets et al., 1994, Michiels et al., 1995) that have been implicated in the regulation of cytoskeletal changes and the control of morphology, adhesion and motility of cells (Hall, 1992; Tominaga et al., 1993; Takaishi et al., 1993). The original finding suggested that retroviral insertions generated truncated *tiam-1* proteins that could interfere with the normal modulation of *rho*-like GTPases (Habets et al., 1994; Michiels et al., 1995)

TPL-1, TPL-2

Analysis of T-cell lines established from MoMuLV-induced rat T-cell lymphoma after extended time in culture revealed the occurrence of two proviral insertion sites in addition to the original one. They were named *tpl-1* and *tpl-2*. The *tpl-1* proviral insertion turned out to be in the direct 5' vicinity of the *ets-1* gene. However, a transcriptional activation or any other evidence for an activation of the *ets-1* gene (Bear et al., 1989, Bellacosa et al., 1994) by the proviral insertion was not found and thus it was suggested that the proviral insertion in the *tpl-1* locus either affects another unknown gene or that the insertion in the *tpl-1* locus produces a subtle effect possibly on cell cycle progression that have not yet been recognized. In contrast, proviral insertions in the *tpl-2* locus occur in the last intron of a gene that encodes a protein kinase and provoke the overexpression of C-terminally truncated forms of this protein (Makris et al., 1993, Patriotis et al., 1993). Transfection experiments suggested that *tpl-2* may function in the MAP-kinase pathway (Patriotis et al., 1994).

Synergistic Effects and Oncogene Cooperation

The multistep process of tumorigenesis requires the subsequent activation of oncogenes or the inactivation of tumor suppressor genes whose products cooperate in a synergistic fashion to malignantly transform cells. This was first demonstrated in an elegant experiment with primary embryo fibroblasts that are in contrast to the widely used not able to proliferate in culture after a certain number of passages. Transfection of an activated *myc* gene or an activated Ha-*ras* gene alone did not alter the growth or survival of the cells. However, the cotransfection of both activated oncogenes produced clones that could proliferate continuously. Moreover these cells also grew as aggressive fibrosarcomas in syngeneic animals (Land et al., 1983). This landmark experiment was the basis of the concept of oncogene cooperation. In this model at least two independent events that act in a synergistic manner are necessary to form a malignantly transformed cell which can be regarded as a bona fide cancer cell. This concept has been further validated in particular in very elegant transgenic mouse models where the tumor incidence, latency period and in some instances also metastatic behavior was potentiated if two transoncogenes were bred into one mouse strain (Adams and Cory, 1991, Hunter, 1991). The fact that in transgenic mice tumorigenesis can be accelerated by the introduction of a synergistically-acting oncogene has stimulated experiments with transgenic mice that allowed the isolation of new and unknown oncogenes on the basis of their ability to accelerate the incidence or latency period on tumor formation (Berns, 1991). The first such experiments was done using the Eμ myc transgenic mouse (see above, Adams et al., 1985). When these animals are infected with MoMuLV they rapidly succumb with B-cell lymphoma in which the *pim 1*, *bmi 1* and the *gfi 1* genes are targeted (van Lohuizen et al., 1991, Haupt et al., 1991) suggesting that these genes can cooperate with *myc*. Vice versa, MoMuLV infected Eμ *pim-1* transgenic mice that are weakly predisposed to the development of T-cell lymphoma produce these tumors now within a considerably shorter latency period and the analysis of common viral integration sites in

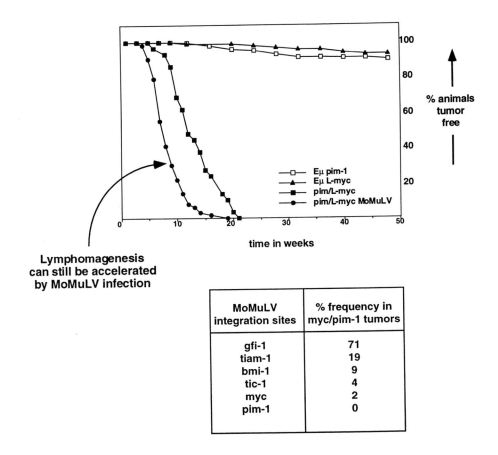

Figure 6. Tripartite oncogene cooperation between pim-1, L-myc and gfi-1. Shown is the percentage of tumor free animals (survival) against their age in weeks of transgenic mice carrying particular trans-oncogenes, here: L-myc or pim-1 or both, deregulated by the Eµ element in comparison with double L-myc/pim-1 transgenics after infection with MoMuLV. Eµ L-myc and Eµ pim-1 single transgenic mice are weakly predisposed to develop T-cell lymphoma (closed triangles and open squares). Double pim-1/L-myc transgenics generated by crossbreeding develop tumors much faster (closed squares). Upon infection with MoMuLV these double transgenic show again an acceleration of tumorigenesis (closed circles). The common integration site found in over 70% of tumors from these mice is gfi-1.

the genomic DNA of these tumors revealed that c- and N-*myc* genes are the primary targets of proviral insertion (van Lohuizen et al., 1989b).

To demonstrate that the cooperation between *pim-1* and *myc* family genes is not only a particular feature of retrovirally-infected mice, the Eµ *myc* and the Eµ *pim-1* mice were crossed directly to show the synergistic cooperation of both genes. The presence of both activated oncogenes was so strong that double *pim-1/myc* transgenic mice develop malignant preB/B- cell lymphoma *in utero* (Verbeek et al., 1991). However, it was also noted that these malignancies were still clonal or oligoclonal, suggesting that additional genetic events had occurred to assure the outgrowth of these fully malignant tumors (Verbeek et al., 1991). It was not obvious how to detect the genetic mutations responsible for these additional events. Double *pim-1/myc* transgenic mice die *in utero* and therefore were not amenable to further experimentation. Thus, other *myc* family trans-oncogenic animals were used. The L-*myc* gene is a close homologue of c-*myc* and is tumorigenic when deregulated in transgenic mice (Möröy et al., 1990). Moreover, the L-*myc* gene can cooperate with the *pim-1* gene in transgenic mice albeit with a lower efficiency than c-*myc* (Möröy et al., 1991). Hence, Eμ L-*myc*/Eμ *pim-1* double transgenic mice were ideal as experimental models to identify a third oncogene cooperation partner for *myc* and *pim-1* (Zörnig et al., 1996). Indeed, it was possible to infect *pim/L-myc* double transgenics with MoMuLV and to still accelerate tumorigenesis (Fig. 6 and Zörnig et al., 1996). The common viral integration site that was identified in the vast majority of the tumors emerging from the infected double transgenic mice was the *pal-1* locus containing the *gfi-1* gene which was also found to be transcriptionally activated without disruption of the coding region (Zörnig et al., 1996, Scheijen et al., 1997). Crossing experiments with *gfi-1* transgenic mice and either Eμ *pim-1* or Eμ L-*myc* animals showed accelerated tumor formation in both cases (Schmidt et al., 1998). This indicated that the *gfi-1* gene represents a true collaborator for myc and *pim-1* genes and can be seen as a third partner of *pim-1* and *myc* in a tripartite oncogene cooperation model.

Conclusion

To date, cancer is regarded as a multistep process and our ability in the future to interfere with this process effectively and on all levels of progression will depend on a detailed knowledge of the mechanisms that make a cell a cancer cell. In this respect, retroviruses can give us a wealth of information. Some retroviruses bear oncogenes and allow a direct analysis of their activation. Other retroviruses can cause cancer without bearing the mutated genes that initiate or promote malignancy; they target the appropriate gene at the genomic level. Based on this particular ability, retroviruses have been used as tools to identify a large number of genes involved in various stages of tumorigenesis and to decipher the wiring of oncogene cooperation and the synergistic actions of oncogenes and suppressor genes. What makes this tool so powerful is that it allows the correlation of the induction of a particular phenotype and the possibility to directly with a genetic mutation through the proviral integration. This will allow us in the future to refine and complete our understanding of genetic alterations required for malignant diseases. In addition, the degree of complementation and redundancy of different signaling pathways and any synergistic effects of oncogene cooperation in tumorigenesis will hopefully become evident.

Acknowledgment

Work from the authors was supported by grants of the Deutsche Forschungsgemeinschaft (DFG, SFB 215-D10, DFG 435/11-1), the Dr. Mildred Scheel Stiftung für Krebsforschung and the Fonds der chemischen Industrie. Special thanks to H. Karsunky for critically reading the manuscript. We apologize to all colleagues whose work has been indirectly cited due to space constraints.

References

Adams, J.M. and Cory, S. (1991). Transgenic models of tumor development. Science 254, 1161-1167.

Adams, J.M., Harris, A.W., Pinkert, C.A., Corcoran, L.M., Alexander, W.S., Cory, S., Palmiter, R.D. and Brinster, R.L. (1985). The c-*myc* oncogene driven by immunoglobulin enhancers induces lymphoid malignancy in transgenic mice. Nature 318, 533-538.

Allen, J.D., Verhoeven, E., Domen, J., van der Valk, M. and Berns, A. (1997). Pim-2 transgene induces lymphoid tumors, exhibiting potent synergy with c-*myc*. Oncogene 15, 1133-1141.

Bartek, J., Bartkova, J. and Lukas, J. (1996). The retinoblastoma protein pathway and the restriction point. Curr. Opin. Cell. Biol. 8, 805-814.

Bartholomew, C. and Ihle, J.N. (1991). Retroviral insertions 90 kilobases proximal to the *Evi*-1 myeloid transforming gene activate transcription from the normal promoter. Mol. Cell. Biol. 11, 1820-1828.

Bartholomew, C., Morishita, K., Askew, D., Buchberg, A., Jenkins, N.A., Copeland, N.G. and Ihle, J.N. (1989). Sequence organization of the human *int*-2 gene and its expression in teratocarcinoma cells. Oncogene 4, 529-534.

Bear, S.E., Bellacosa, A., Lazo, P.A., Jenkins, N.A., Copeland, N.G., Hanson, C., Levan, G. and Tsichlis, P.N. (1989). Provirus insertion in *Tpl*-1, an *Ets*-1-related oncogene, is associated with tumor progression in Moloney murine leukemia virus-induced rat thymic lymphomas. Proc. Natl. Acad. Sci. USA 86, 7495-7499.

Bellacosa, A., Datta, K., Bear, S.E., Patriotis, C., Lazo, P.A., Copeland, N.G., Jenkins, N.A. and Tsichlis, P.N. (1994). Effects of provirus integration in the *Tpl*-1/*Ets*-1 locus in Moloney murine leukemia virus-induced rat T-cell lymphomas: levels of expression, polyadenylation, transcriptional initiation, and differential splicing of the *Ets*-1 mRNA. J. Virol. 68, 2320-2330.

Ben-David, Y., Giddens, E.B. and Bernstein, A. (1990). Identification and mapping of a common proviral integration site *Fli*-1 in erythroleukemia cells induced by Friend murine leukemia virus. Proc. Natl. Acad. Sci. USA 87, 1332-1336.

Berns, A. (1991) Separating the wheat from the chaff. Curr. Biol. 1, 28-29

Berns, A., van der Lugt, N., Alkema, M., van Lohuizen, M., Domen, J., Acton, D., Allen, J., Laird, P.W., Jonkers, J. (1994). Mouse model systems to study multistep tumorigenesis. Cold Spring Harb. Symp. Quant. Biol .59, 435-447.

Bodrug, S.E., Warner, B.J., Bath, M.L., Lindeman, G.J., Harris, A.W., Adams, J.M. (1994). Cyclin D1 transgene impedes lymphocyte maturation and collaborates in lymphomagenesis with the *myc* gene. EMBO J. 13, 2124-2130.

Boguski, M.S. and McCormick, F. (1993). Proteins regulating Ras and its relatives. Nature 366, 643-654.

Bolognesi, D.P., Montelavo, R.C., Frank, H. and Schäfer, W. (1978). Assembly of type Concornaviruses: A model. Science 199, 183-186.

Buchberg, A.M., Bedigian, H.G., Taylor, B.A., Brownell, E., Ihle, J.N., Nagata, S., Jenkins, N.A. and Copeland, N.G. (1988). Localization of *Evi*-2 to chromosome 11: linkage to other proto-oncogene and growth factor loci using interspecific backcross mice. Oncogene Res. 2, 149-165.

Buchberg, A.M., Cleveland, L.S., Jenkins, N.A. and Copeland, N.G. (1990). Sequence homology shared by neurofibromatosis type-1 gene and IRA-1 and IRA-2 negative regulators of the RAS cyclic AMP pathway. Nature 347, 291-293.

Chretien, S., Moreau-Gachelin, F., Apiou, F., Courtois, G., Mayeux, P.-, Dutrillaux, B., Cartron, J.P., Gisselbrecht, S. and Lacombe, C. (1994). Putative oncogenic role of the erythropoietin receptor in murine and human erythroleukemia cells. Blood 83, 1813-1821.

Corcoran, L.M., Adams, J.M., Dunn, A.R. and Cory, S. (1984). Murine T lymphomas in which the cellular myc oncogene has been activated by retroviral insertion. Cell 37, 113-122.

Cuypers, H.T., Selten, G., Quint, W., Zijlstra, M., Maandag, E.R., Boelens, W., van Wezenbeek, P., Melief, C. and Berns, A. (1984). Murine leukemia virus-induced T-cell lymphomagenesis: integration of proviruses in a distinct chromosomal region. Cell 37, 141-150.

Davis, B.D., Dulbecco, R., Eisen, H.N. and Ginsberg, H.S. (1980). Microbiology: including immunology and molecular genetics, third edition, HarperandRow, 1231-1261.

Delattre, O., Zucman, J., Plougastel, B., Desmaze, C., Melot, T., Peter, M., Kovar, H., Joubert, I., De Jong, P., Rouleau, G., Aurias, A. and Thomas, G. (1992). Gene fusion with an ETS DNA-binding domain caused by chromosome translocation in human tumours. Nature 359, 162-165.

Dolcetti, R., Rizzo, S., Viel, A., Maestro, R., De Re, V., Feriotto, G. and Boiocchi, M. (1989). N-myc activation by proviral insertion in MCF 247-induced murine T-cell lymphomas. Oncogene 4, 1009-1014.

Domen, J., van der Lugt, N.M., Laird, P.W., Saris, C.J., Clarke, A.R., Hooper, M.L. and Berns, A. (1993a). Impaired interleukin-3 response in Pim-1-deficient bone marrow-derived mast cells. Blood 82, 1445-1452.

Domen, J., van der Lugt, N.M., Acton, D., Laird, P.W., Linders, K. and Berns, A. (1993b). Pim-1 levels determine the size of early B lymphoid compartments in bone marrow. J. Exp. Med. 178, 1665-1673.

Donehower, L.A. and Varmus, H.E. (1984). A mutant murine leukemia virus with a single missense codon in pol is defective in a function affecting integration. Proc. Natl. Acad. Sci. U S A 81, 6461-6465.

Evan, G.I., Wyllie, A.H., Gilbert, C.S., Littlewood, T.D., Land, H., Brooks, M., Waters, C.M., Penn, L.Z. and Hancock, D.C. (1992). Induction of apoptosis in fibroblasts by c-myc protein. Cell 69, 119-128.

Fujiwara,T. and Mizuuchi, K. (1988). Retroviral DNA integration: structure of an integration intermediate. Cell 54, 497-504.

Gilks, C.B., Bear, S.E., Grimes, H.L. and Tsichlis, P.N. (1993). Progression of Interleukin-2 (IL-2)-dependent rat T cell lymphoma lines to IL-2-independent growth following aktivation of a gene (gfi-1) encoding a novel zinc finger protein. Mol. Cell. Biol. 13; 1759-1768.

Grimes, H.L., Chan, T.O., Zweidler-McKay, P.A., Tong, B.and Tsichlis, P.N. (1996). The Gfi-1 proto-oncoprotein contains a novel transcriptional repressor domain, SNAG, and inhibits G1 arrest induced by Interleukin-2 withdrawal. Mol. Cell. Biol. 16, 6263-6272.

Haas, K., Staller, P., Geisen, C., Bartek, J., Eilers, M. and Möröy, T. (1997). Mutual requirement of CDK4 and Myc in malignant transformation: evidence for cyclin D1/CDK4 and p16INK4A as upstream regulators of Myc. Oncogene 15, 179-192.

Habets, G.G., Scholtes, E.H., Zuydgeest, D., van der Kammen, R.A., Stam, J.C., Berns, A. and Collard, J.G. (1994). Identification of an invasion-inducing gene, Tiam-1, that encodes a protein with homology to GDP-GTP exchangers for Rho-like proteins. Cell 77, 537-549.

Hall, A. (1992). Ras-related GTPases and the cytoskeleton. Mol. Biol. Cell. 3, 475-479.

Hall, M. and Peters, G. (1996). Genetic alterations of cyclins, cyclin-dependent kinases, and Cdk inhibitors in human cancer. Adv. Cancer Res. 68, 67-108.

Hartley, J.W., Wolford, N.K., Old, L.J. and Rowe, W.P. (1977). A new class of murine leukemia virus associated with development of spontaneous lymphomas. Proc. Natl. Acad. Sci. U S A 74, 789-792.

Hayward, W.S., Neel, B.G. and Astrin, S.M. (1981). Activation of a cellular onc gene by promoter insertion in ALV-induced lymphoid leukosis. Nature 290, 4 75-480.

Haupt, Y., Alexander, W.S., Barri, G., Klinken, S.P. and Adams, J.M. (1991). Novel zinc finger gene implicated as myc collaborator by retrovirally accelerated lymphomagenesis in Eµ myc tranogenic mice. Cell 65, 753-763.

Haupt, Y., Bath, M.L., Harris, A.W. and Adams, J.M. (1993). bmi-1 transgene induces lymphomas and collaborates with myc in tumorigenesis. Oncogene 8, 3161-3164.

Henriksson, M. and Lüscher, B. (1996). Proteins of the Myc network: essential regulators of cell growth and differentiation. Adv. Cancer Res. 68, 109-182.

Hinds, P.W., Dowdy, S.F., Eaton, E.N., Arnold, A. and Weinberg, R.A. (1994). Function of a human cyclin gene as an oncogene. Proc. Natl. Acad. Sci. USA 91, 709-713.

Hino, M., Tojo, A., Misawa, Y., Morii, H., Takaku, F. and Shibuya, M. (1991). Unregulated expression of the erythropoietin receptor gene caused by insertion of spleen focus-forming virus long terminal repeat in a murine erythroleukemia cell line. Mol. Cell. Biol. 11, 5527-5533.

Hoatlin, M.E., Kozak, S.L., Lilly, F., Chakraborti, A., Kozak, C.A. and Kabat, D. (1990). Activation of erythropoietin receptors by Friend viral gp55 and by erythropoietin and down-modulation by the murine Fv-2r resistance gene. Proc. Natl. Acad. Sci. USA 87, 9985-9989.

Hunter, T. (1991). Cooperation between oncogenes. Cell 64, 249-270

Jenkins, N.A., Copeland, N.G., Taylor, B.A. and Lee, B.K. (1982). Organization, distribution, and stability of endogenous ecotropic murine leukemia virus DNA sequences in chromosomes of Mus musculus. J. Virol. 43, 26-36.

Jonkers, J. and Berns, A. (1996) Retroviral insertional mutagenesis as a strategy to identify cancer genes. Bioch. Biophys. Acta. 1287, 29-57

Kerkhoff, E. and Ziff, E.B. (1995). Cyclin D2 and Ha-Ras transformed rat embryo fibroblasts exhibit a novel deregulation of cell size control and early S phase arrest in low serum. EMBO J. 14, 1892-1903.

Lacombe, C., Chretien, S., Lemarchandel, V., Mayeux, P., Romeo, P.H., Gisselbrecht, S. and Cartron, J.P. (1991). Spleen focus-forming virus long terminal repeat insertional activation of the murine erythropoietin receptor gene in the T3Cl-2 friend leukemia cell line. J. Biol. Chem. 266, 6952-6956.

Laird, P.W., van der Lugt, N.M., Clarke, A., Domen, J., Linders, K., McWhir, J., Berns, A. and Hooper, M. (1993). In vivo analysis of Pim-1 deficiency. Nucleic Acids Res. 21, 4750-4755.

Lammie, G.A., Smith, R., Silver, J., Brookes, S., Dickson, C. and Peters, G. (1992). Proviral insertions near cyclin D1 in mouse lymphomas: a parallel for BCL1 translocations in human B-cell neoplasms. Oncogene 7, 2381-2387.

Land, H., Parada, L.F. and Weinberg, R.A. (1983). Tumorigenic conversion of primary embryo fibroblasts requires at least two cooperating oncogenes. Nature 304, 596-602.

Largaespada, D.A., Shaughnessy, J.,Jr., Jenkins, N.A. and Copeland, N.G. (1995). Retroviral integration at the Evi-2 locus in BXH-2 myeloid leukemia cell lines disrupts Nf1 expression without changes in steady-state Ras-GTP levels. J. Virol. 69, 5095-5102.

Li, J.P., D'Andrea, A.D., Lodish, H.F. and Baltimore, D. (1990). Activation of cell growth by binding of Friend spleen focus-forming virus gp55 glycoprotein to the erythropoietin receptor. Nature 343, 762-764.

Liao, X., Buchberg, A.M., Jenkins, N.A. and Copeland, N.G. (1995). Evi-5, a common site of retroviral integration in AKXD T-cell lymphomas,maps near Gfi-1 on mouse chromosome 5. J. Virol. 69, 7132-7137.

Liao, X., Du, Y., Morse, H.C. 3rd., Jenkins, N.A. and Copeland, N.G. (1997). Proviral integrations at the Evi-5 locus disrupt a novel 90 kDa protein with homology to the Tre-2 oncogene and cell-cycle regulatory proteins. Oncogene 14, 1023-1029.

Lovec, H., Sewing, A., Lucibello, F.C., Muller, R. and Möröy, T. (1994a). Oncogenic activity of cyclin D1 revealed through cooperation with Ha-ras: link between cell cycle control and malignant transformation. Oncogene 9, 323-326.

Lovec, H., Grzeschiczek, A., Kowalski, M.B. and Möröy, T. (1994b). Cyclin D1/bcl-1 cooperates with myc genes in the generation of B-cell lymphoma in transgenic mice. EMBO J. 13, 3487-3495.

Lowy, D. (1986) Genetics of retrovirus tumorigenicity. In: Concepts of viral Pathogenesis II (Notkins, A.L.andOldstone, M.B.A. eds.,Springer Verlag), 132-140.

Lüscher, B. and Eisenman, R. N (1989) New light on Myc and Myb. Part II. Myb. Genes and Dev. 4, 2235-2241.

Makris, A., Patriotis, C., Bear, S.E. and Tsichlis, P.N. (1993). Genomic organization and expression of Tpl-2 in normal cells and Moloney murine leukemia virus-induced rat T-cell lymphomas: activation by provirus insertion. J. Virol. 67, 4283-4289.

Matsugi, T., Morishita, K. and Ihle, J.N. (1990). Identification, nuclear localization, and DNA-binding activity of the zinc finger protein encoded by the evi-1 myeloid transforming gene. Mol. Cell. Biol. 10, 1259-1264.

May, W.A., Gishizky, M.L, Lessnick, S.L., Lunsford, L.B., Lewis, B.C., Delattre, O., Zucman, J., Thomas, G. and Denny, C.T. (1993). Ewing sarcoma 11;22 translocation produces a chimeric transcription factor that requires the DNA-binding domain encoded by FLI1 for transformation. Proc. Natl. Acad. Sci. USA 90, 5752-5756.

Meeker, T.C., Grimaldi, J.C., O'Rourke, R., Louie, E., Juliusson, G. and Einhorn, S. (1989). An additional breakpoint region in the BCL-1 locus associated with the t(11;14)(q13;q32) translocation of B-lymphocytic malignancy. Blood 74, 1801-1806.

Meichle, A., Philipp, A. and Eilers, M. (1992). The functions of Myc proteins. Biochim. Biophys. Acta 1114, 129-146.

Meylink, F., Curran, T., Miller, A.D. and Verma, I.M. (1985). Removal of a 67-base-pair sequence in the noncoding region of the protooncogene fos converts it to a transforming gene. Proc. Natl. Acad. Sci. USA 82, 4987-4991.

Michiels, F., Habets ,G.G., Stam, J.C., van der Kammen, R.A. and Collard, J.G. (1995). A role for Rac in Tiam1-induced membrane ruffling and invasion. Nature 375, 338-340.

Möröy T., Fisher P., Guidos C., Ma A., Zimmerman K., Tesfaye A., DePinho R., Weissman I., Alt F.W. (1990). IgH enhancer deregulated expression of L-myc: abnormal T lymphocyte development and T cell lymphomagenesis. EMBO J 9, 3659-3666

Möröy, T., Verbeek, S., Ma, A., Achacoso, P., Berns, A. and Alt, F. (1991). Eμ N- and Eμ L-*myc* cooperate with Eμ *pim*-1 to generate lymphoid tumors at high frequency in double-transgenic mice. Oncogene 6, 1941-1948.

Moreau-Gachelin, F., Ray, D., de Both, N.J., van der Feltz, M.J., Tambourin, P. and Tavitian, A. (1990). *Spi*-1 oncogene activation in Rauscher and Friend murine virus-induced acute erythroleukemias. Leukemia 4, 20-23.

Moreau-Gachelin, F., Tavitian, A. and Tambourin, P. (1988). *Spi*-1 is a putative oncogene in virally induced murine erythroleukaemias. Nature 331, 277-280.

Morishita, K., Parganas, E., Matsugi, T. and Ihle, J.N. (1992). Expression of the *Evi*-1 zinc finger gene in 32Dc13 myeloid cells blocks granulocytic differentiation in response to granulocyte colony-stimulating factor. Mol. Cell. Biol. 12, 183-189.

Morishita, K., Parker, D.S., Mucenski, M.L., Jenkins, N.A., Copeland, N.G. and Ihle, J.N. (1988). Retroviral activation of a novel gene encoding a zinc finger protein in IL-3-dependent myeloid leukemia cell lines. Cell 54, 831-840.

Motokura, T. and Arnold, A. (1993). PRAD1/cyclin D1 proto-oncogene: genomic organization, 5' DNA sequence, and sequence of a tumor-specific rearrangement breakpoint. Genes Chromosomes Cancer 7, 89-95.

Mucenski, M.L., Gilbert, D.J., Taylor, B.A., Jenkins, N.A. and Copeland, N.G. (1987). Common sites of viral integration in lymphomas arising in AKXD recombinant inbred mouse strains. Oncogene Res. 2, 33-48.

Mucenski, M.L., Taylor, B.A., Ihle, J.N., Hartley, J.W., Morse III, H.C., Jenkins, N.A. and Copeland, N.G. (1988). Identification of a common ecotropic viral integration site, *Evi*-1, in the DNA of AKXD murine myeloid tumors. Mol. Cell. Biol. 8, 301-308.

Mukhopadhyaya, R. and Wolff, L. (1992). New sites of proviral integration associated with murine promonocytic leukemias and evidence for alternate modes of c-*myb* activation. J. Virol 66, 6035-6044.

Nazarov, V. and Wolff, L. (1995). Novel integration sites at the distal 3' end of the c-*myb* locus in retrovirus-induced promonocytic leukemias. J. Virol 69, 3885-3888.

Neil, J.C. and Onions, D.E. (1985). Feline leukemia viruses: molecular biology and pathogenesis. Anticancer Res. 5, 49-63.

O'Donnell, P.V., Fleissner, E., Lonial, H., Koehne, C.F. and Reicin, A. (1985). Early clonallty and high-frequency proviral integration into the c-myc locus in AKR leukemias. J. Virol. 55, 500-503.

Ohno, T., Rao, V.MN. and Reddy, E.S.P. (1993). EWS/Fli-1 chimeric protein is a transcriptional activator. Cancer Res. 53, 5859-5863.

Panganiban, A.T. and Temin, H.M. (1984). The retrovirus *pol* gene encodes a product required for DNA integration: identification of a retrovirus int locus. Proc. Natl. Acad. Sci. USA 81, 7885-7889.

Panganiban, A.T. and Temin, H.M. (1984). Circles with two tandem LTRs are precursors to integrated retrovirus DNA. Cell 36, 673-679.

Patriotis, C., Makris, A., Bear, S.E. and Tsichlis, P.N. (1993). Tumor progression locus 2 (Tpl-2) encodes a protein kinase involved in the progression of rodent T-cell lymphomas and in T-cell activation. Proc. Natl. Acad. Sci. USA 90, 2251-2255.

Patriotis, C., Makris, A., Chernoff, J. and Tsichlis, P.N. (1994). Tpl-2 acts in concert with Ras and Raf-1 to activate mitogen-activated protein kinase. Proc. Natl. Acad. Sci. USA 91, 9755-9759.

Saris, C.J.M., Domen, J. and Berns, A. (1991). The *pim*-1 oncogene encodes two related protein-serine/threonine kinases by alternativ initiation at AUG and CUG. EMBO J. 10, 655-664.

Scheijen, B., Jonkers, J., Acton, D. and Berns, A. (1997). Characterization of *pal*-1, a common proviral insertion site in Murine Leukemia Virus-induced lymphomas of c-*myc* and *pim*-1 transgenic mice. J. Virol. 71; 9-16.

Schmidt, T., Zörnig, M., Beneke, R. and Möröy, T. (1996). MoMuLV proviral integrations identified by Sup-F selection in tumours from infected *myc*/*pim* bitransgenic mice correlate with activation of the *gfi-1* gene. Nuc. Acid Res. 24; 2528-2534.

Schmidt, T., Karsunky, H., Gau, E., Zevnik, B., Elsasser, H. P. and Möröy, T. (1998). Zinc finger protein Gfi-1 has low oncogenic potential but cooperates strongly with *pim* and *myc* genes in T-sell lymphomagenesis. Oncogene, *in press*

Schwartzberg, P., Colicelli, J. and Goff, S.P. (1984). Construction and analysis of deletion mutations in the *pol* gene of Moloney murine leukemia virus: a new viral function required for productive infection. Cell 37, 1043-1052.

Sels, F.T., Langer, S., Schulz, A.S., Silver, J., Sitbon, M. and Friedrich, R.W. (1992). Friend murine leukemia virus is integrated at a common site in most primary spleen tumours of erythroleukemic animals. Oncogene 7, 643-652.

Selten, G., Cuypers, H.T., Zijlstra, M., Melief, C. and Berns A (1984). Involvement of c-*myc* in MuLV-induced T cell lymphomas in mice: frequency and mechanisms of activation. EMBO J. 3, 3215-3222.c

Selten, G., Cuypers, H.T. and Berns, A. (1985). Proviral activation of the putative oncogene Pim-1 in MuLV induced T-cell lymphomas. EMBO J. 4, 1793-1798.

Selten, G., Cuypers, H.T., Boelens, W., Robanus-Maandag, E., Verbeek, J., Domen, J., van Beveren, C. and Berns, A. (1986). The primary structure of the putative oncogene *pim*-1 shows extensive homology with protein kinases. Cell 46, 603-611.

Shaw, G. and Kamen, R. (1986). A conserved AU sequence from the 3′untranslated region of GM-CMSF mediates selective mRNA degradation. Cell 46, 659-667.

Shen-Ong, G.L. and Wolff, L. (1987). Moloney murine leukemia virus-induced myeloid tumors in adult BALB/c mice: requirement of c-*myb* activation but lack of v-*abl* involvement. J. Virol 61, 3721-3725.

Steiner P., Philipp A., Lukas J., Godden-Kent D., Pagano M., Mittnacht S., Bartek J. and Eilers M. (1995). Identification of a Myc-dependent step during the formation of active G1 cyclin-cdk complexes. EMBO J 14, 4814-4826.

Takaishi, K., Kikuchi, A., Kuroda, S., Kotani, K., Sasaki, T. and Takai, Y. (1993). Involvement of rho p21 and its inhibitory GDP/GTP exchange protein (rho GDI) in cell motility. Mol. Cell. Biol. 13, 72-79.

Temin, H.M. (1980). Origin of retroviruses from cellular moveable genetic elements. Cell 21, 599-600.

Temin, H.M. (1981). Retroviruses. Cell 27, 1-3.

Tominaga, T., Sugie, K., Hirata, M., Morii, N., Fukata, J., Uchida, A., Imura, H. and Narumiya, S. (1993). Inhibition of PMA-induced, LFA-1-dependent lymphocyte aggregation by ADP ribosylation of the small molecular weight GTP binding protein, rho. J. Cell. Biol. 120, 1529-1537.

Tremblay, P.J., Kozak, C.A. and Jolicoeur, P. (1992). Identification of a novel gene, Vin-1, in murine leukemia virus-induced T-cell leukemias by provirus insertional mutagenesis. J. Virol. 66, 1344-1353.

Tsujimoto, Y., Jaffe, E., Cossman, J., Gorham, J., Nowell, P.C. and Croce, C.M. (1985). Clustering of breakpoints on chromosome 11 in human B-cell neoplasms with the t(11;14) chromosome translocation. Nature 315, 340-343.

van der Lugt, N.M., Domen, J., Linders, K., van Roon, M., Robanus-Maandag, E., te Riele, H., van der Valk, M., Deschamps, J., Sofroniew, M., van Lohuizen, M., et al (1994). Posterior transformation, neurological abnormalities, and severe hematopoietic defects in mice with a targeted deletion of the *bmi*-1 proto-oncogene. Genes Dev. 8, 757-769.

van der Lugt, N.M., Domen, J., Verhoeven, E., Linders, K., van der Gulden, H., Allen, J. and Berns, A. (1995). Proviral tagging in Eμ-*myc* transgenic mice lacking the Pim-1 proto-oncogene leads to compensatory activation of Pim-2. EMBO J. 14, 2536-2544.

van der Putten, H., Quint, W., van Raaij, J., Maandag, E.R., Verma, I.M. and Berns, A. (1988). M-MuLV-induced leukemogenesis: integration and structure of recombinant proviruses in tumors. Cell 24, 729-739.

van Lohuizen, M., Breuer, M. and Berns, A. (1989a). N-*myc* is frequently activated by proviral insertion in MuLV-induced T cell lymphomas. EMBO J. 8, 133-136.

van Lohuizen, M., Verbeek, S., Krimpenfort, P., Domen, J., Saris, C., Radaszkiewicz, T. and Berns, A. (1989b). Predisposition to lymphomagenesis in *pim*-1 transgenic mice: cooperation with c-*myc* and N-*myc* in murine leukemia virus-induced tumors. Cell 56, 673-682.

van Lohuizen, M., Verbeek, S., Scheijen, B., Wientjens, E., van der Gulden, H. and Berns, A. (1991b). Identification of cooperating oncogenes in Eμ-*myc* transgenic mice by provirus tagging. Cell 65, 737-752.

Varmus, H.E. (1988). Retroviruses. Science 240, 1427-1435.

Varmus, H.E. (1982). Form and function of retroviral proviruses.Science 216, 812-820

Verbeek, S., van Lohuizen, M., van der Valk, M., Domen, J., Kraal, G. and Berns, A. (1991). Mice bearing the Eμ-*myc* and Eμ-*pim*-1 transgenes develop pre-B-cell leukemia prenatally. Mol. Cell. Biol. 11, 1176-1179.

Vogelstein, B. and Kinzler, K.W. (1993). The multistep nature of cancer. Trends Genet. 9, 138-141.

Weiss, R., Teich, N., Varmus, H. and Coffin, J. (1982). RNA Tumor Viruses: Molecular Biology of Tumor Viruses, 2nd Ed. Cold Spring Harbor Laboratory, Cold Spring Harbor, New York.

Withers, D.A., Harvey, R.C., Faust, J.B., Melnyk, O., Carey, K. and Meeker, T.C. (1991). Characterization of a candidate bcl-1 gene. Mol. Cell. Biol. 11, 4846-4853.

Wolff, L., Koller, R. and Davidson, W. (1991). Acute myeloid leukemia induction by amphotropic murine retrovirus (4070A): clonal integrations involve c-*myb* in some but not all leukemias. J. Virol. 65, 3607-3616.

Xu, G., Lin, B., Tanaka, K., Dunn, D., Wood, D., Gesteland, R., White, R., Weiss, R. and Tamanoi, F. (1990). The catalytic domain of the neurofibromatosis type 1 gene product stimulates ras GTPase and complements ira mutants of S. cerevisiae. Cell 63, 835-841.

Xu, G., O'Connell, P., Viskochil, D., Cawthon, R., Robertson, M., Culver, M., Dunn, D., Stevens, J., Gesteland, R., White, R. and Weiss, R. (1990). The neurofibromatosis type 1 gene encodes a protein related to GAP. Cell 62, 599-608.

Zörnig, M., Schmidt, T., Karsunky, H., Grzeschiczek, A. and Möröy, T. (1996). Zinc finger protein *gfi*-1 cooperates with *myc* and *pim*-1 in T-cell lymphomagenesis by reducing the requirements for IL-2. Oncogene 12, 1789-1801.

Zweidler-McKay, P.A., Grimes, H.L., Flubacher, M.M. and Tsichlis, P.N. (1996). Gfi-1 encodes a nuclear zinc finger protein that binds DNA and functions as a transcriptional repressor. Mol. Cell. Biol. 16, 4024-4034.

THE INDUCTION AND SUPPRESSION OF APOPTOSIS BY VIRUSES

Ester M. Hammond[1] and Roger J.A. Grand[2]

[1]Dept. of Radiation Oncology, Stanford University School of Medicine
[2]CRC Institute for Cancer Studies, University of Birmingham

1. Introduction

Apoptosis is a form of programmed cell death (PCD) which occurs in most, perhaps all, multicellular organisms. In vertebrates it is of particular importance during development, in homeostasis and in the functioning of the immune system. It is characterised by a set of morphological changes which are common to most cells undergoing apoptosis. Cells detach from their neighbours with accompanying distortion of the cell membrane. Condensation of the cytoplasm occurs together with very obvious condensation of chromatin. The cell splits to give a set of membrane- bound apoptotic bodies such that the cellular contents are not released to the surrounding environment. Apoptosis can be initiated by a great variety of stimuli such as DNA damage (by irradiation or chemicals), injury to plasma membranes, stimulation of cell surface receptors of the tumour necrosis factor (TNF) family (for example CD95/Fas), deprivation of cytokine survival factors (for example IGF-1) and viruses. In all cases the cellular response is broadly comparable.

The mechanism of apoptosis has been highly conserved evolutionarily, such that similar effectors and regulators have been identified in the nematode *Caenorhabditis elegans* and in *Homo sapiens*. It has recently become apparent that the major effectors of apoptosis, driving the cell to the formation of apoptotic bodies, are a set of cysteine proteases, termed caspases. The first member of this family of proteins to be identified in mammals was interleukin-1β converting enzyme (ICE/caspase 1) which is homologous to the product of *C.elegans ced-3* gene. This has been shown to encode a protease essential for apoptosis and correct development of the nematode. At least fourteen caspases are expressed in mammalian cells and together they appear to form a proteolytic cascade such that certain components serve as substrates and are activated by caspases further up the cascade. Thus, for example, pro-caspase 3, is cleaved by autoprotealysis and one more caspases (e.g. caspases 8) in trans giving active caspase 3, which can then degrade proteins such as DNA-dependent protein kinase (DNA-PK) and pRb. Caspase activity is essential for most of the morphological changes associated with apoptosis as well as DNA degradation.

The primary regulators of apoptosis in mammalian cells are members of the Bcl-2 family of proteins (Bcl-2, Bcl-$_{XL}$, Bax and many others) which can assume both a positive and negative role. Bcl-2 itself is homologous to the product of the *C.elegans ced-9* gene and suppresses apoptosis. All members of this family possess either pro-apoptotic or anti-apoptotic properties with the relative proportions of the two sets determining the fate of the cell. Of particular relevance to the subsequent discussion have been the ob-

351

servations that Bcl-2 homologues are encoded by a number of viral genes (for example adenovirus early region 1B [E1B] 19K, Epstein-Barr virus (EBV) BHRF1 and African swine fever virus (ASFV) LMW5-HL).

The relationship of viruses to the apoptotic process is complex. Obviously, an early initiation of apoptosis very soon after infection would lead to cell death before viral replication had taken place. Thus, many viruses express anti-apoptosis factors (which may or may not be structurally homologous to Bcl-2) as "early" proteins, inhibiting the cellular response as soon as possible after initiation of viral protein expression. Viruses also express proteins which may either cause apoptosis directly or sensitize cells to other apoptosis-inducing stimuli. Ostensibly, these might be expected to act "late" in infection such that apoptosis and cell lysis would occur at a time appropriate for the release of viral progeny. In fact many viral apoptosis-inducing proteins are, like the anti-apoptosis factors, expressed as "early" proteins. An additional important advantage, from the viral point of view, of inducing apoptosis during infection is that it facilitates evasion of the host's immune inflammatory responses, since there is no release of cellular contents to the surrounding environment. Rather, they are all contained within apoptotic bodies which are phagocytosed by neighboring cells. The relationship of virus infection and the host's immune response to apoptosis has been discussed in great detail by Razvi and Welsh (1995) and will only be considered here in passing.

The aim of this chapter is to consider in some detail how viruses induce and/or suppress apoptosis, concentrating mainly on those viruses which can also transform cells and cause cancers in mammals or those that have provided invaluable insights into the mechanism of apoptosis. From some viewpoints apoptosis can be seen as an opposing process to transformation *in vivo* as cells which fail to apoptose correctly can then grow inappropriately, perhaps giving rise to tumors. It is hoped that a consideration of the ways in which viral oncogenes regulate apoptosis, both positively and negatively, will provide insights into some of the mechanisms by which virally-induced and naturally occurring tumors might arise.

The relationship of viruses to apoptosis is an area of great interest at present. Various aspects of the subject have been described in detail in recent reviews (Shen and Shenk, 1995; Razvi and Welsh, 1995; Young et al., 1997; Teodoro and Branton, 1997a; O'Brien, 1998) as well as two recent issues of Seminars in Virology (Smith, 1998; Miller and White, 1998). Several of these studies are all-encompassing, (Razvi and Welsh, 1995; Teodoro and Branton, 1997a; O'Brien, 1998; Smith, 1998; Miller and White, 1998) describing all viruses which have been shown to either induce or suppress apoptosis – readers interested in non-oncogenic viruses are referred to these works.

2. Tumor Suppressor Gene Products p53 and pRb
in Virally-Induced Apoptosis

The concept of tumor suppressor genes is now accepted as one of the most important ideas in cancer biology. It is, however, slightly sobering to consider that almost all of the detailed biochemical analysis of the proteins encoded by these genes has been carried out since 1980. With a field of research moving so quickly it is probably not possible to present an up-to-date review in book form. However, some discussion of the properties of p53 and pRb, the two tumor suppressor genes which have been studied in most detail, is necessary for a full understanding of the mechanism of induction and suppression of apoptosis by viruses. Readers requiring a detailed account of the properties of p53 and pRb are referred to the many recent excellent reviews (for example, Wang et al., 1994; Weinberg, 1995; Gottlieb and Oren, 1996; Ko and Prives, 1996; Beijersbergen and Bernards, 1996; Levine, 1997; Herwig and Strauss, 1997; Mulligan and Jacks, 1998).

a. p53 and apoptosis

p53 is a nuclear phosphoprotein which regulates transcription primarily by sequence-specific DNA binding. Mutations in the *p53* gene occur in a large proportion of human tumors (Hollstein et al., 1991), giving rise to a protein with lost or modified activity. The significance of p53 loss or mutation for tumor development is confirmed by the high rate of tumor incidence in individuals with Li-Fraumeni Syndrome (Li and Fraumeni, 1969; Li et al., 1988) and in p53 'knockout' mice (Donehower et al., 1992). The most important point of action of p53 seems to occur after its induction in response to external stress classically resulting in DNA damage (Maltzman and Czyzyk, 1984) when it can induce cell cycle arrest and subsequent DNA repair or initiate the cell death mechanism (Lane, 1992). Thus, p53 does not play a significant role under "normal" circumstances but can be called upon in times of crisis when the well-being of the cell or animal is threatened, particularly by agents which will cause damage to the genome. This hypothesis is now largely accepted and is given added credence by the observation that $p53^{-/-}$ mice develop normally and are viable for an appreciable time (Donehower et al., 1992).

(I) TRANSCRIPTIONAL REGULATORY PROPERTIES OF p53

As already noted, p53 is a regulator of cell growth being able to block cells in G1 phase of the cell cycle after exogenous expression (Baker et al., 1990; Diller et al., 1990; Mercer et al., 1990; Michalovitz et al., 1990; Martinez et al., 1991) or as a result of induction following DNA damage (Kastan et al., 1991; Kuerbitz et al., 1992). In addition, p53 can induce differentiation (Shaulsky et al., 1991) or apoptosis (Yonish-Rouach et al., 1991; Shaw et al., 1992; Lowe et al., 1993; Clarke et al., 1993) under appropriate conditions.

The most obvious biochemical property of p53 is its ability to regulate transcription. It binds, as a tetramer, to specific upstream DNA regulatory sequences (consensus site: 2 copies of 5'-Pu Pu Pu C (A/T) (T/A) G Py Py Py-3' separated by up to 13 base pairs [El-Diery et al., 1992]) increasing transcription of genes such as *p21, GADD45, mdm2, bax* and *IGF-BP3*. Proteins encoded by these genes all play a role in cell cycle arrest or apoptosis as well as having "house-keeping" functions. In addition, a large set of p53-inducible genes have been identified (termed PIGs – [p53-induced genes] [Polyak et al., 1997]). The functions of some of these proteins are, as yet, unknown but the remainder comprise a diverse group although, probably significantly, many play a role in the generation of, or response to, oxidative stress (Polyak et al., 1997). A number of other genes contain p53 DNA binding elements but the biological significance of some of these is not obvious (see for example Selivanova and Wiman, 1995). In addition, p53 can suppress transcription through interaction with, and inhibition of, Tata binding protein (TBP) (Seto et al., 1992; Mack et al., 1993). The transcriptional repression domain of p53 and TBP binding site have both been mapped to the C-terminus (Subler et al., 1994; Shaulian et al., 1995; Horikoshi et al., 1995). Genes repressed by p53 in this way include *c-fos, c-jun* and *Rb*. These transcriptional regulatory properties of p53 are considered to be of importance for the ability of p53 both to cause cell cycle arrest and to trigger apoptosis (see below).

The best-understood activity of p53 is its ability to arrest the cell cycle in G1. Thus in response to DNA damage increased levels of p53 cause changes in transcription. A primary target for activation is the *p21* gene (El-Diery et al., 1993; 1994; Xiong et al., 1993; Harper et al., 1993; 1995). Increased p21 acts as a cycle dependent kinase (CDK) inhibitor, binding to, and inhibiting, cyclin E/CDK2, cyclin D/CDK4 and cyclin A/CDK2 complexes (Dulic et al., 1994). This has the effect of preventing phosphorylation of the pRb family of proteins and S phase entry (blocking cells in G1) so that damaged DNA is not replicated. p21 also binds to PCNA (a subunit of DNA polymerase δ) such that if DNA damage (and p53 up-regulation) occurs in S phase p21 can inhibit DNA replication directly (Waga et al., 1994). A gene encoding a p53 homologue, p73, has been cloned (Kaghad et al., 1997). p73 has many properties in common with p53 being able to regulate expression of p21 and to induce apoptosis (Jost et al., 1997). As yet, however, no evidence is available on the relative contributions of p53 and p73 to transcriptional regulation and apoptosis induction.

(II) INDUCTION OF APOPTOSIS BY P53

The mechanism by which p53 induces apoptosis is still not clear – the evidence so far presented being somewhat equivocal. Whilst the ability of p53 to induce cell cycle arrest depends on its transcriptional activation properties (Crook et al., 1994; Pietenpol et al., 1994) this may not be the case for induction of apoptosis. p53-dependent apoptosis can occur in the presence of inhibitors of transcription and translation (Caelles et al., 1994; Wagner et al., 1994) and can be induced by transcriptionally defective p53 (Haupt et al., 1995a & b). However, in other systems it has been suggested that induction of apoptosis by adenovirus early region 1A protein (Ad E1A) requires transcriptionally active p53 (Sabbatini et al., 1995a; Attardi et al., 1996). Interestingly, it has been shown that when p53-induced apoptosis is blocked by Ad E1B 19K protein or Bcl-2 it is the transcription repression rather than transcriptional activation properties of p53 which are neutralized (Shen and Shenk, 1994; Sabbatini et al., 1995b). Consistent with this view, evidence indicates that the proline-rich domain of p53 (Walker and Levine, 1996) which is involved in transcriptional repression is essential for apoptosis (Sakamuro et al., 1997; Venot et al., 1998). However, it is possible that apoptosis could be a result of both the repression and specific activation function of this region as it is able to activate MDM2, p21 and Bax promoters but not those of the recently identified p53-

induced gene 3 (PIG3, Polyak et al., 1997) (Venot et al., 1998). No doubt resolution of these apparent contradictions will soon be forthcoming but it seems reasonable to suppose that cell type and apoptotic stimulus will have an effect on the induction process.

Since Bax expression is regulated by p53 (Miyashita et al., 1994) it has been supposed that an increase in Bax level in response to up-regulated p53 could initiate apoptosis. Whilst this may happen in some cases *in vitro* it is clearly not the whole story as p53 can induce apoptosis in the absence of Bax *in vivo* (Knudson et al., 1995) and Bax is not always activated by p53 during apoptosis (Canman et al., 1995). It is also worth noting that p53 can repress Bcl-2 expression (Miyashita et al., 1994) which might provide an alternative means by which the balance of the Bcl-2 family of apoptosis regulators is tipped in favour of cell death. It can be seen that the mechanism of apoptosis induction by p53 is still unresolved. Certainly there is little evidence, at present, to confirm whether any of these effects of p53 are responsible for the observed virally-induced apoptosis.

As cell cycle arrest and apoptosis are both possible results of p53 induction it is interesting to consider what factors are involved in making the decision. This is of some relevance to a consideration of what happens following up-regulation of p53 in response to viral infection since cell cycle arrest (and inhibition of DNA synthesis) is no more beneficial to the virus than early apoptosis. It appears that if p53 induction results from viral protein expression (e.g. Ad E1A, see below) the most likely outcome will be apoptosis, although in reality viruses will also express appropriate apoptosis-suppressing proteins. The preference for apoptosis and up-regulation of p53 is determined, at least for the small DNA tumor viruses, by the ability of the viral early proteins to bind pRb (see section 4a) and consequently de-regulate E2F (see section 2e and f). This is attributable to specific protein:protein interactions between Ad E1A, SV40 T and HPV E7 with pRb which, together with other protein binding, result in cell cycle initiation. In cells where pRb and E2F function normally it is more likely that p53 induction will result in cell cycle arrest (discussed in Ko and Prives, 1996; White, 1996; Levine, 1997). It is worth noting that Ad E1A and activated c-Myc both appear to induce p53-mediated apoptosis by over-riding G1 cell cycle arrest (Hermeking and Eick, 1994).

(III) REGULATION OF p53 PROTEIN EXPRESSION

In normal cycling cells the level of expression of p53 is very low as a consequence of the protein having a half life of only a few minutes (Oren et al., 1981). p53 is usually degraded by the proteasome following ubiquitination (Maki et al., 1996). In a number of situations dramatic increases in p53 protein level are observed and in most, perhaps all, cases this is attributable to stabilization of the protein rather than an increase in transcription. As already mentioned, p53 expression is elevated in response to DNA damage and other external stresses, to viral oncoproteins such as SV40 Tag, Ad E1A and the larger Ad E1B protein and to naturally occurring mutations.

Of particular significance in any consideration of the properties of p53 is its relationship with MDM2. MDM2 can act as an oncogene transforming immortalized rodent fibroblasts (Fakharzadeh et al., 1991) and primary rat fibroblasts in association with mutant *ras* (Finlay, 1993). It is also over-expressed in a number of human cancers.

MDM2 binds to p53 close to the N-terminus at a site required for the latter's transacti-vation function, thus inhibiting its biological activity (Momand et al., 1992; Oliner et al., 1993; Lin et al., 1994; 1995; Kussie et al., 1996; Bottger et al., 1996). Expression of MDM2 is also regulated by p53 such that its level is increased following DNA damage. Thus an auto-regulatory feedback loop between p53 and MDM2 is present in normal cells such that p53 can cause an increase in expression of MDM2 and MDM2 over-expression can then inhibit p53 transactivational activity (Barak et al., 1993; Perry et al., 1993; Wu et al., 1993; Chen et al., 1994).

It is now considered that one of the major roles of MDM2 is to target p53 for protea-some-mediated degradation (Haupt et al., 1997; Kubbutat et al., 1997) so that, in effect, p53 regulates transcription of the protein which controls its own degradation. Lane and Hall (1997) have suggested a number of important implications resulting from this observation. They consider that the high levels of mutant p53 usually observed in tu-mors are due to a lack of MDM2 rather than a direct consequence of idiosyncratic changes in the primary structure of p53. Thus MDM2 is not expressed or is present only at a very low level because the mutant p53 present is unable to up-regulate transcription of the *mdm2* gene. Support for this idea is provided by the demonstration that high levels of transcriptionally inactive mutant p53 are unable to induce expression of MDM2 which would normally target p53 for degradation (Midgley and Lane, 1997). Similarly, when p53, which cannot bind MDM2, is expressed against a *wt* cellular background (i.e. one which will process p53 normally) it is stabilized and accumulates at high level (Midgley and Lane, 1997).

Furthermore, it seems likely that increased p53 seen as a result of DNA damage is due to the activation of enzymes which interfere with the MDM2/p53 complex. Consis-tent with this suggestion is the observation that phosphorylation of Ser15 on p53 results in reduced binding to MDM2 and that the kinase responsible is activated by DNA dam-age (Shieh et al., 1997). DNA-PK can phosphorylate p53 at Ser15 and 37 and this has been shown to cause a conformational change which is probably responsible for inhibi-tion of binding to MDM2 (Wang and Eckhart, 1992; Lees-Miller et al., 1992; Shieh et al., 1997). Similarly, it has recently been demonstrated that ATM and ATR can also phosphorylate p53 on Ser15 (Banin et al., 1998; Canman et al., 1998). In addition, phosphorylation of MDM2, also by DNA-PK, contributes to reduction in its affinity for p53 (Mayo et al., 1997).

As discussed below it appears that the larger Ad E1B proteins and perhaps SV40 Tag increase p53 expression by interfering directly with proteasome targeting by MDM2. Ad E1A increases p53 levels by a different mechanism which is dependent on an increase in p53 half-life due to the induction of p19[ARF], a protein encoded by the INK4a/ARF locus (de Stanchina et al., 1998). p19[ARF] can bind to MDM2 and/or p53 inhibiting MDM2-mediated degradation of p53 and apoptosis (Pomerantz et al., 1998; Zhang et al., 1998; Kamijo et al., 1998) (see below).

(IV) VIRAL PROTEINS ACTING DIRECTLY ON P53

Whilst many viruses express proteins which act to inhibit apoptosis by supplementing host cell Bcl-2-like activity or by directly inhibiting caspase activity, the small DNA tumor viruses (Ad, HPV and SV40) adopt an alternative or, in the case of Ad, additional strategy of directly neutralizing the activity of p53. In the case of Ad and SV40 this is by direct protein-protein binding whilst HPV expresses a protein which facilitates proteasomal degradation of p53.

p53 was originally identified as an interacting species with SV40 Tag (Lane and Crawford, 1979; Linzer and Levine, 1979) and was later shown to bind Ad5 E1B 58K protein (Sarnow et al., 1982). Sites of interaction for the two viral proteins are however quite distinct with SV40 Tag binding p53 in the central DNA binding domain and Ad E1B 58K binding to the N-terminal activation domain (reviewed Levine, 1993; Ko and Prives, 1996). As well as inhibiting the transactivating activity of p53 (Mietz et al., 1992; Yew and Berk, 1992; Yew et al., 1994) Tag and Ad E1B 58K increase the level of expression of the protein in transfected cells. Thus, it appears that expression of both viral proteins in transformed cells leads to the accumulation of transcriptionally inactive p53 which is incapable of inducing apoptosis. The high levels of p53 observed in response to the larger Ad E1B proteins and perhaps SV40 Tag seem to be a direct result of interference with MDM2-mediated targeting of p53 to the proteasome. The binding sites on p53 for MDM2 and Ad5 E1B 58K protein overlap at the N-terminus of the molecule and it therefore seems likely that interaction of p53 with the viral protein physically obstructs MDM2 binding and consequent degradation. This would account for the exceptionally long half-life (in excess of 2 days) observed for p53 in cells expressing Ad12 E1B 54K protein but no other Ad proteins (Grand et al., 1996). The situation with SV40 is rather more complex since the SV40 Tag binding site on p53 is remote from that for MDM2 to such an extent that ternary complexes comprising the three proteins can be detected (Henning et al., 1997). Since MDM2, as well as p53, is stabilized in SV40-infected and transformed cells it is possible that no component of the complex is degraded by the proteasome (Henning et al., 1997). Whilst there is some confusion as to whether the transcriptional activity of p53 is necessary for apoptosis induction (see for example Sabbatini et al., 1995b; Haupt et al., 1995b) it seems clear that binding to the DNA tumor virus proteins is sufficient to neutralize any activity required. However, it is worth noting that whilst Ad2/5 E1B 58K protein will suppress Ad E1A-induced apoptosis it is not as efficient as Ad E1B 19K protein (Rao et al., 1992).

Although Ad E1B 58K protein neutralizes the activity of p53 in Ad-transformed cells it has a quite different mode of action during adenoviral infection. In that case it forms part (with E4 orf 6) of the viral machinery regulating RNA metabolism (Babiss and Ginsberg, 1984; Babiss et al., 1985). The Ad E1B 55K – E4 orf6 complex appears to bind a cellular factor required for mRNA export and transports it to the site of viral replication and transcription (Ornelles and Shenk, 1991). This has the effect of encouraging viral mRNA processing and limiting host cell mRNA metabolism, leading to a reduction in cellular p53 levels by proteasomal degradation. In addition it has recently been shown that Ad5 E1B 58K protein and the E4 orf6 product combine to actively target p53 (both mutant and wt) for degradation (Moore et al., 1996; Querido et al., 1997a; Steegenga et al., 1998). E4 orf6 alone is able to bind to p53 blocking its transcriptional activation functions (Dobner et al., 1996; Nevels et al., 1997) and its ability to induce apoptosis (Moore et al., 1996).

Human papilloma viruses have evolved a novel method of neutralizing increased p53 levels which could initiate apoptosis. The HPV16 and 18 E6 proteins bind directly to p53 (Werness et al., 1990; Scheffner et al., 1990) and target it for proteasomal degradation (Scheffner et al., 1990). HPV16 and 18 E6 function in a complex with the cellular factor E6 AP (E6-associated protein) as a ubiquitin protein ligase promoting ubiquitination of p53 and subsequent proteolysis (Scheffner et al., 1993). Ubiquitin is transferred from an E1 ubiquitin-activating enzyme to an E2 ubiquitin-conjugating enzyme and then to E6-AP, the E3 ubiquitin ligase (Scheffner et al., 1995). E6 proteins from other HPV serotypes which are less oncogenic than types 16 and 18 are less effective in stimulation of p53 degradation but can still give rise to immortalized cell lines with reduced p53 levels (Band et al., 1993; Crook et al., 1994). It should be noted that HPV E6 is able to inhibit the transactivation and transrepression functions of p53 quite distinct from enhancing its rate of proteolysis and to block DNA binding by p53 (Mietz et al., 1992; Lechner and Laimins, 1994; Thomas et al. 1995; Pim et al. 1994). Thus it can be seen that whilst a single HPV protein is employed in the neutralization of ability of p53 to induce apoptosis a number of different activities are involved. (See chapter 6 in this volume).

(b) *The retinoblastoma family of proteins*

(I) RB AND THE CELL CYCLE

The retinoblastoma (*Rb1*) gene which encodes the retinoblastoma protein (pRb) is absent or mutated in retinoblastomas and other tumor cells. pRb acts as an inhibitor of cell proliferation and when re-introduced into most retinoblastoma cell lines it suppresses growth, arresting cells in G1 (Huang et al., 1988; Ewen et al., 1993). Phosphorylation of pRb varies through the cell cycle with the protein being hypophosphorylated (relatively dephosphorylated) in G0 and G1, hyperphosphorylated in S and G2, and dephosphorylated once more in M phase (Buchkovich et al., 1989; De Caprio et al., 1989; Chen et al., 1989). On the basis of these data it has been concluded that pRb acts as a regulator of the cell cycle with its activity being phosphorylation-dependent. The ability of pRb to control the cell cycle is governed by its binding to the E2F/DP1 family of transcription factors (Chellappan et al., 1991; Hiebert et al., 1992; Helin et al., 1992; 1993; reviewed Dyson, 1998) such that hypophosphorylated pRb interacts with E2F but when it becomes hyperphosphorylated dissociation occurs. Free E2F then activates transcription of genes required for cell cycle progression such as cdc2, c-myc, B-myb, thymidine kinase and dihydrofolate reductase by binding to a DNA sequence similar to that in the promoter of the adenovirus E2 gene (TTTCGCGC).

Phosphorylation of pRb is largely, perhaps entirely, mediated by cyclin-dependent kinases (Lees et al., 1991). The G1 cyclins probably direct the appropriate kinases to pRb in some cases by direct protein:protein interaction. Thus cyclin D components form complexes with pRb (Ewen et al., 1993; Dowdy et al., 1993) which is phosphorylated by the associated CDK4 and CDK6 (Meyerson and Harlow, 1993; Kato et al., 1993). In addition it appears that cyclin E – CDK2 complexes may phosphorylate pRb. Thus, simplistically it can be seen that signals deriving from mitogen activation of surface receptors encourage phosphorylation of pRb through up-regulation of cyclin D. Phosphorylated pRb dissociates from E2F which stimulates transcription of genes important for cell cycle progression (Weinberg, 1995). Of course, reality is rather more complex with at least five E2F components having been isolated and two other Rb homologues (p107 and p130). p107 and p130 have amino acid sequence similarities to pRb particularly in the functionally important A and B domains (pocket domains) (Ewen et al., 1991; Li et al., 1993; Hannon et al., 1993). p107 and p130 bind E2F4 and E2F5 preferentially whilst pRb itself tends to interact with E2F1, E2F2 and E2F3 (Cao et al., 1992; Dyson et al., 1993; Lees et al., 1993; Schwarz et al., 1993; Ginsburg et al., 1994; Beijersbergen et al., 1994). The significance of these different interactions is not yet totally clear but the E2F4 or 5:p107 and E2F4 or 5:p130 interactions (like those of E2F and pRb) are also cell cycle-dependent. In addition to binding to the E2F proteins, p107 and p130 can also bind to cyclins A and E-CDK2 complexes (Faha et al., 1992; Li et al., 1993; Ewen et al., 1992; Hannon et al., 1993), probably through the "spacer" domain between A and B regions.

Interactions of p107 and p130 with E2F do not co-incide temporally with pRb:E2F binding. p107 binding to E2F4 occurs primarily during S phase (Schwarz et al., 1993), probably indicating a more important role for the protein as a transcriptional repressor in quiescent cells. Since pRb associates with E2F mainly in G1 and S it has been suggested that p107 and p130 are primarily responsible for the regulation of E2F activity in the progression from G0/G1 to S. This is considered to be the stage at which Ad E1A exerts its effect on the cell cycle inducing progress of quiescent cells into S phase (Braithwaite et al., 1983; Quinlan and Grodzicker, 1987; discussed in Bayley and Mymryk, 1994). Recent studies have shown different specificities of the different E2F components such that, for example, E2F1,2,3 and 4 but not E2F5 can activate DNA polymerase α and cyclin E transcription, whereas cyclin A and cdc2 are stimulated by E2F1 and E2F2 but not by E2F3,4 or 5 (DeGregori et al., 1997).

Associated with the cyclins interacting with pRb, p107 and p130 are appropriate CDKs. Formation of these complexes also appears to be cell cycle dependent (Devoto et al., 1992; Lees et al., 1992; Schwarz et al., 1993; Dowdy et al., 1993). Since the activity of pRb is regulated by CDKs, it is also dependent indirectly on the actions of CDK inhibitor proteins such as $p27^{Kip1}$, $p15^{INK4B}$, and $p16^{INK4A}$ and $p21^{CIP1}$ (reviewed Wang et al., 1994; Weinberg, 1995; Chin et al., 1998). Thus, for example, $p15^{INK4B}$ expression is induced by TGFβ and inhibits the activity of CDK4 and CDK6 which phosphorylate pRb when associated with cyclin D. Similarly, induction of p53, for example by DNA damage, results in the up-regulation of $p21^{CIP1}$ expression (El-Deiry et al., 1993; Dulic et al., 1994) and subsequent CDK2 and CDK6 inhibition. This favours the build up of hypophosphorylated pRb and stabilization of the pRb-E2F complex. A summary of the relationship between pRb, E2F and the cell cycle is given in Figure 1.

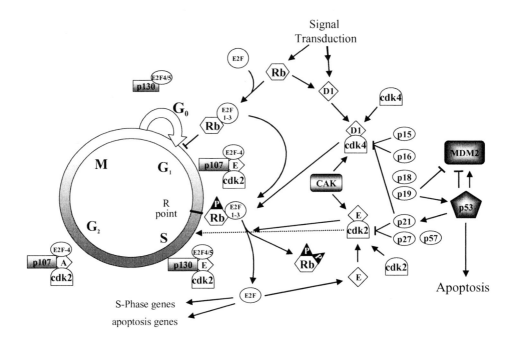

Figure 1. Relationship between the Rb family of proteins, E2F and the cell cycle. Phosphorylation of pRb by cyclin/D CDK4 causes dissociation from E2F and subsequent transcription of genes required for DNA synthesis. Inhibitors of cdk activity – the INK4 and p21 families are shown. CDK, cyclin dependent kinase; CAK, CDK activating kinase; R, restriction point in the cell cycle, the black triangles with a 'P' denote phosphate groups on Rb. Based on a figure in Herwig and Strauss (1997).

(II) PRB AND APOPTOSIS

Although the fore-going discussion offers a rather simplified version of reality it can be seen that the pRb family of proteins are the focus of a complex set of protein:protein interactions which can regulate cell cycle progression. So, how is pRb directly relevant to virally-induced apoptosis? Original studies using Rb$^{-/-}$ mice showed that foetuses die at E12-E13 with extensive apoptosis in the nervous system (Clarke et al., 1992; Jacks et al., 1992; Lee et al., 1992). Thus, whilst many cell divisions occur prior to day 13 of gestation in the absence of pRb, at a particular stage in development lack of the protein becomes of overriding importance giving rise to serious abnormalities as seen, for example, in the nervous system, the eye and in the haemopoietic system (Clarke et al., 1992; Jacks et al., 1992; Lee et al., 1992). It appears that the apoptosis is probably attributable to the unrestrained activity of E2F. Support for this proposition is supplied by the observation that enforced overexpression of E2F results in DNA synthesis and apoptosis (Qin et al., 1994; Shan and Lee, 1994; Wu and Levine, 1994; Kowalik et al., 1995). Interestingly, it is only the E2F1 component (not E2F2-5) which is able to induce apoptosis and this is due to its ability to stimulate transcription of a particular gene or set of genes (DeGregori et al., 1997). Further supporting evidence is provided by the observation that re-introduction of pRb into Rb $^{-/-}$ cells inhibits apoptosis (Haas-Kogan et al., 1998).

Apoptosis induced by loss of pRb/excess E2F is largely p53-dependent. Thus, if Rb is inactivated by genetic targeting or by expression of HPV16 E7 (see below), for example in the lens of the eye of transgenic mice, apoptosis occurs resulting in inappropriate development. However, if Rb is inactivated or HPV E7 is expressed in p53$^{-/-}$ mice (or mice in which p53 is degraded due to expression of HPV16 E6), the apoptosis-inducing effects of the Rb knock-out are suppressed, although there is an appreciable increase in tumor incidence (Howes et al., 1994; Morgenbesser et al., 1994; Pan and Griep, 1994; 1995). These data are consistent with the ability of E2F1 to induce apoptosis *in vitro*, as already mentioned. Furthermore, E2F1$^{-/-}$ mice suffer from certain limited developmental abnormalities which are attributable to aberrant cell proliferation probably caused by lack of appropriate apoptosis (Field et al., 1996; Yamasaki et al., 1996). Perhaps surprisingly, these animals develop "normally" and are viable, suggesting that under most circumstances the role of E2F1 can be taken over by other E2F proteins and that E2F1-mediated apoptosis is not of central importance, whilst pRb and p53 are functioning normally. Confirmation that E2F1-induced apoptosis is p53-dependent has also been provided by *in vitro* experiments (Hiebert et al., 1995; Kowalik et al., 1998). Accumulation of p53 in response to E2F-1 is blocked by MDM2 (Kowalik et al., 1998). Interestingly over-expression of dE2F and dDP in the *Drosophila* eye causes S phase entry, abnormal development and apoptosis in the eye disc (Du et al., 1996). Obviously, in this case induction of apoptosis occurs in the absence of p53 but it is not clear how enhanced cell cycle progression/DNA synthesis results in cell death.

As discussed above, in mammalian cells hypophosphorylated pRb binds E2F and acts to arrest the cell cycle and inhibit DNA synthesis. When dissociated from pRb E2F stimulates passage into S phase. However, pRb is also necessary for p53-induced cell cycle arrest in G1 following DNA damage (Demers et al., 1994; Hickman et al., 1994; Slebos et al., 1994; White et al., 1994) and can, under some circumstances, overcome p53-mediated apoptosis (Qin et al., 1994; Haupt et al., 1995a). In normal cells p53 regulates expression of p21 which inhibits CDK-mediated phosphorylation of pRb imposing cycle arrest in G1. However, when pRb is absent p21 is unable to affect the cell cycle (i.e. inhibit the activity of E2F) with the result that death may result from "inappropriate growth signals" (discussed by White, 1994; 1996; Kasten and Giordano, 1998; Choisy-Rossi and Yonish-Rouach, 1998). These "inappropriate growth signals" may involve transcriptional activation by E2F, as discussed above (DeGregori et al., 1997). In addition, it has been shown that the E2F-DP1 complex itself can bind to p53 and increase its expression inducing apoptosis (Hiebert et al., 1995; Kowalik et al., 1998). Quite how these "inappropriate growth signals" trigger the apoptotic pathway effect through a direct increase in p53 expression is still unclear but is probably a function of its activity as a transcriptional regulator. It is interesting to note, however, that pRb and p21 are substrates for caspases during apoptosis, suggesting that their elimination may favour the rapid completion of the process (Janicke et al., 1996; An and Dou, 1996; Gervais, et al., 1998).

(III) INTERACTION OF SMALL DNA TUMOR VIRUS ONCOPROTEINS WITH pRB

pRb is the other major tumor suppressor gene product besides p53 involved in the induction of apoptosis by the small DNA tumor viruses. In this case, however, the mechanism of subversion is similar for Ad, SV40, HPV and polyoma (although in the latter case there is little evidence to suggest that this leads to apoptosis). Ad E1A, SV40 Tag, HPV16/18 E7 and polyoma large T antigen all interact with pRb (Whyte et al., 1988; DeCaprio et al., 1988; Dyson et al., 1989). The viral proteins bind to the A and B subdomains on pRb (amino acids 393 to 572 and 646 to 772 respectively). The binding sites for pRb on Ad E1A have been mapped to conserved regions 1 and 2 (Egan et al., 1988; Whyte et al., 1989), on SV40 T to a site between amino acids 105 and 114 (Ewen et al., 1989) and to a site between amino acids 18-37 on HPV16 E7 (Dyson et al., 1989). Each of these viral proteins contains the LXCXE motif which is considered to be essential for interaction and which is also present in D cyclins (Sherr, 1993), BRG family (Strober et al., 1996), HDAC1 (De Pinho et al., 1998), HPB1 (Tevosian 1997), ELF1 (Wang et al., 1994) and CBP (Chen et al., 1996a). During normal regulation of the cell cycle hypophosphorylated pRb binds to members of the E2F/DP1 family of transcription factors through the A and B pockets, as discussed above. Interaction of the viral oncoproteins with pRb results in disruption of the complex with E2F, facilitating entry into the cell cycle (Chellappan et al., 1992). Ad E1A, SV40 Tag and HPV16 E7 also bind the p107 and p130 members of the pRb family which form complexes with E2F4 and 5. Again viral protein interaction facilitates cell cycle progression (Shirodkar et al., 1992; Lees et al., 1992; Schwarz et al., 1993) by dissociating the host protein complex. Binding sites on the viral proteins for p107 and p130 are similar to those determined for pRb (e.g. CR1 and CR2 for Ad E1A).

In most studies of Ad E1A, SV40 Tag and HPV E7 from high risk virus serotypes it has been shown that there is a direct correlation between binding to the pRb family of proteins and transforming and immortalizing activity as discussed in detail in Chapters 2, 3 and 6. However, it appears that disruption of the normal function of these cellular proteins is of considerable significance for the induction of apoptosis under normal circumstances in certain cell lineages. Therefore, it seems that a major role of p53 is to act as a failsafe mechanism to induce apoptosis in cells which undergo de-regulated cell cycle progression due to loss of pRb function (considered in detail by White, 1994).

As discussed in the previous section, from a consideration of data obtained from transgenic mice studies it may be concluded that when only pRb is inactivated either by viral proteins or genetic targeting apoptosis can result, depending on the cellular background. Loss of p53 imparts a strong predisposition to tumor development. Loss or inactivation of both gene products by binding to viral oncoproteins gives rise to a relatively normal phenotype with little apparent inappropriate apoptosis and a relatively low tumor incidence (Mulligan and Jacks, 1998).

It can be seen that these data are relevant to a discussion of infection and transformation and apoptosis induction by the DNA tumor virus oncoproteins. Each virus expresses a protein which binds the pRb family members releasing free E2F. This step seems to be essential for both processes, giving rise to cell cycle progression and DNA synthesis. In the normal course of events, this would be detected within the cell and apoptosis induced by a p53-dependent mechanism. However, Ad, SV40 and HPV all have mechanisms for dealing with p53 as described above – SV40 Tag and the larger Ad E1B protein forming an inactivating complex, HPV E6 targeting it for degradation and the smaller Ad E1B protein and perhaps SV40 Tag mimicking the Bcl-2 anti-apoptotic mechanism. Under these circumstances cell transformation is the probable outcome.

3. Induction of Apoptosis by Viruses

Many virus types are able to induce apoptosis in host cells and these are summarised in Table 1. We will consider here, in some detail, only the small DNA tumor viruses, which have been studied in most detail, and HIV.

a. *Induction of apoptosis by adenoviruses*

The introduction and repression of apoptosis by adenoviruses serves as the paradigm for the complex love-hate relationship between viruses and cell death. The means by which adenoviruses cause apoptosis has been an area of study for the last three decades and although our understanding of the subtle relationship between the viral proteins involved in the initiation and delay of the process and the cellular effector proteins is now considerable there are still large areas where our knowledge is superficial at best.

Observations that infection of human cells in culture with certain adenovirus 12 mutants produced large clear plaques due to the cytocidal effects of the virus were contemporaneous with the first major reports of apoptosis as a novel form of cell death (Saunders and Fallon, 1966; Takemori et al., 1968; 1969; Kerr et al., 1972). These *cyt* mutants were also shown to cause the degradation (*deg*) of cellular and viral DNA following infection (Ezoe et al., 1981). A large number of comparable Ad2 and Ad5 mutants which also caused cytopathic effects and DNA degradation were isolated somewhat later (Chinnadurai, 1983; Takemori et al., 1984; White et al., 1984; Pilder et al., 1984). Whilst there were certain differences between the cytocidal (*cyt*$^+$), degradation of DNA (*deg*$^+$) and large plaque (*lp*$^+$) mutants, all were mapped to the Ad E1B gene encoding the 19K protein (Lai Fatt and Mak, 1982; Chinnadurai, 1983; Subramanian et al., 1984; Takemori et al., 1984; White et al., 1984) which has now been shown to be functionally and structurally homologous to Bcl-2 (see below).

Thus, whilst one of the proteins involved in protection of adenovirus-infected cells from apoptosis has been well-known for many years it is only much more recently that the proteins and mechanism responsible for induction of the *cyt*$^+$, *lp*$^+$ and *deg*$^+$ phenotypes (i.e. apoptosis) have been characterized. It is now clear, however, that in the absence of the E1B proteins, Ad E1A induces apoptosis in infected or transfected cells (White et al., 1991; Rao et al., 1992). Apoptosis may be inhibited in transfected cells by

Table 1. Viral proteins involved in the initiation or inhibition of apoptosis

Virus	Initiators of apoptosis	Inhibitors of apoptosis	Reference
Adenovirus	E1A, E4, E3	E1B-19k, E1B-55k, E3-14.7k, RID (E3 10.4/14.5k)	Rao et al., 1992; Debbas and White, 1993; Marcellus et al., 1996; Tollefson et al., 1996; Dimitrov et al., 1997
Simian Virus 40	T ag	T ag	Allemand et al., 1995; Tzeng et al., 1996; McCarthy et al., 1994; Conzen et al., 1997
Human Cytomegalovirus		IE1, IE2	Zhu et al., 1995
Cowpox virus		crm A	Dbaido and Hannun, 1998
Human papilloma virus	E7, E2	E6	Pan and Griep, 1994, 1995
Vaccinia virus		SPI-2	Dobbelstein and Shenk, 1996
Epstein Barr virus		BHRF1, LMP1	Khanim et al., 1997
Baculovirus		p35, IAP	Clem et al., 1996; Seshagiri and Miller, 1997
Human/ Simian immunodeficiency virus1	Tat		New et al., 1998
Human T lymphotropic virus-1	Tax		Chen et al., 1997
Chicken anaemia virus	Apoptin (VP3)		Danen van Oorschot et al., 1997
Parvovirus	NSP		Morey et al., 1993
African Swine fever virus		LMW5-HL, A224L	Afonso et al., 1996
CELO adenovirus		GAM-1	Chiocca et al., 1997
Hepatitis B Virus Hepatitis C Virus		pX Core protein	Pagano et al., 1997
Myxomavirus		T2, MIIL	Schreiber et al., 1997
Herpes virus saimiri		ORF 16	Nava et al., 1997
Bovine Papilloma virus		E5, E8	Sparkowski et al., 1996
Herpes simplex virus		☐34.5 gene	He et al., 1997
Gamma herpesvirus		vFLIPs	Thome et al., 1997
Kaposi's sarcoma associated human herpesvirus type 8		KSbcl-2	Sarid et al., 1997
Porcine reproductive and respiratory syndrome virus	p25		Suarez et al., 1996

either the smaller (19K) or larger (58K in Ad2/5 and 54K in Ad12) E1B proteins, although the former of these is essential during viral infection. In addition, Ad E4 and Ad E3 products appear to have somewhat subsidiary roles in the induction and/or suppression of apoptosis during viral infection.

Using mutational analysis it has been established that Ad E1A is responsible for initiation of the cytopathic effects following adenovirus infection (White and Stillman, 1987; White et al., 1991). In addition, transfection of Ad E1A into human and rodent cells results in apoptosis which can be inhibited by Ad E19K protein or Bcl-2 (Rao et al., 1992). The observation that cells expressing E1A rapidly apoptose goes some way to explaining the difficulties experienced by a number of labs in the isolation of Ad E1A-transformed cell lines. Following transfection of E1A into primary rodent and human cells, transformed foci are formed at relatively high frequency – however, the foci then abort so that isolation of stable transformed cell lines occurs rarely with rodent cells and virtually never with human cells. As might be expected in view of the preceeding discussion co-transfection of either of the Ad E1B genes together with Ad E1A results in a dramatic increase in the formation of stable rodent transformants. Interestingly, it is no easier to produce human cell lines with Ad E1A together with either one of the genes encoding Ad E1B 19K or Ad E1B 54K proteins than with Ad E1A alone (Gallimore et al., 1986). In that case expression of both Ad E1B genes is essential. Quite why Ad E1B 19K protein will inhibit Ad E1A-induced apoptosis following transfection into rodent but not human cells is not clear.

The ability of Ad E1A to induce apoptosis appears to reside primarily, although not solely, in its ability to increase the level and activity of p53. Thus, transient transfection of rodent cells results in an appreciable increase in p53 expression which can then go on to initiate apoptotic pathways as discussed above (Lowe and Ruley, 1993; Debbas and White, 1993). In addition, infection of human cells with mutant adenoviruses which express only E1A and the smaller E1B protein also causes marked increase in p53 levels, although in this case apoptosis is limited by E1B expression (Grand et al., 1994). The mechanism of p53 induction by Ad E1A is now beginning to be understood. It has long been established that the ability of E1A to affect recipient cells resides in its interaction with important cellular regulatory proteins such as pRb, the related p107 and p130, p300/CBP and TBP (discussed in detail in chapter 3). The binding sites on E1A for these and other cellular components have been mapped to conserved regions 1, 2 and 3 (Moran and Mathews, 1987). Thus, for example, pRb binds to conserved regions (CR) 1 and 2, whilst the major site of interaction for TBP is in CR3. Mutational analysis has shown that sequences in CR1 and at the N terminus of E1A are essential for its ability to increase the level of cellular p53 in 'normal' human cells and induce apoptosis (White et al., 1991; Mymryk et al., 1994; Sanchez-Prieto et al., 1995; Querido et al., 1997b; Chiou and White, 1997; Nakajima et al., 1998). In all cell types examined, the ability of E1A to interact with p300 was essential for p53 induction. However, this was not the case in rodent or Hela cells in which HPV E6 and E7 proteins are present (Chiou and White, 1997; Querido et al., 1997b). Therefore it appears that similar Ad E1A sequences are required for accumulation of p53 as are required for the induction of DNA synthesis (White et al., 1991; Mymryk et al., 1994; Querido et al., 1997b).

Accumulation of p53 in response to Ad E1A is probably not due to increase in transcription but to an extension of protein half-life (Lowe and Ruley, 1993; Grand et al., 1996; Chiou and White, 1997). In the presence of E1A half-life is extended from a few minutes to approximately 2 hours (Grand et al., 1996) with this additional p53 being transcriptionally active (Grand et al., 1996; Querido et al., 1997b). The means by which E1A regulates p53 levels are only now becoming apparent. It has been shown (de Stanchina et al., 1998) that activation (and increased expression) of p53 by E1A is attributable to an increase in level of p19^{ARF}, a product of the INK4A locus which is frequently disrupted in human cancers (Haber, 1997; Chin et al., 1998). The observations that induction of p53 by DNA damage does not involve p19^{ARF} (Kamijo et al., 1997) and that there are differences in phosphorylation of p53 in response to DNA damage and E1A (de Stanchina et al., 1998) suggests that alternative pathways are involved in the two responses. Clues to the mechanism of induction of p19^{ARF} have recently been provided by the observation that activation of p19^{ARF} expression is dependent on the transcriptional activity of E2F-1 (Bates et al., 1998). Thus, it has been shown that Ad E1A, by binding to pRb, gives rise to deregulated E2F-1 activity, induction of p19^{ARF} and stabilization of p53 through binding of p19^{ARF} to p53/MDM2 (Pomerantz et al., 1998; Zhang et al., 1998; Kamijo et al., 1998). It is not clear precisely how p53 is stabilized but it has been suggested that p19^{ARF} interferes with p53 polyubiquitination (Pomerantz et al., 1998) and/or leads to retention in the nucleolus (discussed in Sherr, 1998).

The interaction between E1A and pRb has been known for over a decade (Whyte et al., 1988) and has been seen to be of critical importance in cell transformation both with adenoviruses and with Ad E1 DNA (Whyte et al., 1989; Egan et al., 1989). Following infection or DNA transfection E1A binds to the A and B subdomains of pRb through sequences in CR1 and more importantly CR2 (Whyte et al., 1989; Howe et al., 1990; Dyson et al., 1992). This interaction effectively dissociates pRb from E2F, leaving E2F free to activate transcription of its normal target genes (see for example, Bagchi et al., 1990; Bandara and La Thangue, 1991; Raychaudhuri et al., 1991) including p19^{ARF} as discussed above.

During *wt* adenovirus infection the activity of p53 is neutralized by the E1B proteins and by rapid down-regulation of the protein through degradation and inhibition of mRNA processing – all of which combine to give levels of p53 insufficient to elicit an apoptotic response. Following transfection transformed foci expressing only E1A apoptose and abort but those where the E1B proteins are present (inhibiting p53 and apoptosis) will grow on to form permanent cell lines. The significance of Ad E1A binding to the pRb homologues p107 and p130 is not immediately apparent – indeed it is not certain whether such interactions are essential for the induction of either apoptosis or transformation but it is likely that the release of all E2F components will favour cell cycle progression and, certainly in the context of pRb inactivation, cell death or the formation of transformed cell lines.

Whilst Ad E1A-induced p53-dependent apoptosis has been most closely studied, it has also been noted that Ad E1A can cause apoptosis in the absence of p53 following Ad infection (Subramanian et al., 1995a; Teodoro et al., 1995; Chiou and White, 1997). The observation that the larger Ad E1A 13S but not the 12S protein induces cell death in Ad-infected p53 null cells (Teodoro et al., 1995) suggested that a further Ad protein is involved and more recent investigations have implicated an E4 product (Marcellus et al., 1996; Lavoie et al., 1998; Shtrichman and Kleinberger, 1998). Thus Ad5 E4 orf4 can induce apoptosis in recipient cells in the absence or presence of p53 and this apoptotic response can be inhibited by Bcl-2 (Lavoie et al., 1998; Shtrichman and Kleinberger, 1998). It has been suggested that initiation of apoptosis may be due to the production of "conflicting signals" within the cell perhaps caused by interaction of E4 orf4 with protein phosphatase 2A (Shtrichman and Kleinberger, 1998; Kleinberger and Shenk, 1993). Interestingly, "apoptosis" induced by E4 orf4, whilst inhibitable by Bcl-2, does not appear to involve caspase 3 and is suggested to be a novel form of cell death (Lavoie et al., 1998).

As mentioned in the introduction, it appears that viruses go to considerable lengths to inhibit apoptosis in the initial steps of infection to allow virus replication to proceed in an intact cell unhindered by the host immune system. However, later in infection, at least by non-enveloped viruses, host cell lysis is desirable - to facilitate release of the progeny viruses. It has been suggested that apoptosis might play a role in this process. The adenovirus system again serves as a model. Mutational analysis has shown that an 11.6K protein encoded by the E3 region (termed 'adenovirus death protein' [ADP]) is essential for nuclear lysis and release of progeny late in infection, although it is not necessary for the observed cytopathic effects (Tollefson et al., 1992; 1996a; 1996b). ADP is expressed early in infection but at very high levels in the later stages (Tollefson et al., 1992) and appears to control lysis of the cell's nuclear membrane where it is located (Scaria et al., 1992) by an, as yet, unknown mechanism. ADP might promote cell death by inhibiting the anti-apoptotic activities of E1B 19K protein and the cellular Bcl-2 family (Tollefson et al., 1996b). However, few of the diagnostic features of apoptosis (for example condensed chromatin, blebbed membranes or DNA degradation) could be distinguished in wt Ad infected cells immediately prior to lysis (Tollefson et al., 1996b).

b. *Induction of apoptosis by SV40 and HPV*

Oncoproteins encoded by SV40 and HPV have many properties in common with adenovirus E1A and E1B – in particular their ability to interact with and modulate the activity of the same set of cell cycle regulators (discussed in detail in Chapters 2 and 6, respectively). For example, Tag and HPV16/18 E7, like E1A, bind strongly to pRb and the related p107 and p130 whilst the larger Ad E1B proteins, Tag and HPV16/18 E6 can affect the level and/or activity of p53. On the basis of these observations it might be expected that proteins encoded by these viruses would be able to modulate apoptosis in recipient cells in a similar manner to adenovirus E1.

In initial studies using transgenic mice it was demonstrated that whilst expression of intact SV40 Tag leads to rapid tumor induction, the N terminal fragment of Tag (which does not contain the p53 binding site) causes, in some cases, slow-growing tumors and appreciable levels of apoptosis in the brain choroid plexus (Saenz Robies et al., 1994; Symonds et al., 1994; McCarthy et al., 1994). In the absence of p53 the Tag fragment causes rapid tumor induction and no appreciable apoptosis (Symonds et al., 1994). It seems reasonable to suppose that the ability of this truncated protein to induce apoptosis can be attributed to its sequestration of pRb and subsequent disruption of the pRb E2F complex. p53-dependent apoptosis then takes place as discussed in sections 2 and 4a. Full-length Tag forms a complex with p53, inhibiting its activity and inhibiting p53-dependent apoptosis. Other studies have suggested that in some tissues of transgenic mice intact SV40 Tag can give rise to apoptosis at certain stages during development (Allemand et al., 1995; Tzeng et al., 1996). In these cases it seems likely that there is a "developmental contribution" to induction such that under certain circumstances Tag is not able to totally neutralize the ability of p53 to induce an apoptosis pathway or perhaps p53-independent apoptosis occurs.

As well as being implicated in the induction of cell death SV40 Tag also possesses "anti-apoptosis" capabilities. This is most obviously attributable to its ability to bind p53 (Lane and Crawford, 1979; Linzer and Levine, 1979). Thus, as mentioned above expression of *wt* SV40 Tag in transgenic mice leads to tumor induction rather than apoptosis. Direct demonstration that SV40 Tag can prevent apoptosis induced by over-expression of ICE but not ICH-1$_L$ has been presented (Jung and Yuan, 1997). More interestingly, perhaps it has recently been shown that SV40 Tag is able to act as a viability factor quite distinct from any ability to form a complex with p53 (Conzen et al., 1997). This property has been mapped to a sequence between amino acids 525 and 541 which has greater than 60% homology to a region of Ad5 E1B 19K protein which is necessary for protection of infected cells from Ad E1A-induced apoptosis. Most persuasively, mutation of two of the conserved amino acids in this region (528 and 539) resulted in loss of SV40 Tag's ability to protect from p53-induced apoptosis (Conzen et al., 1997). Thus, it appears that, like the adenovirus E1B gene, SV40 T encodes two distinct mechanisms for protection of infected cells from apoptosis.

Investigations carried out on human papillomaviruses have focussed primarily on the abilities of the E6 and E7 proteins to modulate apoptosis. As with the Ad E1 proteins and with SV40 Tag it appears that regulation of the activity, or in this case level of expression, of p53 and activity of pRb is of most obvious importance. HPV16 and 18 E7 binds to the pRb family members through a site within amino acids 18-37 which includes the motif LXCXE (Dyson et al., 1989). As with SV40 T ag this is presumed to dissociate and free E2F. In a particularly significant series of experiments HPV16/18 E7 has been targeted to the eye of transgenic mice and found to trigger extensive apoptosis in the retina and lens (Howes et al., 1994; Pan and Griep, 1994). If the E7 protein was expressed against a p53-null background, produced either by co-expression of HPV16/18 E6 or by genetic "knockout", little apoptosis was apparent and tumors developed (Pan and Griep, 1994; Howes et al., 1994; Nakamura et al., 1997). *In vitro* HPV E7 is also able to sensitize recipient cells to apoptosis-inducing stimuli (such as irradiation) presumably by complex formation with and subsequent degradation of pRb, consistent with the *in vivo* experiments (Puthenveettil et al., 1996). Interestingly, it has been suggested that HPV E7 might target pRb for degradation by the 26S proteasome through an interaction with the S4 subunit (Berezutskaya and Bagchi, 1997). If this were the case it would favour the presence of free E2F in the cell.

In the mouse models HPV16/18 E6 is able to overcome p53-induced apoptosis by targeting it, by ubiquitination, for proteasomal degradation. Similar data has been presented to suggest that this also occurs in transfected cell lines (for example, Thomas et al., 1996; Puthenveettil et al., 1996). In addition, it has been shown that E6 can impair irradiation-induced p53 transcriptional activity presumably by reducing protein levels (Gu et al., 1994).

Interestingly, it has been suggested that HPV16/18 E6 has anti-apoptosis activity quite distinct from its ability to modulate p53 levels and that HPV16/18 E7 can induce p53-independent apoptosis (Pan and Griep, 1994; 1995). In these transgenic mouse studies p53-dependent apoptosis occurred during the early stages of foetal development (up to 18 days gestation), whereas later apoptosis was p53 dependent and independent (Pan and Griep, 1995).

Other PV proteins have also been implicated in the induction of apoptosis. For example, BPV1 and HPV18 E2 can increase p53 transcriptional activity by repressing transcription of E6 but can also cause apoptosis directly (Desaintes et al., 1997). Evidence has also been presented to indicate a role for BPV1-E5 and BPV4-E8 in suppression of apoptosis (discussed in O'Brien, 1998).

c. *Apoptosis following HIV infection*

Cytotoxic T lymphocytes (CTLs) provide a major line of defence, in vertebrates, against cells that could pose a threat to the host. Normally CTLs can recognise and induce apoptosis in virally-infected or transformed cells by two mechanisms (reviewed in Razvi and Welsh, 1995; Vaux and Strasser, 1996). Firstly they can express Fas ligand as a result of target cell recognition which will bind to the Fas surface receptor on the target cell. Secondly they can deliver granules containing pro-apoptotic molecules (e.g. perforin and granzymes) to the target cell. In HIV-infected individuals there is a marked reduction in T cell function leading to immune deficiency (see for example Fauci, 1993). Many of these defects are attributable to the induction of apoptosis by HIV in various populations of cells involved in the immune response to viral infection (reviewed Ameisen et al., 1995).

T cells isolated from asymptomatic HIV-infected individuals are relatively unresponsive to mitogens or T cell receptor (TCR) stimulation, failing to proliferate in the same way as normal cells. At a later stage in the progress of the disease there is a considerable reduction in numbers of CD4[+] T cells due to apoptosis (Terai et al, 1990; Laurent-Crawford et al., 1991; Groux et al., 1992). These CD4[+] T cells seem to be particularly susceptible to cell death, undergoing apoptosis in response to signals which would cause proliferation in normal cells. In addition, there is a loss of CD8[+] T cells during the development of AIDS with high levels of CD4[+] and CD8[+] cell apoptosis observed in the lymph nodes of infected individuals (considered in detail in Pantaleo et al., 1994). Whilst apoptosis of CD4[+] cells, following HIV infection might be expected, the observation that CD8[+] T cells were also particularly prone to apoptosis was unexpected as these are not considered to be a usual target for infection. However, it now appears that much cell death is induced by an indirect mechanism such that bystander cells comprise the major set of apoptotic cells in animal models (Mosier et al., 1993; Bonyhadi et al., 1993; Aldrovani et al., 1993) and HIV-infected individuals (Finkel et al., 1995).

Our knowledge of the mechanism by which HIV induces apoptosis in target T cells is still somewhat confused. Earlier reports suggested that interaction of the HIV envelope protein (Env gp120) on infected T cells with CD4 on uninfected cells was sufficient to induce apoptosis (Cohen et al., 1992; Oyaizu et al., 1994) although viral replication was not necessary (Maldarelli et al., 1995). Similarly, cross-linking of CD4 with antibodies or gp120/gp120 antibody complexes could cause cell death in uninfected T cells (Banda et al., 1992; Oyaizu et al., 1994; Newell et al., 1990). However, more recent evidence suggests that HIV proteins can promote apoptosis through the Fas-FasL pathway (see section 3). Cross-linking of CD4 with gp120 together with TCR activation results in marked increase in apoptosis mediated by Fas/FasL with greatly increased levels of FasL which can bind directly to Fas on gp120-bound cells and on bystander cells (Westendorp et al., 1995; Accornero et al., 1997).

In addition to gp120, the HIV-1 Tat protein also appreciably enhances T cell apoptosis following TCR stimulation, cross-linking of CD4 with CD4 antibody or gp120 together with gp120 antibody (Westendorp et al., 1995). Stimulation of T cells with Tat and antibody to the TCR causes an increase in level of FasL mRNA and presumably activation of the Fas-FasL apoptotic pathway. Tat is a multifunctional protein which acts primarily as a transcription factor and has been shown to be able to down-regulate Bcl-2, at both the transcriptional and translational levels under low-serum conditions (Sastry et al., 1996). In addition, expression of Tat correlates well with increased Bax expression (Sastry et al., 1996). Obviously, these changes in protein expression will favour apoptosis.

Expression of the 14.6K nuclear Vpr protein also appears to induce apoptosis either alone or in the context of HIV infection (Stewart et al., 1997). Vpr has previously been shown to induce G2 cell cycle arrest (Bartz et al., 1996; He et al., 1995; Jowett et al., 1995) probably by inhibition of the activity of cdc2. Recent mutational analysis has established a correlation between the ability of Vpr to produce cell cycle arrest and to induce apoptosis, although no requirement for cdc2 kinase activity was observed (Stewart et al., 1997). It has also been noted that HIV-1 protease is able to induce apoptosis in transfected cells by specific cleavage of host cell Bcl-2 initially between amino acids F112 and A113 (Strack et al., 1996). Loss of Bcl-2 results in activation of NFκB, a transcription factor required for HIV replication (Strack et al., 1996).

The major area of controversy in any consideration of the induction of apoptosis by HIV-1 in the infected host is the role of Fas/FasL. This has recently been discussed in detail by Kaplan and Sieg (1998) – therefore only a brief summary of the arguments needs to be given here. There is little doubt that expression of Fas and FasL can be enhanced *in vitro* following HIV infection or exposure to HIV proteins causing apoptosis (Badley et al., 1996; Westendorp et al., 1995). In addition, an increase in T cells expressing Fas is seen in HIV-1 infected hosts as the disease progresses (Debatin et al., 1994; Aries et al., 1995). Kaplan and Sieg (1998), however, have argued that these data do not necessarily mean that CD4[+] and CD8[+] CTLs die in the infected host by Fas-mediated apoptosis. Furthermore, as they note some reports have concluded that there is no involvement of the Fas pathway in HIV-induced T cell apoptosis (Katsikis et al., 1996; 1997) nor is there an involvement of Fas signaling in apoptosis in peripheral blood cells from HIV-1 infected individuals (Katsikis et al., 1996; Baumler et al., 1996). Additional evidence against the involvement of Fas/FasL is provided by the finding that FasL expression and activity is suppressed in HIV-1 infected individuals – despite the presence of FasL mRNA in the appropriate T cells (Sieg et al., 1997). It is possible that the ligand is lost from the surface of these cells as it has been reported that elevated levels of FasL are present in the blood following HIV-1 infection (Bahr et al., 1997). It is also interesting to note that there is an increase in T cells expressing Fas in the infected host (Aries et al., 1995; Katsikis et al., 1995; Gehri et al., 1996; Silvestris et al., 1996). If Fas/FasL-mediated apoptosis were (totally) responsible for depletion of CD4$^+$ T cells Kaplan and Sieg (1998) have suggested that Fas/FasL-expressing cells would not be expected to accumulate. In spite of these arguments it seems that most researchers would agree that CD4$^+$ T cells are depleted by apoptosis in HIV-infected individuals and that this apoptosis is attributable, directly or indirectly, to the activities of the viral proteins.

Significantly, perhaps, data presented by Kolesnitchenko et al. (1997) have suggested that HIV gp120-mediated killing by CD4$^+$ binding is not attributable to apoptosis. In these studies it was shown that gp120-induced killing did not involve Fas and was not inhibited by increased levels of Bcl-2 or Ad E1B 19K protein. In addition, diagnostic cleavage of PARP by caspases was not observed (Kolesnitchenko et al., 1997). In contrast, the same authors confirmed that Tat expression sensitized cells to Fas-mediated killing (Li et al., 1995; Westendorp et al., 1995) which had some of the classical characteristics of apoptosis. Whilst Kolesnitchenko et al. (1997) have suggested that gp120-mediated (non-apoptotic) killing accounts for an appreciable proportion of cell death attributable to HIV, previous reports have reached the opposite conclusion (Katsikis et al., 1995; Estaquier et al., 1995).

As has already been noted, most viruses encode sets of proteins which are able to initiate and suppress apoptosis (Table 2). This also seems to be the case for HIV-1, although evidence in favour of the anti-apoptotic components is rather weak at present. However, the observation, made on the basis of *in vitro* experiments, that HIV-1-infected cells, unlike bystander cells, are resistant to HIV-induced cell death strongly suggests a viral mechanism for suppression of apoptosis (Nardelli et al., 1995; Finkel et al., 1995). The Tat protein which induces apoptosis in uninfected cells is able to protect T cells from apoptosis when endogenously expressed (McCloskey et al., 1997). This may be attributable to up-regulation of Bcl-2. Other viral proteins have also been suggested as possible anti-apoptotic factors. HIV-1 Vpr can supress apoptosis induced through TCR by inhibition of NFκB activity by means of the induction of the inhibitor IκB (Ayyavoo et al., 1997). It has also been shown that monocytes isolated from HIV-infected patients had very low levels of FasL on their surface compared to similar cells from normal individuals. The virally-induced reduction in FasL would be expected to reduce apoptosis, although the mechanism of its regulation remains unknown (Sieg et al., 1997). It is also interesting to note that peptides derived from p17 and p24 Gag proteins may inhibit lysis of target cells presenting the epitope, reducing cell death (Klenerman et al., 1994).

The importance of the multiplicity of HIV gene products that are able to induce cell death is not clear. Nor has it yet been established unequivocally which of these are most relevant to infection *in vivo*. However, it appears that there is an increased surface expression of Fas on cells of HIV-infected individuals and there is an increase in FasL level and surface expression of Fas following HIV infection of human monocytic cells and macrophages (Katsikis et al., 1995; Badley et al., 1996). However, there is not universal acceptance of the idea that Fas-FasL pathway is involved in the direct killing of HIV-infected T cells *in vivo* (Katsikis et al., 1996; Noraz et al., 1997).

It should also be borne in mind that a recent report (Sylwester et al., 1997) has suggested that the main cause of T cell death following HIV infection is due to the formation of syncytia. Whilst earlier studies (Leonard et al., 1988; Kiernan et al., 1990) had indicated that these cell fusions accounted for relatively little death, it now appears that syncytia, in infected cultures, can reach considerable size, are self-perpetuating and are the main source of new virus (Sylwester et al., 1997). Support for the idea that syncytia play an important role, *in vivo,* in cell death is provided by the observation that they are relatively common in adenoid and axillary lymph node biopsies (Frankel et al., 1996).

4. Induction of Apoptosis by Cytokine Signaling

a. *TNF receptor and Fas*

The cytokines are a family of proteins that regulate cellular proliferation and differentiation by binding to their specific receptors on target cells. Two such receptors, both members of the tumour necrosis factor (TNF) sub-family, TNFR and Fas have also been characterized extensively due to their ability to induce apoptosis (Nagata and Golstein 1995). In both cases the ligands, TNF and FasL, are synthesized as type II-membrane proteins which are cleaved by a membrane metalloproteinase to generate soluble cytokine (Gearing et al., 1994). However, membrane-bound TNF is more active than the soluble form and in mice soluble FasL has no activity at all (Grell et al., 1995). These results indicate that FasL and TNF mediate their functions through cell-cell interactions and that the purpose of shedding TNF or FasL is to attenuate the process (Nagata 1997). The functional cytokines exist as trimers (Tanaka et al., 1995) and it is in these forms that they interact with the receptors, Fas (APO-1/CD95) and tumour necrosis factor receptor (TNFR) 1/2 respectively. Both receptors are type 1-membrane proteins that have been shown to contain death domains (DD). The death domain is a conserved protein-protein interaction sequence motif of about 90 amino acids. In the absence of their death domains the interaction of the ligand, or agonist antibody, with receptor no longer initiates apoptosis (Feinstein et al., 1995).

Ligand binding induces trimerisation of the receptor and this causes the recruitment of several proteins that form a complex around the cytoplasmic moiety of the receptor.

The complex is known as the death initiating signaling complex or DISC. The components of the DISC differ slightly between the Fas and TNF receptors although they have a similar effect. Upon Fas activation FADD (Fas-associating protein with death domain, also known as MORT-1) binds to Fas via interactions between the death domains present on both molecules (Kischkel et al., 1995). The N-terminal portion of FADD has another conserved domain known as a death effector domain (DED), it is this domain that interacts with the next molecule in the cascade. Using the yeast two hybrid system, caspase 8 was identified (Boldin et al., 1996). This caspase, previously known as FLICE (FADD-like ICE) or MACH (MORT 1-associated *ced*-3 homologue) was found also to contain a DED domain in the N-terminal region through which it interacts with FADD.

After trimerisation of the TNFR1 receptor, TRADD (TNFR1-associated death domain protein) is recruited to the DISC by interaction of the death domains present in both molecules (Hsu et al., 1995). This protein unlike FADD does not contain a death effector domain. However, the death domain present on TRADD binds to the death domain in FADD (Hsu et al., 1996). From this point, the signaling machinery is similar to that used after Fas activation leading to the activation of the caspases. However, there is a second death pathway induced by TNFR1 activation. RIP (receptor interacting protein) contains a death domain coupled to a kinase domain. Through interaction of the death domains, RIP binds to TRADD (Hsu et al., 1996). RIP does not contain a death effector domain but does induce apoptosis when overexpressed, indicating the recruitment of another molecule. A further death-domain-containing adapter was isolated, RAIDD (RIP-associated Ich-1/ced-3 homologous protein with a death domain). RAIDD binds to RIP through the interaction of death domains and recruits caspase 2 (Duan and Dixit, 1997). Figure 2 shows the signaling pathway through the Fas receptor.

b. *Protection against TNF-induced apoptosis by adenovirus E3 proteins*

The RID (receptor internalization degradation) complex represents an anti-apoptotic mechanism conserved in all the major adenovirus serotypes. The complex, formerly known as E3-10.4K/14.5K is composed of two polypeptides encoded by the Ad E3 region. The complex is formed from one 14.5K (RIDβ) protein and two 10.4K (RIDα) proteins. Together they contain four membrane spanning domains (Stewart et al., 1995). The RID complex has been shown to function to protect many but not all mouse cell lines from lysis by TNF (Gooding et al., 1991). The mechanism of this action is unknown. Recently however the RID complex was also shown to protect cells treated with a monoclonal antibody that triggers Fas-induced apoptosis (Tollefson et al., 1998). Some of the data presented by Tollefson et al., (1998) are summarized in Table 2.

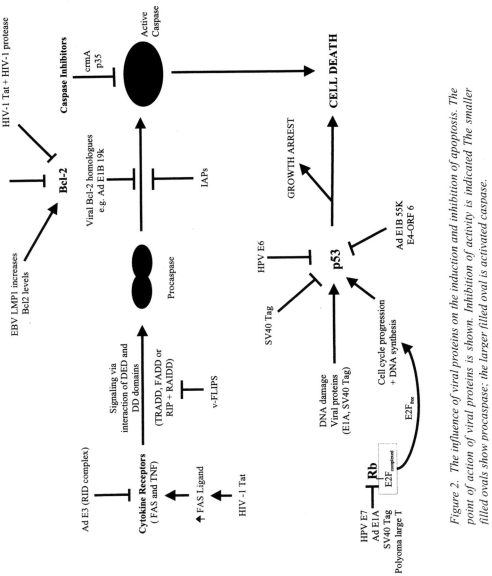

Figure 2. The influence of viral proteins on the induction and inhibition of apoptosis. The point of action of viral proteins is shown. Inhibition of activity is indicated The smaller filled ovals show procaspase; the larger filled oval is activated caspase.

Table 2. Apoptosis following infection with mutant adenovirus with deletions in the E3 and E1B genes

Virus used to infect mcf-7-Fas cells	Approximate % apoptosis (detected by visualization of the nucleus)
Wild type	1%
Del. RIDα	1%
Del. RIDβ	1%
Del. E1B 19k	10%
Del. RIDα, RIDβ, E1B 19k	90%

Immunoflourescence studies have demonstrated that after infection with wild-type adenovirus the Fas receptor was internalized and subsequently degraded inside lysosomes, presumably via endosome transport. Mutant adenovirus deleted for RIDα and β showed no effect on the localization of FasR. The same research group previously reported the internalization of the epidermal growth factor receptor by the same complex (Tollefson et al., 1991; see also Elsing and Bugert, 1998). This led to the speculation that the RID complex had a general effect on cell surface receptors. This has been shown not to be the case. The RID complex has no effect on the distribution of the transferrin receptor, the class I antigens of the major histocompatibility complex (MHC) or LTβR (Tollefson et al., 1998, Shisler et al., 1997).

By effectively removing Fas from the surface of infected cells the host cell is protected from attack by leukocytes such as CTLs, which express Fas L. It has been speculated that adenovirus infection may be linked with auto-immune disease. Mice bearing a mutation known as *lpr* (lymphoproliferation) develop lymphadenopathy and suffer from autoimmune disease. The *lpr* mice have a mutation in Fas. The lymphadenopathy seen in these mice has been attributed to the accumulation of cells, which in normal mice would apoptose (Watanabe-Fukunga et al., 1992). In the case of adenovirus infection the action of the RID complex could result in the presence of Fas-negative T lymphocytes which are capable of self-reactivity. Such cells would therefore contribute to an auto-immune disease. In support of this theory, which is as yet only correlative, multiple sclerosis patients have been identified as having higher anti-adenovirus antibody titres than matched controls (Compston et al., 1986).

The protection against TNF-mediated apoptosis offered by the RID complex involves no alteration in the cell surface distribution of the TNF receptor (Gooding et al., 1991). Therefore the RID complex would appear to employ different mechanisms to protect from Fas and TNF-induced apoptosis. Studies have shown that the RID complex and E3-14.7K block TNF-induced cPLA$_2$ translocation and subsequent arachidonic acid release (Dimitrov et al., 1997). Following normal translocation from the cytosol to cell membranes cPLA$_2$ cleaves arachidonic acid from membrane phospholipids (Channon and Leslie, 1990). The arachidonic acid can then be metabolised to form prostaglandins, leuktrines and lipoxyns, all of which amplify inflammation. Therefore as a result of these proteins not only is the cell death response ablated but so is inflammation. In support of this suggestion mice infected with adenovirus deleted for E3-10.4k and 14.5K show a dramatically increased inflammatory response (Sparer et al., 1996). Recently Chen et al., (1998) have demonstrated an interaction between adenovirus 14.7K and caspase 8 and have speculated that it is responsible for the inhibition of Fas L-induced apoptosis. E3-14.7K is not a member of the v-FLIPs (discussed later) and the nature of the interaction with caspase 8 is unknown. In accordance with previous reports caspase activation is required for cPLA$_2$ release (Wissing et al., 1997). Therefore, by targeting caspase 8 at the apex of the caspase cascade cPLA$_2$ translocation would be attenuated.

c. *Protection against TNF-induced apoptosis by pox virus*

A more blatant method of inhibiting the stimulation of the TNF receptor has been employed by some of the pox viruses. Members of this group have been demonstrated to secrete proteins with significant homology to the TNF receptor. Examples include S-T2 from Shope fibroma virus (SPV) which causes benign fibromas in rabbits, M-T2 from myxoma virus and Crm B and C from cowpox virus. The TNF receptor and members of the super-family contain multiple cysteine rich domains (CRDs) at their N-termini. Each CRD is approximately 40 amino acids in length and contains six cysteines in a conserved pattern. It is these CRDs that have been "copied" by the poxviruses. Both S-T2 and M-T2 contain four CRDs along with the appropriate signal sequence. The proteins do not however contain transmembrane domains and are therefore secreted from infected cells. Both S-T2 and Crm C have been demonstrated to bind to TNFα (Smith et al., 1991, Smith et al., 1996). Of interest is the finding that M-T2 appears to have a dual function as mutant versions unable to bind TNFα are still capable of inhibiting apoptosis (Schreiber et al., 1997). A protein with CRDs has also been reported in human cytomegalovirus (HCMV) implying that this phenomenon is not restricted to pox viruses (Cha et al., 1996).

5. The BCL-2 Protein Family

The first mammalian cell death regulator isolated was Bcl-2, the protein product of the proto-oncogene *bcl-2*. This gene was discovered as a consequence of its chromosomal translocation (t14:18) in human follicular center B-cell lymphoma (Tsujimoto et al., 1984). This translocation results in *bcl-2* being situated in close proximity to the enhancer element of immunoglobulin heavy chain at 14q32. Experiments in two cytokine-dependent hematopoietic cell lines demonstrated that enforced expression of Bcl-2 promoted survival but not proliferation after growth factor (IL-3) deprivation (Vaux et al., 1988). This observation and many like it demonstrated that Bcl-2 is a mammalian antagonist of apoptosis and that cell death and cell division are subject to distinct genetic control.

Table 3 Domain structure of the Bcl-2 family of proteins

Bcl-2 related protein	BH1	BH2	BH3	BH4	TM	Apoptosis
Bcl-2	+	+	+	+	+	Antagonist
Bcl-X$_L$	+	+	+	+	+	Antagonist
Bcl-w	+	+	+	+	+	Antagonist
Mcl-1	+	+	+	+	+	Antagonist
Bfl 1	+	+	+	+	(+)	Antagonist
A1	+	+	+	+	+	Antagonist
Boo	+	+	-	+	+	Antagonist
Bax	+	+	+	-	+	Agonist
Bak	+	+	+	-	+	Agonist
Bad	+	+	+	-	-	Agonist
Bcl-Xs	-	-	+	+	+	Agonist
Bik/Nbk	-	-	+	-	+	Agonist
Bim	-	-	+	-	+	Agonist
Bok	+	+	+	-	+	Agonist
Hrk	-	-	+	-	+	Agonist
Bid	-	-	+	-	-	Agonist
Ad E1B-19k	+	-	+	-	-	Antagonist
AFSV LMW5	+	+	+	-	-	Antagonist
EBV-BHRF1	+	+	+	-	+	Antagonist
HSV ORF 16	+	+	+	-	+	Antagonist

BH: Bcl-2 homology domain; TM: transmembrane domain.

a. *Structure of Bcl-2 family of proteins*

The 26K protein Bcl-2 is homologous to ced-9, the *C.elegans* suppressor of apoptosis. Whilst ced-9 is the only gene of this type found in *C.elegans* there is a family of Bcl-2-related proteins present in mammals (summarised in Table 3). Ced-9 appears to be bifunctional in its inhibition of apoptosis. In the first case ced-9 is capable of competitively inhibiting ced-3 via direct protein-protein interaction. Ced-9 is also a substrate for ced-3 and can be cleaved at two sites near its N-terminus (Xue and Horvitz, 1997). One of the cleavage products resembles Bcl-2 and baculovirus p35 in function and appears to inhibit apoptosis via a similar mechanism (Xue and Horvitz, 1997). In the majority of cases members of the Bcl-2 family possess a C-terminal transmembrane (TM) region which influences their subcellular distribution. In addition, they possess Bcl-2 homology (BH) regions (BH1,2,3 and 4), which determine their capacity to interact with each other and with other unrelated proteins. Differential splicing is a common feature of the *bcl-2* family genes. *bcl-2* itself is spliced to give two products Bcl-2α and Bcl-2β. These differ in the presence of the TM domain, which is absent in Bcl-2β due to the failure to remove an intron (Tsujimoto and Croce, 1986: Tanaka et al., 1993). Differential splicing of both *bcl-x* and *bax* has also been demonstrated (Fang et al., 1994; Oltvai et al., 1993). Viral proteins exhibiting varying degrees of homology with Bcl-2 have also been identified. These include Ad E1B-19K, EBV BHRF1, ASFV LMW5-HL and HSV ORF 16. The current members of the Bcl-2 family including viral homologues are summarized in Table 3.

The identification of proteins with homology to Bcl-2 was facilitated by the finding that many homo or heterodimerise. Therefore, it was possible to use immunoprecipitation or yeast two hybrid experiments to isolate them. Initially Bax was identified as a Bcl-2 binding protein (Oltvai et al., 1993). Bcl-2 also dimerises with Bak which, like Bad, commits cells to apoptosis (Kiefer et al., 1995). Bak was also identified independently by its ability to bind Ad E1B-19K (Farrow et al., 1995). It has become clear that the presence of all of the signature BH1, 2 and 3 domains is not required for interactions between family members. The protein Bik for example, which contains only BH3 is capable of binding Bcl-2, Ad E1B-19K, Bcl-x$_L$ and Bcl-x$_s$ (Boyd et al., 1995). 53BP2 was originally identified as a p53-binding protein (Kernohan et al., 1997) but has since been shown to interact with Bcl-2 (Naumovski and Cleary, 1996). Bcl-2 can block p53-induced apoptosis but does not prevent p53-mediated cell cycle arrest. Over-expression of 53BP2 impedes cell cycle progression at G2/M (Naumovski and Cleary, 1996). Since the same residues are required to bind p53 as are required to bind Bcl-2, 53BP2 might be the intermediate protein that allows Bcl-2 to block only one aspect of p53 function (Kernohan et al., 1997). The examples described above represent just some of the interactions between the Bcl-2 family of proteins. Whether all the interactions demonstrated occur in any single cell is unclear and seems unlikely. It is now generally accepted that the ratio of heterodimer versus homodimer pairs is critical to the determination of the cell's fate. An attractive possibility is that specific dimer pairs are subject to regulation by phosphorylation/dephosphorylation. In support of this, Guan et al., (1996) have shown that Bcl-2 in the human colon line, HT-29, is phosphorylated on seven serine residues. This phosphorylation could prevent the binding of Bcl-2 to Bax and thus tip the balance towards apoptosis (Hadlar et al., 1994). More recently it was shown that Bcl-2 was phosphorylated on serine 20 and that this phosphorylation was required for its anti-apoptic activity (Ito et al., 1997). Bad has also been demonstrated to be phosphorylated on serines in response to survival factors (Zha et al., 1996). It should be noted, however, that suppression or induction of apoptosis by the Bcl-2 family can, in some cases, be independent of their interactions (Cheng et al., 1997; Simonian et al., 1996).

Considering the presence of a TM domain in Bcl-2 it is not surprising that it has been shown to be localized to intracellular membranes. Bcl-2 is present on the outer mitochondrial membrane, nuclear membrane and the endoplasmic reticulum (ER) (Monaghan et al., 1992; Jacobson et al., 1993; Krajewski et al., 1993). Other reports have concluded that the majority of Bcl-2 is present on the cytosolic face of the ER (Zehava and Cleary, 1990) or on the outer mitochondrial membrane (Reed, 1994; Yang and Korsmeyer, 1996). Presumably the exact localization is cell type specific. Interestingly in the mitochondrion Bcl-2 appears to be localized to the contact sites between the inner and outer membranes. In lymphoid cells, Bcl-2 expression correlates stoichiometrically with that of peripheral benzodiazepine receptor (PBR) which is a putative component of the permeability transition (PT) pore (Zoratti and Szabo, 1995; Kroemer et al., 1997). Bcl-2 has also been localized to the chromosomes during the prophase, metaphase and anaphase stages of mitosis. This localization does not persist through to telophase (Lu et al., 1994; Willingham and Bhalla, 1994), which has led to the speculation that Bcl-2 is in some way involved in chromatin cleavage. Bcl-x_L, Bcl-x_s and mcl-1 have all been demonstrated to be localized predominantly in the mitochondrion (Gonzalez-Garcia et al., 1994; Krajewski et al., 1994).

As shown in Table 3 the Bcl-2 family members differ in their effects on apoptosis. They either suppress apoptosis or induce/enhance it. This is reflected by the results of knockout mice experiments. Bcl-2-null mice survive embryonic development but eventually die due to a complex set of problems including massive involution of the thymus and spleen as well as polycystic kidney disease (Kamada et al., 1995). Polycystic kidney disease is believed to result from excessive apoptosis during metanephric development. Bcl-$_{xL}$-null mice die at embryonic day (E) 13 due to massive apoptotic cell death in the nervous and hematopoetic systems (Motoyama et al., 1995). Bax-null mice develop normally and have few phenotypic features. They show thymocyte and splenic B-cell hyperplasia as well as excessive numbers of granulosa cells in atretic ovarian follicles in females and infertility in males due to the lack of mature sperm and the apoptotic cell death of precursors (Knudson et al., 1995). The results seen with this knockout mouse were surprising as Bax has been classified as an apoptosis agonist and so excessive cell death would be expected during development. This implies a more complex mode of action for Bax probably depending on cellular partners. The exact mode of action of Bcl-2, its partners and homologues has not yet been elucidated and, as with many of the proteins involved in apoptosis seems to be largely dependent on the cell type and environment. What is clear however is that the interactions between the Bcl-2 family members and their location within the cell play a pivotal role in function. For example it has been demonstrated that mutations introduced in the BH1 or BH2 domains of Bcl-2 at a number of conserved positions prevents not only the suppression of apoptosis by Bcl-2 but also the binding to Bax (Yin et al., 1994).

It is unlikely that Bcl-2 suppresses apoptosis by a single mechanism. Bcl-2 co-immunoprecipitates R-ras and the serine/threonine kinase Raf-1 (Fernandez-Sarabia and Bischoff, 1993; Wang et al., 1994). Raf-1 and R-ras bind each other in a GTP-dependent manner which results in the activation of the microtubule-associated protein kinase cascade. Through these associations, Bcl-2 may serve to target Raf-1 to the mitochondria. The structure of Bcl-$_{xL}$ bears significant similarity to the pore-forming domains of several bacterial toxins, in particular colicins A and E1 and diptheria toxin (Muchmore et al., 1996). Like these bacterial proteins, Bcl-$_{xL}$ is capable of inserting into synthetic lipid vesicles to form ion-conductance channels (Minn et al., 1997). The channel forming region of Bcl-xL, between BH 1 and BH2 represents a variable region in the Bcl-2 family members. This suggests that different members may produce channels with variations in the charge or conformation that may determine ion selectivity and/or conductance. Bcl-2 has previously been shown to affect subcellular Ca^{2+} levels at the ER, nucleus and mitochondria (Lam et al., 1994; Martin et al., 1996; Baffy et al., 1993). However Ca^{2+} levels have also been shown to both increase and decrease during apoptosis (Reynolds and Eastman, 1996; Baffy et al., 1993).

The recent identification of the mammalian homologue of *C.elegans* ced-4 (Apaf-1) has thrown more light on the mode of action of Bcl-2 (Zou et al., 1997). Ced-4 is essential for apoptosis and interacts with ced-9, Bcl-$_{xL}$ and with members of the caspase family - ced-3, caspase 2 and caspase 8 (Chinnaiyan et al., 1997; Irmler et al., 1997; Seshagiri and Miller, 1997). It has been speculated that when ced-4 is bound to ced-9 it is unable to stimulate ced-3 and hence initiate the caspase cascade. This is presumed to be due to a change in the conformation of ced-4 (Newton and Strasser, 1998 and references therein). It has not been firmly established whether Apaf-1 represents ced-4 in mammals, but it seems likely that several molecules of this type will be identified as were the ced-9 and ced-3 homologues. Recently, a novel negative regulator of cell death , Boo, has been identified (Song et al., 1999). Boo has homology to Bcl-2, having BH1, 2 and 4 domains. It forms a complex with Apaf-1 and caspase 9 which can be disrupted by Bik and Bak. Boo appears to be tissue specific, its expression being limited to the ovaries and epididymis, suggesting that other Boo-like Bcl-2 homologues may be limited in their expression. The reader is directed towards several excellent reviews for more information concerning the function of the Bcl-2 family (Newton and Strasser, 1998; Rao and White, 1997).

b. *Viral Bcl-2 homologues*

As discussed above (Section 4(a)) the function of Ad E1B 19K protein became evident from a study of the phenotypes of a large number of adenovirus mutants. These viruses, exhibiting the *cyt/deg* phenotype were seen to cause rapid lysis of the infected cell and degradation of both host and viral DNA (Ezoe et al., 1981). Thus, Ad E1B 19K inhibits virally-induced apoptosis and therefore DNA degradation. E1B-19K has been classified as a Bcl-2 homologue despite the limited sequence homology between the two proteins. What homology does exist is restricted to key residues and domains (Chiou et al., 1994). In addition to the BH domains E1B 19K and Bcl-2 share the so called NH domains (NH1 and NH2). Domain swapping and mutation studies have demonstrated that these regions, in particular NH1, are significant in survival promotion (Subramanian et al., 1995b). Functional studies have shown that 19K is indeed a true Bcl-2 homologue. The two genes are interchangeable. E1B 19K does not upregulate endogenous Bcl-2 therefore indicating that it functions in the same manner as Bcl-2 (Huang et al., 1997). Ad E1B 19K has also been shown to have a similar cellular localization to Bcl-2, despite the lack of a TM domain (Rao and White, 1997). Huang et al., (1997) conducted experiments to determine if Bcl-2, Bcl-$_{xL}$ and E1B 19K were functionally equivalent. The findings were that all three were capable of mediating protection against growth factor deprivation, staurosporine, ceramide, peroxide, cycloheximide, dexamethasone, γ-irradiation, cisplatin and etoposide.

Like Bcl-2, Ad E1B 19K has several cellular binding partners. It has been shown to interact with Bax (Chen et al., 1996b; Han et al., 1996), Bak (Farrow et al., 1995) and Bik (Han et al., 1996) as well as the NIPs (nineteen k interacting proteins). NIPs 1,2 and 3 are a group of unrelated proteins which bind both E1B 19K and Bcl-2 (Boyd et al., 1995). NIP3 contains a transmembrane domain, which is presumably responsible for the mitochondrial location of the protein. NIP3 has been shown to rapidly induce apoptosis, although this effect is abrogated if the TM domain is altered (Chen et al., 1997).

Unlike Ad E1B 19K EBV-BHRF1 shows distinct homology with Bcl-2, enough in fact for it to be identified as a putative Bcl-2 homologue purely by sequence alignments (Clarke et al., 1994; Khanim et al., 1997). BHRF1 is dispensable for virus-induced cell growth and transformation *in vitro* and virus replication (Kieff, 1995). Instead, BHRF1 seems to be involved in the EBV lytic cycle and the subsequent release of viral progeny. However, like Bcl-2 and E1B 19K BHRF1 protects cells infected with adenovirus E1B 19K mutants from apoptosis (Tarodi et al., 1994) and is located in the mitochondria. BHRF1 also protects cells from serum depletion, ionophore treatment (Henderson et al., 1993), DNA damage (Tarodi et al., 1994) and in intestinal epithelial cells TNFα or Fas stimulation(Kawanishi, 1997). Whilst BHRF1 is not consistently expressed in EBV-associated tumours it has been linked to oral 'hairy' leukoplakia. This is a benign lesion of the oral tongue mucosa. Examination of the gene expression patterns found in these lesions has indicated that none of the latent genes are expressed but that BHRF1 is (Rickinson et al., 1996). It has been suggested that the role of BHRF1 is to delay apoptosis during the lytic life cycle so that complete viral replication is ensured. It is however possible that certain mutations in BHRF1 may contribute to oncogenesis. As with Bcl-2, BHRF1 has been demonstrated to interact with p23 R-ras (Theodorakis et al., 1996). BHRF1 mutants were generated which although unable to bind to R-ras were still capable of suppressing p53-induced apoptosis. Surprisingly these mutants demonstrated a gain of function phenotype, they induced cell proliferation and showed more efficient co-operation with E1A in transformation assays (Theodorakis et al., 1996). Other cellular partners of BHRF1 include Bik, NIPs 1,2 and 3 but, interestingly, not Bax.

As with many of the viruses studied EBV relies on more than one mechanism to protect infected cells from apoptosis. Both EBNA5 and BZLF1 have a role to play in apoptosis prevention. These proteins bind to p53. ENBA5 can also interact with pRb whilst BZLF1 seems to modulate NF-κB (Szekely et al., 1993; Daibata et al., 1996). Also of importance is latent membrane protein 1 (LMP1). As its name suggests this is a multi-membrane spanning protein expressed during latency. It has been postulated that apoptosis can be a useful phenomenon to viruses during the lytic cycle although if latency is to be achieved cell death must be suppressed. This theory provides the rationale behind producing an anti-apoptotic factor such as LMP1 only during latency. This 63kDa phosphoprotein is oncogenic in rodent fibroblasts and is essential for the transformation of B cells *in vitro* by EBV. Research using infected B cells has shown that LMP1 prevents apoptosis (Gregory et al., 1991) and that this is principally due to an induction of Bcl-2 expression (Henderson et al., 1991). Other anti-apoptotic factors induced by LMP1 expression include Bcl_{xl}, Mcl1 and A20. A20 is an anti-apoptotic zinc finger protein which is known to protect cells from TNFα (Kieff, 1995). Up-regulation of both CD40 and CD54 has also been attributed to LMP1 expression. As is usually the case LMP1 seems to exert its effect via more then one mechanism and these seem to be at least in part dependent on cell type and situation. For example, the induction of Bcl-2 in response to LMP1 previously reported is not detected in epithelial cells (Lu et al.,

1996). LMP1 has been demonstrated to up-regulate p53 expression but simultaneously inhibit p53-mediated apoptosis (Okan et al., 1995). This may be due to the activation of the transcription factor NF-κB by LMP1 which, in turn induces expression of A20 (Lu et al., 1996). LMP1 contains two carboxy terminal activating domains (CTAR 1 and 2) which seem to have distinct functions. CTAR1 interacts with TRADD as well as the TRAFs, principally TRAF 1 and 3 but also TRAF 2 (Song et al., 1996). It has been speculated that these interactions are responsible for the recruitment of cellular IAPs (Uren et al., 1996). The interaction with TRAFs is mediated through a conserved PXQXT motif, which is also found in CD40 and other members of the TNF super-family. LMP1 is strongly related to the TNF family receptors, although a critical differ-ence is that LMP1 is constitutively active and requires no ligand binding. CTAR2 is required for the activation of c-Jun kinase (JNK) which in turn causes an induction of AP1. AP1, a transcription factor composed of both c-Jun and Fos, is then involved in growth control.

Although not oncogenic in humans African swine fever virus (AFSV) is also of in-terest here as it encodes a Bcl-2 homologue. LMW5-HL contains both a BH1 and 2 domain but lacks a TM motif. LMW5-HL has been shown to suppress apoptosis (Afonso et al., 1996; Brun et al., 1996). It has also been demonstrated that by mutating a single amino acid in the BH1 domain of LMW5-HL this protective effect was abro-gated. An identical mutation in Bcl-2 prevents heterodimerisation between Bcl-2 and Bax or Bcl-xs indicating that LMW5-HL has similar cellular partners to Bcl-2 (Yin et al., 1994; Zhang et al., 1995). ASFV also encodes a homologue of IAP although this is not thought to influence apoptosis (Neilan et al., 1997).

6. The Caspases in Virally-Induced Apoptosis

a. *Mode of action of caspases*

In some cases viruses require only that apoptosis be delayed in order that replication can be completed. In these cases the strategy employed is often to inhibit the final stages of apoptosis. The caspases are the demolition experts of the cell, responsible for the cleav-age of specific substrates. The term caspase, standing for cysteinyl aspartate specific proteinase, has been adopted recently to group thirteen mammalian enzymes, although the original "caspase" is ced-3 from C.elegans. Interleukin 1β-converting enzyme (ICE) was found to have significant homology to ced-3 and was the first mammalian caspase to be identified. Subsequently, caspase 3 has been identified as the most similar mam-malian enzyme to ced-3. The homology between ICE and ced-3 gave the first clue to the extensive role of proteases in apoptosis.

The thirteen enzymes have been grouped on the basis of certain conserved features:
- The mature enzymes exist as heterodimers composed of two subunits, which are ultimately associated to form a single catalytic domain.

- The enzyme is synthesised as a pro-enzyme from which both subunits are produced as a result of proteolytic cleavage. This cleavage is mediated by other caspases, or in some situations by auto-proteoltyic cleavage.
- All of the enzymes appear to have an absolute requirement for aspartic acid in the P1 position in both macro-molecular and peptide substrates (where P4P3P2P1/P11 indictates the position of residues relative to the cleavage site).
- The caspases show different preferences for the amino acids present at P4.

Since the original classification of the caspases this group of enzymes has been divided further into two classes, based on the length of their N-terminal prodomains (Humke et al., 1998). For example, caspases 8 and 9 have long prodomains whilst 1 and 3 have relatively short prodomains. It has also been noted that the group with longer prodomains tend to function upstream in the caspase cascade (e.g. caspase 8) with the second group acting at a more distal point (Song et al., 1999). The need for so many caspases in mammalian cells is unknown, although several possible explanations have been given. It is possible that the caspases may be synthesised in a tissue specific manner, although this is not generally believed to be a widespread phenomenon. Most of the caspases can be detected at the mRNA level in a single cell, for example the Jurkat or HL60 cell lines (Alnemri, 1997; Martins et al., 1997). However, knockout mice lacking caspase 3 suffer only from a defect in cell death in the central nervous system, indicating that in some cases tissue specific expression may occur (Kuida et al., 1996). The caspases also differ in substrate specificity thus supporting the need for multiple family members. The variable amino acids preferred at P4 by the enzymes are probably responsible for this, for example caspase 1 prefers large, hydrophobic amino acids in the P4 position whilst caspase 3 seems to prefer an aspartic acid in this position (Thornberry, 1997). Therefore by having multiple enzymes the cell is ensured of being able to efficiently and rapidly cleave a wide range of substrates, for example caspase 3 is a potent PARP protease but a poor lamin protease (Takahashi et al., 1996). The caspases have been shown to act sequentially thus producing a proteolytic cascade, e.g. the cleavage and activation of caspase 3 by caspase 8 following TNF or Fas signaling (Enari et al., 1996). It has been suggested that different caspases function in specific subcellular compartments i.e. one group in the cytoplasm and another in the nucleus (Martins et al., 1997). A similar situation could also occur in the different organelles of the cell. In support of the cell's need for multiple caspases is the observation that many of them have been shown to exist in different forms, thus producing yet more alternatives. These alternative forms are produced as a result of differential splicing (caspases 1,2 and 8), post-translational modification and/or proteolytic processing (Martins et al., 1997; Faleiro et al., 1997). It is interesting to note that many potential caspase cleavage sites remain intact in protein substrates even at very late times in apoptosis. This observation suggests that other factors beside simple substrate recognition sites are important in determining the rate and dimensions of the products of capsase activation.

Many comprehensive reviews detail the substrates of the caspase that have been characterized. There are those that become activated as a result of proteolytic cleavage, for example the caspases themselves (Thornberry, 1997), those that become inactivated by the caspases e.g. Rb, MDM2 and the catalytic subunit of DNA protein kinase (DNA-

PKcs) (Janicke et al., 1996; Erhardt et al., 1997 and Song et al., 1996). The substrates in class three are the structural proteins, the disassembly of which is required for the cell to collapse in an organised fashion e.g. lamins and keratins (Rao et al., 1996; Caulin et al., 1997). Finally, there are a number of caspase substrates, which are cleaved for no readily apparent reason.

b. *Viral inhibitors of caspases*

The finding that some viruses encode proteins, which specifically inactivate caspases, highlights their functional significance during apoptosis. These proteins are designed to inhibit the execution stage of apoptosis and will be discussed in turn.

(I) CRM A

Pox viruses, including both smallpox and cowpox, are known to infect their respective hosts in an acute manner rarely giving rise to a persistent or latent phase. The natural host response to infection is to mediate an inflammatory response, activate natural killer cells and induce apoptosis. The cowpox virus, one of the more studied pox viruses for historical reasons, has been demonstrated to facilitate infection by the inhibition of the host inflammatory response and the inhibition of apoptosis (Ray et al., 1992). The cowpox gene responsible for this is *Crm a*, standing for cytokine response modifier. *Crm a* encodes a 38K member of the serpin (serine protease inhibitors) family of proteases which is expressed in the cytoplasm of the host cell throughout infection. Crm A is an unusual serpin as it functions as a cysteine rather than a serine protease. Serpin inhibitors generally form 1:1 complexes with the target proteins thus rendering them inactive (Komiyama et al., 1994). Crm a is a potent and specific inhibitor of the caspases, although it does not inhibit all the caspases with the same efficiency - for example it is a more potent inhibitor of caspase 1 protease than caspase 3 (Nicholson et al., 1995). The preferred Crm a recognition sequence is known to be LVAD/C i.e. Crm a is cleaved here by the caspase leaving the cleavage products to form a complex with the caspase thus rendering it inactive.

Crm a has been shown to protect cells induced to apoptose by a variety of stimuli, for example growth factor withdrawal, Fas activation and cytotoxic T cells (Quan et al., 1995). A particularly elegant piece of work was carried out by Gagliardini et al., (1994) who showed that sensory neurones micro-injected with an expression vector containing Crm a were significantly less likely to die after NGF withdrawal than were un-injected cells. As previously mentioned the caspases have been demonstrated to act in a cascade in some situations with an amplification effect, for example TNF or Fas activation, see figure 2. Crm a is a more potent protease inhibitor of caspase 8 than 3 or 7. Having considered the caspase cascade triggered by for example Fas activation it is clear why caspase 8 makes a better physiological target for Crm a than the more downstream caspases. It should be noted however that the ability of Crm a to inhibit apoptosis is dependent on cell type and stimulus i.e. Crm a-sensitive and non-sensitive apoptotic pathways exist even within the same cell. Other pox viruses known to express proteins that inhibit apoptosis at this stage include vaccinia virus which encodes a protein highly homologous to Crm a which inhibits both TNF and Fas-induced apoptosis (Dobbelstein and Shenk, 1996). Rabbit pox virus (RPV) encodes the SPI-1 protein which prevents premature death of infected porcine kidney or human A549 epithelial cells (Brooks et al., 1995).

(II) BACULOVIRUS

The presence of genes, which have specifically evolved to target caspases in the genomes of baculoviruses, provides further evidence of the pivotal role the caspases have to play during apoptosis. The first inhibitor of apoptosis identified in a baculovirus genome was p35 from *Autographica californica* nuclear polyhedrosis virus (AcMNPV). Mutants of this particular baculovirus were identified that induced massive apoptosis in host cells within 12 hours of infection, thus prohibiting the completion of viral replication (Clem et al., 1991, Clem and Miller 1993). This phenotype was termed "annihilator". The induced apoptosis appears to be due to the shut down of the host cell RNA synthesis by the baculovirus (Clem and Miller, 1994). Normally it is vital, for the virus to reproduce and hence survive, that this apoptosis is suppressed. This mutant phenotype led to the isolation of p35 which subsequent research has shown functions in a similar way to Crm a (Hershberger et al., 1992; 1994). There are however significant differences between p35 and Crm a, for example p35 seems to be a much broader caspase inhibitor but unlike Crm a does not protect cells from cytotoxic T cell attack via granzyme B (Bump et al., 1995, reviewed in Clem et al., 1996). However, like Crm a purified recombinant p35 inactivates caspases at equimolar concentrations, as demonstrated with purified recombinant caspases 1,2,3 and 4. The p35 is cleaved by the caspases at the sequence DQMD/G to generate 20 and 10K fragments. The 10K fragment then forms a complex with the caspase rendering it inactive and therefore unable to activate other caspases and so amplify the apoptotic signal (Bump et al., 1995; Bertin et al., 1996).

p35 is not the only baculovirus protein capable of suppressing the distal stages of apoptosis. Baculoviruses have been identified which were capable of complementing the cell death inhibition properties missing in p35 mutant viruses (Crook et al., 1993, Clem and Miller, 1994). This led to the discovery of a family of genes known simply as the inhibitors of apoptosis (IAPs). The two founding members of this family are both from baculovirus; Cp-IAP for *Cydia pomonella* granulosis virus (CpGp) and Op-IAP from *Orgyia pseudotsugata* polyhedrosis virus. Since these initial observations family members have been identified in *Drosophila* and humans. These proteins have been grouped together due to an apparent conserved function and structure. They contain a common motif which has been called the baculovirus IAP repeat (BIR). The number of BIRs varies between 2 and 3 with baculovirus IAPs having 2. All members of the IAP family, except NAIP and survivin, also have a C_3HC_4 (RING) zinc finger in their carboxy termini (Saurin et al., 1996). This RING domain has no known function at present although a role in transcriptional regulation seems probable. It has been noted that artificial IAPs containing BIR domains but not the RING still inhibit apoptosis whilst in the converse situation (i.e. a RING domain but no BIRs) apoptosis is induced. This suggests that at least in baculovirus the RING domain functions as a negative regulator of cell death suppression (Roy et al., 1997). Two cellular IAPs have been identified by their interaction with the TNF receptor associated factors (TRAFs) (Rothe et al., 1995). This led to the speculation that IAPs may inhibit the caspases downstream of TNF or Fas signaling pathways. Recently human IAPs, c-IAP-1 and c-IAP-2, have been demonstrated directly to inhibit caspases 3, 7, and 9 (Deveraux et al., 1998) but not 8,1 or 6 (Roy et al., 1997). Baculovirus IAPs can block activation of sf caspase 1 from insect cells (Seshagiri and Miller, 1997). This may indicate that multiple IAPs exist within an organism to target the different caspases (Manji et al., 1997).

(III) V-FLIPS

The v-FLIPs (viral FLICE (caspase 8) inhibitory proteins) have been identified as a group of viral products that interfere with apoptosis mediated through proteins containing death receptors. Cells expressing these proteins are therefore protected from apoptosis induced by CD95, TRAMP and TRAIL-R. Sophisticated screening of DNA databases originally identified this group of proteins. Searches for sequences which had significant homology to the DED domains in FADD, caspase 8 (FLICE) and caspase 10 (Mch 4) from both human and mouse led to the isolation of ORF E8 from equine herpesvirus-2 (EHV-2). This 23kDa protein was found to contain 2 motifs with highly significant homology to DEDs (Thome et al., 1997). v-FLIPs have been reported in the genomes of bovine herpesvirus 4 (BORFE2), herpesvirus saimiri (ORF 71), human herpesvirus 8 and the tumourigenic human molluscipoxvirus. A putative second v-FLIP has been identified in molluscipoxvirus (MCV) known as MC160. MC160 has homology with MC159 and DEDs but, at present, it is not clear whether it functions in a similar manner. Humans infected with MCV display hyperplastic cutaneous lesions, which last for months and sometimes years but do not give rise to an inflammatory response (Gottlieb and Myskowski, 1994). Of interest is the finding that neither EHV-2 nor MCV encode a Bcl-2 homologue or any caspase inhibitors. This points to the v-FLIPs being the only source of anti-apoptotic activity in these viruses.

By means of co-immunoprecipitation and yeast-2-hybrid experiments it has been demonstrated that EHV-2 E8 binds to the pro-domain of caspase 8 whilst MC159 interacts with FADD (Thome et al., 1997; Bertin et al., 1997). As a result of this the formation of a functional DISC is prevented. This is turn leads to a failure to activate caspase 8. As a consequence, for example, Raji cells expressing E8 are made less susceptible to apoptosis via the TNF pathway but are still effectively killed after staurosporine treatment. The v-FLIPs appear to be expressed late in the viral lytic cycle, sometimes only 24 hours before lysis. It has been speculated that these anti-apoptotic proteins are needed when the viral load reaches its maximum levels (Thome et al., 1997).

(IV) OTHER CASPASE INHIBITORS

The avian CELO adenovirus can transform cells and induce tumours in newborn hamsters (Cotten et al., 1993). As with human adenoviruses expression of this viral transforming protein also seems capable of inhibiting apoptosis. However, despite the complete sequencing of the CELO genome no sequence has been identified with homology to Ad E1B 19K, Bcl-2 or any other well-characterised anti-apoptotic protein. Recently

GAM-1 (Gallus anti morte) was demonstrated to function in a comparable way to E1B 19K or Bcl-2. The gene was identified by transfecting fragments of the CELO genome into primary human fibroblasts, a procedure which itself induces apoptosis, cells were then monitored for increased survival (Chiocca et al., 1997). Since its isolation, GAM-1 has been found to encode a 30K nuclear protein which is capable of blocking TNFα signaling. As previously mentioned GAM-1 has no homology with Bcl-2 i.e. it has no BH domains or a Bax interaction motif. The cellular localization of GAM-1 means that it is unlikely to possess a function similar to Crm a (i.e. as a direct inhibitor of the caspases). It has been speculated that GAM-1 may function at the transcriptional level, possibly in a way similar to LMP1 upregulating Bcl-2.

Human cytomegalovirus (HCMV) is a herpesvirus and a widespread human pathogen. Whilst the infections are asymptomatic in healthy individuals they pose serious problems for fetuses and immunocompromised patients. HCMV infection represents the leading cause of viral birth defects and gives rise to life threatening conditions in AIDS and transplant patients (Britt et al., 1991). As with all viral infections some genes are expressed earlier than others, the so-called immediate early genes appearing first. In the case of HCMV, two of these IE1 and IE2 (immediate early 1 and 2) are of interest with respect to apoptosis (Mocarski et al., 1993). These two genes are transcribed from one transcriptional unit and have 80 amino acids in common at their N-termini. However mutational studies have indicated that it is the regions of the proteins C-terminal to this that are of interest. Despite this it is largely unknown how exactly IE1 and 2 function. They have both been shown to inhibit apoptosis caused by TNFα or adenovirus infection with an E1B 19K deleted virus (Zhu et al., 1995). However, neither IE1 nor 2 protect cells from UV irradiation-induced apoptosis. Parallels can be drawn at this point between the DNA tumour viruses e.g. adenovirus and HCMV. Like adenovirus, HCMV exhibits a lengthy replication cycle and life-long persistent infection. It is perhaps for these reasons that the anti-apoptotic machinery is expressed early and at high levels. As was found with the CELO adenovirus discussed above no other obvious anti-apoptotic proteins have been identified in the HCMV genome. IE1 and 2 are both nuclear proteins and have no homology with any of the Bcl-2 family. Therefore, again it seems likely that they function by regulating transcription. In support of this it has been shown that IE2 can bind TBP, TFIIB and Sp1 (Lukac et al., 1994), whilst IE1 activates transcription via some but not all NF κB sites. IE1 and 2 seem to co-operate to activate their target promoters, which are as yet unknown. Initial studies from Zhu et al., (1995) demonstrated that regulation of Bcl-2, Bax, Bag-1 and caspase 1 were unlikely. More conclusively, IE2 interacts with p53 and pRb. This again is reminiscent of the Ad E1 proteins. This interaction with p53 is capable of inhibiting the ability of p53 to transcriptionally transactivate, demonstrated with the use of a reporter construct (Speir et al., 1994). The possible downstream effects of this are numerous and certainly include the inhibition of p53-mediated apoptosis. However Zhu et al., (1995) also showed that IE1 and 2 were still capable of inhibiting apoptosis in the p53-negative cell line Saos2 indicating that they must inhibit apoptosis at more than one point in the apoptotic pathway.

Like adenovirus and baculovirus HSV-1 is a large DNA virus and would be expected to encode anti-apoptotic factors. Indeed HSV-infected tissue culture cells display no apoptotic characteristics indicating that apoptosis has been inhibited (Koyama and Miwa 1997). Commonly it has been postulated that γ34.5 and the transcription factor ICP4 from HSV represent the anti-apoptotic genes (Chou and Roizman 1992, Chou et al., 1990 and Teodoro and Branton, 1997a). However, more recent evidence does not support these suggestions. As an alternative, a new candidate has been isolated, a serine threonine protein kinase known as US3. US3 is a specific protein kinase, phosphorylating only within an arginine rich consensus sequence (Purves et al., 1986). Infection with HSV deleted for US3 promotes apoptosis in infected cells, and this is abolished on the return of the US3 gene product (Leopardi et al., 1997). It is at present unknown what the downstream targets of this kinase are. The possibility exists that this protein will represent a new class of viral anti-apoptotic factors.

7. Concluding Remarks

This chapter was never intended to be all encompassing, instead focussing on those aspects of the subject which we found to be particularly interesting. However, even on the basis of our rather lopsided appraisal of viruses and apoptosis, it is possible to draw several interesting, although perhaps rather obvious, conclusions. Firstly, following viral infection there is considerable pressure on the host cell to apoptose rapidly as a way of combating the virus. Secondly, most viruses express one or more proteins to inhibit apoptosis, although often only temporarily, so that optimal production of progeny can occur at an appropriate time. Thirdly, at a late stage during infection a process akin to, but perhaps distinct from, apoptosis occurs so that cell lysis can take place releasing the viral progeny. Quite how this process is regulated remains one of the most interesting unanswered questions in this area of research. However, on the basis of recent data obtained from a study of adenoviruses it appears that specific proteins such as adenovirus death protein (ADP) (Tollefson et al., 1996a and b) may play an inportant role initiating a "death response" which does not require or involve condensation of the nucleus or DNA degradation (discussed in Wold and Tollefson, 1998). Whether comparable proteins are expressed by other viruses remains to be seen. Similarly, investigation of the extent to which this virus-induced cell lysis relies on the cells "normal" apoptotic mechanism should provide valuable information of possible alternative forms of cell death.

From the data presented in this chapter it should be apparent that the study of virus-induced apoptosis has provided considerable insight into how the mechanism of apoptosis is regulated, both positively and negatively. Furthermore, these investigations have considerably increased our knowledge of many aspects of normal cellular functioning. It is hoped and expected that studies in the near future will be equally valuable, providing new information which will be valuable in increasing our understanding of viruses, apoptosis and cancer.

Acknowledgements

We are most grateful to Dr Philip Lecane for help with the figures; Drs Jane Steele, Andrew Turnell, Peter Weber and Grant Stewart for invaluable discussion. We thank the Cancer Research Campaign U.K. for funding over the years.

References

Accornero, P., Radrizzani, M., Delia, D., Gerosa, F., Kurrle, R. and Colombo, M.P. (1997) Differential susceptibility to HIV-GP120-sensitized apoptosis in CD4+ T-cell clones with different T-helper phenotypes: role of CD95/CD95L interactions. Blood 89, 558-569.

Afonso, C.L., Neilan, J.G., Kutish, G.F. and Rock, D.L. (1996) An African swine fever virus Bcl-2 homolog, 5-HL, suppresses apoptotic cell death. J. Virol. 70, 4858-4863.

Aldrovani, G.M. (1993) The SCID-Hu mouse as a model for HIV-1 infection. Nature 363, 732-736.

Allemand, L., Grimber, G., Komprobst, M., Bennoun, M., Molina, T., Briand, P. and Joulin, V. (1995) Compensatory apoptosis in response to SV40 large T antigen expression in the liver. Oncogene 11, 2583-2590.

Almasan, A., Yin, Y., Kelly, R., Lee, E.Y.H.P., Bradley, A., Li, W., Bertino, J.R. and Wahl, G.M.. (1995) Deficiency of retinoblastoma protein leads to inappropriate S-phase entry, activation of E2F-responsive genes, and apoptosis. Proc. Natl. Acad. Sci. (USA) 92, 5436-5440.

Alnemri, E.S. (1997) Mammalian cell death proteases: A family of highly conserved aspartate specific cysteine proteases. J. Cell. Biochem. 64, 33-42.

Ameisen, J.C., Estaquier, J., Idziorek, T. and De Bels, F. (1995) The relevance of apoptosis to AIDS pathogenesis. Trends Cell Biol. 5, 27-31.

An, B. and Dou, Q.P. (1996) Cleavage of retinoblastoma protein during apoptosis: an interleukin 1 beta converting enzyme-like protease as candidate. Cancer Res. 53, 438-442.

Anouja, F., Wattiez, R., Mousset, S., Caillet Fauquet, P. (1997) The cytotoxicity of the parvovirus minute virus of mice nonstructural protein NS1 is related to changes in the synthesis and phosphorylation of cell proteins. J. Virol. 71, 4671-4678.

Aries, S.P., Schaaf, B., Muller, C., Dennin, R.H. and Dalhoff, K. (1995) Fas (CD95) expression on CD4+ T cells from HIV-infected patients increases with disease progression. J. Mol. Med. 73, 591-593.

Attardi, L.D., Lowe, S.W., Brugarolas, J. and Jacks, T. (1996) Transcriptional activation by p53, but not induction of the p21 gene, is essential for oncogene-mediated apoptosis. EMBO J. 15, 3693-3701.

Ayyavoo, V., Mahboubi, A., Mahalingam, S., Ramalingam, R., Kudchodkar, S., Williams, W.V., Green, D.R. and Weiner, D.B. (1997) HIV-1 Vpr suppresses immune activation and apoptosis through regulation of nuclear factor kappa B. Nat. Med. 3, 1117-1123.

Babiss, L.E. and Ginsberg, H.S. (1984) Adenovirus type 5 early region 1B gene product is required for efficient shutoff of host protein synthesis. J. Virol. 50, 202-212.

Babiss, L.E., Ginsberg, H.S. and Darnell, J.E. (1985) Adenovirus E1B proteins are required for accumulation of late viral messenger RNA and for effects on cellular messenger RNA translation and transport. Mol. Cell. Biol. 10, 2552-2558.

Badley, A.D., McElhinny, J.A., Leibson, D.H., Lynch, D.H., Alderson, M.R. and Paya, C.V. (1996) Upregulation of Fas ligand expression by human immunodeficiency virus in human macrophages mediates apoptosis of uninfected T lymphocytes. J. Virol. 70, 199-206.

Baffy, G., Miyashita, T., Williamson, J.R. and Reed, J.C. (1993) Apoptosis induced by withdrawl of interleukin-3 (IL-3) from an IL-3-dependent hematopoietic-cell line is associated with repartitioning of intracellular calcium and is blocked by enforced Bcl-2 oncoprotein production. J. Biol. Chem. 268, 6511-6519.

Bagchi, S., Raychaudhuri, P. and Nevins, J.R. (1990) Adenovirus E1A proteins can dissociate heteromeric complexes involving the E2F transcription factors: a novel mechanism for E1A transactivation. Cell 62, 659-669.

Bahr, G.M., Capron, A., Dewulf, J., Nagata, S., Tanaka, M., Bourez, J. and Mouton, Y. (1997) Elevated serum level of Fas ligand correlates with the asymptomatic stage of human immunodeficiency virus infection. Blood 90, 896-896.

Baker, S.J., Markowitz, S., Fearon, E.R., Willson, J.K. and Vogelstein, B. (1990) Suppression of human colorectal cell growth by wild type p53. Science 249, 912-915.

Band, V., Dalal, S., Delmolino, L. and Androphy, E.J. (1993) Enhanced degradation of p53 protein in HPV-6 and BPV-1 E6-immortalized human mammary epithelial cells. EMBO J. 12, 1847-1852.

Banda, N.K., Bernier, J., Kurshava, D.K., Kurrle, R., Haigwood, N., Sekaly, R.P. and Finkel, T.H. (1992) Crosslinking CD4 by human immunodeficiency virus gp120 primes T cells for activation-induced apoptosis. J. Exp. Med. 176, 1099-1106.

Bandara, L.R. and LaThangue, N.B. (1991) Adenovirus E1a prevents the retinoblastoma gene from complexing with a cellular transcription factor. Nature 351, 494-497.

Banin, S., Moyal, L., Shieh, S.Y., Taya, Y., Anderson, C.W., Chessa, L., Smorodinsky, N.I., Prives, C., Reiss, Y., Shiloh, Y. and Ziv, Y. (1998) Enhanced phosphorylation of p53 by ATM in response to DNA damage. Science 281, 1674-1677.

Barak, Y., Juven, T., Haffner, R. and Oren, M. (1993) MDM2 expression is induced by wild-type p53 activity. EMBO J. 12, 461-468.

Bartz, S.R., Rogel, M.E. and Emerman, M. (1996) Human immunodeficiency virus type 1 cell cycle control: Vpr is cytostatic and mediates G_2 accumulation by a mechanism which differs from DNA damage checkpoint control. J. Virol. 70, 2324-2331.

Bates, S., Phillips, A.C., Clark, P.A., Stoff, F., Peters, G., Ludwig, R.L. and Vousden, K.H. (1998) p14[ARF] links the tumour suppressors RB and p53. Nature 395, 124-125.

Baumler, C., Bohler, T., Herr, I., Benner, P., Krammer, P. and Debatin, K. (1996) Activation of CD95 (APO-1/Fas) system in T cells from HIV-1-infected children. Blood 88, 1741-1746.

Bayley, S.T. and Mymryk, J.S. (1994) Adenovirus E1A proteins and transformation. Int. J. Onc. 5, 425-444.

Beijersbergen, R.L. and Bernards, R. (1996) Cell cycle regulation by the retinoblastoma family of growth inhibitory proteins. Biochim. Biophys. Acta 1287, 103-120.

Beijersbergen, R.L., Kerkhoven, R.M., Zhu, L., Cartee, L., Voorhoeve, P.M. and Bernards, R. (1994) E2F-4 a new member of the E2F gene family has oncogenic activity and associates with p107 in vivo. Genes Dev. 8, 2680-2690.

Berezutskaya, E. and Bagchi, S. (1997) The human papillomavirus E7 oncoprotein functionally interacts with the S4 subunit of the 26S proteasome. J. Biol. Chem. 272, 30135-30140.

Berezutskaya, E., Yu, B., Morozov, A., Raychaudhuri, P. and Bagchi, S. (1997) Differential regulation of the pocket domains of the retinoblastoma family proteins by the HPV16 E7 oncoprotein. Cell Growth Diff. 8, 1277-1286.

Bertin, J., Mendrysa, S.M., LaCount, D.J., Gaur, S., Krebs, J.F., Armstrong, R.C., Tomaselli, K.J. and Friesen, P.D. (1996) Apoptotic supression by baculovirus P35 involves cleavage by and inhibition of virus-induced CED-3/ICE-like protease. J. Virol. 70, 6251-6259.

Bertin, J., Armstrong, R.C., Ottilie, S., Martin, D.A., Wang, Y., Banks, S., Wang, G.H., Senkevich, T.G., Alnemri, E.S., Moss, B., Lenardo, M.J., Tomaselli, K.J. and Cohen, J.I. (1997) Death effector domain-containing herpesvirus and poxvirus proteins inhibit both Fas- and TNFR1-induced apoptosis. Proc. Natl. Acad. Sci. (USA) 94, 1172-1176.

Boldin, M.P., Goncharov, T.M., Goltsev, Y.V. and Wallach, D. (1996) Involvement of MACH, a novel MORT1/FADD-interacting protease, in FAS/APO-1-induced and TNF receptor-induced cell-death. Cell 85, 803-815.

Bonyhadi, M.L., Rabin, L., Salimi, S., Brown, D.A., Kosek, J., McCune, J.M. and Kaneshima, H. (1993) HIV induces thymus depletion in vivo. Nature 363, 728-732.

Böttger, V., Böttger, A., Howard, S.F., Picksley, S.M., Chène, P., Garcia-Echeverria, C., Hochkeppel, H.K. and Lane D.P. (1996) Identification of novel mdm2 binding peptides by phage display. Oncogene 13, 2141-2147.

Boyd, J. M., Malstrom, S., Subramanian, T., Venkatesh, L. K., Schaeper, U., Elangovan, B., D'Sa, E. C. and Chinnadurai, G. (1995) Adenovirus E1B 19kDa and Bcl-2 proteins interact with a common set of cellular proteins. Cell 79, 341-351.

Braithwaite, A.W., Cheetham, B.F., Li, P., Parish, C.R., Waldron-Stevens, L.K. and Bellett, A.D. (1983) Adenovirus induced alterations of the cell growth cycle – a requirement for expression of E1A but not E1B. J. Virol. 45, 192-199.

Britt, W.J., Pass, R.F., Stagno, S. and Alford, C.A. (1991) Pediatric cytomegalovirus-infection. Transplantation Procs. 23, 115-117.

Brooks, M.A., Ali, A.N., Turner, P.C. and Moyer, R.W. (1995) A rabbitpox virus serpin gene controls host-range by inhibiting apoptosis in restrictive cells. J. Virol. 69, 7688-7698.

Brun, A., Rivas,C., Esteban, M., Escribano, J.M. and Alonso, C. (1996) African swine fever virus gene A179L, a viral homologue of BCL-2, protects cells from programmed cell death. Virology 225, 227-230.

Buchkovich, K., Duffy, L.A. and Harlow, E. (1989) The retinoblastoma protein is phosphorylated during specific phases of the cell cycle. Cell 58, 1097-1105.

Bump, N.J., Hackett, M., Hugunin, M., Seshagiri, S., Brady, K., Chen, P., Ferenz, C., Franklin, S., Ghayur, T., Li, P., Licari, P., Mankovich, J., Shi, L.F., Greenberg, A.H., Miller, L.K. and Wong, W.W. (1995) Inhibition of ICE family proteases by Baculovirus antiapoptotic protein p35. Science 269, 1885-1888.

Caelles, C., Heimberg, A. and Karin, M. (1994) p53-dependent apoptosis in the absence of transcriptional activation of p53-target genes. Nature 370, 220-223.

Canman, C., Gilmer, T.M., Coutts, S.B. and Kastan, M.B. (1995) Growth factor modulation of p53-mediated growth arrest versus apoptosis. Genes Dev. 9, 600-611.

Canman, C.E., Lim, D.-S., Cimprich, K.A., Taya, Y., Tamai, K., Sakaguchi, K., Appella, E., Kastan, M.B. and Siliciano, J.D. (1998) Activation of the ATM kinase by ionising radiation and phosphorylation of p53. Science 281, 1677-1679.

Cao, L., Faha, B., Dembski, M., Tsai, L.H., Harlow, E. and Dyson, N. (1992) Independent binding of the retinoblastoma protein by the transcription factor E2F. Nature 355, 176-179.

Caulin, C., Salvesen, G.S. and Oshima, R.G. (1997) Caspase cleavage of keratin 18 and reorganization of intermediate filaments during epithelial cell apoptosis, J. Cell. Biol. 138, 1379-1394.

Cha, T.A., Tom, E., Kemble, G.W., Duke, G.M., Mocarski, E.S. and Spaete, R.R. (1996) Human cytomegalovirus clinical isolates carry at least 19 genes not found in laboratory strains. J. Virol. 70, 78-83.

Channon, J.Y. and Leslie, C.C. (1990) A calcium-dependent mechanism for associating a soluble arachidonoyl-hydrolyzing phospholipase-A2 with membrane in the macrophage cell-line RAW 264.7. J. Biol. Chem. 265, 5409-5413.

Chellappan, S., Hiebert, S., Mudryj, M., Horowitz, J.M. and Nevins, J.R. (1991) The E2F transcription factor is a cellular target for the Rb protein. Cell 65, 1053-1061.

Chellappan, S., Kraus, V.B., Kroger, B., Munger, K., Howley, P.M., Phelps, W.C. and Nevins, J.R. (1992) Adenovirus-E1A, Simian virus-40, tumor-antigen and human papillomavirus-E7 protein share the capacity to disrupt the interaction between transcription factor-E2F and the retinoblastoma gene product. Proc. Natl. Acad. Sci. (USA) 89, 4549-4553.

Chen, P.L., Scully, P., Shew, J.Y., Wang, J.Y.J and Lee, W.H. (1989) Phosphorylation of the retinoblastoma gene product is modulated during cell cycle and cellular differentiation. Cell 58, 1193-1198.

Chen, C.Y., Oliner, J.D., Zhan, Q., Fornace, A.J., Vogelstein, B. and Kastan, M.B. (1994) Interactions between p53 and MDM2 in a mammalian cell cycle checkpoint pathway. Proc. Natl. Acad. Sci. (USA) 91, 2684-2688.

Chen, P.L., Riley, D.J., Chen, Y., and Lee, W.-H. (1996a) Retinoblastoma protein positively regulates terminal adipocyte differentiation through direct interaction with C/EBPs. Genes Dev. 10, 2794-2804.

Chen, G., Branton, P.E., Yang, E., Korsmeyer, S.J. and Shore, G.C. (1996b) Adenovirus E1B 19-kDa death suppressor protein interacts with Bax but not with Bad. J. Biol. Chem. 271, 24221-24225.

Chen, G., Ray, R., Dubik, D., Shi, L.F., Cizeau, J., Bleackley, R.C., Saxena, S., Gietz, R.D. and Greenberg, A.H. (1997) The E1B 19K Bcl-2-binding protein Nip3 is a dimeric mitochondrial protein that activates apoptosis. J. Exp. Med. 186, 1975-1983.

Chen, P., Tian, J., Kovesdi, I. and Bruder, J.T. (1998) Interaction of the adenovirus 14.7-kDa protein with FLICE inhibits Fas ligand-induced apoptosis. J. Biol. Chem. 273, 5815-5820.

Cheng, E.H.Y., Nicholas, J., Bellows, D.S., Hayward, G.S., Guo, H.G., Reitz, M.S. and Hardwick, J.M. (1997) A Bcl2 homolog encoded by Kaposi sarcoma-associated virus, human herpesvirus 8, inhibits apoptosis but does not heterodimerize with Bax or Bak. Proc. Natl. Acad. Sci. USA 94, 690-694.

Chin, L., Pomerantz, J. and DePinho, R.A. (1998) The INK4a/ARF tumour suppressor: one gene – two products – two pathways. Trends Biochem. Sci. 23, 291-296.

Chinnadurai, G. (1983) Adenovirus 2 1p+ locus codes for a 19kd tumor antigen that plays an essential role in cell transformation. Cell 33, 759-766.

Chinnadurai, G. (1998) Control of apoptosis by human adenovirus genes. Sem. Virol. 8, 399-408.

Chinnaiyan, A.M., Chaudhary, D., O'Rourke, K., Koonin, E.V. and Dixit, V.M. (1997) Role of CED-4 in the activation of CED-3. Nature, 388, 728-729.

Chiocca, S., Baker, A. and Cotten, M. (1997) Identification of a novel antiapoptotic protein, GAM-1, encoded by the CELO adenovirus. J. Virol. 71,.3168-3177.

Chiou, S.K. and White, E. (1997) p300 binding by E1A cosegregates with p53 induction but is dispensible for apoptosis. J. Virol. 71, 3515-3525.

Chiou, S.K., Tseng, C.C., Rao, L. and White, E. (1994) Functional complementation of the adenovirus E1B 19-kilodalton protein with Bcl-2 in the inhibition of apoptosis in infected cells. J. Virol. 68, 6553-6566.

Choisy-Rossi, C. and Yonish-Rouach, E. (1998) Apoptosis and the cell cycle: the p53 connection. Cell Death Diff. 5, 129-131.

Chou, J., Kern, E.R., Whitley, R.J. and Roizman, B. (1990) Mapping of herpes-simplex virus-1 neurovirulence to γ-134.5, a gene nonessential for growth in culture. Science, 250, 1262-1266.

Chou, J. and Roizman, B. (1992) The γ-134.5 gene of herpes-simplex virus-1 precludes neuroblastoma-cells from triggering total shutoff of protein-synthesis characteristic of programmed cell-death in neuronal cells. Proc. Natl. Acad. Sci. (USA) 89, 3266-3270.

Clarke, A.R., Maandag, E.R., van Roon, M., van der Lug, N.M.T., van der Valk, M., Hooper, M.L., Berns, A. and Te Riele, H. (1992) Requirement for a functional Rb-1 gene in murine development. Nature 359, 328-330.

Clarke, A.R., Purdie, C.A., Harrison, D.J., Morris, R.G., Bird, C.C., Hooper, M.L. and Wyllie, A.H. (1993) Thymocyte apoptosis induced by p53 dependent and independent pathways. Nature 362, 849-852.

Clarke, P., Hickish, T., Robertson, D., Hill, M., Distefan O.F. and Conningham, D (1994) In vivo expression and localization of BHRF-1, an Epstein-Barr-virus (EBV) encoded Bcl-2 homologue. J. Cell. Biochem. S18C, 230.

Clem, R.J. and Miller, L.K. (1993) Apoptosis reduces both the in vitro replication and the in vivo infectivity of a Baculovirus. J. Virol. 67, 3730-3738.

Clem, R.J. and Miller, L.K. (1994) Control of programmed cell-death by the baculovirus genes p35 and IAP. Mol. Cell. Biol. 14, 5212-5222.

Clem, R.J., Fechheimer, M. and Miller, L.K. (1991) Prevention of apoptosis by a Baculovirus gene during infection of insect cells. Science 254, 1388-1390.

Clem, R.J., Hardwick, J.M. and Miller, L.K. (1996) Anti-apoptotic genes of baculoviruses. Cell Death Diff. 3, 9-16.

Compston, D.A.S., Vakarelis, B.N., Paul, E., McDonald, W.I., Batchelor, J.R., Mims, C.A. (1986) Viral-infection in patients with multiple-sclerosis and HLA-DR matched controls. Brain 109, 325-344.

Cohen, D.I., Tani, Y., Tian, H., Boone, E., Samelson, L. and Lane, H.C. (1992) Participation of tyrosine phosphorylation in the cytopathic effect of Human-Immunodeficiency-Virus 1. Science 256, 542-545.

Conzen, S.D., Snay, C.A. and Cole, C.N. (1997) Identification of a novel antiapoptotic functional domain in Simian virus 40 large T antigen. J. Virol. 71, 4536-4543.

Cotten, M., Wagner, E. Zatloukal, K. and Birnstiel, M.L. (1993) Chicken adenovirus (celo virus) particles augment receptor-mediated DNA delivery to mammalian-cells and yield exceptional levels of stable trans-formants. J. Virol. 67, 3777-3785.

Crook, N.E., Clem, R.J. and Miller, L.K. (1993) An apoptosis-inhibiting baculovirus gene with a zinc finger-like motif. J. Virol. 67, 2168-2174.

Crook, T., Fisher, C., Masterson, P.J. and Vousden, K.H. (1994) Modulation of transcriptional regulatory properties of p53 by HPV E6. Oncogene 9, 1225-1230.

Daibata, M., Enzinger, E.M., Monroe, J.E., Kilkuskie, R.E., Field, A.K. and Mulder, C. (1996) Antisense oligodeoxynucleotides against the BZLF1 transcript inhibit induction of productive Epstein-Barr-virus replication. Antiviral Res. 29, 243-260.

Danen Van Oorschot, A.A.A.M., Fischer, D.F., Grimbergen, J.M., Klein, B., Zhuang, S.M., Falkenburg, J.H.F., Backendorf, C., Quax, P.H.A., Van der Eb, A.J. and Noteborn, M.H.M. (1997) Apoptin induces apoptosis in human transformed and malignant cells but not in normal cells. Proc. Natl. Acad. Sci. (USA) 94, 5843-5847.

Dbaibo, G.S. and Hannun, Y.A. (1998) Cytokine response modifier A (CrmA): A strategically deployed viral weapons. Clin. Immunol. and Immunopath. 86, 134-140.

Debatin, K.M., Fahrigfaissner, A., Enenkelstoodt, S., Kreuz, W., Benner, A. and Krammer, P. (1994) High expression of APO-1 (CD95) on T lymphocytes from human immunodeficiency virus-1 infected children. Blood, 83, 3101-3103.

Debbas, M. and White,E. (1993) Wild-type p53 mediates apoptosis by E1A, which is inhibited by E1B. Genes Dev. 7, 546-554.

DeCaprio, J.A., Ludlow, J.W., Figge, J., Shew, J.Y., Huang, C.M., Lee, W.H., Marsillo, E., Paucha, E. and Livingston, D.M. (1988) SV40 large tumor-antigen forms a specific complex with the product of the retinoblastoma susceptibility gene. Cell 54, 275-283.

DeCaprio, J.A., Ludlow, J.W., Lynch, D., Furukawa, Y., Griffin, J., Piwnica-Worms, H., Huang, C.M. and Livingston, D.M. (1989) The product of the retinoblastoma susceptibility gene has properties of a cell cycle regulatory element. Cell 58, 1085-1095.

De Gregori, J., Leone, G., Miro, A., Jakoi, L. and Nevins, J.R. (1997) Distinct roles for E2F proteins in cell growth control and apoptosis. Proc. Natl. Acad. Sci. (USA) 94, 7245-7250.

DePinho, R. (1998) The cancer-chromatin connection. Nature 391, 533-536.

Demers, G.W., Foster, S.A., Halbert, C.L. and Galloway, D.A. (1994) Growth arrest by induction of p53 in DNA damaged keratinocytes is bypassed by human papilloma virus 16 E7. Proc. Natl. Acad. Sci. (USA) 91, 4382-4386.

Desaintes, C., Demeret, C., Goyat, S., Yaniv, M. and Thierry, F. (1997) Expression of the papillomavirus E2 protein in HeLa cells leads to apoptosis. EMBO J. 16, 504-514.

de Stanchina, E., McCurrach, M.E., Zindy, F., Shieh, S.-Y., Ferbeyre, G., Samuelson, A.V., Prives, C., Roussel, M.F., Sherr, C.J. and Lowe, S.W. (1998) E1A signalling to p53 involves the p19ARF tumour suppressor. Genes Dev. 12, 2434-2443.

Deveraux, Q.L., Roy, N., Stennicke, H.R., VanArsdale, T., Zhou, Q., Srinivasula, S.M., Alnemri, E.S., Salvesen, G.S. and Reed, J.C. (1998) IAPs block apoptotic events induced by caspase-8 and cytochrome c by direct inhibition of distinct caspases. EMBO J. 17, 2215-2223.

Devoto, S.H., Mudryj, M., Pines, J., Hunter, T. and Nevins, J.R. (1992) A cyclin A-protein kinase complex possesses sequence-specific DNA binding activity: p33cdk2 is a component of the E2F cyclin A complex. Cell 68, 167-176.

Diller, L., Kassel, J., Nelson, C.E., Gryka, M.A., Litwak, G., Gebhardt, M., Bressac, B., Ozturk, M., Baker, S.J., Vogelstein, B. and Friend, S.H. (1990) p53 functions as a cell cycle control protein in osteosarcomas. Mol. Cell. Biol. 10, 5772-5781.

Dimitrov, T., Krajcsi, P., Hermiston, T.W., Tollefson, A.E., Hannink, M. and Wold, W.S.M. (1997) Adenovirus E3-10.4K/14.5K protein complex inhibits tumor necrosis factor-induced translocation of cytosolic phospholipase A(2) to membranes. J. Virol. 71, 2830-2837.

Dobbelstein, M. and Shenk, T. (1996) Protection against apoptosis by the vaccinia virus SPI-2 (B13R) gene product. J. Virol. 70, 6479-6485.

Dobner, T., Horikoshi, N., Rubenwolf, S. and Shenk, T. (1996) Blockage by adenovirus E4orf6 of transcriptional activation by the p53 tumor suppressor. Science 272, 1470-1473.

Donehower, L.A., Harvey, M., Slagle, B.L., McArthur, M.J., Montgomery, C.A., Butel, J.S. and Bradley, A. (1992) Mice deficient for p53 are developmentally normal but susceptible to spontaneous tumours. Nature 356, 215-221.

Dou, Q.P., An, B., Antoku, K. and Johnson, D.E. (1997) Fas stimulation induces RB dephosphorylation and proteolysis that is blocked by inhibitors of the ICE protease family. J. Cell. Biochem. 64, 586-594.

Dowdy, S.F., Hinds, P.W., Louie, K., Reed, S.I., Arnold, A. and Weinberg, R.A. (1993) Physical interaction of the retinoblastoma protein with human D-cyclins. Cell 73, 499-511.

Du, W., Xie, J.-E. and Dyson, N. (1996) Ectopic expression of dE2F and dDP induces cell proliferation and death in the Drosophila eye. EMBO J. 15, 3684-3692.

Duan, H. and Dixit, V.M. (1997) RAIDD is a new 'death' adaptor molecule. Nature 385, 86-89.

Dulic, V., Kaufmann, W.K., Wilson, S.J., Tilsty, T.D., Lees, E., Harper, J.W., Elledge, S.J. and Reed, S.J. (1994) p53-dependent inhibition of cyclin-dependent kinase activities in human fibroblasts during radiation-induced G1 arrest. Cell 76, 1013-1023.

Dyson, N. (1998) The regulation of E2F by pRB-family proteins. Genes Dev. 12, 2245-2262.

Dyson, N., Howley, P.M., Munger, K. and Harlow, E. (1989) The human papilloma virus-16 E7 oncoprotein is able to bind to the retinoblastoma gene product. Science 243, 934-937.

Dyson, N., Guida, P., McCall, C. and Harlow, E. (1992) Adenovirus E1A makes 2 distinct contacts with the retinoblastoma protein. J. Virol. 66, 4606-4611.

Dyson, N., Dembski, M., Fattaey, A., Ngwu, C., Ewen, M. and Helin, K. (1993) Analysis of p107 associated proteins-p107 associates with a form of E2F that differs from pRB assocated E2F-1. J. Virol. 67, 7641-7647.

Egan, C., Jelsma, T.N., Howe, J.A., Bayley, S.T., Ferguson, B. and Branton, P.E. (1988) Mapping of cellular protein – binding sites on the products of the early region 1A of human adenovirus type 5. Mol. Cell. Biol. 8, 3955-3959.

Egan, C. Bayley, S.T. and Branton, P.E. (1989) Binding of the Rb1 protein to E1A products is required for adenovirus transformation. Oncogene 4, 383-388.

El-Diery, W.S., Kern, S.E., Pietenpol, J.A., Kinzler, K.W. and Vogelstein, B. (1992) Definition of a consensus binding site for p53. Nature Genetics 1, 45-49.

El-Diery, W.S., Tokino, T., Velculescu, V.E., Levy, D.B., Parsons, R., Trent, J.M., Lin, D., Mercer, W.E., Kinzler, K.W. and Vogelstein, B. (1993) WAF1, a potential mediator of p53 tumour suppression. Cell 75, 817-825.

El-Diery, W.S., Harper, J.W., O'Connor, P.M., Velculescu, V.E., Canman, C.E., Jackman, J., Pietenpol, J.A., Burrell, M., Hill, D.E., Wang, Y., Wiman, K.G., Mercer, W.E., Kastan, M.B., Kohn, K.W., Elledge, S.J., Kinzler, K.W. and Vogelstein, B. (1994) WAF1/CIP1 is induced in p53-mediated G1 arrest and apoptosis. Cancer Res. 54, 1169-1174.

Elsing, A. and Burgert, H.G. (1998). The adenovirus E3/10.4K-14.5K proteins down-modulate the apoptosis receptor Fas/Apo-1 by inducing its internalization. Proc. Natl. Acad. Sci. USA 95, 10072-10077.

Enari, M., Talanian, R. V., Wong, W. W. and Nagata, S. (1996) Sequential activation of ICE-like and C32-like proteases during Fas-mediated apoptosis. Nature 380, 723-726.

Erhardt, P., Tomaselli, K. J. and Cooper, G. M. (1997) Identification of the mdm2 oncoprotein as a substrate for C32-like apoptotic proteases. J. Biol. Chem. 272, 15049-15052.

Estaquier, J., Idziorek, T., Zou, W., Emillie, D., Farber, C.M., Bowrez, J.M. and Ameisen, J.C. (1995) T helper type 1/T helper type 2 cytokines and T cell death: preventative effect of interleukin 12 on activation-induced and CD95 (Fas/apo⁻1)-mediated apoptosis of CD4+T cells from human immunodeficiency virus-infected persons. J. Exp. Med. 182, 1759-1767.

Ewen, M.E., Ludlow, J.W., Marsilio, E., DeCaprio, J.A., Millikan, R.C., Cheng, S.H., Paucha, E. and Livingston, D.M. (1989) An N-terminal transformation-governing sequence of SV40 large T-antigen contributes to the binding of both p110 Rb and a second cellular protein, p120. Cell, 58, 257-267

Ewen, M.E., Xing, Y., Lawrence, J.B. and Livingston, D.M. (1991) Molecular cloning, chromosomal mapping and expression of the cDNA for p107, a retinoblastoma gene product related protein. Cell 66, 1155-1164.

Ewen, M.E., Faha, B., Harlow, E. and Livingston, D.M. (1992) Interaction of p107 with cyclin A independent of complex formation with viral oncoproteins. Science 255, 85-87.

Ewen, M.E., Sluss, H.K., Sherr, C.J., Matsushime, H., Kato, J.Y. and Livingston, D.M. (1993) Functional interactions of the retinoblastoma protein with mammalian D-type cyclin. Cell 73, 487-497.

Ezoe, H., Fatt, R.B.L. and Mak, S. (1981) Degradation of intracellular DNA in KB cells infected with CYT mutants of human Adenovirus-type-12. J. Virol. 40, 20-27.

Faha, B., Ewen, M.E., Tsai, L.H., Livingston, D.M. and Harlow, E. (1992) Interaction between human cyclin-A and adenovirus E1A-associated p107 protein. Science 255, 87-90.

Fakharzadeh, S.S., Trusko, S.P. and George, D.L. (1991) Tumourigenic potential associated with enhanced expression of a gene that is amplified in a mouse tumour cell line. EMBO J. 10, 1565-1569.

Faleiro, L., Kobayashi, R., Fearnhead, H. and Lazebnik, Y. (1997) Multiple species of C32 and Mch2 are the major active caspases present in apoptotic cells. EMBO J. 16, 2271-2281.

Fang, W., Rivard, J.J., Mueller, D.L. and Behrens, T.W. (1994) Cloning and molecular characterization of mouse Bcl-X in B-lymphocytes and T-lymphocytes. J. Immunol. 153, 4388-4398.

Farrow, S. N., White, J. R. M., Martinou, I., Raven, T., Pun, K. T., Grinham, C. J., Martinou, J. C. and Brown, R. (1995) Cloning of a Bcl-2 homolog by interaction with adenovirus E1B 19k. Nature 374, 731-733.

Fauci, A.S. (1993) Multifactorial nature of human immunodeficiency virus disease: implications for therapy. Science 262, 1011-1018.

Feinstein, E., Kimchi, A., Wallach, D., Boldin, M. and Varfolomeev, E. (1995) The Death Domain - A module shared by proteins with diverse cellular functions. Trends Biochem. Sci. 20, 342-344.

Fernandez-Sarabia, M. J. and Bischoff, J. R. (1993) Bcl-2 associates with the Ras-related protein R-ras p23. Nature 366, 274-275.

Field, S.F., Tsai, F.-Y., Kuo, F., Zubiaga, A.M., Kaelin, W.G., Jr., Livingston, D.M., Orkin, S.H. and Greenberg, M.E. (1996) E2F-1 functions in mice to promote apoptosis and suppress proliferation. Cell 85, 549-561.

Finkel, T.H., Tudor-Williams, G., Banda, N.K., Cotton, M.F., Curiel, T., Monks, C. Baba, T.W., Ruprecht, R.M. and Kupfer, A. (1995) Apoptosis occurs predominantly in bystander cells and not in productively infected cells of HIV- and SIV-infected lymph nodes. Nature Med. 1, 129-134.

Finlay, C.A. (1993) The MDM2 oncogene can overcome wild-type p53 suppression of transformed cell growth. Mol. Cell. Biol. 13, 301-306.

Frankel, S.S., Wenig, B.M., Burke, A.P., Mannan, P., Thompson, L.D.R., Abbondanzo, S.L., Nelson, A.M., Pope, M. and Steinman, R.M. (1996) Replication of HIV-1 in dendritic cell-derived syncytia at the mucosal surface of the adenoid. Science 272, 115-117

Gagliardini, V., Fernandez, P.A., Lee, R.K.K., Drexler, H.C.A., Rotello, R.J., Fishman, M.C. and Yuan, J. (1994) Prevention of vertebrate neuronal death by the crmA gene. Science 263, 826-828.

Gallimore, P.H., Grand, R.J.A. and Byrd, P.J. (1986) Transformation of human embryo retinoblasts with Simian virus 40, adenovirus and ras oncgenes. Anticancer Res. 499-508.

Gearing, A.J.H., Beckett, P., Christodoulou, M., Churchill, M., Clements, J., Davidson, A.H., Drummond, A.H., Galloway, W.A., Gilbert, R., Gordon, J.L., Leber, T.M., Mangan, M., Miller, K., Nayee, P., Owen, K., Patel, S., Thomas, W., Wells, G., Wood, L.M. and Woolley, K. (1994) Processing of tumor-necrosis-factor-alpha precusor by metalloproteinases. Nature 370, 555-557.

Gehri, R., Hahn, S., Rothen, M., Steuerwald, M., Neusch, R. and Erb, P. (1996) The fas receptor in HIV infection: expression on peripheral blood lymphocytes and role in the depletion of T cells. AIDS 10, 9-16.

Gervais, J.L.M., Seth, P. and Zhang, H. (1998) Cleavage of the cdk inhibitor p21 [Cip1/Waf1] by caspases is an early event during DNA damage-induced apoptosis. J. Biol. Chem. 273, 19207-19212.

Giaccia, A.J. and Kastan, M.B. (1998) The complexity of p53 modulation: emerging patterns from divergent signals. Genes Dev. 12, 2973-2983.

Ginsburg, D., Vairo, G., Chiltendon, T., Xiao, Z.X., Xu, G., Wydner, K.L., DeCaprio, J.A., Lawrence, J.B. and Livingston, D.M. (1994) E2F-4 a new E2F transcription factor family member interacts with p107 and has transforming potential. Genes Dev. 8, 2665-2679.

Gonzalez-Garcia, M., Perez-Ballestero, R., Ding, L. Y., Duan, L., Boise, L. H., Thompson, C. B. and Nunez, G. (1994) Bcl-x$_L$ is the major Bcl-x messenger-RNA form expressed during murine development and its product localizes to mitochondria. Development 120, 3033-3042.

Gooding, L.R., Ranheim, T.S., Tollefson, A.E., Aquino, L., Duerksenhughes, P., Horton, T.M. and Wold, W.S.M. (1991) The 10,400-dalton and 14,500-dalton proteins encoded by region E3 of Adenovirus function together to protect many but not all mouse-cell lines against lysis by tumor-necrosis-factor. J. Virol. 65, 4114-4123.

Gottlieb, S.L. and Myskowski, P.L. (1994) Molluscum Contagiosum. Int. J. Dermatol. 33, 453-461.

Gottlieb, T.M. and Oren, M. (1996) p53 in growth control and neoplasia. Biochim. Biophys. Acta 1287, 77-102.

Grand, R.J.A., Grant, M.L. and Gallimore, P.H. (1994) Enhanced expression of p53 in human cells infected with mutant adenoviruses. Virology 203, 229-240.

Grand, R.J.A., Owen, D., Rookes, S.M. and Gallimore, P.H.. (1996) Control of p53 expression by adenovirus 12 early region 1A and early region 1B 54K proteins. Virology 218, 23-24.

Grand, R.J.A., Parkhill, J., Szestak. T., Rookes, S.M., Roberts, S. and Gallimore, P.H. (1999) Definition of a major p53 binding site on Ad2E1B58K protein and a possible nuclear localization signal on the Ad12E1B54K protein. Oncogene 18, 955-965.

Greenberg, M.E., Ostapenko, D.A. and Mathews, M.B. (1997) Potentiation of human immunodeficiency virus type 1 Tat by human cellular proteins. J. Virol. 71, 7140-7144.

Gregory,C.D., Dive,C., Henderson,S., Smith,C.A., Williams,G.T., Gordon,J. and Rickinson, A.B. (1991) Activation of Epstein-Barr-virus latent genes protects human B-cells from death by apoptosis. Nature 349, 612-614.

Grell, M., Douni, E., Wajant, H., Lohden, M., Clauss, M., Maxeiner, B., Georgopoulos, S., Lesslauer, W., Kollias, G., Pfizenmaier, K. and Scheurich, P. (1995) The transmembrane form of tumor-necrosis-factor is the prime activating ligand of the 80 kda tumor-necrosis-factor receptor. Cell 83, 793-802

Groux, H., Torpier, G., Monté, D., Mouton, Y., Capron, A. and Ameisen, J.C. Activation-induced death by apoptosis in CD4+ T cells from human immunodeficiency virus-infected asymptomatic individuals. (1992) J. Exp. Med. 175, 331-340.

Gu, Z., Pim, D., Labrecque, S., Banks, L. and Matlashewski, G. (1994) DNA damage induced p53 mediated transcription is inhibited by human papillomavirus type 18 E6. Oncogene 9, 629-633.

Guan, R.J., Moss, S.F., Arber, N., Krajewski, S., Reed, J.C. and Holt, P.R. (1996) 30 KDa phosphorylated form of Bcl-2 protein in human colon. Oncogene 12, 2605-2609.

Haas-Kogan, D.A., Kogan, S.C., Levi, D., Dazin, P., T'Ang, A., Fung, Y.K.T. and Israel, M.A. (1995) Inhibition of apoptosis by the retinoblastoma gene product. EMBO J. 14, 461-472.

Haber, D.A. (1997) Splicing into senescence: the curious case of p16 and p19^{ARF}. Cell 91, 555-558.

Hadlar, S., Negrini, M., Monne, M., Sabbioni, S. and Croce, C. M. (1994) Down regulation of bcl-2 by p53 in breast cancer cells. Cancer Res. 54, 2095-2097.

Han, J., Sabbatini, P. andWhite, E. (1996) Induction of apoptosis by human Nbk/Bik, a BH3-containing protein that interacts with E1B 19K. Mol. Cell Biol, 16, 5857-5864.

Hannon, G.J., Demetrick, D. and Beach, D. (1993) Isolation of the Rb related p130 through its interaction with cdk2 and cyclins. Genes Dev. 7, 2378-2391.

Harper, J.W., Adami, G.R., Wei, N., Keyomarsi, K. and Elledge, S.J. (1993) The p21 Cdk interacting protein Cip1 is a potent inhibitor of G1 cyclin dependent kinases. Cell 75, 805-816.

Harper, J.W., Elledge, S.J., Keyomarsi, K.I., Dynlacht, B., Tsai, L.H., Zhang, P.M., Dobrowolski, S., Bai, C., Connellcrowley, L., Swindell, E., Fox, M.P. and Wei, N. (1995) Inhibition of cyclin-dependent kinases by p21. Mol. Biol. Cell. 6, 387-400.

Haupt, Y., Maya, R., Kazaz, A. and Oren, M. (1997) Mdm2 promotes the rapid degradation of p53. Nature 387, 296-299.

Haupt, Y., Rowan, S. and Oren, M. (1995a) p53-mediated apoptosis in HeLa cells can be overcome by excess pRb. Oncogene 10, 1563-1571.

Haupt, Y., Rowan, S., Shaulian, E., Vousden, K.H. and Oren, M. (1995b) Induction of apoptosis in HeLa cells by *trans*-activation-deficient p53. Genes Dev. 9, 2170-2183.

He, B., Chou, J., Brandimarti, R., Mohr, I., Gluzman, Y. and Roizman, B. (1997) Suppression of the phenotype of gamma(1)34.5(-) herpes simplex virus-1: Failure of activated RNA-dependent protein kinase to shut off protein synthesis is associated with a deletion in the domain of the alpha 47 gene. J. Virol. 71, 6049-6054.

He, J., Choe, S., Walker, R., DiMarzio, P., Morgan, D.O. and Landau, N.R. (1995) Human immunodeficiency virus type 1 viral protein R (Vpr) arrests cells in the G2 phase of the cell cycle by inhibiting p34^{cdc2} activity. J. Virol. 69, 6705-6711.

Helin, K., Lees, J.A., Vidal, M., Dyson, N., Harlow, E. and Fattaey, A. (1992) A cDNA encoding a pRB binding protein with properties of the transcription factor E2F. Cell 70, 337-350.

Helin, K., Harlow, E. and Fattaey, A. (1993) Inhibition of E2F-1 transactivation by direct binding of the retinoblastoma protein. Mol. Cell. Biol. 13, 6501-6508.

Henderson, S., Rowe, M., Gregory, C., Croomcarter, D., Wang, F., Longnecker, R., Kieff, E. and Rickinson, A. (1991) Induction of Bcl-2 expression by Epstein-Barr-virus latent membrane protein-1 protects infected B-cells from programmed cell-death. Cell 65, 1107-1115.

Henderson, S., Huen, D., Rowe, M., Dawson, C., Johnson, G. and Rickinson, A. (1993) Epstein-Barr virus-coded BHRF1 protein, a viral homolog of Bcl-2, protects human b-cells from programmed cell-death. Proc. Natl. Acad. Sci. (USA) 90, 8479-8483.

Henning, W., Rohaly, G., Kolzau, T., Knippschild, U., Maacke, H. and Deppert, W. (1997) MDM2 is a target of Simian virus 40 in cellular transformation and during lytic infection. J. Virol. 71, 7609-7618.

Hermeking, H. and Eick, D. (1994) Mediation of c-Myc-induced apoptosis by p53. Science 265, 2091-2093.

Hershberger, P.A., Dickson, J.A. and Friesen, P.D. (1992) Site-specific mutagenesis of the 35-kilodalton protein gene encoded by autographa-californica nuclear polyhedrosis-virus-cell line-specific effects on virus-replication. J. Virol. 66, 5525-5533.

Hershberger, P.A., Lacount, D.J. and Friesen, P.D. (1994) The apoptotic suppressor p53 is required early during baculovirus replication and is targeted to the cytosol of infected-cells. J. Virol. 68, 3467-3477.

Herwig, S. and Strauss, M. (1997) The retinoblastoma protein : a master regulator of cell cycle, differentiation and apoptosis. Eur. J. Biochem. 246, 581-601.

Hickman, E.S., Pickersley, S.M. and Vousden, K.H. (1994) Cells expressing HPV 16 E7 continue cell cycle progression following DNA damage induced by p53 activation. Oncogene 9, 2177-2181.

Hiebert, S.W., Chellappan, S.P., Horowitz, J.M. and Nevins, J.R. (1992) The interaction of RB with E2F coincides with an inhibition of the transcriptional activity of E2F. Genes Dev. 6, 177-185.

Hiebert, S.W., Packham, G., Strom, D.K., Haffner, R., Oren, M., Zambetti, G. and Cleveland, J.L. (1995) E2F-DP-1 induces p53 and overrides survival factors to trigger apoptosis. Mol. Cell. Biol. 15, 6864-6874.

Hollstein, M., Sidransky, D., Vogelstein, B. and Harris, C.C. (1991) p53 mutations and human cancers. Science 253, 49-53.

Horikoshi, N., Usheva, A., Chen, J., Levine, A.J., Weinmann, R. and Shenk, T. (1995) Two domains of p53 interact with the TATA-binding protein, and the adenovirus 13S E1A protein disrupts the association, relieving p53-mediated transcriptional repression. Mol. Cell. Biol. 15, 227-234.

Howe, J.A., Mymryk, J.S., Egan, C., Branton, P.E. and Bayley, S.T. (1990) Retinoblastoma growth suppressor and a 300-kDa protein appear to regulate cellular DNA synthesis. Proc. Natl. Acad. Sci. (USA) 87, 5883-5887.

Howes, K.A., Ransom, N., Papermaster, D.S., Lasudry, J.G.H., Albert, D.M. and Windle, J.J. (1994) Apoptosis or retinoblastoma: alternative fates of photoreceptors expressing the HPV-16 E7 gene in the presence or absence of p53. Genes Dev. 8, 1300-1310.

Hsu, H.L., Xiong, J. and Goeddel, D.V. (1995) The TNF receptor 1-associated protein TRADD signals cell-death and NF-κ -B activation. Cell 81, 495-504.

Hsu, H.L., Huang, J.N., Shu, H.B., Baichwal, V. and Goeddel, D.V. (1996) TNF-dependent recruitment of the protein-kinase RIP to the TNF receptor-1 signaling complex. Immunity 4, 387-396.

Huang, H.J.S., Yee, J.K., Shew, J.Y., Chen, P.L., Bookstein, R., Friedmann, T., Lee, E.Y.H.P. and Lee, W.H. (1988) Suppression of the neoplastic phenotype by replacement of the Rb gene in human cancer cells. Science 242, 1563-1566.

Huang, D.C.S., Cory, S. and Strasser, A. (1997) Bcl-2, Bcl-x(L) and adenovirus protein E1B19kD are functionally equivalent in their ability to inhibit cell death. Oncogene, 14, 405-414.

Humke, Ni, J. and Dixit, V.M. (1998) ERICE, A novel ELICE-activatable caspase. J. Biol. Chem. 273, 15702-15707.

Irmler, M., Hofmann, K., Vaux, D. and Tscho, J. (1997) Direct physical interaction between the Caenorhabditis elegans 'death proteins' CED-3 and CED-4. FEBS Lett.406, 189-190.

Ito, T. Dong, X., Carr, D., and May, W.S. (1997). Bcl-2 phosphorylization required for anti-apoptosis function. J. Biol. Chem. 272, 11671-11673.

Jacks, T., Fazeli, A., Schmitt, E.M., Bronson, R.T. and Weinberg, M.A. (1992) Effects of a Rb mutation in the mouse. Nature 359, 295-300.

Jacobson, M. D., Burne, J. F., King, M. P., Miyashita, T., Reed, J. C. and Raff, M. C. (1993) Bcl-2 blocks apoptosis in cells lacking mitochondrial-DNA. Nature 361, 365-369.

Jänicke, R. U., Walker, P. A., Lin, X. Y. and Porter, A. G. (1996) Specific cleavage of the retinoblastoma protein by an ICE-like protease in apoptosis. EMBO J., 15, 6969-6978.

Jost, C.A., Marin, M.C. and Kaelin, W.G., Jr. (1997) p73 is a human p53-related protein that can induce apoptosis. Nature 389, 191-194.

Jowett, J.B.M., Planelles, V., Poon, B., Shah, N.P., Chen, M. and Chen, I.S.Y. (1995) The human immunodeficiency type 1 Vpr gene arrests infected T cells in the G_2+M phase of the cell cycle. J. Virol. 69, 6304-6313.

Jung, Y.-K. and Yuan, J. (1997) Suppression of interleukin-1b converting enzyme (ICE)-induced apoptosis by SV40 large T antigen. Oncogene 14, 1207-1214.

Kabbutat, M.H.G., Jones, S.N. and Vousden, K.H. (1998) Regulation of p53 stability by mdm2. Nature 387, 299-303.

Kaghad, M., Bonnet, H., Yang, A., Creancier, L., Biscan, J.-C., Valent, A., Minty, A., Chalon, P., Lelias, J.M., Dumont, X., Ferrara, P., McKeon, F., Caput, D. (1997) Monoallelically expressed gene related to p53 at 1p36, a region frequently deleted in neuroblastoma and other human cancers. Cell 90, 809-819.

Kamada, S., Shimono, A., Shinto, Y., Tsujimura, T., Takahashi, T., Noda, T., Kitamura, Y., Kondoh, H. and Tsujimoto, Y. (1995) Bcl-2 deficiency in mice leads to pleiotropic abnormalities-accelerated lymphoid-cell death in thymus and spleen, polycystic kidney, hair hypopigmentation, and distorted small-intestine. Cancer Res. 55, 354-359.

Kamijo, T., Zindy, F., Roussel, M.F., Quelle, D.E., Downing, J.R., Ashmun, R.A., Grosveld, G. and Sherr, R.J. (1997) Tumor suppression at the mouse INK4a locus mediated by the alternative reading frame product p19^{ARF}. Cell 91, 649-659.

Kamijo, T., Weber, J.D., Zambetti, G., Zingy, F., Roussel, M.F. and Sherr, C.J. (1998) Functional and physical interactions of the ARF tumor suppressor with p53 and Mdm2. Proc. Natl. Acad. Sci. (USA) 95, 8292-8297.

Kaplan, D. and Sieg, S. (1998) Role of the Fas/Fas ligand apoptotic pathway in human immunodeficiency virus type 1 disease. J. Virol. 72, 6279-6282.

Kastan, M.B., Onyekwere, O., Sidransky, D., Vogelstein, B. and Craig, R.W. (1991) Participation of p53 protein in the cellular-response to DNA damage. Cancer Res. 51, 6304-6311.

Kasten, M.M. and Giordano, A. (1998) pRb and the Cdks in apoptosis and the cell cycle. Cell Death Diff. 5, 132-140.

Kato, J., Matsushime, H., Hiebert, S.W., Ewen, M.E. and Sherr, C.J. (1993) Direct binding of cyclin-D to the retinoblastoma gene-product (pRb) and pRb phosphorylation by the cyclin D-dependent kinase cdk4. Genes Dev. 7, 331-342.

Katsikis, P.D., Wunderlich, E.S., Smith, C.A. and Herzenberg, L.A. (1995) Fas antigen stimulation induced marked apoptosis of T lymphocytes in human immunodeficiency virus-infected individuals. J. Exp. Med. 81, 2029-2036.

Katsikis, P.D., Garcia-Ojeda, M., Wunderlich, E.S., Smith, C., Yagita, H., Okumura, K., Kayagaki, N., Alderson, M., Herzenberg, L.A. and Herzenberg, L.A. (1996) Activation induced peripheral blood T cell apoptosis is Fas independent in HIV-1 infected individuals. Int. Immunol. 8, 1311-1317.

Katsikis, P.D., Garcia-Ojeda, M.E., Terres-Roca, J.F., Tijoe, I.M., Smith, C.A., Herzenberg, L.A. and Herzenberg, L.A. (1997) Interleukin 1β converting enzyme-like protease involvement in Fas-induced and activation-induced peripheral blood T cell apoptosis in HIV-infection. TNF-related apoptosis-inducing ligand can mediate activation-induced T cell death in HIV-1 infection. J. Exp. Med. 186, 1365-1372.

Kawanishi, M. (1997) Expression of Epstein-Barr virus latent membrane protein 1 protects Jurkat T cells from apoptosis induced by serum deprivation. Virology 228, 244-250.

Kernohan, N.M., Helps, N.R., Lane, D.P. and Cohen, P.T.W. (1997) Characterisation of the in vivo properties of the p53 binding protein 53BP. J. Pathol. 181, A34.

Kerr, J.F.R., Wyllie, A.H. and Currie, A.H. (1972) Apoptosis: a basic biological phenomenon with wide-ranging implications in tissue kinetics. Brit. J. Cancer 26, 239-257.

Khanim, F., Dawson, C., Meseda, C.A., Dawson, J., Mackett, M. and Young, L.S. (1997) BHRF1, a viral homologue of the Bcl-2 Oncogene, is conserved atboth the sequence and functional level in different Epstein-Barr virus isolates. J. Gen. Virol., 78, 2987-2999.

Kiefer, M.C., Brauer, M.J., Powers, V.C., Wu, J.J., Umansky, S.R., Tomei, L.D. and Barr, P.J. (1995) Modulation of apoptosis by the widely distributed Bcl-2 homolog Bak. Nature 374, 736-739.

Kieff, E. (1995) Epstein-Barr-virus - increasing evidence of a link to carcinoma. New Eng. J. Med. 333, 724-726.

Kiernan, R., Marshall, J., Bowers, R., Doherty, R. and McPhee, D. (1990) Kinetics of HIV-1 replication and intracellular accumulation of particles in HTLV-1-transformed cells. AIDS Res. Hum. Retroviruses 6, 743-751

King, K. and Cidlowski, J.A. (1998) Celll cycle regulation and apoptosis. Ann. Rev. Physiol. 60, 601-617.

Kischkel, F.C., Hellbardt, S., Behrmann, I., Germer, M., Pawlita, M., Krammer, P.H. and Peter, M.E. (1995) Cytotoxicity-dependent APO-1 (FAS/CD95)-associated proteins form a death-inducing signaling complex (DISC) with the receptor. EMBO J. 14, 5579-5588.

Kleinberger, T. and Shenk, T. (1993) Adenovirus E4orf4 protein binds to protein phosphatase 2A and the complex down regulates E1A enhanced junB transcription. J. Virol. 67, 7556-7560.

Klenerman, P., Rowland-Jones, S., McAdam, S., Edwards, J., Daenke, S., Lalloo, D., Koppe, B., Rosenberg, W., Boyd, D., Edwards, A, Giangrande, P., Phillips, R.E. and McMichael, A.J. (1994) Cytotoxic T-cell activity antagonized by naturally occurring HIV-1 Gag variants. Nature 369, 403-407.

Knudsen, E.S., Buckmaster, C., Chen, T.T., Feramisco and Wang, J.Y.J. (1998) Inhibition of DNA synthesis by RB: effects on G_1/S transition and S-phase progression. Genes. Dev. 12, 2278-2292.

Knudson, C.M., Tung, K.S.K., Tourtellotte, W.G., Brown, G.A.J. and Korsmeyer, S.J. (1995) Bax-deficient mice demonstrate lymphoid hyperplasia and male germ cell death, Science 270, 96-99.

Ko, L.J. and Prives, C. (1996) p53: puzzle and paradigm. Genes Dev. 10, 1054-1072.

Kolesnitchenko, V., King, L., Riva, A., Tani, Y., Korsmeyer, S.J. and Cohen, D.J. (1997) A major human immunodeficiency virus type 1-initiated killing pathway distinct from apoptosis. J. Virol. 71, 9753-9763.

Komiyama, T., Ray, C.A., Pickup, D.J., Howard, A.D., Thornberry, N.A., Peterson, E.P. and Salvesen, G. (1994) Inhibition of Interleukin-1-b converting-enzyme by the Cowpox virus serpin CrmA - An example of cross-class inhibition. J. Biol. Chem. 269, 19331-19337.

Kowalik, T.F., DeGregori, J., Leone, G., Jakoi, L. and Nevins, J.R. (1998) E2F1 specific induction of apoptosis and p53 accumulation, which is blocked by MDM2. Cell Growth Differen. 9, 113-118.

Kowalik, T.F., DeGregori, J., Schwarz, J.K. and Nevins, J.R. (1995) E2F1 overexpression in quiescent fibroblasts leads to induction of cellular DNA synthesis and apoptosis. J. Virol. 69, 2491-2500.

Koyama, A.H. and Miwa, Y. (1997) Suppression of apoptotic DNA fragmentation in herpes simplex virus type 1-infected cells. J. Virol., 71, 2567-2571

Krajewski, S., Tanaka, S., Takayama, S., Schibler, M.J., Fenton, W. and Reed, J.C. (1993) Investigation of the subcellular-distribution of the Bcl-2 oncoprotein - residence in the nuclear-envelope, endoplasmic- reticulum, and outer mitochondrial-membranes. Cancer Res. 53, 4701-4714.

Krajewski, S., Krajewska, M., Shabaik, A., Wang, H.G., Irie, S., Fong, L. and Reed, J.C. (1994) Immunohistochemical analysis of in vivo patterns of Bcl-x expression. Cancer Res. 54, 5501-5507.

Kroemer, G., Zamzami, N. and Susin, S. A. (1997) Mitochondrial control of apoptosis. Immunol. Today 18, 44-51.

Kubbutat, M.H., Jones, S.N. and Vousden, K.H. (1997) Regulation of p53 stability by Mdm2. Nature 387, 299-303.

Kuerbitz, S.J., Plunkett, B.S., Walsh, W.V. and Kastan, M.B. (1992) Wild-type p53 is a cell cycle checkpoint determinant following irradiation. Proc. Natl. Acad. Sci. (USA) 89, 7491-7495.

Kuida, K., Zheng, T.S., Na, S., Kuan, C.Y., Yang, D., Karasuyama, H., Rakic, P. and Flavell, R.A. (1996) Decreased apoptosis in the brain and premature lethality in C32-deficient mice. Nature 384, 368-372.

Kussie, P.H., Gorina, S., Marechal, V., Elenbaas, B., Moreau, J., Levine, A.J. and Pavletich, N.P. (1996) Structure of the MDM2 protein bound to the p53 tumour suppressor transactivation domain. Science 274, 948-953.

Lai Fatt, R.B. and Mak, S. (1982) Mapping of an adenovirus function involved in the inhibition of DNA degradation. J. Virol. 42, 969-977.

Lam, M., Dubyak, G., Chen, L., Nunez, G., Miesfeld, R. L. and Distelhorst, C. W. (1994) Evidence that Bcl-2 represses apoptosis by regulating endoplasmic reticulum-associated Ca^{2+} fluxes. Proc. Natl. Acad. Sci. (USA), 91, 6569-6573.

Lane, D.P. (1992) p53, guardian of the genome. Nature 358, 15-16.

Lane, D.P. and Crawford, L. (1979) T antigen is bound to a host protein in SV40-transformed cells. Nature 278, 261-263.

Lane, D.P. and Hall, P.A. (1997) MDM2-arbiter of p53's destruction. Trends Biochem. Sci. 22, 373-374.

Laurent-Crawford, A.G., Krust, B., Muller, A., Rwiere, Y., Reg-Culle, M.A., Bechet, J.M., Montagnier, L. and Hovanessian, A.G. (1991) The cytopathic effect of HIV is associated with apoptosis. Virology 185, 829-839.

Lavoie, J.N., Nguyen, M., Marcellus, R.C., Branton, P.E. and Shore, G.C. (1998) E4orf4, a novel adenovirus death factor that induces p53-independent apoptosis by a pathway that is not inhibited by zVAD-fmk. J. Cell Biol. 140, 637-645.

Lechner, M. and Laimins, L. (1994) Inhibition of p53 DNA binding by human papillomavirus E6 proteins. J. Virol. 68, 4262-4273

Lee, E.Y.H.P., Chang, C.Y., Hu, N., Wang, Y.C.J., Lai, C.C., Herrup, K., Lee, W.H. and Bradley, A. (1992) Mice deficient for Rb are nonviable and show defects in neurogenesis and haematopoiesis. Nature 359, 288-294.

Lee, J.O., Russo, A.A. and Pavletich, N.P. (1998) Structure of the retinoblastoma tumour-suppressor pocket domain bound to a peptide from HPV E7. Nature 391, 859-865.

Lees, J.A., Buchkovich, K.J., Marshak, D.R. Anderson, C.W. and Harlow, E. (1991) The retinoblastoma protein is phosphorylated on multiple sites by human CDC2. EMBO J. 10, 4279-4290.

Lees, E., Faha, B., Dulic, V., Reed, S.I. and Harlow, E. (1992) Cyclin-E CDK2 and cyclin-A CDK2 kinases associate with p107 and E2F in a temporally distinct manner. Genes Dev. 6, 1874-1885.

Lees, J.A., Saito, M., Vidal, M., Valentine, M., Look, T., Harlow, E., Dyson, N. and Helin, K. (1993) The retinoblastoma protein binds to a family of E2F transcription factors. Mol. Cell. Biol. 13, 7813-7825.

Lees-Miller, S.P., Skaguchi, K., Ulrich, S.J., Appella, E. and Anderson, C.W. (1992) Human DNA-activated protein kinase phosphorylates serines 15 and 37 in the amino terminal transactivation domain of human p53. Mol. Cell. Biol. 12, 5041-5049.

Leonard, R., Zagury, D., Desportes, I., Bernard, J., Zagury, J.F. and Gallo, R.C. (1988) Cytopathic effect of human immunodeficiency virus in T4 cells is linked to the last stage of virus infection. Proc. Natl. Acad. Sci. (USA) 85, 3570-3574

Leopardi, R., VanSant, C. and Roizman, B. (1997) The herpes simplex virus 1 protein kinase U(s)3 is required for protection from apoptosis induced by the virus. Proc. Natl Acad. Sci. (USA), 94, 7891-7896.

Levine, A.J. (1993) The tumor suppressor genes. Annu. Rev. Biochem. 62, 623-651.

Levine, A.J. (1997) p53, the cellular gatekeeper for growth and division. Cell 88, 323-331.

Li, F. and Fraumeni, J. (1969) Soft-tissue sarcomas, breast cancer, and other neoplasms: a familial syndrome? Ann. Int. Med. 71, 747-753.

Li, F.P., Fraumeni, J.F., Mulvihill, J.J., Blattner, W.A., Dreyfus, M.G., Tucker, M.A. and Miller, R.W. (1988) A cancer family syndrome in 24 kindreds. Cancer Res., 48, 5358-5362

Li, Y., Graham, C., Lacy, S., Duncan, A.M.V. and Whyte, P. (1993) The adenovirus E1A associated 130-Kd protein is encoded by a member of the retinoblastoma gene family and physically interacts with cyclin A and cyclin E. Genes Dev. 7, 2366-2377.

Li, C.J., Friedman, D.J., Wang, C., Metelev, V. and Pardee, A.B. (1995) Induction of apoptosis in uninfected lymphocytes by HIV-1 Tat protein. Science 268, 429-431.

Lin, J., Chen, J., Elezhaas, B. and Levine, A.J. (1994) Several hydrophobic amino acids in the p53 amino terminal domain are required for transcriptional activation, binding to mdm2 and the adenovirus 5 E1B 55kD protein. Genes Dev. 8, 1235-1246.

Lin, J.L., Teresky, A.K. and Levine, A.J. (1995) Two critical hydrophobic amino acids in the amino terminal domain of the p53 proteins are required for the gain of function phenotypes of human p53 mutants. Oncogene 10, 2387-2390.

Linzer, D.I.H. and Levine, A.J. (1979) Characterization of a 54Kd cellular SV40 tumor antigen present in SV40-transformed cells and uninfected embryonal carcinoma cells. Cell 17, 43-52.

Lowe, S.W. and Ruley, H.E. (1993) Stabilization of the p53 tumor suppressor is induced by adenovirus E1A and accompanies apoptosis. Genes Dev. 7, 535-545.

Lowe, S.C., Schmitt, E.M., Smith, S.W., Osborne, B.A. and Jacks, T. (1993) p53 is required for radiation-induced apoptosis in mouse thymocytes. Nature 362, 847-849.

Lu, Q.L., Hanby, A.M., Hajibagheri, M.A.N., Gschmeissner, S.E., Lu, P.J., Taylorpapadimitriou, J, Krajewskl, S, Reed, J.C. and Wright, N.A. (1994) Bcl-2 protein localizes to the chromosomes of mitotic nuclei and is correlated with the cell-cycle in cultured epithelial-cell lines. J. Cell Sci. 107, 363-371.

Lu, J.J.Y., Chen, J.Y., Hsu, T.Y., Yu, W.C.Y., Su, I.J. and Yang, C.S. (1996) Induction of apoptosis in epithelial cells by Epstein-Barr virus latent membrane proteins 1. J. Gen. Virol. 77, 1883-1892.

Lukac, D.M., Manuello, J.R. and Alwine, J.C. (1994) Transcriptional activation by the Human Cytomegalovirus immediate-early proteins - requirements for simple promoter structures and interactions with multiple components of the transcription complex. J. Virol. 68, 5184-5193.

Mack, D.H., Vartikar, J., Pipas, J.M. and Laimins, L.A. (1993) Specific repression of TATA-mediated but not initiator-mediated transcription by wild-type p53. Nature 363, 281-283.

Maki, C.G., Huibregtse, J.M. and Howley, P.M. (1996) *In vivo* ubiquitination and proteasome-mediated degradation of p53. Cancer Res. 56, 2649-2654.

Maldarelli, F., Sato, H., Berthold, E., Orenstein, J. and Martin, M.A. (1995) Rapid induction of apoptosis by cell-to-cell transmission of human immunodeficiency virus type 1. J. Virol. 69, 6457-6465.

Maltzman, W. and Czyzyk, L. (1984) UV irradiation stimulates levels of p53 cellular tumour-antigen in non-transformed mouse cells. Mol. Cell. Biol. 4, 1689-1694.

Manji, G.A., Hozak, R.R., LaCount, D.J. and Friesen, P.D. (1997) Baculovirus inhibitor of apoptosis functions at or upstream of the apoptotic suppressor p35 to prevent programmed cell death. J. Virol. 71, 4509-4516.

Marcellus, R.C., Teodoro, J.C., Wu, T., Brough, D.E., Ketner, G., Shore, G.C. and Branton, P.E. (1996) Adenovirus 5 early region 4 is responsible for E1A induced p53-independent apoptosis. J. Virol. 70, 6207-6215.

Martin, M.C., Fernandez, A., Bick, R.J., Brisbay, S., Buja, M., Snuggs, M., McConkey, D.J., Voneschenbach, A.C., Keating, M.J. and McDonnell, T.J. (1996) Apoptosis suppression by Bcl-2 is correlated with the regulation of nuclear and cytosolic Ca2+. Oncogene 12, 2259-2266.

Martinez, J., Georgoff, I., Martinez, J. and Levine, A.J. (1991) Cellular localisation and cell cycle regulation by a temperature sensitive p53 protein. Genes Dev. 5, 151-159.

Martins, L. M., Kottke, T., Mesner, P. W., Basi, G. S., Sinha, S., Frigon, N., Tatar, E., Tung, J. S., Bryant, K., Takahashi, A., Svingen, P. A., Madden, B. J., McCormick, D. J., Earnshaw, W. C. and Kaufmann, S. H. (1997) Activation of multiple interleukin-1 b converting enzyme homologues in cytosol and nuclei of HL-60 cells during etoposide-induced apoptosis. J. Biol. Chem. 272, 7421-7430.

Mayo, L.D., Turchi, J.J. and Berberich, S.J. (1997) Mdm-2 phosphorylation by DNA-dependent protein kinase prevents interaction with p53. Can. Res. 57, 5013-5016.

McCarthy, S.A., Symonds, H.S. and van Dyke, T. (1994) Regulation of apoptosis in transgenic mice by Simian virus 40 T antigen-mediated inactivation of p53. Proc. Natl. Acad. Sci. (USA) 91, 3979-3983.

McCloskey, T.M., Ott, M., Tribble, E., Khan, S.A., Teichberg, S., Paul, M.O., Pahwa, S., Verdin, E. and Chirmule, N. (1997) Dual role of HIV Tat in regulation of apoptosis in T cells. J. Immunol. 158, 1014-1019.

Mercer, W.E., Shields, M.T., Amin, A., Sauve, G.J., Appella, E., Romano, J.W. and Ullrich, S.J. (1990) Negative growth regulation in a glioblastoma tumour cell line that continually expresses human wild-type p53. Proc. Natl. Acad. Sci. (USA) 88, 1958-1962.

Meyerson, M. and Harlow, E. (1993) Identification of G1 kinase-activity for CDK6, a novel cyclin-D partner. Mol. Cell. Biol. 14, 2077-2086.

Michalovitz, D., Halevy, O. and Oren, M. (1990) Conditional inhibition of transformation and of cell proliferation by a temperature-sensitive mutant of p53. Cell 62, 671-680.

Midgley, C.A. and Lane, D.P. (1997) p53 protein stability in tumour cells is not determined by mutation but is dependent on Mdm2 binding. Oncogene 15, 1179-1189.

Mietz, J.A., Unger, T., Huibregtse, J.M. and Howley, P.M. (1992) The transcriptional transactivation function of wild type p53 is inhibited by SV40 large T antigen and HPV-16 E6 oncoprotein. EMBO J. 11, 5013-5020.

Miller, L.K. and White, E. (1998) (editors) Apoptosis and virus infection. Sem. Virol. 8, 443-523.

Minn, A.J., Velez, P., Schendel, S.L., Liang, H., Muchmore, S.W., Fesik, S.W., Fill, M. and Thompson, C.B. (1997) Bcl-x(L) forms an ion channel in synthetic lipid membranes. Nature 385, 353-357.

Miyashita, T., Krajewski, S., Krajewska, M., Wang, H.G., Lin, H.K., Liebermann, D.A., Hoffman, B. and Reed, J.C. (1994) Tumour suppressor p53 is a regulator of Bcl-2 and Bax gene expression *in vitro* and *in vivo*. Oncogene 9, 1799-1805.

Mocarski, E.S., Bonyhadi, M., Salimi, S., Mccune, J.M. and Kaneshima, H. (1993) Human Cytomegalovirus in a SCID-HU mouse - thymic epithelial-cells are prominent targets of viral replication. Proc. Natl. Acad. Sci. (USA) 90, 104-108.

Momand, J. Zambetti, G.P., Olson, D.C., George, D. and Levine, A.J. (1992) The MDM2 oncogene product forms a complex with the p53 protein and inhibits p53-mediated transactivation. Cell 69, 1237-1245.

Monaghan, P., Robertson, D., Amos, T.A.S., Dyer, M.J.S., Mason, D.Y. and Greaves, M.F. (1992) Ultrastructural-localization of Bcl-2 protein. J. Histochem. Cytochem. 40, 1819-1825.

Moore, M., Horikoshi, N. and Shenk, T. (1996) Oncogenic potential of the adenovirus E4orf6 protein. Proc. Natl. Acad. Sci. (USA) 93, 11295-11301.

Moran, E. and Mathews, M.B. (1987) Multiple functional domains in the adenovirus E1A gene. Cell 48, 177-178.

Morey, A.L., Ferguson, D.J.P. and Fleming, K.A. (1993) Ultrastructural features of fetal erythroid precursors infected with parvovirus B19 *in vitro* – evidence of cell death by apoptosis. J. Pathol. 169, 213-220.

Morgenbesser, S.D., Williams, B.O., Jacks, T. and DePinho, R.A. (1994) p53-dependent apoptosis produced by Rb-deficiency in the developing mouse lens. Nature 371, 72-74.

Mosier, E., Gulizia, R.J., MacIsaac, P.D., Torbett, B.E. and Levy, J.A. (1993) A rapid loss of CD4+ T cells in human-PBL-SCID mice by noncytopathic HIV isolates. Science 260, 689-692.

Mosner, J., Mummenbrauer, T., Buaer, C., Sczakiel, G., Grosse, F. and Deppert, W. (1995) Negative feeback regulation of wild-type p53 biosynthesis. EMBO J. 14, 4442-4449.

Motoyama, N., Wang, F.P., Roth, K.A., Sawa, H., Nakayama, K., Nakayama, K., Negishi, I., Senju, S., Zhang, Q., Fujii, S. and Loh, D.Y. (1995) Massive cell-death of immature hematopoietic-cells and neurones in Bcl-x-deficient mice. Science, 267, 1506-1510.

Muchmore, S.W., Sattler, M., Liang, H., Meadows, R.P., Harlan, J.E., Yoon, H.S., Nettesheim, D., Chang, B.S., Thompson, C.B., Wong, S.L., Ng, S.C. and Fesik, S.W. (1996) X-ray and NMR structure of human Bcl-x$_L$, an inhibitor of programmed cell-death. Nature, 381, 335-341.

Mulligan, G. and Jacks, T. (1998) The retinoblastoma gene family: cousins with overlapping interests. Trends Genet. 14, 223-229.

Mymryk, J.S., Shire, K. and Bayley, S.T. (1994) Induction of apoptosis by adenovirus type 5 E1A in rat cells requires a proliferation block. Oncogene 9, 1187-1193.

Nagata, S. (1997) Apoptosis by death factor. Cell 88, 355-365.

Nagata, S. and Golstein, P. (1995) The Fas death factor. Science 267, 1449-1456.

Nakajima, T., Morita, K., Tsunoda, H., Imajoh-Ohmi, S., Tanaka, H., Yasuda, H. and Oda, K. (1998) Stabilization of p53 by Adenovirus E1A occurs through its amino-terminal region by modification of the ubiquitin-proteasome pathway. J. Biol. Chem. 273, 20036-20045.

Nakamura, T., Pichel, J.G., Williams-Simons, L. and Westphal, H. (1995) An apoptotic defect in lens differentiation caused by human p53 is rescued by a mutant allele. Proc. Natl. Acad. Sci. (USA) 92, 6142-6146.

Nakamura, T., Williams-Simons, L. and Westphal, H. (1997) A human papillomavirus type 18 E6/E7 transgene sensitizes mouse lens cells to human wild-type p53-mediated apoptosis. Oncogene 14, 2991-2998.

Nardelli, B., Gonzalez, C.J., Schechter, M. and Valentine, F.T. (1995) CD4(+) blood lymphocytes are rapidly killed in-vitro by contact with autologous human immunodeficiency virus-infected cells. Proc. Natl. Acad. Sci. (USA) 92, 7312-7316.

Naumovski, L. and Cleary, M.L. (1996) The p53-binding protein 53BP2 also interacts with Bcl-2 and impedes cell-cycle progression at G(2)/M. Mol. Cell. Biol. 16, 3884-3892.

Nava, V.E., Cheng, E.H.Y., Veliunoa, M., Zou, S.F., Clem, R.J., Mayer, M.L. and Hardwick, J.M. (1997) Herpesvirus Saimiri encodes a functional homolog of the human Bcl-2 oncogene. J. Virol. 71, 4118-4122

Neilan, J.G., Lu, Z., Kutish, G.F., Zsak, L., Burrage, T.G. and Borca, M.V. (1997) A BIR motif containing gene of African swine fever virus, 4CL, is nonessential for growth *in vitro* and viral virulence. Virology 230, 252-264.

Nevels, M., Rubenwolf, S., Spruss, T., Wolf, H. and Dobner, T. (1997) The adenovirus E4orf6 protein can promote E1A/E1B-induced focus formation by interferring with p53 tumor suppressor function. Proc. Natl. Acad. Sci. (USA) 94, 1206-1211.

New, D.R., Maggirwar, S.B., Epstein, L.G., Dewhurst, S. and Gelbard, H.A. (1998) HIV-1 Tat induces neuronal death via tumor necrosis factor-alpha and activation of non-N-methyl-D-aspartate receptors by a NF kappa B-independent mechanism. J. Biol. Chem., 273, 17852-17858.

Newell, M.K., Haughn, L.J., Maroun, C.R. and Julius, M.H. (1990) Death of mature T cells by separate ligation of CD4 and the T-cell receptor for antigen. Nature 347, 286-289.

Newton, K. and Strasser, A. (1998) The Bcl-2 family and cell death regulation. Curr. Opin. in Gen. Devel. 8, 68-75.

Nicholson, D.W., Ali, A., Thornberry, N.A., Vaillancourt, J.P., Ding, C.K., Gallant, M., Gareau, Y., Griffin, P.R., Labelle, M., Lazebnik, Y.A., Munday, N.A., Raju, S.M., Smulson, M.E., Yamin, T.T., Yu, V.L. and Miller, D.K. (1995) Identification and inhibition of the ICE/CED-3 protease necessary for mammalian apoptosis. Nature 376, 37-43.

Noraz, N., Gozlan, J., Corbeil, J., Brunner,T. and Spector, S.A. (1997) HIV-induced apoptosis of activated primary CD4$^+$T lymphocytes is not mediated by Fas-Fas ligand. AIDS 11, 1671-1680.

O'Brien, V. (1998) Viruses and apoptosis. J. Gen. Virol. 79, 1833-1845.

Okan, I., Wang, Y.S., Chen, F., Hu, L.F., Imreh, S., Klein, G. and Wiman, K.G. (1995) The EBV-encoded LMP1 protein inhibits p53-triggered apoptosis but not growth arrest. Oncogene 11, 1027-1031.

Oliner, J.D., Pietenpol, J.A., Thiagalingham, S., Gyuris, J., Kinzler, K.W. and Vogelstein, B. (1993) Oncoprotein MDM2 conceals the activation domain of tumor suppressor p53. Nature 362, 857-860.

Oltvai, Z.N., Milliman, C.L. and Korsmeyer, S.J. (1993) Bcl-2 heterodimerizes in-vivo with a conserved homolog, Bax, that accelerates programmed cell-death. Cell 74, 609-619.

Oren, M. (1997) Lonely no more: p53 finds its kin in tumor suppressor heaven. Cell 90, 829-832.

Oren, M., Maltzman, W. and Levine, A.J. (1981) Post-translational regulation of the 54K cellular tumour-antigen in normal and transformed cells. Mol. Cell. Biol. 1, 101-110.

Ornelles, D.A. and Shenk, T. (1991) Localization of the adenovirus early region 1B 55-kilodalton protein during lytic infection – association with nuclear viral inclusions requires the early region-4 34 kilodalton protein. J. Virol. 65, 424-439.

Oyaiza, N., McCloskey, T.W., Coronesi, N., Chirmule, N., Kalyanaraman, V.S. and Pahwa, S. (1993) Accelerated apoptosis in peripheral blood mononuclear cells (PBMCs) from human immunodeficiency virus type-1 infected patients and in CD4 cross-linked PBMCs from normal individuals. Blood 82, 3392-3400.

Oyaizu, N., McCloskey, T.W., Than, S., Hu, R., Kalyanaraman, V.S. and Pahwa, S. (1994) Cross-linking of CD4 molecules up-regulates Fas antigen expression by lymphocytes by inducing interferon-γ and tumor necrosis factor-α secretion. Blood 84, 2622-2631.

Pagano, S., Artini, M., Costanzo, A., Chirillo, P., Falco, M., Natoli, G., Balsano, C. and Levrero, M. (1997) Genetic analysis of HBV pX protein functions: Transcriptional activation, modulation of cell growth and induction of apoptosis. Hepatol. 26, 1796.

Pan, H. and Griep, A.E. (1994) Altered cell cycle regulation in the lens of HPV-16 E6 or E7 transgenic mice: implications for tumour suppressor gene function in development. Genes Dev. 8, 1285-1299.

Pan, H. and Griep, A.E. (1995) Temporally distinct patterns of p53-independent apoptosis during mouse lens development. Genes Dev. 9, 2157-2169.

Pantaleo, G., Graziosi, G., Demarest, J.F., Cohen, O.J., Vaccarezza, M., Gantt, K., Muro-Cacho, C. and Fauci, A.S. (1994) Role of lymphoid organs in the pathogenesis of human immunodeficiency virus (HIV) infection. Immunolog. Rev. 140, 105-130.

Perry, M.E., Piette, J., Zawadzki, J.A., Harvey, D. and Levine, A.J. (1993) The MDM2 gene is induced in response to UV light in a p53 dependent manner. Proc. Natl. Acad. Sci. (USA) 90, 11623-11627.

Pietenpol, J.A., Tokino, T., Thiagalingam, S., El-Diery, W.S., Kinzler, K.W. and Vogelstein, B. (1994) Sequence-specific transcriptional activation is essential for growth suppression by p53. Proc. Natl. Acad. Sci. (USA) 91, 1998-2002.

Pilder, S., Logan, J. and Shenk, T. (1984) Deletion of the gene encoding the adenovirus 5 early region 1B 21,000-molecular weight polypeptide leads to degradation of viral host cell DNA. J. Virol. 52, 664-671.

Pim, D., Storey, A. Thomas, M., Massini, P. and Banks, L. (1994) Mutational analysis of HPV-18 E6 identifies domains required for p53 degradation *in vitro*, abolition of p53 transactivation *in vivo* and immortalisation of primary BHK cells. Oncogene 9, 1869-1876.

Polyak, K., Xia, Y., Zweier, J.L., Kinzler, K.W. and Vogelstein, B. (1997) A model for p53-induced apoptosis. Nature 389, 300-305.

Pomerantz, J., Schreiber-Agus, N., Liegeois, N.J., Silverman, A., Alland, L., Chin, L., Potes, J., Chen, K.,
Orlow, I., Lee, H.-W., Cordon-Cardo, C. and DePinho, R.A. (1998) The *Ink4a* tumor suppressor gene
product, $p19^{ARF}$, interacts with MDM2 and neutralizes MDM2's inhibition of p53. Cell 92, 713-723.

Prives, C. (1998) Signalling to p53: breaking the MDM2-p53 circuit. Cell 95, 5-8.

Purves, F.C., Deana, A.D., Marchiori, F., Leader, D.P. and Pinna, L.A. (1986) The substrate-specificity of the
protein-kinase induced in cells infected with herpesviruses - studies with synthetic substrates indicate
structural requirements distinct from other protein-kinases. Biochim. Biophys. Acta 889, 208-215.

Puthenveettil, J.A., Frederickson, S.M. and Reznikoff, C.A. (1996) Apoptosis in human papillomavirus 16 E7,
but not E6-immortalized human uroepithelial cells. Oncogene 13, 1123-1131.

Qin, X.-Q., Livingston, D.M., Kaelin, W.G. Jr. and Adams, P.D. (1994) Deregulated transcription factor E2F-
1 expression leads to S-phase entry and p53-mediated apoptosis. Proc. Natl. Acad. Sci. (USA) 91, 10918-
10922.

Quan, L.T., Caputo, A., Bleackley, R.C., Pickup, D.J. and Salvesen, G.S. (1995) Granzyme-B is inhibited by
the cowpox virus serpin cytokine response modifier-A. J. Biol. Chem. 270, 10377-10379.

Querido, E., Marcellus, R.C., Lai, A., Charbonneau, R., Teodoro, J., Ketner, G. and Branton, P.E. (1997a)
Regulation of p53 levels by the E1B 55-kilodalton protein and E4orf6 in adenovirus-infected cells. J. Virol. 71, 3788-3798.

Querido, E., Teodoro, J.G. and Branton, P.E. (1997b) Accumulation of p53 induced by the adenovirus E1A
protein requires regions involved in the stimulation of DNA synthesis. J. Virol. 71, 3526-3533.

Quinlan, M.P. and Grodzicker, T. (1987) Adenovirus E1A 12S protein induces DNA synthesis and proliferation in primary epithelial cells in both the presence and absence of serum. J. Virol. 61, 673-682.

Rao, L., Debbas, M., Sabbatini, P., Hockenberry, D., Korsmeyer, S. and White, E. (1992) The adenovirus
E1A proteins induce apoptosis which is inhibited by the E1B 19K-Da and Bcl-2 proteins. Proc. Natl.
Acad. Sci. (USA) 89, 7742-7746.

Rao, L., Perez, D. and White, E. (1996) Lamin proteolysis facilitates nuclear events during apoptosis. J. Cell
Biol. 135, 1441-1455.

Rao, L. and White, E. (1997) Bcl-2 and the ICE family of apoptotic regulators: Making a connection. Curr.
Opin. Genet. Dev. 7, 52-58.

Ray, C.A., Black, R.A., Kronheim, S.R., Greenstreet, T.A., Sleath, P.R., Salvesen, G.S. and Pickup, D.J.
(1992) Viral inhibition of inflammation-cowpox virus encodes an inhibitor of the interleukin-1-beta converting enzyme. Cell 69, 597-604.

Raychaudhuri, P., Bagchi, S., Devoto, S.H., Kraus, V.B., Moran, E. and Nevins, J.R. (1991) Domains of the
adenovirus E1A protein required for oncogenic activity are also required for dissociation of E2F transcription factor complexes. Gene Dev. 5, 1200-1211.

Razvi, E.S. and Welsh, R.M. (1995) Apoptosis in viral infections. Adv. Virus Res. 45, 1-60.

Reed, J. C. (1994) Bcl-2 and the regulation of programmed cell-death. J. Cell Biol. 124, 1-6.

Reynolds, J. E. and Eastman, A. (1996) Intracellular calcium stores are not required for Bcl-2-mediated
protection from apoptosis. J. Biol. Chem. 271, 27739-27743.

Rickinson, A.B., Lee, S.P. and Steven, N.M. (1996) Cytotoxic T lymphocyte responses to Epstein-Barr virus.
Curr. Opin. Immunol. 8, 492-497.

Rothe, M., Sarma, V., Dixit, V.W. and Goeddell, D.V. (1995) TRAF2-mediated activation of NF-KAPPA-B
by TNF recepotr and CD40. Science 269, 1424-1427.

Roy, N., Deveraux, Q.L. Takahashi, R., Salvesen, G.S. and Reed, J.C. (1997) The c-IAP-1 and c-IAP-2
proteins are direct inhibitors of specific caspases. EMBO J. 16, 6914-6925.

Rubenwolf, S., Schutt, H., Nevels, M., Wolf, H. and Dobner, T. (1997) Structural analysis of the adenovirus
type 5 E1B 55-kilodalton – E4orf6 protein complex. J. Virol. 71, 1115-1123.

Sabbatini, P., Lin, J., Levine, A.J. and White, E. (1995a) Essential role for p53-mediated transcription in E1A-
induced apoptosis. Genes Dev. 9, 2184-2192.

Sabbatini, P., Chiou, S.K., Rao, L. and White, E. (1995b) Modulation of p53-mediated transcriptional repression and apoptosis by the adenovirus E1B 19K protein. Mol. Cell. Biol. 15, 1060-1070.

Saenz-Robies, M.T., Symonds, H., Chen, J. and Van Dyke, T. (1994) Induction versus progression of brain tumor development: Differential functions for the pRB- and p53-targeting domains of SV40 T antigen. Mol. Cell. Biol. 14, 2686-2698.

Sakamuro, D., Sabbatini, P., White, E. and Prendergast, G.C. (1997) The polyproline region of p53 is required to activate apoptosis but not growth arrest. Oncogene 15, 887-898.

Samuelson, A.V. and Lowe, S.W. (1997) Selective induction of p53 and chemosensitivity in RB-deficient cells by E1A mutants unable to bind the RB-related proteins. Proc. Natl. Acad. Sci. (USA) 94, 12094-12099.

Sanchez-Prieto, R., Llenoart, M. and Cajal, S. (1995) Lack of correlation between p53 protein level and sensitivity to DNA-damaging agents in keratinocytes carrying adenovirus E1A mutants. Oncogene 11, 675-682.

Sarid, R., Sato, T., Bohenzky, R.A., Russo, J.J. and Chang, Y. (1997) Kaposi's sarcoma-associated herpesvirus encodes a functional Bcl-2 homologue. Nature Med., 3, 293-298.

Sarnow, P., Shih Ho, Y., Williams, J. and Levine, A.J. (1982) Adenovirus E1B-58Kd tumor antigen and SV40 large tumor antigen are physically associated with the same 54Kda cellular protein in transformed cells. Cell 28, 387-394.

Sastry, K.J., Martin, M.C., Nehete, P.N., McConnell, K., El-Naggar, A.K. and McDonnell, T.J. (1996) Expression of human immunodeficiency virus type I tat results in down-regulation of bcl-2 and induction of apoptosis in hematopoietic cells. Oncogene 13, 487-493.

Saunders, J.W. and Fallon, J.S. (1966) Cell death in morphogenesis in: Major problems in developmental biology (Lock M., editor) 25th Symposium of the Society for Developmental Biology, New York Academic Press, pp. 289-314.

Saurin, A.J., Borden, K.L.B., Boddy, M.N. and Freemont, P.S. (1996) Does this have a familiar ring? Trends Biochem. Sci. 21, 208-214.

Scaria, A., Tollefson, A.E., Saha, S.K. and Wold, W.S.M. (1992) The E3-11.6K protein of adenovirus is an Asn-glycosylated integral membrane protein that localizes to the nuclear membrane. Virology 191, 743-753.

Scheffner, M., Werness, B.A., Huibregtse, J.M., Levine, A.J. and Howley, P.M. (1990) The E6 oncoprotein encoded by human papillomavirus types 16 and 18 promotes the degradation of p53. Cell 63, 1129-1136.

Scheffner, M., Huibregste, J., Vierstra, R. and Howley, P. (1993) The HPV-16 E6 and E6-AP complex functions as an ubiquitin-protein ligase in the ubiquitination of p53. Cell 75, 495-505.

Scheffner, M., Nuber, U. and Huibregtse, J.M. (1995) Protein ubiquitination involving an E1-E2-E3 enzyme ubiquitin thioester cascade. Nature 373, 81-83.

Schreiber, M., Sedger, L. and McFadden, G. (1997) Distinct domains of M-T2, the myxoma virus tumor necrosis factor (TNF) receptor homolog, mediate extracellular TNF binding and intracellular apoptosis inhibition. J. Virol. 71, 2171-2181.

Schwarz, J.K., Devoto, S.H., Smith, E.J., Chellappan, S.P., Jakoi, L. and Nevins, J.R. (1993) Interactions of the p107 and Rb proteins with E2F during the cell proliferation response. EMBO J. 12, 1013-1020.

See, R.H. and Shi, Y. (1998) Adenovirus E1B 19,000-molecular-weight protein activates c-Jun N-terminal kinase and c-Jun-mediated transcription. Mol. Cell. Biol. 18, 4012-4022.

Selivanova, G. and Wiman, K.G. (1995) p53: a cell cycle regulator activated by DNA damage. Adv. Can. Res. 66, 143-180.

Serrano, M., Lin, A.W., McCurrach, M.E., Beach, D. and Lowe, S.W. (1997) Oncogenic ras provokes premature cell senescence associated with accumulation of p53 and p16[INK4a]. Cell 88, 593-602.

Seshagiri, S. and Miller, L.K. (1997) Baculovirus inhibitors of apoptosis (IAPs) block activation of Sf-caspase-1. Proc.Natl. Acad. Sci. (USA) 94, 13606-13611.

Seto, E., Usheva, A., Zambetti, G.P., Momand, J., Horikoshi, N., Weinmann, R., Levine, A.J. and Shenk, T. (1992) Wild-type p53 binds to the TATA-binding protein and represses transcription. Proc. Natl. Acad. Sci. (USA) 89, 12028-12032.

Shaulsky, G., Goldfinger, N., Peled, A., Rotter, V. (1991) Involvement of wild-type p53 in pre-B-cell differentiation in vitro. Proc. Natl. Acad. Sci. (USA) 88, 8982-8986.

Shan, B. and Lee, W. (1994) Deregulated expression of E2F-1 induces S phase entry and leads to apoptosis. Mol. Cell. Biol. 14, 8166-8173.

Shaulian, E., Haviv, I., Shaul, Y. and Oren, M. (1995) Transcriptional repression by the C-terminal domain of p53. Oncogene 10, 671-680.

Shaw, P., Bovey , R., Tardy, S., Sahli, R., Sordat, b. and Costa, J. (1992) Induction of apoptosis by wild-type p53 in a human colon tumour-derived cell line. Proc. Natl. Acad. Sci. (USA) 89, 4495-4499.

Shen, Y. and Shenk, T. (1994) Relief of p53 mediated transcriptional repression of the adenovirus E1B 19k-Da protein or the cellular Bcl-2 protein. Proc. Natl. Acad. Sci. (USA) 91, 8940-8944.

Shen, Y. and Shenk, T. (1995) Viruses and apoptosis. Curr. Opin. Genet. Develop. 5, 105-111.

Shenk, T. and Flint, J. (1991) Transcriptional and transforming activities of the adenovirus E1A proteins. Advances in Cancer Res. 57, 47-85.

Sherr, C.J. (1993) Mammalian G1 cyclins. Cell 73, 1059-1065.

Sherr, C.J. (1998) Tumor surveillance via the ARF-p53 pathway. Genes Dev. 12, 2984-2991.

Shieh, S.Y., Ikeda, M., Taya, Y. and Prives, C. (1997) DNA damage-induced phosphorylation of p53 alleviates inhibition by MDM2. Cell 91, 325-334.

Shirodkar, S., Ewen, M., DeCaprio, J.A., Morgan, J., Livingston, D.M. and Chittenden, T. (1992) The transcription factor E2F interacts with the retinoblastoma product and a p107-cyclin A complex in a cell-cycle-regulated manner. Cell 68, 157-166.

Shisler, J., Yang, C., Walter, B., Ware, C.F. and Gooding, L.R. (1997) The adenovirus E3-10.4K/14.5K complex mediates loss of cell surface Fas (CD95) and resistance to fas-induced apoptosis. J. Virol. 71, 8299-8306.

Shtrichman, R. and Kleinberger, T. (1998) Adenovirus type 5 E4 open reading frame 4 protein induces apoptosis in transformed cells. J. Virol. 72, 2975-2982.

Sieg, S., Smith, D., Yildirim, S. and Kaplan, D. (1997) Fas ligand deficiency in HIV disease. Proc. Natl. Acad. Sci. (USA) 94, 5860-5865.

Silicano, J.D., Canman, C.E., Taya, Y., Sakaguchi, K., Appella, E. and Kastan, M.B. (1997) DNA damage induced phosphorylation of the amino terminus of p53. Genes Dev. 11, 3471-3481.

Silvestris, F., Cafforio, P., Frassanito, M., Tucci, M., Romito, A., Nagata, S. and Dammacco, F. (1996) Overexpression of Fas antigen on T cells in advanced HIV-1 infection: differential ligan constantly induces apoptosis. AIDS 10, 131-141.

Simonian, P.L., Grillot, D.A.M., Merino, R. and Nunez, G. (1996) Bax can antagonize Bcl-x(L) during etoposide and cisplatin-induced cell death independently of its heterodimerization with Bcl-x(L). J. Biol. Chem. 271, 22764-22772.

Slebos, R.J.C., Lee, M.H., Plunkett, B.S., Kessis, T.D., Williams, B.O., Jacks, T., Hedrick, L., Kastan, M.B. and Cho, K.R. (1994) p53-dependent G1 arrest involves pRb related proteins and is disrupted by human papillomavirus 16 E7 oncoprotein. Proc. Natl. Acad. Sci. (USA) 91, 5320-5324.

Smith, G.L. (1998) (editor) Apoptosis and virus infection. Sem. Virol. 8, 359-442.

Smith, C.A., Davis, T., Wignall, J.M., Din, W.S., Farrah, T., Upton, C., McFadden, G. and Goodwin, R.G. (1991) T2 open reading frame from the Shope Fibroma virus encodes a soluble form of the TNF receptor. Biochem. Biophys. Res. Comms. 176, 335-342.

Smith, C.A., Hu, F.Q., Smith, T.D., Richards, C.L., Smolak, P., Goodwin, R.G. and Pickup, DJ. (1996) Cowpox virus genome encodes a second soluble homologue of cellular TNF receptors, distinct from CrmB, that binds TNF but not LT alpha. J. Virol. 223, 132-147.

Smith, M.L. and Fornace, A.J. Jr. (1997) p53-mediated protective responses to UV irradiation. Proc. Natl. Acad. Sci. (USA) 94, 12255-12257.

Song, Q. Z., Burrows, S. R., Smith, G., Leesmiller, S. P., Kumar, S., Chan, D. W., Trapani, J. A., Alnemri, E., Litwack, G., Lu, H., Moss, D. J., Jackson, S. and Lavin, M. F. (1996) Interleukin-1-b-converting enzyme-like protease cleaves DNA-dependent protein-kinase in cytotoxic T-cell killing. J. Exp. Med. 184, 619-626.

Song, Q., Kuang, Y., Dixit, V.M. and Vincenz, C. (1999) Boo, a novel negative regulator of cell death, interacts with Apaf-1. EMBO J. 18, 167-178.

Sparer, T.E., Tri, R.A., Dillehay, D.L., Hermiston, T.W., Wold, W.S.M. and Gooding, L.R. (1996) The role of Human adenovirus early region-3 proteins (GP19K, 10.4K, 14.5K, and 14.7K) in a murine pneumonia model. J. Virol. 70, 2431-2439.

Sparkowski, J., Mense, M., Anders, J. and Schlegel, R. (1996) E5 oncoprotein transmembrane mutants dissociate fibroblast transforming activity from 16-kilodalton protein binding and platelet-derived growth factor receptor binding and phosphorylation. J. Virol. 70, 2420-2430.

Speir, E. Modali, R., Huang, E.S., Leon, M.B., Shawl, F., Finkel, T. and Epstein, S.E. (1994) Potential role of Human Cytomegalovirus and p53 interaction in coronary restenosis. Science, 265, 391-394.

Steegenga, W.T., Riteco, N., Jochemsen, A.G., Fallaux, F.J. and Bos, J.L. (1998) The large E1B protein together with the E4orf6 protein target p53 for active degradation in adenovirus infected cells. Oncogene 16, 349-357.

Stewart, A.R., Tollefson, A.E., Krajcsi, P., Yei, S.P. and Wold, W.S.M. (1995) The Adenovirus E3 10.4K and 14.5K proteins, which function to prevent cytolysis by tumor-necrosis-factor and to down-regulate the epidermal growth-factor receptor, are localized in the plasma-membrane. J. Virol. 69, 172-181.

Stewart, S.A., Poon, B., Jowett, J.B.M. and Chen, I.S.Y. (1997) Human immunodeficiency virus type 1 Vpr induces apoptosis following cell cycle arrest. J. Virol. 71, 5579-5592.

Strack, P.R., West Frey, M., Rizzo, C.J., Cordova, B., George, H.J., Meade, R., Ho, S.P., Corman, J., Tritch, R. and Korant, B.D. (1996) Apoptosis mediated by HIV protease is preceded by cleavage of Bcl-2. Proc. Natl. Acad. Sci. (USA) 93, 1996, 9571-9576.

Strober, B.E., Dunaief, J.L., Guha, S. and Goff, S.P. (1996) Functional interactions between the hBRM/hBRG1 transcriptional activators and the pRB family of proteins. Mol. Cell. Biol. 16, 1576-1583.

Suarez, P., DiazGuerra, M., Prieto, C., Esteban, M., Castro, J.M., Nieto, A. and Ortin, J. (1996) Open reading frame 5 of porcine reproductive and respiratory syndrome virus as a cause of virus-induced apoptosis. J. Virol. 70, 2876-2882.

Subler, M.A., Martin, D.W. and Deb, S. (1994) Overlapping domains on the p53 protein regulate its transcriptional activation and repression functions. Oncogene 9, 1351-1359.

Subramanian, T., Kuppuswamy, M., Mak, S. and Chinnadurai, G. (1984) Adenovirus cyt+ locus, which controls cell transformation and tumorigenicity, is an allele of 1p+ locus, which codes for a 19-kilodalton tumor antigen. J. Virol. 52, 336-343.

Subramanian, T., Tarodi, B. and Chinnadurai, G. (1995a) p53-independent apoptotic and necrotic cell deaths induced by adenovirus infection: suppression by E1B 19K and Bcl-2 proteins. Cell Growth Diff. 6, 131-137.

Subramanian, T., Boyd, J.M. and Chinnadurai, G. (1995b) Functional substitution identifies a cell survival promoting domain common to Adenovirus E1B 19 kDa and Bcl-2 proteins. Oncogene 11, 2403-2409.

Sylwester, A., Murphy, S., Shutt, D. and Soll, R.D. (1997) HIV-induced T cell syncytia are self-perpetuating and the primary cause of T cell death in culture. J. Immunol. 158, 3996-4007.

Symonds, H., Krall, L., Remington, L., Saenz-Robles, M., Lowe, S., Jacks, T. and Van Dyke, T. (1994) p53-dependent apoptosis suppresses tumor growth and progression in vivo. Cell 78, 703-711.

Szekely, L., Selivanova, G., Magnusson, K.P., Klein, G. and Wiman, K.G. (1993) EBNA-5, an Epstein-Barr virus-encoded nuclear antigen, binds to the retinoblastoma and p53 proteins. Proc. Natl. Acad. Sci. (USA) 90, 5455-5459.

Takahashi, A., Alnemri, E. S., Lazebnik, Y. A., Fernandesalnemri, T., Litwack, G., Moir, R. D., Goldman, R. D., Poirier, G. G., Kaufmann, S. H. and Earnshaw, W. C. (1996) Cleavage of lamin-A by Mch2-alpha but not C32-multiple interlekin 1-beta-converting enzyme-related proteases with distinct substrate recognition properties are active in apoptosis, Proc. Natl. Acad. Sci. (USA) 93, 8395-8400.

Takemori, N., Riggs, J.L. and Aldrich, C. (1968) Genetic studies with tumorigenic adenoviruses. 1. Isolation of cytocidal (cyt) mutants of adenovirus type 12. Virology 36, 575-586.

Takemori, N., Riggs, J.L. and Aldrich, C. (1969) Genetic studies with tumorigenic adenoviruses II. Heterogeneity of cyt mutants of adenovirus type 12. Virology 38, 8-15.

Takemori, N., Cladaras, C., Bhat, B., Conley, A.J. and Wold, W.S.M. (1984) cyt gene of adenovirus 2 and 5 is an oncogene for transforming function in early region E1B and encodes the E1B 19,00- molecular-weight polypeptide. J. Virol. 52, 793-805.

Tanaka, S., Saito, K. and Reed, J. C. (1993) Structure-function analysis of the Bcl-2 oncoprotein - addition of a heterologous transmembrane domain to portions of the Bcl-2-beta protein restores function as a regulator of cell-survival. J. Biol. Chem., 268, 10920-10926.

Tanaka, M., Suda, T., Takahashi, T. and Nagata, S. (1995) Expression of the functional soluble form of human Fas ligand in activated lymphocytes. EMBO J. 14, 1129-1135.

Tarodi, B., Subramanian, T. and Chinnadurai, G. (1994) Epstein-Barr-virus BHRF1 protein protects against cell-death induced by DNA-damaging agents and heterologous viral-infection. Virology 201, 404-407.

Teodoro, J. G. and Branton, P. E. (1997a) Regulation of apoptosis by viral gene products. J. Virol. 71, 1739-1746.

Teodoro, J.G. and Branton, P.E. (1997b) Regulation of p53-dependent apoptosis, transcriptional repression, and cell transformation by phosphorylation of the 55-kilodalton E1B protein of human adenovirus type 5. J. Virol. 71, 3620-3627.

Teodoro, J.G., Shore, G.C. and Branton, P.E. (1995) Adenovirus E1A proteins induce apoptosis by both p53-dependent and p53-independent mechanisms. Oncogene 11, 467-474.

Terai, C., Kornbluth, R.S., Pauza, C.D., Richman, D.D. and Carson, D.A. (1990) Apoptosis as a mechanism of cell death in cultured T lymphoblasts acutely infected with HIV-1. J. Clin. Invest. 87, 1710-1715.

Tevosian, S.G. (1997) HBP1: a HMG box transcriptional repressor that is targeted by the retinoblastoma family. Genes Dev. 11, 383-396.

Theodorakis, P., D Sa Eier, C., Subramanian, T. and Chinnadurai, G. (1996) Unmasking of a proliferation-restraining activity of the anti-apoptosis protein EBV BHRF1. Oncogene 12, 1707-1713.

Thomas, M., Massini, P., Jenkins, J. and Banks, L. (1995) HPV-18 E6 mediated inhibition of p53 DNA binding activity is independent of E6-induced degradation. Oncogene 10, 261-268.

Thomas, M., Matlashewski, G., Pim, D. and Banks, L. (1996) Induction of apoptosis by p53 is independent of its oligomeric state and can be abolished by HPV-18 E6 through ubiquitin mediated degradation. Oncogene 13, 265-273.

Thomas, A. and White, E. (1998) Suppression of the p300-dependent *mdm2* negative-feeback loop induces the p53 apoptotic function. Genes Dev. 12, 1975-1985.

Thomas, J.T., Laimins, L.A. and Ruesch, M.N. (1998) Perturbation of cell cycle control by E6 and E7 oncoproteins of human papillomaviruses. Papillomavirus Rep. 9, 59-64.

Thome, M., Schneider, P., Hofmann, K., Fickenscher, H., Meinl, E., Neipel, F., Mattmann, C., Burns, K., Bodmer, J.L., Schroter, M., Scaffidi, C., Krammer, P.H., Peter, M.E. and Tscho, J. (1997) Viral FLICE-inhibitory proteins (FLIPs) prevent apoptosis induced by death receptors. Nature 386, 517-521.

Thornberry, N.A. (1997) The caspase family of cysteine proteases. Brit. Med. Bull. 53, 478-490.

Thornberry, N.A., Bull, H.G., Calaycay, J.R., Chapman, K.T., Howard, A.D., Kostura, M.J., Miller, D.K., Molineaux, S.M., Weidner, J.R., Aunins, J., Elliston, K.O., Ayala, J.M., Casano, F.J., Chin, J., Ding, G.J.F., Egger, L.A., Gaffney, E.P., Limjuco, G., Palyha, O.C., Raju, S.M., Rolando, A.M., Salley, J.P., Yamin, T.T., Lee, T.D., Shively, J.E., Maccross, M., Mumford, R.A., Schmidt, J.A. and Tocci, M.J. (1992) A novel heterodimeric cysteine protease is required for Interleukin-1-b processing in monocytes. Nature 356, 768-774.

Tollefson, A.E., Stewart, A.R., Yei, S.P., Saha, S.K. and Wold, W.S.M. (1991) The 10,400-Dalton and 14,500-Dalton proteins encoded by region-E3 of Adenovirus form a complex and function together to down-regulate the epidermal growth-factor receptor. J. Virol. 65, 3095-3105.

Tollefson, A.E., Scaria, A., Saha, S.K. and Wold, W.S.M. (1992) The 11,600-MW protein encoded by region E3 of adenovirus is expressed early but is greatly amplified at late stages of infection. J. Virol. 66, 3633-3642.

Tollefson, A.E., Scaria, A., Hermiston, T.W., Ryerse, J.S., Wold, L. and Wold, W.S.M. (1996a) The adenovirus death protein (E3-11.6K) is required at very late states of infection for efficient cell lysis and release of adenovirus from infected cells. J. Virol. 70, 2296-2306.

Tollefson, A.E., Ryerse, J.S., Scaria, A., Hermiston, T.W. and Wold, W.S.M. (1996b) The E3-11.6kDa adenovirus death is required for efficient cell death: characterizsation of cells infected with adp mutants. Virology 220, 152-162.

Tollefson, A.E., Hermiston, T.W., Lichtenstein, D.L., Colle, C.F., Tri, R.A., Dimitrov, T., Toth, K., Wells, C.E., Doherty, P.C. and Wold, W.S.M. (1998) Forced degradation of Fas inhibits apoptosis in adenovirus-infected cells. Nature 392, 726-730.

Tsujimoto, Y., Finger, L.R., Yunis, J., Nowell, P.C. and Croce, C.M. (1984) Cloning of the chromosome breakpoint of neoplastic B-cells with the T(14-18) chromosome-translocation. Science 226, 1097-1099.

Tsujimoto, Y. and Croce, C.M. (1986) Molecular-genetics of human B-cell neoplasia. Curr. Microbiol. Immunol. 132, 183-192.

Tsujimoto, Y. and Croce, C.M. (1988) Recent progress on the human Bcl-2 gene involved in follicular lymphoma - characterization of the protein products. Curr. Topics Microbiol. Immunol. 141, 337-340.

Tzeng, Y.J., Gottlob, K., Santarelli, R. and Graessmann, A. (1996) The SV40 T-antigen induces premature apoptotic mammary gland involution during late pregnancy in transgenic mice. FEBS Lett 380, 215-218.

Uren, A.G., Pakusch, M., Hawkins, C.J., Puls, K.L. and Vaux, D.L. (1996) Cloning and expression of apoptosis inhibitory protein homologues that function to inhibit apoptosis and/or bind tumor necrosis factor receptor-associated factors. Proc. Natl. Acad. Sci. (USA) 93, 4974-4978.

Vaux, D.L. and Strasser, A. (1996) The molecular biology of apoptosis. Proc. Natl. Acad. Sci. (USA) 93, 2239-2244.

Vaux, D.L., Cory, S. and Adams, J.M. (1988) Bcl-2 gene promotes hematopoietic-cell survival and cooperates with c-myc to immortalize pre-B-cells. Nature 335, 440-442.

Venot, C., Maratrat, M., Dureuil, C., Conseiller, E., Bracco, L. and Debussche, L. (1998) The requirement for the p53 proline-rich functional domain for mediation of apoptosis is correlated with specific PIG3 gene transactivation and with transcriptional repression. EMBO J. 17, 4668-4679.

Waga, S., Hannon, G.J., Beach, D. and Stillman, B. (1994) The p21 inhibitor of cyclin dependent kinases controls DNA replication by interaction with PCNA. Nature 369, 574-578.

Wagner, A.J., Kokontis, J.M. and Hay, N. (1994) MYC-mediated apoptosis requires wild type p53 in a manner independent of cell cycle arrest and the ability of p53 to induce $p21^{waf1/cip1}$. Genes Dev. 8, 2817-2830.

Walker, K.K. and Levine, A.J. (1996) Identification of a novel p53 functional domain which is necessary for efficient growth suppression. Proc. Natl. Acad. Sci. (USA) 93, 15335-15340.

Wang, H. G., Miyashita, T., Takayama, S., Sato, T., Torigoe, T., Krajewski, S., Tanaka, S., Hovey, L., Tromair, J., Ra, U. R. and Reed, J. C. (1994) Apoptosis regulation by interaction of Bcl-2 protein and raf-1 kinase. Oncogene 9, 2751-2756.

Wang, J.Y.J., Knudsen, E.S. and Welch, P.J. (1994) The retinoblastoma tumour suppressor protein. Adv. Can. Res. 64, 25-85.

Wang, Y. and Eckhart, W. (1992) Phosphorylation sites in the amino-terminal region of mouse p53. Proc. Natl. Acad. Sci. (USA) 89, 4231-4235.

Watanabe-Fukunaga, R., Brannan, C. I., Copeland, N. G., Jenkins, N. A. and Nagata, S. (1992) Lymphoproliferation disorder in mice explained by defects in Fas antigen that mediates apoptosis. Nature 356, 314-317.

Weinberg, R.A. (1995) The retinoblastoma protein and cell cycle control. Cell 81, 323-330.

Weintraub, S.J., Prater, C.A. and Dean, D. (1992) Retinoblastoma protein switches the E2F site from a positive to a negative element. Nature 358, 259-261.

Werness, B.A., Levine, A.J. and Howley, P.M. (1990) Association of human papillomavirus types 16 and 18 E6 proteins with p53. Science 248, 76-79.

Westendorp, M.O., Frank, R., Ochsenbauer, C., Stricker, K., Dhein, J., Walczak, H., Debatin, K.-M. and Krammer, P.H. (1995) Sensitization of T cells to CD95-mediated apoptosis by HIV-1 Tat and gp120. Nature 375, 497-500.

Whalen, S.G., Marcellus, R.C., Whalen, A., Ahn, N.G., Riccardia, R.P. and Branton, P.E. (1997) Phosphorylation within the transactivation domain adenovirus E1A protein by mitogen-activated protein kinase regulates expression of early region 4. J. Virol. 71, 3545-3553.

White. E. (1994) p53, guardian of Rb. Nature 371, 2122.

White. E. (1996) Life, death, and the pursuit of apoptosis. Genes Dev. 10, 1-15.

White, E. and Cipriani, R., Sabbatini, P. and Denton, A. (1991) Adenovirus-E1B 19-kilodalton protein overcomes the cytotoxicity of E1A proteins. J. Virol. 65, 2968-2978.

White, E., Grodzicker, T. and Stillman, B.W. (1984) Mutations in the adenovirus early region 1B 19,000-molecular weight tumor antigen cause the degradation of chromosomal DNA. J. Virol. 52, 410-419.

White, E. and Stillman, B. (1987) Expression of adenovirus-E1B mutant phenotypes is dependent on the host-cell and on synthesis of E1A protines. J. Virol. 61, 426-435.

Whyte, P., Buchkovich, K.J., Horowitz, J.M., Friend, S.H., Raybuck, M., Weinberg, R.A. and Harlow, E. (1988) Association between an oncogene and an anti-oncogene: the adenovirus E1A proteins bind to the retinoblastoma gene product. Nature 334, 124-129.

Whyte, P., Williamson, N.M. and Harlow, E. (1989) Cellular targets for transformation by the adenovirus E1A proteins. Cell 56, 67-75.

Willingham, MC. and Bhalla, K. (1994) Transient mitotic phase localization of Bcl-2 oncoprotein in human carcinoma-cells and its possible role in prevention of apoptosis J. Histochem. Cytochem.42, 441-450.

Wissing, D., Mouritzen, H., Egeblad, M., Poirier, G.G. and Jaattela, M. (1997) Involvement of caspase-dependent activation of cytosolic phospholipase A(2) in tumor necrosis factor-induced apoptosis. Proc. Natl. Acad. Sci. (USA) 94, 5073-5077.

Wold, W.S.M. and Tollefson, A.E. (1998) Adenovirus E3 proteins : 14.7K, RID, and gp19K inhibit immune-induced cell death, adenovirus death protein promotes cell death. Sems. in Virol. 8, 515-523.

Wu, X. and Levine, A.J. (1994) P53 and E2F-1 cooperate to mediate apoptosis. Proc. Natl. Acad. Sci. (USA) 91, 3602-3606.

Wu, X., Bayle, J.H., Olson, D. and Levine, A.J. (1993) The p53-MDM2 autoregulatory feedback loop. Genes Dev. 7, 1126-1132.

Xiong, Y., Hannon, G.J., Zhang, H., Casso, D., Kobayashi, R. and Beach, D. (1993) p21 is a universal inhibitor of cyclin kinases. Nature 366, 701-704.

Xue, D. and Horvitz, H.R. (1997) Caenorhabditis elegans CED-9 protein is a bifunctional cell-death inhibitor. Nature 390, 305-308.

Yamasaki, L., Jacks, T., Bronson, R., Goillot, E., Harlow, E. and Dyson, N.J. (1996) Tumor induction and tissue atrophy in mice lacking E2F-1. Cell 85, 537-548.

Yang, E. and Korsmeyer, S.J. (1996) Molecular thanatopsis: A discourse on the BCL2 family and cell death. Blood 88, 386-401.

Yew, P.R. and Berk, A.J. (1992) Inhibition of p53 transactivation required for transformation by adenovirus early 1B protein. Nature 357, 82-85.

Yew, P.R., Liu, X. and Berk, A.J. (1994) Adenovirus E1B oncoprotein tethers a transcriptional repression domain to p53. Genes Dev. 8, 190-202.

Yin, X.M., Oltvai, Z.N. and Korsmeyer, S.J. (1994) BH1 and BH2 domains of Bcl-2 are required for inhibition of apoptosis and heterodimerization with Bax. Nature 369, 321-323.

Yonish-Rouach, E., Resnitzky, D., Lotem, J., Sachs, L., Kimchi, A. and Oren, M. (1991) Wildtype p53 induces apoptosis of myeloid leukaemia cells that is inhibited by interleukin-6. Nature 352, 345-347.

Young, L.S., Dawson, C.W. and Eliopoulos, A.G. (1997) Viruses and apoptosis. Brit. Med. Bull. 53, 509-521.

Zackesenhaus, E., Bremner, R., Jiang, Z., Gill, R.M., Muncaster, M., Sopta, M., Phillips, R.A. and Gallie, B.L. (1993) Unravelling the function of the retinoblastoma gene. Adv. Can. Res. 61, 115-141.

Zehava, C.L. and Cleary, M.L. (1990) Membrane topology of the Bcl-2 protooncogenic protein demonstrated invitro. J. Biol Chem..265, 4929-4933.

Zha, J.P., Harada, H., Yang, E., Jockel, J. and Korsmeyer, S.J. (1996) Serine phosphorylation of death agonist BAD in response to survival factor results in binding to 14-3-3 not Bgl-X(L). Cell 87, 619-628.

Zhang, H.C., Saeed, B. and Ng, S.C. (1995) Combinatorial interaction of human Bcl-2 related proteins - maing of regions important for Bcl-2/Bcl-XS interaction. Biochem. Biophys. Res. Comms. 208, 950-956.

Zhang, Y., Xiong, Y. and Yarbrough, W.G. (1998) ARF promotes MDM2 degradation and stabilizes p53: ARF-INK4a locus deletion impairs both the Rb and p53 tumour suppressor pathways. Cell 92, 725-734.

Zhu, H., Shen,Y.Q. and Shenk, T. (1995) Human Cytomegalovirus IE1 and IE2 proteins block apoptosis. J. Virol. 69, 7960-7970.

Zindy, F., Eischen, C.M., Randle, D., Kamijo, T., Cleveland, J.L., Sherr, C.J. and Roussel, M.F. Myc signalling via the ARF tumor suppressor regulates p53-dependent apoptosis and immortalization. Genes Dev. 12, 2424-2433.

Zoratti, M. and Szabo, I. (1995) The mitochondrial permeability transition. Biochim. Biophys. Acta - reviews on biomembranes 1241, 139-176.

Zou, H., Henzel, W.J., Liu, X.S., Lutschg, A. and Wang, X.D. (1997) Apaf-1, a human protein homologous to *C.elegans* CED-4, participates in cytochrome c-dependent activation of caspase-3. Cell 90, 405-413.

EVASION OF THE IMMUNE SYSTEM BY TUMOR VIRUSES

Nicola Philpott and G. Eric Blair

School of Biochemistry and Molecular Biology, University of Leeds

Introduction

Virally-induced tumors usually contain integrated viral or, in the case of retroviruses, proviral DNA in their cellular genomes and normally express viral proteins. Such proteins can be processed and complexes of processed viral peptides with MHC class I molecules may be expressed on the surface of tumor cells. Thus, tumor cells expressing viral proteins can stimulate and/or become the targets of specific T cell immune responses, as well as being susceptible to eradication by natural killer cells and lymphokine-activated killer cells. This virus-specific immunity is crucial in prevention of the outgrowth of viral-associated tumors. As a consequence, viruses are under evolutionary pressure within this hostile environment with their survival dependent on evasion of the host immune system. A variety of strategies have been developed by these pathogens to avoid immune recognition by inhibiting the presentation of antigens on the surface of infected cells. Therefore, before describing such mechanisms, the MHC class I antigen-presentation pathway will be outlined below.

The MHC class I antigen presentation pathway

Most nucleated cells express both cellular and foreign antigens on their surface. Cytotoxic T lymphocytes are able to distinguish between self and non-self antigens via a process known as immunosurveillance and hence only kill infected or aberrant cells. Antigens are presented to CTLs as peptides bound to MHC class I molecules and the pathway by which the peptides and MHC class I molecules become associated is discussed below.

Host and foreign proteins are degraded into peptides in the cell cytosol via the ubiquitin/proteasome system. The antigens are ubiquitinated (Chen and Hochstrasser, 1995; Deveraux et al., 1994) and then the multisubunit, 26S proteasome degrades the proteins within its core, in an ATP-dependent manner (Driscoll and Goldberg, 1990). Upon induction by interferon-γ, the low molecular weight proteins (LMP), LMP2 and LMP7 displace homologous subunits on the 26S proteasome (Fruh et al., 1994; Belich et al., 1994; Akiyama et al., 1994). Following degradation, peptides are translocated into the endoplasmic reticulum (ER) via transporter-associated with antigen processing (TAP) proteins. TAP1 and TAP2 exist as a heterodimer that pumps peptides across the ER membrane (Levy et al., 1991). The initial binding of peptides to TAP proteins does not require ATP (Androlewicz et al., 1994; Van Endert et al., 1994). Meanwhile, also in the ER, β-microglobulin subunits are bound to newly-synthesized MHC class I heavy

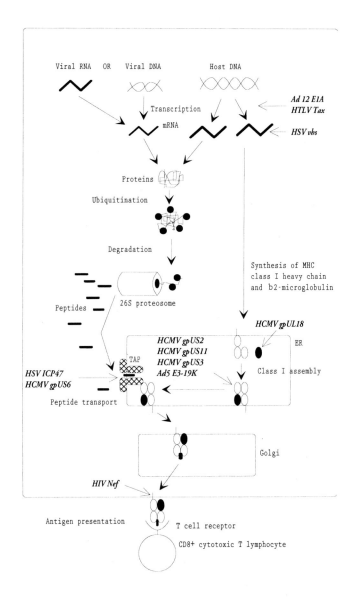

Figure 1 MHC class I antigen presentation pathway. Viral and host DNA is transcribed and mRNA is translated to produce cellular and viral polypeptides. Following the ubiquitination of both self and foreign proteins the ubiquitin is removed by the 26S proteasome. Proteins are degraded in the core of the 26S proteasome and then translocated across the ER membrane by TAP proteins which are associated with newly synthesised MHC class I molecules. Peptides bind the MHC class I molecule which is then transported to the cell membrane via the Golgi network. Antigenic peptides are presented to CTLs on the surface of the cell. Viral proteins that interfere with the antigen processing pathway are shown in italics.

chains. TAP proteins associate with these empty MHC class I molecules on the luminal side of the ER membrane. The appropriate peptide is loaded onto the MHC class I molecule and this causes the release of the MHC class I-peptide complex from its interaction with the TAP proteins (Suh et al., 1994; Ortmann et al., 1994). The heterotrimeric molecule is then transported through the Golgi network to the cell surface (Figure 1).

Immune Evasion by Viruses

There are many different mechanisms by which tumor viruses, such as herpesviruses, retroviruses, papovaviruses and adenoviruses escape immune surveillance and these mechanisms are discussed in more detail below. The mechanisms of immune evasion exhibited by the pox virus, vaccinia, will also be discussed. Despite the fact that vaccinia virus has not been shown to be tumorigenic, the variety of pathways that it utilises in order to avoid immune recognition have been well documented.

Poxviruses

VACCINIA VIRUS

Vaccinia virus, as well as other pox viruses, is capable of expressing a range of proteins which assist the virus in evading the host immune response. These include proteins which inhibit apoptosis, counteract interleukins, oppose chemokines, suppress interferons, interfere with complement and activate steroid synthesis.

Following viral replication within the host cell, the intracellular mature virus (IMV) becomes wrapped in membranes and as intracellular enveloped virus (IEV) it moves towards the cell surface. The IEV then fuses with the plasma membrane and is exuded from the cell as extracellular enveloped virus (EEV). Some EEV particles remain on the cell membrane and are targeted by antibodies of the host humoral immune response. The antibodies block virion release by sequestering the EEV particles on the cell surface (Vanderplasschen et al., 1997) and the virus simulataneously escapes antibody-induced neutralisation.

The cell-mediated immune response occurs when viral peptides associating with MHC class I molecules are presented on the cell surface and recognised by cytotoxic T lymphocytes. The CTLs are then capable of eradicating target cells by one of the following pathways. Firstly, the CTLs produce cytotoxic granules containing perforin and granzymes. The perforin creates pores in the cell membrane, and granzymes then enter the target cells through the pores and induce apoptosis. The second mechanism by which CTLs induce cell death is via the interaction between Fas and Fas ligand to promote apoptosis directly. Both systems require the activity of either interleukin-1β-converting enzyme (ICE) or related cysteine proteases (caspases).

Inhibiting apoptosis

In an attempt to evade this CTL-induced cell killing, vaccinia virus expresses serine protease inhibitors (serpins) which inhibit caspases including ICE. Serpins function as inhibitors of serine proteinases by forming equimolar stable protein complexes. However, it is thought that these serpins do not contribute to reduced antigen presentation or inhibition of target cell killing by CTLs *in vitro* (Smith et al., 1997). Vaccinia virus also induces subtle changes in antigen expression to CTLs (Coupar et al., 1986), by a mechanism which is not fully understood.

The serpin SPI-2 of vaccinia virus is a potent inhibitor of ICE both *in vitro* and *in vivo* and hence blocks ICE-mediated apoptosis (Komiyama et al., 1994; Miura et al., 1993). It has also been suggested that SPI-2 prevents apoptosis by interfering with the binding of anti-Fas antibodies or the function of tumor necrosis factor (Enari et al., 1995; Los et al.,1995; Tewari and Dixit, 1995; Heinkelein et al., 1996; Dobbelstein and Shenk, 1996; Kettle et al., 1997). In addition, there is evidence to indicate that SPI-2 inhibits other cysteine proteinases such as caspase 8 (Muzio et al., 1997). Furthermore, SPI-2 has been shown to block DNA degradation mediated by CTLs and also binds and inhibits the serine proteinase granzyme B which is involved in this DNA fragmentation (Tewari et al., 1995; Quan et al., 1995). Another serpin, SPI-1, is also thought to inhibit apoptosis by blocking DNA fragmentation, either on its own (Ali et al., 1994; Brooks et al., 1995) or in conjunction with SPI-2 (Macen et al., 1996). Finally, Vaccinia virus prevents apoptosis via a family of viral proteins known as vFLIPS (viral FLICE [FADD (Fas-associated death domain-containing protein)-like interleukin-1 beta-converting enzyme]-inhibitory proteins). These proteins bind Fas and TNF cell surface receptors (reviewed in McFadden and Barry, 1998) and hence prevent the binding of natural ligands inhibiting cell death.

Counteracting cytokines

The cytokines are a family of messenger proteins that have important functions in both natural and specific immunity to infection. However, their activation must be tightly regulated in order to prevent disease. Vaccinia virus has evolved mechanisms to interfere with the immune responses which are mediated by both interleukin-1β (IL-1β) and tumor necrosis factor (TNF).

There are two mechanisms by which poxviruses inhibit the normal activity of IL-1β. Firstly, the viral intracellular protein SPI-2 prevents conversion of the IL-1β precursor into mature IL-1β, via inhibition of caspase 1 (Ray et al., 1992; Kettle et al., 1997), although it should be noted that very few strains of vaccinia virus express SPI-2. The second, more effective way of inhibiting IL-1β, is by the secretion of a soluble IL-1β receptor (IL-1βR) which is expressed in the majority of vaccinia virus strains (Spriggs et al., 1992; Alcami and Smith, 1992). Viral IL-1βR has a higher affinity for human IL-1β and is more abundant than cellular IL-1βR. Hence the viral receptor prevents IL-1β associating with cellular IL-1R and suppresses its activity *in vitro*. Furthermore, it has been recently reported that viral IL-1βR inhibits the febrile response. This occurs via the viral receptor controlling host temperature through its interaction with the endogenous pyrogen IL-1β (Alcami and Smith, 1996).

Some strains of vaccinia virus also express a TNF receptor (TNFR), which is either cell surface bound or secreted from the host. By binding TNF, the TNFR could potentially inhibit the normal function of TNF (Smith et al. 1997; McFadden and Barry, 1998).

Chemokines are soluble cytokines that mediate their effects through specific G protein-coupled receptors which are expressed on cells of the immune system (Alcami et al., 1998a). There are four different groups of chemokine, based on the number and arrangement of their conserved cysteine residues: CC chemokines, for example RANTES and macrophage inflammatory protein (MIP)-1α; CXC chemokines such as IL-8; the C chemokine lymphotactin; and CX_3C chemokine neurotactin. All chemokines function by attracting leukocytes to regions of inflammation and are inhibited by pox viruses and herpesviruses by several different mechanisms. Viral pathogens such as the β-herpesvirus, human cytomegalovirus, often encode their own versions of chemokines or chemokine receptors, and these are important components of the immune evasion phenomenon (see below). Vaccinia viruses, however, appear only to alter the function of CC chemokines (Alcami et al., 1998b). This occurs due to the expression of a soluble 35 kDa viral protein known as vCKBP (viral chemokine-binding protein), which acts as a chemokine receptor by binding and consequently inhibiting chemokine activity. Graham et al. (1997) reported that vCKBP of vaccinia virus binds the chemokines RANTES and IL-8 (despite the fact that IL-8 is a CXC chemokine). vCKBP also binds macrophage inflammatory protein-1α (MIP-1α), a CC chemokine (Alcami et al., 1998a).

Interferons (IFN) play a central role in the host immune response. There are three classes of IFN, denoted IFN-α, -β and -γ. IFN-α and IFN-β (type I IFN) have four principal functions: inhibition of viral replication, inhibition of cell proliferation, increasing the lytic potential of NK cells and the modulation of MHC molecule expression. The functions of IFN-γ (type II IFN) include activation of macrophages, neutrophils and NK cells, increasing MHC molecule expression, promoting cell differentiation and activation of vascular endothelial cells.

IFN-γ released by B lymphocytes triggers the expression of the protein kinase, PKR and 2′,5′oligoadenylate synthetase by the host cell. These two cellular enzymes are activated by binding double-stranded (ds) RNA, which is often produced during virus infection. Upon activation, both cellular enzymes contribute to the inhibition of protein synthesis and hence prevent virus replication (Figure 2). Pox viruses have evolved ways of interfering with these defence mechanisms, as described below (reviewed in Smith et al., 1998).

Vaccinia virus expresses two proteins known as E3L and K3L, both of which neutralise the cellular response to IFN release. The 25 kDa, E3L protein functions by binding ds RNA so that the cellular proteins are unable to interact with it and, as a result, activation of both PKR (Lee and Esteban, 1994) and 2′-5′oligoadenylate synthetase is inhibited. The 10.5 kDa protein, K3L interferes with the host cell response to IFN by blocking phosphorylation of eukaryotic translation initiation factor 2α

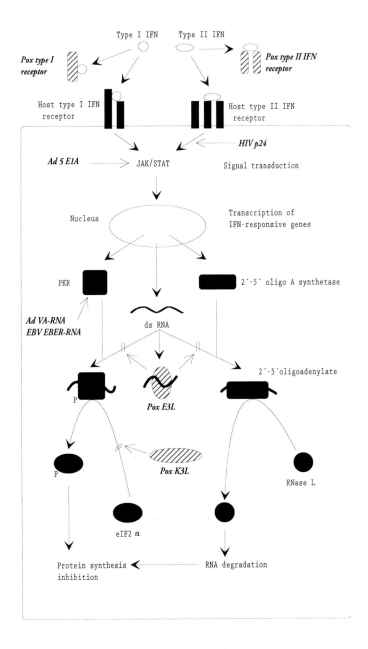

Figure 2. Inhibition of interferon activity in virally-infected cells. Viral proteins that block the cellular responses to interferon, such as pox virus proteins E3L and K3L, are shown in italics. IFN = interferon; JAK = protein tyrosine kinases; STAT = signal transducers and activators of transcription; PKR = dsRNA-dependent protein kinase; eIF2α = eukaryotic initiation factor 2α.

(eIF2α) by PKR. Protein synthesis is therefore sustained, due to the lack of eIF2α phosphorylation.

Vaccinia virus also expresses two extracellular, secreted glycoproteins that inhibit the IFN response. They both function as IFN receptors (IFNR), the first by binding IFN-γ and the second by associating with either IFN-α or IFN-β. The 43 kDa, viral IFN-γR interacts with IFN-γ and therefore prevents it associating with the host IFN-γR on the cell surface. Ultimately, this hinders the antiviral activity of IFN-γ (Alcami and Smith, 1995). The viral IFN-α/βR interacts with both IFN-α and IFN-β with very high affinity and hence blocks their binding to their cellular receptors (Symons et al., 1995). As well as signal transduction being inhibited, the phosphorylation of JAK kinases is prevented (Colamonici et al., 1995), and this leads to reduced transcription of IFN-responsive genes, such as PKR.

Suppressing complement

In order to counteract the complement system which creates immunity to both microorganisms and viruses, the vaccinia virus secretes the vaccinia complement control protein (VCP) (Isaacs and Moss, 1994). VCP associates with complement proteins C3b and C4b and as a consequence blocks activation of the complement cascade by both classical and alternative pathways (Kotwal et al., 1990; Isaacs et al., 1992; McKenzie et al., 1992). VCP is an important virulence factor which blocks both complement and antibody-induced neutralisation of virus.

In addition, vaccinia virus expresses a protein from the B5R gene, which contributes to evasion of the complement system. The B5R protein is a member of the regulation of complement activation (RCA) superfamily. It is expressed on the outer envelope of the virus and has been shown to be essential for viral virulence (Engelstad and Smith, 1993; Wolffe et al., 1993). However, its mechanism of action is not fully understood.

Activating steroid synthesis

Finally, vaccinia virus expresses a protein with sequence similarity to the cellular 3β-hydroxysteroid dehydrogenase enzyme (Goebel et al., 1990; Smith et al., 1991; Blasco et al., 1991). It has been suggested that the function of this viral enzyme is to catalyse the synthesis of immunosuppressive glucocorticoids (Cupps and Fauci, 1982) and hence contribute to viral immune evasion.

Immune Evasion by Tumor Viruses

Herpesviruses

The survival and propagation of herpesviruses depends on their ability to evade the host immune system. There are several features of this immune evasion: the virus must first be able to infect the host and establish residence with minimal effect; secondly, it must establish latent or persistent infection and maintain an intact viral genome in the host for decades; finally, it has to become reactivated and enter the reproductive cycle to produce sufficient virus progeny for the infection of new hosts.

A general mechanism by which herpesviruses avoid immune clearance is that of latency, the ability of the virus genomes to persist within host cells. During latency a very restricted subset of virus genes are expressed, thereby minimizing the potential for immune recognition of foreign antigens. However, latent viral infection usually occurs at a different site to the primary infection and this is discussed in more detail later.

There are three types of herpesvirus, the α-, β- and γ-herpesviruses. In this Chapter the immune evasion strategies utilized by α-herpesviruses, β-herpesviruses and γ-herpesviruses have been discussed, exemplified by Herpes Simplex virus, Human Cytomegalovirus and Epstein Barr virus (Chapter 8), respectively.

At present, only γ-herpesviruses have been associated with tumors. Human herpesvirus-8 (HHV-8), for example infects lymphocytes and is the etiologic agent of Kaposi's sarcoma of AIDS patients (see Chapters 9 and 10). For this reason it is also known as Kaposi's sarcoma-associated herpesvirus (KSHV). In addition HHV-8 has been associated with some B cell lymphomas and the lymphoproliferative disorder, multicentric Castleman's disease.

A) HERPES SIMPLEX VIRUSES

Herpes Simplex viruses (HSVs) are neurotropic α-herpesviruses that induce the primary infection of human mucosal epithelium. Despite the fact that strong humoral immune responses are exerted in order to combat HSV infection, most of the evidence appears to suggest that cellular immunity is more important (Schmid and Rousse, 1992; York and Johnson, 1994). Antibodies effectively neutralize primary HSV infection but because the virions spread quickly and efficiently between cells, and because there are no targets for antibodies during latency, this method of immune response becomes very ineffective. After the primary humoral response to HSV infection by antibodies, macrophages and natural killer cells limit the viral spread, while the specific immune responses develop (Domke-Optiz and Swatzkym, 1990). The specific immunity exerted by CD8+ and CD4+ T lymphocytes, are essential for clearance of both primary and recurring HSV infection (Martin et al., 1987; Nash et al., 1987).

During primary infection of mucosa, sensory ganglia become invaded by HSV and latency is established. Very little viral protein synthesis occurs during latency and neurones express few MHC class I molecules, protecting cells from the cellular immune system.

One of the first defence mechanisms used by the immune system to combat viral infection is the complement cascade. Activation of the complement system may occur via two pathways; either through binding of the complement factor C1 to the Fc domain of immunoglobulins or to a foreign surface in the absence of antibody. The enzyme C3 convertase is synthesised during both pathways. C3 convertase production leads to the deposition of complement factor C3b on the cell surface causing the subsequent assembly of the membrane attack complex (MAC) and cell lysis.

HSV-1, among other α-herpesviruses, has been shown to express a protein, known as glycoprotein C (gC). gC binds complement factor C3 fragments and could therefore potentially act as their receptor (Seidel-Dugan et al., 1990; Cines et al., 1982). As a consequence of these cell surface receptors sequestering complement factor fragments, HSV-infected cells are unaffected by complement-mediated neutralization (McNearney et al., 1987; Hidaka et al., 1991). However, to date, there is no evidence to suggest that this occurs *in vivo*. Similarly, HSV-1 glycoproteins E and I (gE and gI, respectively) bind the Fc domains of both monomeric and antigen-associated IgG molecules (Johnson and Feenstra, 1987; Johnson et al., 1988). The expression of Fc receptors on HSV-infected cells has been shown to protect the cells *in vitro* against both antibody and complement. However, again there is no evidence for this *in vivo* (Frank and Friedman 1989; Dubin et al. 1991; York and Johnson; 1994).

Early in HSV-infection, cells are sensitive to lysis by natural killer (NK) cells. However, at later stages of infection cells become resistant to both NK and lymphokine-activated killer (LAK) cells (Fitzgerald-Bocarsly et al., 1989; Confer et al., 1990). This is thought to be due to the fact that both NK and T lymphocytes have to be in close proximity to an infected cell in order to eradicate it. However, in so doing the NK and lymphocytes become vulnerable to infection by HSV due to the ease with which HSV spreads between cells (York and Johnson, 1993). Once infected by HSV, the immunocyte becomes inactivated, probably via structural or early proteins of the virus.

The CD8+ CTL frequency is often low in individuals infected by HSV. A possible reason for this could be the cessation of class I antigen presentation soon after HSV-infection (Tigges et al., 1992; Koelle et al., 1993). The viral component known as virion host shutoff (vhs) protein is responsible for the rapid degradation of host mRNA. The vhs protein of HSV-2 is much more active than its HSV-1 equivalent and hence MHC class I molecule biosynthesis is inhibited even more rapidly in HSV-2- than in HSV-1-infected cells (Fenwick and Everett, 1990; Hill et al., 1994; Tigges et al., 1996). Despite this, vhs protein cannot account for the total inhibition of antigen presentation, particularly at early stages of infection. Consequently, other HSV proteins must also be responsible for the observed reduction in MHC class I presentation (York et al., 1994).

A more plausible explanation for the reduction in MHC class I presentation on the cell surface of HSV-infected cells is that MHC class I molecules are sequestered in the endoplasmic reticulum or *cis*-Golgi compartment (Hill et al., 1994; York et al., 1994). The 88 amino acid, viral immediate-early protein, ICP47 is responsible for this retention. It functions by interacting with the peptide-binding site of the transporter associated with antigen presentation (TAP) protein and thereby blocks peptide binding to TAP (Tomazin et al., 1996). Consequently, this inhibits TAP-mediated peptide translocation across the ER membrane (Fruh et al., 1995; Hill et al., 1995). ICP47 is among the first HSV proteins to be expressed and, because it binds with such high affinity to TAP and with a slow dissociation rate, the vast majority of the 75 HSV polypeptides escape presentation (York et al., 1994). It should be noted that the mechanisms by which ICP47 inhibits TAP-mediated translocation of peptides, were observed in human cell lines whilst peptide presentation in mouse fibroblasts was inhibited by HSV ICP47 to a lesser extent (Tomazin et al., 1996).

In addition, HSV-1 is able to prevent the inhibition of protein synthesis that is mediated by interferons (Figure 2). He et al. (1997) proposed a mechanism which involves the viral protein, $\gamma_1 34.5$, binding human protein phosphatase 1α. This interaction is thought to redirect the activity of the phosphatase to dephosphorylate eIF2α either by itself or in conjunction with other cellular proteins. Hence, although the double-stranded RNA-dependent protein kinase, PKR is activated, protein synthesis is not inhibited.

A major factor which causes the virus to remain undetected by the immune system is the fact that HSV proteins are not expressed within neuronal cells during latency. Hence there is minimal antigen production and very low presentation of viral peptides at the cell surface.

B) HUMAN CYTOMEGALOVIRUS

β-herpesviruses such as human cytomegalovirus (HCMV) also adopt immune evasion strategies (Davis-Poynter and Farrell, 1998; Dairaghi et al., 1998), however, their oncogenic potential in humans remains uncertain. Since HCMV only has putative oncogenicity in humans and rarely induces symptoms of disease in the immunocompetent host, it remains debatable as to whether HCMV is a human tumor virus or is simply a passenger in human tumor cells (Alford and Britt, 1993; Radsak et al., 1998).

HCMV, like its murine counterpart (MCMV), is capable of down-regulating expression of MHC class I molecules (Del Val et al., 1989; Del Val et al., 1992; Beersma et al., 1993; Warren et al., 1994). The consequent inhibition of antigen presentation is caused by a variety of CMV proteins interfering with every step of the MHC class I/peptide presentation pathway. The mechanism of each is outlined below.

Gilbert et al. (1996) reported that the viral protein pp65 is able specifically to block the presentation of peptides derived from the immediate early viral protein, IE-1. The pp65 protein inhibits IE-1 presentation from early stages of infection, by phosphorylating threonine residues in the IE-1 protein. This phosphorylation is thought to occur prior to the peptides' interaction with MHC class I molecules.

HCMV has been shown to block the passage of peptides across the ER membrane via TAP proteins. It is thought that the product of the viral US6 gene (gpUS6) is responsible for this inhibition (Hengel et al., 1997; Ahn et al., 1997). The gpUS6 glycoprotein interacts with a TAP 1 and 2, MHC class I, tapasin, calreticulin complex which is involved in peptide loading of the MHC class I molecule (Sadasivan et al., 1996). As a consequence, peptides are able to bind TAP but are prevented from moving into the ER lumen.

The two viral glycoproteins gpUS2 and gpUS11 are both independently capable of reducing the stability of the MHC class I molecule, by inducing its degradation (Jones et al., 1995; Wiertz et al., 1996a and 1996b). This degradation is thought to occur in the proteasome. The gpUS11 glycoprotein is localised in the ER and functions by extruding newly synthesised, glycosylated MHC class I molecules into the cytosol, where they are deglycosylated by N-glycanase and then degraded by the proteasome. The gpUS2 protein induces a similar translocation function via the Sec61 pore complex, which is usually involved in the movement of proteins into the ER. This retrograde translocation causes the premature dislocation of MHC class I heavy chains into the cell cytoplasm (Rapoport et al., 1996). Like the MHC class I molecule, gpUS2 is subjected to deglycosylation followed by proteasomal degradation.

The viral glycoprotein gpUS3 has been shown to bind and simultaneously mediate the retention of MHC class I in the ER lumen of the infected cell (Ahn et al., 1996; Jones et al., 1996). In addition, it has been proposed that gpUS3 contributes to more efficient degradation of MHC class I molecules which is mediated by gpUS2 and gpUS11 (Ahn et al., 1996).

HCMV expresses an MHC class I-like glycoprotein known as gpUL18 which is capable of associating with endogenous β2-microglobulin (β2-m) (Browne et al., 1990). It therefore replaces the down-regulated cellular MHC class I molecules in expressing β2-m on the surface of infected cells. This action means that the cell avoids attack from NK cells which usually target cells that express low levels of MHC class I molecules (Reyburn et al., 1997). As well as interacting with peptides (Fahnestock et al., 1995), gpUL18 is also able to bind a receptor on the surface of NK cells and thereby mimic the presence of MHC class I complexes (Phillips et al., 1996; Sivori et al., 1996; Cosman et al., 1997).

As well as interfering with the peptide presentation pathway, HCMV expresses its own versions of host chemokines and chemokine receptors. Of particular interest are the putative G protein-coupled receptors (GCRs) that it expresses. The viral GCR, expressed from the US28 ORF has been shown to bind CC chemokines such as RANTES, MCP-1 and MIP-1α (Neote et al., 1993; Gao and Murphy 1994; Schall et al., 1994). US28 binds the ligands with a higher affinity than cellular GCRs. The protein product of the HCMV UL33 ORF is another potential GCR since it has high sequence similarity to cellular receptors. However, the particular chemokines to which it binds are unknown (Margulies et al., 1996). The US27 ORF shows sequence similarity to US28 and the cellular fMLP (fMet-Leu-Phe) receptor, but despite this, the function of US27 is unclear.

C) EPSTEIN BARR VIRUS

Epstein Barr Virus (EBV) is a γ-herpesvirus which productively infects stratified epithelium in the nasopharynx and establishes latency within B lymphocytes (Kieff, 1996 and chapter 8 in this book). Its genome and gene products have been detected in a variety of human tumor cells. EBV has been associated with human cancers such as Burkitt's lymphoma (BL), nasopharyngeal carcinoma (NPC), and Hodgkin's disease (HD), as well as post-transplant proliferative disorders (PTLD), pleiomorphic T cell lymphomas, gastric adenocarcinomas and smooth muscle cell tumors in AIDS patients (reviewed in Niedobitek et al., 1997).

Although EBV infection is highly immunostimulatory, the host immune system never completely eliminates the virus. Early in EBV infection expression of IgG and IgM antibodies is activated as part of the humoral immune response (Khanna et al., 1995). This is followed later by anti-EBV cellular responses such as T lymphocyte activation which maintains or restricts latently infected B cells (Thorley-Lawson et al., 1977;

Thorley-Lawson, 1980). Hence both CD8+ and CD4+ cytotoxic T lymphocytes (CTLs) play a central role in controlling the spread of EBV. Disturbances in EBV-specific immunity at different levels may contribute to the development of EBV-associated tumors.

There are at least three ways in which EBV-positive BL tumors escape immunosurveillance by CTLs. Firstly, restricted latent viral gene expression; secondly, reduced expression of MHC class I molecules; thirdly, down-regulation of adhesion molecules. All three features are discussed below.

It has been hypothesised that viral persistence occurs due to non-dividing, latently infected cells being resistant to the potent immune response. The CTL response particularly, would be stimulated by EBV-infected B cells that are released from this latent reservoir (Rowe and Masucci, 1995).

Latent EBV-infected cells express at least six virus-encoded nuclear antigens, EBNA-1 to 6, three latent membrane proteins, LMP 1, 2A and 2B, and two untranslated mRNAs, EBER-1 and -2. EBER RNAs bear similarity to the virus-associated RNA molecules of adenoviruses. EBER-1 is able to bind the cellular protein kinase PKR and inhibit its function and as a consequence the cell is unable to block viral protein synthesis (Figure 2) (Elia et al., 1996).

In Burkitt's lymphoma (BL) cells the EBV nuclear antigen-1 (EBNA-1) is the only viral protein expressed and clearly this reduces the efficiency of immune surveillance by CTLs (Sample et al., 1991; Marchini et al., 1992). The main function of EBNA-1 is to maintain the EBV episome, through interaction with the origin of replication of the EBV genome (Yates et al., 1984).

The EBNA-1 phosphoprotein fails to undergo processing and antigen presentation, due to the presence of a Gly-Ala repeat region situated between its N- and C-terminal domains (Levitskaya et al., 1995). The Gly-Ala region acts in *cis* to prevent presentation by MHC class I molecules. Proteins containing the Gly-Ala sequence have been shown to be more resistant to proteasome-mediated degradation than proteins without the Gly-Ala repeat (Sharipo et al., 1998). It appears that after ubiquitination Gly-Ala - containing proteins are unable to form stable complexes with the proteasome. One possible reason for this is that the Gly-Ala sequence forms stable β-sheet structures that are resistant to unfolding. Hence entry to the proteasome would be blocked because substrates have to be unfolded in order to gain access to enzymatic sites in the catalytic core of the proteasome. Alternatively, the Gly-Ala repeat may interfere with the targetting of the protein to the proteasome either by directly masking a substrate-specific binding site or by altering the activity of molecular chaperones involved in the unfolding process (Sharipo et al., 1998).

The immune escape of BL cells also includes the down-regulation of MHC class I molecules as well as other components of the antigen processing pathway. Reduced expression of several HLA class I molecules, in particular HLA-A11 antigen, have been found to occur at the level of transcription (Rooney et al., 1985; 1986; Torsteinsdottir et al., 1986; 1988).

Despite the fact that BL cells express MHC class I molecules on the cell surface, these molecules are often present in the absence of peptide. This is possibly due to reduced transcription of the TAP genes, leading to low TAP 1 and TAP 2 protein expression and hence, inefficient peptide processing (Khanna et al., 1994; Rowe et al., 1995). Moreover, a decrease in CTL adherence to infected cells has been detected. This could be caused by a reduction in the expression of lymphocyte function-associated antigens 1 and 3, and intercellular adhesion molecule (ICAM)-1, on the transformed cell surface (Gregory et al. 1988; Khanna et al., 1993).

The BZLF2 gene product of EBV is a membrane-bound glycoprotein that is capable of binding MHC class II molecules. BZLF2 has been shown to block EBV infection of B lymphocytes but not epithelial cells (Li et al., 1995) and can inhibit class II antigen presentation. However, the principal function of BZLF2 may be as a determinant of cell tropism rather than as an immune evasion molecule, although at present this is unclear.

Apoptosis is a crucial feature of the immune system and a method by which CTLs eradicate virally-infected cells. It is therefore advantageous for the virus to express proteins that inhibit apoptosis or prolong host cell survival (Hill and Masucci, 1998). Two proteins that carry out this process are BHRF1 and the viral latent membrane protein-1 (LMP1). BHRF1 and other viral anti-apoptosis proteins such as adenovirus E1B-19 kDa (White, 1996), possess sequence similarity to bcl-2, a cellular protein which prevents apoptosis (Austin et al., 1988). BHRF1 is expressed by EBV during lytic infection and has been shown to protect EBV-negative BL cells from apoptosis-inducing stresses (McCarthy et al., 1996). Latently infected B cells express LMP1 which up-regulates expression of cellular bcl-2 and A20, both of which can extend cell persistence *in vivo* (Henderson et al., 1991; Miller et al., 1995).

Burkitt's Lymphoma is not the only EBV-associated tumor to display impaired T cell immunity. A reduction in EBV-specific CTLs has also been reported in EBV-positive Hodgkin's Disease (HD) cells (Frisan et al., 1995). Again the precise mechanisms of this virally-induced immune suppression are unknown (Niedobitek et al., 1997). However, it has been suggested that LMP1 enhances expression of the pleiotropic cytokine interleukin 10 (IL10) (Nakagomi et al., 1994). IL10 is capable of inhibiting cytokine synthesis and also blocking T cell proliferation. It can also confer increased resistance to tumor antigen-specific CTLs (Salazar-Onfray et al., 1995).

Finally, it has been suggested that EBV has evolved ways to avoid expressing immunodominant CTL epitopes such as those in EBNA-4 (de Campos-Lima et al., 1993; 1994) and, as a consequence, the virally-infected cells evade immune surveillance.

Retroviruses

A) HUMAN IMMUNODEFICIENCY VIRUS

The human immunodeficiency virus type-1 (HIV-1) can cause latent or productive infection depending on cell type and activation state. HIV-1 is capable of persisting for years within the host without affecting the normal immune responses to the virus. However, despite the vigorous responses exerted by the host, the virus is still able to persist and CTLs do not succeed in completely eradicating the HIV infection. During the progression of HIV to acquired immune deficiency syndrome (AIDS), an increase in viral replication has been observed, as well as a suppression in the HIV-specific responses (Carmichael et al., 1993). HIV suppresses the immune response via a number of different mechanisms, as discussed below.

The level of circulating MHC class I molecules increases with the progression of HIV-infection (Puppo et al., 1990). It has been suggested that these soluble class I antigens could interfere with immune function and therefore contribute to immune deficiency.

In contrast, a decrease in MHC class I cell surface expression occurs several days post-infection. The peripheral host CD4+ T cells which exhibit this reduced MHC class I expression are, therefore, rarely targetted by class I CTLs (Kerkau et al., 1989; Scheppler et al., 1989). It has been suggested that the HIV *Nef* protein contributes to this reduced expression by causing the rapid internalization of MHC class I molecules, which accumulate in endosomes and are subsequently degraded (Schwartz et al., 1996). Mechanisms responsible for the stable association between MHC-binding peptides and MHC class I molecules may be affected by acute HIV infection which leaves MHC class I antigens empty (Kerkau et al., 1992).

Several HIV proteins are presented on the surface of infected cells at a very low density (Tsomides et al., 1994). Inevitably, this reduces the effectiveness of immune surveillance by CTLs and hence CTL-mediated lysis of infected cells is not triggered. Moreover, it is thought that some peptides are not immunogenic due to crucial mutations within CTL epitopes. *In vivo* evidence indicates that alterations in peptide anchor residues can lead to reduced MHC binding, variations in non-anchor residues can inhibit T cell recognition and altered flanking residues can affect the processing of epitopes within the HIV *Nef* protein (Couillin et al., 1994). Furthermore, mutations in HIV-*gag* epitopes can influence CTL recognition (Phillips et al., 1991). These mutants express antagonistic peptides that also inhibit the immune recognition of target cells which present the unmutated epitope (Klenerman et al., 1994).

In addition, during the onset of AIDS, MHC class II expression on the surface of circulating monocytes is less than in healthy individuals (Haegy et al., 1984). This could be due to the expression of the viral core protein p24 which prevents IFN-γ activating the transcription of the HLA-DR genes (Nong et al., 1991).

Antibodies expressed by infected individuals, to the HIV envelope protein, env, are thought to cross-react with MHC class II antigens on human B cells (Golding et al., 1988). These antibodies could interfere with the class II-mediated response to infection (Blackburn et al., 1991; Zaitseva et al., 1992).

The human T-lymphotropic virus type 1 (HTLV-1) transcriptional activator, Tax, is capable of interfering with multiple cellular transcription pathways and is therefore thought to mediate the uncontrolled growth of HTLV-1-infected T cells which leads to adult T-cell leukemia (Yoshida et al., 1982). Tax induces the phosphorylation and subsequent degradation of IκBα (Kanno et al., 1994; 1995), releasing active NF-κB heterodimers which are able to activate transcription of MHC class I genes. By increasing the cellular expression of MHC class I molecules, the cell is able to avoid lysis by natural killer cells. Tax also stimulates expression of the cellular oncogene *c-fos* (Fujii et al., 1988) which also activates transcription of MHC class I genes.

Papovaviruses

A) SIMIAN VIRUS 40

Like human polyomaviruses, Simian Virus 40 (SV40) expresses six viral proteins; the large T antigen - a multi functional 94 kDa nuclear oncoprotein, the small T antigen, an agnoprotein and VP1, VP2 and VP3 (Alwine, 1982; Hay et al., 1982; Ng et al., 1985). In addition, mouse polyomaviruses also code for a middle T antigen which contributes to transformation by these viruses. Several studies have detected SV40 DNA or large T antigen in human brain tumors (reviewed in Barbanti-Brodano et al., 1998).

The SV40 large T antigen induces a strong cellular immune response, which leads to the rejection of developing T antigen-induced tumors (Tevethia, 1980 and 1990). Development of the tumors appears to inversely correlate with the ability to induce T antigen-specific CTLs which, in turn are controlled by the MHC haplotype (Abramczuk et al., 1984; Pan et al., 1987). Furthermore, progression of T antigen-induced tumors depends on selective loss of MHC class I molecules.

Mice of the H-2^d haplotype have been shown to have a particularly low susceptibility to SV40 T antigen-induced tumorigenesis (Gooding, 1982; Flyer et al., 1983; Pan et al., 1987). However, SV40-transformed H-2^d cells are thought to induce tumor growth without inhibiting MHC class I antigen presentation or losing T antigen expression. The mechanism for this is currently not clear (Kagi et al., 1996). In contrast, H-2^b MHC class I molecules were down-regulated in tumors of T antigen-expressing transgenic H-2^b mice (Ye et al., 1994) and also in T antigen-positive SV40-transformed cells which had been passaged *in vivo* in immunocompetent C57BL/6 mice (Flyer et al., 1983). Furthermore, the escape from CTL immunosurveillance in H-2^b mice can be caused by loss of antigenic determinants from within T antigen or loss of T antigen expression (Newmaster et al., 1998).

B) HUMAN PAPILLOMAVIRUSES

The human papilloma viruses (HPVs) are small DNA viruses that infect epithelial cells. Both *in vitro* and *in vivo* studies have reported the involvement of particular HPVs in the development of epithelial malignancies, and over 90 % of cervical carcinomas are positive for HPV infection. At least 90 different HPVs have been identified (DeVilliers, 1989) and they are divided into two classes according to their target of infection - stratified squamous or mucosal epithelia. HPVs that infect mucosal epithelia are further subdivided depending on their tumorigenicity.

The high risk HPVs, such as types 16 and 18, are capable of inducing intraepithelial neoplasia that may progress to anogenital carcinoma (zur Hausen, 1991). Antibodies to both early and late HPV proteins have been detected in many patients with either benign or malignant HPV-associated lesions. This suggests that humoral immune responses do play a role in suppressing HPV-induced tumor progression. It is thought, however that cell-mediated responses also have great influence in controlling HPV-related diseases.

This is because, in addition to developing more frequent and severe benign HPV-related infections, patients with defects in T-cell immunity have a higher frequency of malignant conversions in HPV-positive lesions (Wright and Sun, 1996).

A high proportion of cervical carcinomas have been shown to have reduced levels of MHC class I molecules (Cromme et al., 1993). This would inhibit effective cytotoxic T lymphocyte activity against potential viral antigens (Conner and Stern, 1990). However, a direct correlation between the occurrence of HPV DNA and the down-regulation of MHC class I molecules in cancer cells has not been detected. *In vitro* experiments indicate that the presence of the HPV-16 genome appears to have no effect on MHC class I or class II expression, although HPV-16 may affect MHC class II expression in response to IFN-γ, but the mechanism is unknown (Bartholomew et al., 1995). Furthermore, the mechanism of MHC class I down-regulation in HPV-positive cervical tumors is currently unclear although it is thought to be caused by a post-transcriptional event (Cromme et al., 1993).

Bartholomew et al. (1997) reported that the glucocorticoid hormone, hydrocortisone, consistently down-regulated the cell surface expression of class I MHC antigens in HPV-positive cervical tumor cells but caused up-regulation in HPV-negative cells. Similar results were also reported with the steroid hormone progesterone. Both hormones have been shown to require the presence of functional glucocorticoid or progesterone receptors (respectively) to suppress HLA expression. However, there is no glucocorticoid receptor element within the regulatory regions of MHC class I genes, and consequently a direct effect on gene expression is unlikely. It has been suggested that hydrocortisone functions by altering the balance of NF-κB dimers within the cell. The presence of hydrocortisone has been shown to cause an increase in the level of KBF1 (a p50 homodimer) which is thought to negatively regulate HLA class I transcription. In addition, a reduction in level of the NF-κB transcriptional activator, (the p65/p50 heterodimer) was observed in the presence of hydrocortisone. However, the precise mechanisms are currently unclear.

The HPV early proteins E6 and E7 (like the E1B and E1A proteins of subgenus A adenoviridae) are capable of cell transformation and growth dysregulation via their association and subsequent inactivation of the tumor suppressor proteins, p53 and pRB (see chapter). It is also becoming apparent that the E6 and E7 oncoproteins induce tumor growth via additional molecular interactions (Alani and Munger, 1998). However there is no evidence to suggest that, like E1B and E1A, the HPV E6 and E7 proteins contribute to evasion of the immune system (Cromme et al., 1993).

Human adenoviruses

HUMAN ADENOVIRUSES AS AN EXPERIMENTAL SYSTEM FOR TRANSFORMATION AND ONCOGENICITY

Human adenoviruses cause a variety of lytic and persistent respiratory, enteric and other infections. They are divided into subgenera A to F according to a number of properties, including their site of infection and their oncogenicity in newborn rodents (Tooze, 1984). There are at least forty-seven different adenovirus (Ad) serotypes and all are capable of transforming primary rat cells *in vitro*. Subgenus A adenoviruses such as Ad 12 induce tumors with high frequency and short latency, whereas subgroup B adenoviruses are only weakly oncogenic (Trentin et al., 1962; Williams et al., 1995). Adenoviruses of subgenera C, D, E and F are non-oncogenic (such as the well-studied serotypes Ad 2 and Ad 5 of subgenus C). The ability of Ad 12 of subgenus A to form tumors in immunocompetent newborn rodents correlates with its ability to down-regulate the cell surface expression of MHC class I molecules, while expression of MHC class I in non-oncogenic Ad 5-transformed cells is normal or up-regulated. As a consequence, the human adenoviruses provide an ideal model system to study the regulation of MHC class I expression by oncogenic viruses.

TRANSFORMATION BY, AND ONCOGENICITY OF, HUMAN ADENOVIRUSES

Human adenoviruses were first discovered in latently-infected adenoids (Rowe et al., 1953). They are non-enveloped, double-stranded DNA viruses of approximately 70 nm in diameter. The external capsid is composed of 252 capsomer proteins, 240 hexons and 12 pentons which are positioned at the 12 vertices of the virion (Ginsberg et al., 1966). Each penton is associated with a fibre protein which projects outwards from the capsid and ends in a knob (Wilcox et al., 1963). The double-stranded DNA molecule has a size of approximately 36 kb (van der Eb et al., 1969; Green et al., 1967) and is packaged within the virion with basic, virus-coded polypeptides (Epstein, 1959).

As mentioned above, adenoviruses of all subgenera are capable of transforming primary rodent cells. The transforming activity of the DNA has been strictly correlated with the expression of the adenovirus early genes, E1A and E1B, (Bernards, et al. 1983; Schrier, et al. 1983). E1A is adjacent to E1B in the left-most 11% of the viral genome and co-operates with E1B or activated *ras* to transform rodent cells. Transformation of cells is thought to occur as a result of the adenovirus proteins E1B-19K and E1B-55K suppressing the induction of apoptosis which is caused by E1A proteins (Debbas and White, 1993). E1A is capable of inducing apoptosis in both a p53-dependent and a p53-independent manner and both pathways are inhibited by E1B-19K. E1B-55K prevents apoptosis by binding p53 (Sarnow et al., 1982), hence blocking the transcriptional regulatory function of p53. Both transformed rodent cells and virally-infected human cells are able to evade the host immune system via a number of mechanisms and these are discussed below.

REGULATION OF MHC CLASS I GENE EXPRESSION IN ADENOVIRUS-TRANSFORMED CELLS

The suppression of MHC class I expression in Ad 12-transformed cells is an effect mediated by the adenovirus E1A oncogene and as a consequence much research has been carried out in an attempt to understand the mechanisms which lead to this down-regulation.

During the early phases of infection and also in transformed cells, alternative splicing of the E1A transcript produces at least five mRNA molecules denoted 9S, 10S, 11S, 12S and 13S in Ad 2- and Ad 5-infected cells. An additional 9.5S E1A mRNA molecule is also generated by alternative RNA splicing in Ad 12-infected cells (Brockmann et al., 1994). In Ad 2- or Ad 5-infected cells, the mRNAs are translated into nuclear phosphoproteins of 55, 171, 217, 243 and 289 amino acid residues, respectively (Berk and Sharp, 1978; Chow, et al. 1979; Perricaudet et al., 1979; Kitchingman and Westphal, 1980; Stephens and Harlow, 1987; Ulfendahl et al., 1987). The two major phosphoproteins, the 12S and 13S products, also known as 243R and 289R, are required for the E1A gene to show full transforming capacity.

The tumorigenic potential of Ad 12-E1A is mediated by sequences within the first exon (Jelinek et al., 1994; Telling and Williams, 1994). Ad 5-E1A and Ad 12-E1A differ at 2 separate regions within this first exon and these sites are thought to contribute to the tumorigenic phenotype of Ad 12-E1A. The first encompasses the conserved region (CR) 2 and the 20 amino acid spacer region between the CR2 and the CR3 which is unique to Ad 12. The second extends from the N-terminus of E1A to the left border of the CR2 (Figure 3A). These regions are also thought to contribute to a decrease in class I expression (Pereira et al., 1995). Furthermore, mutation of the alanine-rich region of Ad 12-E1A reduces, but does not abolish, tumorigenicity (Telling and Williams, 1994; Pereira et al., 1995).

Although E1A proteins are predominantly nuclear and must produce their effects on gene expression and cell growth in the nucleus, there is little evidence that E1A proteins act by direct binding to DNA (Ferguson et al. 1985; Chatterjee et al. 1988; Zu et al. 1992). Conversely, there is considerable evidence to suggest that they bind specifically to cellular proteins that play significant roles in controlling gene expression and cell growth. In doing so this alters or inhibits normal cellular functions. E1A proteins act both by affecting a wide variety of transcription factors and by mediating several different *trans*-activating pathways, in order to activate a variety of gene promoters. Cell proliferation increases and differentiation is suppressed. E1A also represses the efficient transcription of a variety of viral and cellular genes including the MHC class I genes (Ackrill and Blair, 1988; Friedman and Ricciardi, 1988).

AD 12 E1A-MEDIATED TRANSCRIPTIONAL REPRESSION OF MHC CLASS I GENES

Much research carried out previously has focused on expression of the MHC class I, H-$2K^b$ gene of b-haplotype mice. Kimura et al. (1986) first identified enhancer-like sequences in the H-$2K^b$ 5′-flanking region.

The reduction in MHC class I gene expression by E1A occurs exclusively in primary rodent cells transformed by the oncogenic, subgenus A adenoviruses, such as Ad 12. This down-regulation of MHC class I genes, in Ad 12-transformed primary rat and mouse cells has been observed at the mRNA level and correlates with the presence of the 13S Ad 12-E1A gene product (Bernards et al., 1983; Schrier et al., 1983). 13S-mediated down-regulation occurs at the level of transcription (Ackrill and Blair, 1988; Friedman and Ricciardi, 1988; Meijer et al., 1989; 1991). It has been proposed that Ad 12-E1A transcriptionally regulates MHC class I gene expression via at least two sites within the 5′-flanking region of the mouse H-$2D^b$ gene (Philpott and Blair, unpublished) and three sites in the 5′-flanking region of the mouse H-$2K^b$ (Figure 3B):

1) The proximal class I regulatory element (CRE) region at -213bp to -159bp (Kralli et al., 1992; Schouten et al., 1995; Logeat et al., 1991; Ge et al., 1992; Meijer et al., 1992; Kushner et al., 1996).

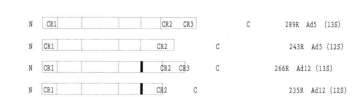

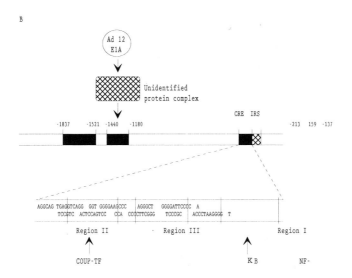

Figure 3. (Top: A) Schematic diagram of E1A polypeptides. The conserved regions (CR) 1, 2 and 3 within the 12S and 13S proteins of Ad 5 and Ad 12 adenoviruses are shown. The black regions located after the CR2 in the Ad 12 polypeptides corresponds to the alanine-rich region that is absent in Ad 5 E1A proteins. (Bottom: B) Regulatory elements of the H-2K^b MHC class I, 5′-flanking region. The class I regulatory element (CRE) is composed of three regions I, II and III. Regions I binds NF-κB and Region II is a nuclear hormone receptor half-site that binds COUP-TF. The IRS corresponds to the interferon response sequence. The black regions correspond to elements that mediate down-regulation of MHC class I gene expression in Ad 12-transformed cells.

2) The 260bp distal region from -1,440bp to -1,180bp (Proffitt et al., 1994).

3) The most upstream, 316bp regulatory sequence at -1,837bp to -1,521bp (Katoh et al., 1990; Ozawa et al., 1993; Tang et al., 1995).

Most research has focused on the control of transcriptional regulation by the conserved enhancer sequence, designated the class I regulatory element (CRE). Katoh et al. (1990) demonstrated that distal elements in the 5′ DNA flanking region of the class I gene repress promoter activity in Ad 12-transformed cells, while a proximal region, which is part of the CRE, activates it.

CRE

The CRE consists of three distinct domains that bind different transcription factors, termed Region I, Region II and Region III (Shirayoshi et al., 1987). Region I is highly conserved between mouse and human MHC class I genes and it binds transcription factors of the NF-κB/c-rel family. Region II forms a half-site for the nuclear hormone receptor superfamily of transcription factors, eg. human RXR-β, mouse H2RIIBP and COUP-TF. Region III contains an NF-κB-like binding site.

NF-κB transcription factors are active as heterodimers consisting of a p65 (relA) and a p50 (NF-κB1-p50) subunit (Baldwin, 1996). In the unstimulated cell, NF-κB is retained in the cytoplasm bound to the inhibitory subunit I-κB. The NF-κB1 gene encodes two functionally distinct proteins, the p50 polypeptide subunit of NF-κB and p105 which is a member of the IκB family. The p50 subunit is generated cotranslationally by a proteasome-mediated process that ensures the production of both p50 and p105 (Lin et al., 1998). Upon cellular stimulation the I-κB, p105 protein becomes phosphorylated and is degraded by the 26S proteasome. The p50 subunit is then able to form heterodimers with p65 and this leads to the nuclear expression of NF-κB. The p50 subunit is also able to dimerise but is transcriptionally inactive in this form.

Regions I and II have both been shown to bind different levels of transcription factors in Ad 5- compared to Ad 12-transformed cells (Ackrill and Blair, 1989; Ge et al., 1992; Meijer et al., 1992). Region I binds several factors, including NF-κB (a p65/p50 heterodimer) and KBF1 (a p50/p50 homodimer), that contribute to regulation of expression of MHC class I genes *in vivo* (Logeat et al., 1991). It has consistently been observed that both dimers bind their cognate DNA sites to a much lesser extent in Ad 12- compared to Ad 5-transformed cells (Ackrill and Blair, 1989; Ge et al., 1992; Meijer et al., 1992).

In Ad 5-transformed cells the E1A 13S product has been found to increase the degradation of I-κB and hence stimulate uptake of NF-κB by the nucleus. In addition it is thought to activate the p65 subunit *in vivo* (Schmitz et al., 1996). The mechanism by which Ad 12-E1A 13S reduces the levels of NF-κB DNA binding activity in the nucleus remains unclear. It has been suggested that Ad 12-E1A 13S interferes with the proteolytic processing of the 105 kDa product of the NF-κB1 gene, by the 26S proteasome. This interference would alter the p50/p105 ratio in favour of p105. Excess p105 would then dimerise with p50 or p65 and sequesters NF-κB in the cytosol, culminating in the formation of few p65/p50 or p50/p50 complexes. The low concentrations of the NF-κB heterodimer (p50/p65) and the KBF1 homodimer (p50/p50) would result in less binding to the the Region I element and hence reduced expression of MHC class I genes. In Ad 5 E1A-transformed cells, p50 is more abundant than p105, so p50/p50 and p50/p65 dimers are favoured, NF-κB is , therefore, constitutively active and high expression of MHC class I results (Schouten et al., 1995).

Other experiments have indicated that an alteration in the level of phosphorylation of the p50 subunit is critical for NF-κB binding to Region I. Dephosphorylation of p50 reduces DNA binding and the level of p50 phosphorylation is greatly reduced in Ad 12-, compared to Ad 5-transformed cells, leading to the decreased binding activity of NF-κB in Ad 12-transformed cells (Kushner and Ricciardi, 1999).

Besides the Region I element, other elements within the MHC class I promoter have been designated as targets for regulation by Ad 12-E1A. Ad 12-transformed cells appear to exhibit more extensive *in vitro* binding of nuclear factors to Region II than Ad 5 E1-transformed cells (Ackrill and Blair, 1989). Increased binding of these factors to Region II was reported to account for repression of class I transcription (Ge et al., 1992; Kralli et al., 1992). One factor that binds to Region II in Ad 12 E1-transformed cells has been identified as COUP-TF (Liu et al., 1994), although over-expression of COUP-TF in Ad 5-transformed cells did not result in reduced levels of MHC class I molecules.

In summary, while it appears that there is a potentially important 'cross-talk' between Regions I and II in Ad 12-transformed cells leading to reduced MHC class I transcription, there is still much to learn about the identity of transcription factors involved (in the case of Region II) and the precise mechanism of transcriptional modulation (in the case of Region I).

-1837 bp/-1521 bp region

It has been reported that binding of an, as yet, unidentified factor to a CAA repeat element located between -1837 bp and -1521 bp upstream of the cap site, contributes to repression of the H-2K^b gene in Ad 12 E1-transformed 3Y1 cells. The H-2K^b gene has CAA repeated sequences in regions -1,736bp to -1,689bp and -1,616bp to -1,535bp and both are necessary for full negative regulation of this gene by the 13S product of E1A, (Katoh et al., 1990; Ozawa et al., 1993). In addition, a TATA-like sequence (TATAA) in the far upstream region of the 5′-flanking sequence (-1,773bp to -1,767bp) appears to be a key element in the negative regulation of expression of the H-2K^{bm1} gene by E1A, in conjunction with either upstream or downstream CAA repeats (Tang et al., 1995). This TATA-like element is sensitive to orientation. Tang et al. (1995) observed that Ad 12-E1A-dependent negative regulation is dependent upon the presence of the specific sequence TAT(A/T)AA at -1,773bp to -1,767bp. This negative regulatory region may well extend back to -1,811bp and contain several elements capable of binding proteins that participate in the down-regulation of MHC class I by E1A (Katoh et al., 1990).

-1180 bp/-1440 bp region

Finally, a 260bp sequence from -1,180bp to -1,440bp has been shown to play a major role in Ad 12-E1A-mediated down-regulation of the H-2K^b promoter (Proffitt et al., 1994). It has been suggested that more than one element is targeted over this region and that these elements may function co-operatively to achieve maximal down-regulation. The precise mechanism of class I repression via this region is not known, but cellular factors are probably involved either by induction or activation by Ad 12-E1A. However, analysis of DNA-protein complexes binding to this region have shown that Ad 12-E1A, but not Ad 5-E1A proteins, form a component of the complex that binds this region of the H-2K^b gene (Philpott and Blair, unpublished).

How does Ad 12-E1A down-regulate MHC class I transcription, when Ad 5-E1A does not? Kushner et al. (1996) observed that the regions of Ad 12-E1A implicated in class I down-regulation and tumorigenesis are also responsible for the strong binding activity of factors to the Region II element and diminished binding activity of NF-κB to the Region I element of the class I enhancer in Ad 12 E1-transformed rat cells. Furthermore, Ge et al. (1994) reported that in the presence of Ad 12-E1A, regardless of the presence of Ad 5-E1A, class I enhancer activity is down-regulated in Ad 5/Ad 12 hybrid cell lines indicating that the Ad 12-E1A phenotype is dominant.

REPRESSION OF OTHER MHC GENES IN AD 12-TRANSFORMED CELLS

Ad 12 has been shown to reduce expression of other MHC genes at the level of transcription. The transporter associated with antigen presentation (TAP) proteins 1 and 2, as well as the low molecular weight protein (LMP) 2 and 7 are all down-regulated in Ad 12-transformed cells but not in Ad 5-transformed cells (Rotem-Yehudar et al., 1994; 1996). Proffit and Blair (1997) reported that the bidirectional promoter, shared by the TAP1 and LMP2 genes, is repressed in Ad 12-, but not Ad 5-transformed cells. Interestingly the TAP1-LMP2 bidirectional promoter contains an NF-κB site which is conserved between the mouse, rat and human genes (Proffit and Blair; 1997). Therefore, these genes could potentially be repressed by Ad 12-E1A via a mechanism similar to that which regulates the NF-κB element of Region I of the CRE in MHC class I genes (see above). Pleiotropic down-regulation of all four genes would cause a reduction in cell surface expression of peptide-containing MHC class I molecules.

REPRESSION OF OTHER GENES LOCATED IN OR LINKED TO THE MHC LOCUS IN AD 12-TRANSFORMED CELLS

Genes that are not involved in the antigen presentation pathway are also modulated in Ad 12-transformed cells. Eyler et al. (1997) observed that the gene product of *Waf*-1, which is involved in cell cycle control and the complement factors, C3 and C2, are all down-regulated in Ad 12-transformed cells. These genes are all located on mouse chromosome 17 in a region that includes the MHC, but it is not yet known whether expression of these genes is directly regulated by the E1A gene products of Ad 12.

E3-MEDIATED DOWN-REGULATION OF MHC CLASS I CELL SURFACE EXPRESSION

Adenovirus transformation requires only the E1A and E1B genes (Tooze, 1984). However, another early gene, E3, encodes important regulatory proteins that affect the pathogenicity of adenoviruses *in vivo*. While not required for oncogenesis, studies on the E3 gene have provided extensive information on the interaction of adenoviruses with the cellular immune system (Blair and Hall, 1998).

A 19 kDa, E3 glycoprotein of adenoviruses from subgenera B, C D and E, has the ability to bind MHC class I molecules within the ER lumen. As a consequence of this interaction, the MHC class I molecules are sequestered inside the ER and are not translocated to the cell surface (Paabo et al., 1986; Burgert and Kvist, 1985; Tanaka and Tevethia, 1988). E3-19K consists of a 107 amino acid (aa) N-terminal domain, situated in the lumen of the ER. This is followed by a 20 - 24 aa transmembrane region and finally a 15 aa cytoplasmic, C-terminal domain, which contains an ER retention signal. It is thought that the E3-19K protein binds below the antigen-binding cleft of the $\alpha 1$ and $\alpha 2$-helix region of the MHC class I molecule (Beier et al., 1994; Feuerbach et al., 1994; Flomenberg et al., 1994). Sester and Burgert (1994) suggested that the region of E3-19K, spanning aa 1 to 84, binds the $\alpha 1$ and $\alpha 2$ domains of the MHC class I molecule, with the 84 to 98 aa region binding the $\alpha 3$ domain. This MHC class I retention in the ER lumen contributes to lower cell surface expression of MHC, reduced antigen presentation and, therefore, CTL immune evasion (Sparer and Gooding, 1998). Interestingly, oncogenic adenoviruses such as Ad 12 (of subgenus A) (Sprengel et al., 1994) and Ad 40 (subgenus F) (Davison et al., 1993) do not encode an E3-19K protein and therefore cannot perform E3-mediated retention of MHC class I molecules. It appears that MHC class I trafficking is only blocked in adenoviruses of subgenera B, C, D and E (Paabo et al., 1986). However, as described above, the E1A gene of the subgenus A virus, Ad 12, mediates transcriptional repression of MHC class I genes, highlighting the importance to the virus of preventing CTL recognition of virally-infected and transformed cells.

It is possible that E3-19K also binds other proteins in the ER leading to their functional inhibition. Feuerbach and Burgert (1993) found that E3-19K coprecipitated with two proteins of 100 and 110 kDa, which are thought to be chaperones, but to date their specific identity is unknown.

E3 AND E1A GENE PRODUCTS MEDIATE CELLULAR RESPONSES TO CYTOKINES

Cytokines are an integral component of the host immune system. Therefore, in order to evade the immune response, adenoviruses have evolved mechanisms to block the cellular response to cytokines, such as tumor necrosis factor-α (TNF-α), interferons (IFNs) and interleukin-6 (IL-6) (Blair and Hall, 1998).

TNF-α is released by activated macrophages and lymphocytes in response to inflammatory stimuli. It is capable of inhibiting the replication of a number of viruses, as well as up-regulating MHC class I cell surface expression. TNF-α has been shown to activate NF-κB binding to sites in the Ad 2 E3 promoter (Deryckere and Burgert, 1996). The subsequent increase in E3-19K expression can then cause retention of MHC class I molecules in the ER. In addition, the 14.7, 14.5 and 10.4 kDa E3 proteins are able to confer resistance to TNF-α (Gooding et al., 1990; Hoffman et al., 1992). It has been suggested that the resistance to TNF-α-induced cell lysis is caused by either the E3-14.7K protein or the E3-10.4/14.5K complex, inhibiting TNF-α-activation of cytosolic phospholipase A2 (cPLA2). Cytosolic PLA2 functions by cleaving arachidonic acid (AA) from membrane phospholipids (Krajcsi et al., 1996). It has been proposed that E3-14.7 acts by down-regulating TNF-α receptors on the cell surface and that the E3-10.4/14.5K complex prevents TNF-α-induced translocation of cPLA2 to the plasma membrane. However, the precise mechanisms are not fully understood.

As mentioned above, there are 3 classes of IFN, -α, -β and -γ. IFN-α and IFN-β are synthesised by most cells and function by associating with common cell surface receptors. This triggers the phosphorylation of two signal transduction and activation of transcription (STAT) proteins, which stimulate the transcription of IFN-responsive genes, such as the gene encoding the protein kinase PKR. When activated by dsRNA, PKR phosphorylates eIF-2α, ultimately causing inhibition of viral protein synthesis. During adenovirus replication, two virus-associated RNA molecules (VA RNA$_I$ and VA RNA$_{II}$) are synthesised. VA RNA$_I$ binds to PKR and blocks its binding to dsRNA, consequently, it remains inactive and viral protein synthesis is able to proceed (Ghadge et al., 1991) (Figure 2).

During normal cellular function, IFN-α activates the transcription factor, IFN-stimulated gene factor 3 (ISGF3) which consists of three subunits, p48, STAT1α and STAT2 (Ihle, 1996). In Ad 5-transformed cells, E1A proteins interfere with the activation of ISGF3 by two different mechanisms. Firstly, by interacting with p300, E1A prevents its binding to STAT2 and hence the ISGF3-mediated transactivation of IFN-responsive genes. Secondly, E1A-containing cells express lower levels of p48 and also block the activation of STAT1α by tyrosine phosphorylation (Leonard and Sen, 1996). In Ad 12-transformed cells, there is no interference by Ad 12-E1A of IFN-mediated activation of ISGF3 (Yusof and Blair, unpublished).

IL-6 is produced by cells in response to IL-1 and induces B cell differentiation, T cell activation, haemopoiesis and synthesis of acute phase proteins. E1A proteins counteract the cellular responses to IL-6 (Takeda et al., 1994) and, via their conserved region 1 (CR1) domains, they also interfere with the transcription of IL-6 (Janaswami et al., 1992). E1A is thought to interfere with IL-6 signal transduction by inhibiting the binding of transcription factors to regulatory elements in IL-6 responsive genes and also by reducing the levels of STAT proteins (Hirano, 1992).

Conclusions

In order to survive often for long periods of time in the infected cell, viruses have evolved unique strategies to avoid eradication by the host immune system. The variety of mechanisms utilized by different viruses depends upon viral life-cycle, the area of the host immune system used to combat infection, the cell-type infected and kinetics of infection. One mechanism by which many viruses, such as HSV, avoid recognition is that of latency. During latency very little viral protein synthesis occurs and few viral peptides bound to MHC class I molecules are expressed on the cell surface. Similarly, EBV-positive BL cells express only one protein (EBNA-1) and this too reduces the efficiency of immune surveillance by CTLs. Interference with host cytokines has also been attributed to an abrogation of the immune response. Vaccinia virus, for example, synthesises its own versions of cytokine receptors which competitively inhibit the functions of host cytokines.

An essential part of the immune response is the MHC class I antigen-presentation pathway and, as a result, many of the DNA tumor viruses carry out specific functions which block the passage of either MHC class I molecules to the cell surface or viral antigens through the cell. This, consequently, leads to low cell surface expression of peptide-bound MHC class I molecules and hence the cell avoids immunosurveillance by cytotoxic T lymphocytes. Low levels of MHC class I expression have been described in many virally-infected cells, such as in HPV positive cervical carcinomas, although the mechanism of down-regulation is unclear. More specifically, adenoviruses appear to reduce MHC class I expression at the level of transcription (Ad 12) or via MHC class I retention in the ER (Ad 5). HCMV expresses proteins that mediate the degradation of MHC class I molecules by the 26S proteasome.

The ability of DNA tumor viruses to acquire functions which contribute to evasion of the host immune system protects infected cells from eradication and could therefore potentially result in the formation of more evasive, highly proliferative tumors.

Acknowledgements

Research in the authors' laboratory is supported by Yorkshire Cancer Research. Nicola Philpott was a University of Leeds research student. We thank Drs. Stephanie Wright , David Kushner and Mark Harris for comments on this chapter.

References

Abramczuk, J., Pan, S., Maul, G. and Knowles, B. (1984) Tumor induction by Simian Virus 40 in mice is controlled by long term persistence of the viral genome and the immune response of the host. J. Virol. 49:540-548.

Ackrill, A. M. and Blair, G. E. (1988) Regulation of major histocompatibility complex class I gene expression at the level of transcription in highlyoncogenic adenovirus transformed rat cells. Oncogene 3:483-487.

Ackrill, A. M. and Blair, G. E. (1989) Nuclear proteins binding to an enhancer element of the major histocompatibility class I promoter: differences between highly oncogenic and non-oncogenic adenovirus-transformed rat cells. Virology 172:643-646.

Ahn, K., Angulo, A., Ghazal, P., Petterson, P. A., Yang, Y. and Fruh, K. (1996) Human cytomegalovirus inhibits antigen presentation by a sequential multistep process. Proc. Natl. Acad. Sci. USA. 93:10990-10995.

Ahn, K., Gruler, A., Galocha, B., Jones, T. R., Wiertz, E. J. H. J., Ploegh, H. L., Petterson, P. A., Yang, Y. and Fruh, K. (1997) The ER-lumenal domain of the HCMV glycoprotein US6 inhibits peptide translocation by TAP. Immunity 6:613-621.

Akiyama, K., Kagawa, S., Tamura, T., Shimbara, N., Takashina, M., Kristensen, P., Hendil, K. B., Tanaka, K. and Ichihara, A. (1994) Replacement of proteasome subunits X and Y by LMP7 and LMP2 induced by interferon-gamma for aquirement of the functional diversit responsible for antigen processing. FEBS Lett. 343:85-88.

Alani, R. M. and Munger, K. (1998) Human papillomaviruses and associated malignancies. J. Clin. Oncol. 16:330-337.

Alcami, A. and Smith, G. L. (1992) A soluble receptor for interleukin-1β encoded by vaccinia virus: a novel mechanism of virus modulation of the host response to infection. Cell 71:153-167.

Alcami, A. and Smith, G. L. (1995) Vaccinia, cowpox and camelpox viruses encode soluble interferon-γ receptors with novel broad specicies specificity. J. Virol. 69:4633-4639.

Alcami, A. and Smith, G. L. (1996) A mechanism for the inhibition of fever by a virus. Proc. Natl. Acad. Sci. USA. 93:11029-11034.

Alcami, A., Symons J. A., Khanna, A. and Smith, G. L. (1998a) Poxviruses: capturing cytokines and chemokines. Sem. Virol. 5:419-427.

Alcami, A., Symons J. A., Collins, P. D., Williams, T. J. and Smith, G. L. (1998b) Blockade of chemokine activity by a soluble chemokine binding protein from vaccinia virus. J. Immunol. 160:624-633.

Alford, C. and Britt, W. (1993) Cytomegalovirus, In: The human herpesviruses. Roizman, B., Whitley, R. and Lopez, C. eds. Raven Press, New York, p.227-255.

Ali, A. N., Turner, P. C., Brooks, M. A. and Moyer, R. W. (1994) The SPI-1 gene of rabbitpox virus determines host range and is required for hemorrhagic pock formation. Virology 202:305-314.

Alwine, J. C. (1982) Evidence for simian virus 40 late transcriptional control: Mixed infections of wild-type simian virus 40 and a late leader deletion mutant exhibit trans effects on late viral RNA synthesis. J. Virol. 42:798-803.

Androlewicz, M. J., Ortmann, B., Van Endert, P. M., Spies, T. and Cresswell, P. (1994) Characteristics of peptide and major histocompatibility complex class I/beta2-microglobulin binding to the transporters associated with antigen processing (TAP1 and TAP2). Proc. Natl. Acad. Sci. USA. 91:12716-12720.

Austin, P. J., Flemington, E., Yandava, C. N., Strominger, J. S. and Speck, S. H. (1988) Complex transcription of the Epstein-Barr virus BamHI fragment H right-ward open reading frame (BHRF1) in latently and lytically infected B lymphocytes. Proc. Natl. Acad. Sci. USA. 85:3678-3682.

Baldwin, A. S., Jr. (1996) The NF-κB and I-κB proteins: New discoveries and insights. Annu. Rev. Immunol. 14:649-681.

Barbanti-Brodano, G., Martini, F., De Mattei, M., Lazzarin, L., Corallini, A. and Tognon, M. (1998) BK and JC human polyomaviruses and simian virus 40. Adv. Virus Res. 50:69-99.

Bartholomew, J., Glenville, S., Sarkar, S., Burt, D. J., Stanley, M. A., Ruiz-Cabello, F., Chengang, J., Garrido, F. and Stern, P. L. (1997) Integration of high-risk human papillomavirus DNA is linked to the down-regulation of class I human leukocyte antigens by steroid hormones in cervical tumor cells. Cancer Res. 57:937-942.

Bartholomew, J., Tinsley, J. M. and Stern, P. L. (1995) MHC expression in HPV-associated cervical cancer. In: Modulation of MHC antigen expression and disease. Blair, G. E., Pringle, C. R. and Maudsley, D. J., eds. Cambridge University Press. p.233-250.

Beersma, M. F. C., Bijlmakers, M. J. E. and Ploegh, H. L. (1993) Human cytomegalovirus down-regulates HLA class I expression by reducing the stability of class I H chains. J. Immunol. 151:4455-4464.

Beier, D. C., Cox, J. H., Vining, D. R., Cresswell, P. and Engelhard, V. H. (1994) Association of human class I MHC alleles with the adenovirus E3/19K protein. J. Immunol. 152:3862-3872.

Belich, M. P., Glynne, R. J., Senger, G., Sheer, D. and Trowsdale, J. (1994) Proteasome components with reciprocal expression to that of the MHC-encoded LMP proteins. Curr. Biol. 4:769-776.

Berk, A. J. and Sharp, P. A. (1978) Structure of the adenovirus 2 early mRNAs. Cell 14:695-711.

Bernards, R., Schrier, P. I., Houweling, A., Bos, J. L., van der Eb, A. J., Zijlstra, M. and Melief, C. J. M. (1983) Tumorigenicity of cells transformed by adenovirus 12 by evasion of T cell immunity. Nature 305:776-779.

Blackburn, R., Clerici, M., Mann, D., Lucey, D. R., Goedert, J., Golding B., Shearer, G. M. and Golding, H. (1991) Common sequence in HIV 1 gp41 and HLA class II beta chains can generate crossreactive autoantibodies with immunosuppressive potential early in the course of HIV 1 infection. Adv. Exp. Med. Biol. 303:63-69.

Blair, G. E. and Hall, K. T. (1998) Human adenoviruses: evading detection by cytotoxic T lymphocytes. Sem. Virol. 8:387-397.

Blasco, R., Cole, N. B. and Moss, B. (1991) Sequence analysis, expression and deletion of a vaccinia virus gene encoding a homolgue of profilin, a eukaryotic actin-binding protein. J. Virol. 65:4598-4608.

Brockmann, D., Feng, L., Kroner, G., Tries, B. and Esche, H. (1994) Adenovirus type 12 early region 1A expresses a 52R protein repressing the trans-activating activity of transcription factor c-jun/AP-1. Virology 198:717-723.

Brooks, M. A., Ali, A. N., Turner, P. C. and Moyer, R. W. (1995) A rabbitpox virus serpin gene controls host range by inhibiting apoptosis in restrictive cells. J. Virol. 69: 7688-7698.

Browne, H., Smith, G., Beck, S. and Minson, T. (1990) A complex between the MHC class I homologue encoded by human cytomegalovirus and beta 2 microglobulin. Nature 347:770-772.

Burgert, H.-G. and Kvist, S. (1985) An adenovirus type-2 glycoprotein blocks cell surface expression of human histocompatibility class I antigens. Cell 41:987-997.

Carmichael, A., Jin, X., Sissons, P. and Borysiewicz, L. (1993) Quantitative analysis of the human immunodeficiency virus type 1 (HIV-1)-specific cytotoxic T lymphocytes (CTL) response at different stages of HIV-1 infection: differential CTL responses to HIV-1 and Epstein Barr virus in late disease. J. Exp. Med. 177:249.

Chatterjee, P. K., Bruner, M., Flint, S. J. and Harter, M. L. (1988) The DNA binding properties of an adenovirus 289R E1A protein. EMBO. J. 7:835-841.

Chen, P. and Hochstrasser, M. (1995) Biogenesis, structure and function of the yeast 20S proteasome. EMBO J. 14:2620-2630.

Chow, L. T., Brooker, T. R. and Lewis, J. B. (1979) Complex splicing pattern of RNAs from early regions of adenovirus-2. J. Mol. Biol. 124:265-303.

Cines, D. B., Lyss, A. P. and Bina, M. (1982) Fc and C3 receptors induced by herpes simplex virus on cultured human endothelial cells. J. Clin. Invest. 69:123-128.

Colamonici, O. R., Domanski, P., Sweitzer, S. M., Larner, A. and Buller, R. M. L. (1995) Vaccinia virus B18R gene encodes a type I interferon-binding protein that blocks interferon alpha transmembrane signaling. J. Biol. Chem. 270:15974-15978.

Confer, D. L., Vercellotti, G. M., Kotasek, D., Goodman, J. L., Ochoa, A. and Jaccob, H. S. (1990) Herpes simplex virus-infected cells disarm killer lymphocytes. Proc. Natl. Acad. Sci. USA. 87:3609-3613.

Conner, M. E. and Stern, P. L. (1990) Loss of MHC class I expression in cervical carcinomas. Int. J. Cancer 46:1029-1035.

Cosman, D., Fanger, N., Borges, L., Kubin, M., Chin, W., Peterson, L. and Hsu, M.-L. (1997) A novel immunoglobulin superfamily receptor for cellular and viral MHC class I molecules. Immunity 8:273-282.

Couillin, I., Culmann-Peniolelli, B., Gomard, E., Choppin, J., Levy, J.-G. and Saragosti, S. (1994) Impaired cytotoxic T lymphocyte recognition due to genetic variations in the main immungenetic region of the human immunodeficiency virus 1 Nef protein. J. Exp. Med. 180:1129.

Coupar, B. E. H., Andrew, M. E., Both, G. W. and Boyle, D. B. (1986) Temporal regulation of influenza hemagglutinin expression in vaccinia virus recombinants and effects on the immune response. Eur. J. Immunol. 16:1479-1487.

Cromme, F. V., Snijders, P. J. F., van den Brule, A. J. C., Kenemans, P., Meijer, C. J. L. M. and Walboomers, J. M. M. (1993) MHC class I expression in HPV 16 positive cervical carcinomas is post-transcriptionally controlled and independent from c-myc overexpression. Oncogene 8:2969-2975.

Cupps, T. R. and Fauci, A. S. (1982) Corticosteroid-mediated immunoregulation in man. Immunol. Rev. 65:133-155.

Dairaghi, D. J., Greaves, D. R. and Schall, T. J. (1998) Abduction of chemokine elements by herpesviruses. Sem. Virol. 8:377-385.

Davison, A. J., Telford, E. A. R., Watson, M. M., McBride, K. and Mautner, V. (1993) The DNA sequence of adenovirus type 40. J. Mol. Biol. 234:1308-1316.

Davis-Poynter, N. J. and Farrell, H. E. (1998) Human and murine cytomegalovirus evasion of cytotoxic T lymphocyte and natural killer cell-mediated immune responses. Sem. Virol. 8:369-376.

Debbas, M. and White, E. (1993) Wild-type p53 mediates apoptosis by E1A, which is inhibited by E1B. Genes Dev. 7:546-554.

de Campos-Lima, P. O., Gavioli, R., Zhang, Q. J., Wallace, L. E., Dolcetti, R., Rowe, M., Rickinson, A. B. and Masucci, M. G. (1993) HLA-A11 epitope loss isolates of Epstein-Barr virus from a highly A11+ population. Science 260:98-100.

de Campos-Lima, P. O., Levitsky, V., Brooks, J., Lee, S. P., Hu, L. F., Rickinson, A. B. and Masucci, M. G. (1994) T cell responses and virus evolution: loss of HLA A11-restricted CTL epitopes in Epstein-Barr virus isolates from highly A11-positive populations by selective mutation of anchor residues. J. Exp. Med. 179:1297-1305.

Del Val, M., Hengel, H., Hacker, H., Hartlaub, U., Ruppert, T., Lucin, P. and Koszinowski, U. H. (1992) Cytomegalovirus prevents antigen presentation by blocking the transport of peptide loaded major histocompatibility complex class I molecules into the medial-golgi compartment. J. Exp. Med. 176:729-738.

Del Val, M., Munch, K., Reddehase, M. J. and Koszinowski, U. H. (1989) Presentation of cytomegalovirus immediate-early antigen cytolytic T lymphocytes is selectively prevented by viral genes expressed in the early phase. Cell 58:305-315.

Deryckere, F. and Burgert, H.-G. (1996) Tumor necrosis factor α induces the adenovirus early 3 promoter by activation of NF-κB. J. Biol. Chem. 271:30249-30255.

Deveraux, Q., Ustrell V., Pickart, C. and Rechsteiner, M. (1994) A 26S protease subunit that binds ubiquitin conjugates. J. Biol. Chem. 169:7059-7061.

DeVilliers, E. M. (1989) Heterogeneity of the human papillomavirus group. J. Virol. 63:4898-4903.

Dobblestein, M. and Shenk, T. (1996) Protection against apoptosis by the vaccinia virus SPI-2 (BI3R) gene product. J. Virol. 70:6479-6485.

Domke-Optiz, I. and Swatzkym, R. (1990) Natural resistance to herpes simplex virus infections: the macrophage-interferon axis. In Boston, A. L. ed. Herpes viruses, the immune system, and AIDS. Kluwer, Dordrecht, p.171-202.

Driscoll, J. and Goldberg, A.L. (1990) The proteasome (multicatalytic protease) is a component of the 1500-kDa proteolytic complex which degrades ubiquitin-conjugated proteins. J. Biol. Chem. 265:4789-4792.

Dubin, G., Socolof, E., Frank, I. and Friedman, H. M. (1991) Herpes simplex virus type 1 Fc receptor protects infected cells from antibody-dependent cellular toxicity. J. Virol. 65:7046-7050.

Elia, A., Laing, K., Schofield, A., Tilleray, V. and Clemens, M. (1996) Regulation of the double-stranded RNA-dependent protein kinase PKR by RNAs encoded by a repeated sequence in the Epstein-Barr virus genome. Nucl. Acids Res. 24:4471-4478.

Enari, M., Hug, H., Nagata, S. (1995) Involvement of an ICE-like protease in Fas-mediated apoptosis. Nature 375:78-81.

Engelstad, M. and Smith, G. L. (1993) The vaccinia virus 42 kDa envelope protein is required for envelopment and egress of extracellular virus and for virulence. Virology 194:627-637.

Epstein, M. A. (1959) Observations on the fine structure of type 5 adenovirus. J. Biophys. Biochem. Cytol. 6:523-524.

Eyler, Y. L., Siwarski, D. F., Huppi, K. E. and Lewis, A. M., Jr. (1997) Down-regulation of Waf1, C2, C3 and major histocompatibility class I loci within an 18cM region of chromosome 17 in adenovirus-transformed mouse cells. Mol. Carcinog. 18:213-220.

Fahnestock, M. J., Johnson, J. I., Feldman, R. M., Neveu, J. M., Lane, W. S. and Bjorkman, P. J. (1995) The MHC class I homologue encoded by human cytomegalovirus binds endogenous peptides. Immunity 3:583-590.

Fenwick, M. L. and Everett, R. D. (1990) Transfer of UL41, the controlling viron-associated host shutoff, between strains of herpes simplex virus. J. Gen. Virol. 71:411-418.

Ferguson, B., Krippl, B., Andrisani, O., Jones, N., Westphal, H. and Rosenberg, M. (1985) E1A 13S and 12S mRNA products made in Escherichia coli both function as nucleus-localised transcription activators but do not directly bind DNA. Mol. Cell. Biol. 5:2653-2661.

Feuerbach, D. and Burgert, H. G. (1993) Novel proteins associated with MHC class I antigens in cells expressing the adenovirus protein E3/19K. EMBO. J: 12:3153-3161.

Feuerbach, D., Etteldorf, S., Ebenau-Jehle, C., Abastado, J. P., Madden, D. and Burgert, H. G. (1994) Identification of amino acids within the MHC class I molecule important for the interaction with adenovirus protein E3/19K. J. Immunol. 153:1626-1636.

Fitzgerald-Bocarsly, P., Felman, M., Curl, S., Schnell, J. and Denny, T. (1989) Positively selected Leu-11a (CD16+) cells require the presence of accessory cells or factors for the lysis of herpes simplex virus-infected fibroblasts but not herpes simplex virus-infected Raji. J. Immunol. 143:1318-1326.

Flomenberg, P., Gutierrez, E. and Hogan, K. T. (1994) Identification of class I MHC regions which bind to the adenovirus E3-19k protein. Mol. Immunol. 31:1277-1284.

Flyer, D. C., Pretell, J., Campbell, A. E., Liao, W. S. L., Tevathia, M. J., Taylor, J. M. and Tevithia, S. S. (1983) Biology of simian virus 40 (SV40) transplantation antigen (TAg). Tumorigenic potential of mouse cells transformed by SV40 in high responder C57BL/6 mice and correlation with the persistance of SV40 TAg, early proteins and viral sequences. Virology 131:207-220.

Frank, I. and Friedman, H. M. (1989) A novel function of the herpes simplex virus type 1 Fc receptor: participation in bipolar bridging of antiviral immunolglobulin G. J. Virol. 63:4479-4488.

Friedman, D. J. and Ricciardi, R. P. (1988) Adenovirus type 12 E1A represses accumulation of MHC class I mRNAs at the level of transcription. Virology 165:303-305.

Frisan, T., Sjoberg, J., Dolcetti, R., Boiocchi, M., De Re, V., Carbone, A., Brautbar, C., Battat, S., Biberfeld, P., Eckman, M., Ost, A., Christensson, B., Sundstrom, C., Bjorkholm, M., Pisa, M. and Masucci, M.G. (1995) Local suppression of Epstein-Barr virus (EBV)-specific cytotoxicity in biopsies of EBV-positive Hodgkin's disease. Blood 86:1493-1501.

Fruh, K., Gossen, M., Wang, K., Bujard, H., Peterson, P. A. and Yang, Y. (1994) Displacement of housekeeping proteasome subunits by MHC-encoded LMPs: a newly discovered mechanism for modulating the multicatalytic proteinase complex. EMBO J. 13:3236-3244.

Fruh, K., Ahn, K., Djaballah, H., Sempe, P., van Endert, P. M., Tampe, R. Peterson, P. A. and Yang, Y. (1995) A viral inhibitor of peptide transporters for antigen presentation. Nature 375:415-418.

Fujii, M., Sassone-Corsi, P. and Verma, I. (1988) c-fos promoter trans-activation by the tax1 protein of human T-cell leukemia virus type I. Proc. Natl. Acad. Sci. USA. 85:8526-8530.

Gao, J. L. and Murphy, P. M. (1994) Human cytomegalovirus open reading frame US28 encodes a functional chemokine receptor. J. Biol. Chem. 269:28539-28542.

Ge, R., Kralli, A., Weinmann, R. and Ricciardi, R. P. (1992) Down-regulation of the major histocompatibility class I enhancer in adenovirus 12-transformed cells is accompanied by an increase in factor binding. J. Virol. 66:6969-6978.

Ge, R., Liu, X., Ricciardi, R. P. (1994) E1A oncogene of adenovirus 12 mediates trans-repression of MHC class I transcription in Ad5/Ad12 somatic hybrid transformed cells. Virology 203:389-392.

Ghadge, G. D., Swaminathan, S., Katze, M. G. and Thimmapaya, B. (1991) Binding of the adenovirus VAI RNA to the interferon induced 68-kDa protein kinase correlates with its function. Proc. Natl. Acad. Sci. USA. 88:7140-7144.

Gilbert, M. J., Riddell, S. R., Plachter, B. and Greenberg, P. D. (1996) Cytomegalovirus selectively blocks antigen processing and presentation of its immediate-early gene product. Nature 383:720-722.

Ginsberg, H. S., Pereira, H. G., Valentine, R. C. and Wilcox, W. C. (1966) A proposed terminology for the adenovirus antigens and virion morphological subunits. Virology 28:782-783.

Goebel, S. J., Johnson, G. P., Perkus, M. E., Davis, S. W., Winslow, J. P. and Paoletti, E. (1990) The complete DNA sequence of vaccinia virus. Virology 179:247-266.

Golding, H., Robey, F. A., Gates III, F. T., Linder, W., Beining P. R., Hoffman, T. and Golding, B. (1988) Identification of homologous regions in human immunodeficiency virus 1 gp41 and human MHC class II beta 1 domain. J. Exp. Med. 167:914-923.

Gooding, L. R. (1982) Characterisation of a progressive tumor from C3H fibroblasts transformed in vitro with SV40 virus. Immunoresistance in vivo correlates with phenotypic loss of H-2K^b. J. Immunol. 129:1306-1312.

Gooding, L. R., Sofola, I. O., Tollefson, A. E., Duerkson-Hughes, P. and Wold, W. S. (1990) The adenovirus E3-14.7K protein is a general inhibitor of tumor necrosis factor-mediated cytolysis. J. Immunol. 145:3080-3086.

Graham, K. A., Lalani, A. S., Macen, J. L., Ness, T. L., Barry, M., Liu, L., Lucas, A., Clark Lewis, I., Moyer, R. W. and McFadden, G. (1997) The T1/35kDa family of poxvirus-secreted proteins bind chemokines and modulate leukocyte influx into virus-infected tissues. Virology 229:12-24.

Green, M., Pina, M., Kimes, R., Wensink, P. C., Machattie, L. A. and Thomas, C. A. (1967) Adenovirus DNA, I. Molecular weight and conformation. Proc. Natl. Acad. Sci. USA. 57:1302-1309.

Gregory, C. P., Murray, R., Edwards, C. F. and Rickinson, A. B. (1988) Down regulation of cell adhesion molecules LFA-3 and ICAM-1 in Epstein-Barr virus-positive Burkitt's lymphoma underlies tumor escape from virus specific T cell surveillance. J. Exp. Med. 167:1811-1824.

Haegy, W., Kelley, V. E., Strom, T. B., Mayer, K., Shapiro, H. M., Mandel, R. and Finberg, R. (1984) Decreased expression of human class II antigens on monocytes from patients with aquired immune deficiency syndrome. J. Clin. Invest. 74:2089-2096.

Hay, N., Skolnick-David, H. and Aloni, Y. (1982) Attenuation in the control of SV40 gene expression. Cell 29:183-193.

He, B., Gross, M. and Roizman, B. (1997) The $\gamma_1$34.5 protein of herpes simplex virus 1 complexes with protein phosphatase 1α to dephosphorylate the α subunit of the eukaryotic translation initiation factor 2 and preclude the shutoff of protein synthesis by double-stranded RNA-activated protein kinase. Proc. Natl. Acad. Sci. 94:843-848.

Heinkelein, M., Pilz, S. and Jassoy, C. (1996) Inhibition of CD95 (Fas/Apo1)-mediated apoptosis by vaccinia virus WR. Clin. Exp. Immunol. 103:8-14.

Henderson, S., Rowe, M., Gregory, C., Croom-Carter, D., Wang, F., Longnecker, R., Kieff, E. and Rickinson, A.B. (1991) Induction of bcl-2 expression by Epstein-Barr virus latent membrane protein-1 projects B cells from programmed cell death. Cell 65:1107-1115.

Hengel, H., Koopmann, J. O., Flohr, T., Muranyi, W., Goulmy, E., Hammerling, G. J., Koszinowski, U. and Momburg, F. (1997) A viral ER-resident glycoprotein inactivates the MHC-encoded peptide transporter. Immunity 6:623-632.

Hidaka, Y., Sakai, Y., Toh, Y. and Mori, R. (1991) Glycoprotein C of herpes simplex virus type 1 is essential for the virus to evade antibody-independent complement-mediated virus inactivation and lysis of virus-infected cells. J. Gen. Virol. 72:915-921.

Hill, A. B., Barnett, B. C., McMichael, A. J. and McGeoch, D. J. (1994) HLA class I molecules are not transported to the cell surface in cells infected with herpes simplex virus types 1 and 2. J. Immunol. 152:2736-2741.

Hill, A., Jugovic, P., York, I., Russ, G., Bennink, J., Yewdell, J., Pleogh, H. and Johnson, D. (1995) Herpes simplex virus turns off the TAP to evade host immunity. Nature 375:411-415.

Hill, A. B. and Masucci, M. G. (1998) Avoiding immunity and apoptosis: manipulation of the host environment by herpes simplex virus and Epstein-Barr virus. Sem Virol. 8:361-368.

Hirano, T. (1992) The biology of interleukin-6. Chem. Immunol. 51:153-156.

Hoffman, P., Yaffe, M. B., Hoffman, B. L., Yei, S., Wold, W. S. and Carlin, C. (1992) Characterisation of the adenovirus E3 protein that down-regulates the epidermal growth factor receptor. J. Biol. Chem. 267:13480-13487.

Ihle, J. N. (1996) STATs: signal transduction and activation of transcription. Cell 84:331-334.

Isaacs, S. N., Kotwal, G. J. and Moss, B. (1992) Vaccinia virus complement-control protein prevents antibody-dependent complement-enhanced neutralization of infectivity and contributes to virulence. Proc. Natl. Acad. Sci. USA. 89:628-632.

Isaacs, S. N. and Moss, B. (1994) Inhibition of complement activation by vaccinia virus. In: McFadden, G. ed. Viroceptors, virokines and related immune modulators encoded by DNA viruses. Austin: R. G. Landes Company; p.55-66.

Janaswami, P. M., Kalvakolanu, D. V. R., Zhang, Y. and Sen, G. C. (1992) Transcriptional repression of interleukin-6 gene by adenoviral E1A proteins. J. Biol. Chem. 267:24886-24891.

Jelinek, T., Pereira, D. S. and Graham, F. L. (1994) Tumorigenicity of adenovirus-transformed rodent cells is influenced by at least two regions of adenovirus type 12 early region 1A. J. Virol. 68:888-896.

Johnson, D. C. and Feenstra, V. (1987) Identification of a novel herpes simplex virus type 1-induced glycoprotein which complexes with gE and binds immunoglobulin. J. Virol. 61:2208-2216.

Johnson, D. C., Frame, M. C., Ligas, M. W., Cross, A. M. and Stow, N. D. (1988) Herpes simplex virus immunoglobulin G Fc receptor activity depends on a complex of two viral glycoproteins, gE and gI. J. Virol. 62:1347-1354.

Johnson, D. C. and Hill, A. B. (1998) Herpesvirus evasion of the immune system. Curr. Top. Microbiol. Immunol. 232:149-177.

Jones, T. R., Hanson, L. K., Sun, L., Slater, J. S., Stenberg, R. M. and Campbell, A. E. (1995) Multiple independent loci within the human cytomegalovirus unique short region down-regulate expression of major histocompatibility complex class I heavy chains. J. Virol. 69:4830-4841.

Jones, T. R., Wiertz, E. J. H. J., Sun, L., Fish, K. N., Nelson, J. A. and Ploegh, H. L. (1996) Human cytomegalovirus US3 impairs transport and maturation of major histocompatibility complex class I heavy chains. Proc. Natl. Acad. Sci. USA. 93:11327-11333.

Kagi, D., Ledermann, B., Burki, K., Zinkernagel, R. M. and Hengartner, H. (1996) Molecular mechanisms of lymphocyte-mediated cytotoxicity and their role in immunological protection and pathogenesis *in vivo*. Annu. Rev. Immunol. 14:207-232.

Kanno, T., Brown, K., Franzoso, G. and Siebenlist, U. (1994) Kinetic analysis of human T-cell leukemia virus type 1 Tax-mediated activation of NF-κB. Mol. Cell. Biol. 14:6443-6451.

Kanno, T., Brown, K. and Siebenlist, U. (1995) Evidence in support of a role for human T-cell leukemia virus type 1 Tax in activating NF-kappa B via stimulation of signaling pathways. J. Biol. Chem. 270:11745-11748.

Katoh, S., Ozawa, K., Kondoh, S., Soeda, E., Israel, A., Shiroki, K., Fujinaga, K., Itakura, K., Gachelin, G. and Yokoyama, K. (1990) Identification of sequences responsible for positive and negative regulation by E1A in the promoter of H-2K^{bm1} class I MHC gene. EMBO. J: 9:127-135.

Kerkau, T., Gernert, S., Kneitz, C. and Schimple, A. (1992) Mechanism of MHC class I downregulation in HIV infected cells. Immunobiology 184:402.

Kerkau, T., Schmitt-Landgraf, R., Schimple, A. and Wecker, E. (1989) Downregulation of HLA class I antigens in HIV-1-infected cells. AIDS Res. Hum. Retroviruses 5:613.

Kettle, S., Alcami, A., Khanna, A., Ehret, R., Jassoy, C. and Smith, G. L., (1997) Vaccinia virus serpin B13R (SPI-2) inhibits interleukin-1β converting enzyme and protects virus-infected cells from TNF- and Fas-mediated apoptosis but does not prevent IL-1β-induced fever. J. Gen. Virol. 78:677-685.

Khanna, R., Burrows, S. R., Argaet, V. and Moss, D. J. (1994) Endoplasmic reticulum signal sequence facilitated transport of peptide epitopes restores immunogenicity of an antigen processing defective tumor cell line. Int. Immunol. 6:639-645.

Khanna, R., Burrows, S. R. and Moss, D. J. (1995) Immune regulation in Epstein-Barr virus-associated diseases. Microbiol. Rev. 59:387-405.

Khanna, R., Burrows, S. R., Suhrbier, A., Jacob, C. A., Griffin, H., Misko, I. S., Sculley, T. B., Rowe, M., Rickinson, A. B. and Moss, D. J. (1993) EBV peptide epitope sensitization restores human cytotoxic T cell recognition of Burkitt's lymphoma cells. Evidence for a critical role for ICAM-2. J. Immunol. 150:5154-5162.

Kieff, E. (1996) Epstein-Barr virus and its replication. In: Fields, B. N., Knipe, D. M. and Howlet, P. M. eds. Fields virology. Raven-Lippincott, Philadelphia, p.2343-2396.

Kimura, A. Israel, A., Le Bail, O., Kourilsky, P. (1986) Detailed analysis of the mouse H-2K^b promoter: enhancer-like sequences and their role in the regulation of class I gene expression. Cell 44:261-272.

Kitchingman, G. R. and Westphal, H. (1980) The structure of adenovirus 2 early nuclear and cytoplasmic RNAs. J. Mol. Biol. 137:23-48.

Klenerman, P., Rowland-Jones, S., McAdam, S., Edwards, J., Daenke, S, Lallo, D., Koppe, B., Rosenberg, W., Boyd, D., Edwards, A., Giangrande, P., Phillips, R. E. and McMichael, A. J. (1994) Cytotoxic T-cell activity antagonized by naturally occurring HIV-1 Gag variants. Nature 369:403-407.

Koelle, D. M., Tigges, M. A., Burke, R. L., Symington, F. W., Riddell, S. R. Abbo, H. and Corey, L. (1993)Herpes simplex virus infection of human fibroblasts and keratinocytes inhibits recognition by cloned CD8+ cytotoxic T lymphocytes. J.Clin. Invest. 91:961-968.

Komiyama, T., Ray, C. A., Pickup, D. J., Howard, A. D., Thornberry, N. A., Peterson, E. P. and Salvesen, G. (1994) Inhibition of interleukin-1 beta converting enzyme by the cowpox virus serpin CrmA: An example of cross-class inhibition. J. Biol. Chem. 269:19331-19337.

Kotwal, G. J., Isaacs, S. N., McKenzie, R., Frank, M. M. and Moss, B. (1990) Inhibition of the complement cascade by the major secretory protein of the vaccinia virus. Science 250:827-830.

Krajcsi, P., Dimitrov, T., Hermiston, T. W., Tollefson, A. E., Ranheim, T. S., Vande Pol, S. B., Stephenson, A. H. and Wold, W. S. (1996) The adenovirus E3-14.7K protein and the E3-10.4K/14.5K complex of proteins, which independently inhibit tumor necrosis factor (TNF)-induced apoptosis, also independently inhibit TNF-induced release of arachidonic acid. J. Virol. 70:4904-4913.

Kralli, A., Ge, R., Graeven, U., Ricciardi, R. P. and Weinmann, R. (1992) Negative regulation of the major histocompatibility class I enhancer in adenovirus type 12-transformed cells via a retinoic acid response element. J. Virol. 66:6979-6988.

Kushner, D. B., Pereira, D. S., Liu, X., Graham, F. L. and Ricciardi, R. P. (1996) The first exon of Ad12 E1A excluding the transactivation domain mediates differential binding of COUP-TF and NF-κB to the MHC class I enhancer in transformed cells. Oncogene 12:143-151.

Kushner, D.B. and Ricciardi, R.P. (1999). Reduced phosphorylation of p50 is responsible for diminished NF-kappaB binding to the major histocompatibility complex class I enhancer in adenovirus 12-transformed cells. Mol. Cell Biol. 19, 2169-2179.

Lee, S. B. and Esteban, M. (1994) The interferon-induced double-stranded RNA-activated protein kinase induces apoptosis. Virology 199:491-496.

Leonard, G. T. and Sen, G. C. (1996) Effects of adenovirus E1A protein on interferon signalling. Virology 224:25-33.

Levitskaya, J., Coram, M., Levitsky, V., Imreh, S., Steigerwald-Mullen, P. M., Klein, G., Kurilla, M. H. and Masucci, M. G. (1995) Inhibition of antigen processing by the internal repeat region of the Epstein-Barr virus nuclear antigen-1. Nature 375:685-688.

Levy, F., Gabathuler, R., Larsson, R. and Kvist, S. (1991) ATP is required for *in vitro* assembly of MHC class I antigens but not for transfer of peptides across the ER membrane. Cell 67:265-274.

Lin, L., DeMartino, G. and Greene, W. (1998) Cotranslational Biogenesis of NF-κB p50 by the 26S proteasome. Cell 92:819-828.

Liu, X., Ge, R., Westmoreland, S., Cooney, A., Tsai, S. and Ricciardi, R. P. (1994) Negative regulation by the R2 element of the MHC class I enhancer in adenovirus-12 transformed cells correlates with high levels of COUP-TF binding. Oncogene 9:2183-2190.

Li, Z., Turk, S. M. and Hutt-Fletcher, L. M. (1995) The Epstein-Barr virus (EBV) BZLF2 gene product associates with the gH and gL homologs of EBV and carries an epitope critical to infection of B cells but not epithelial cells. J. Virol. 69:3987-3994.

Logeat, F., Israel, N., Ten, R., Blank, V., Le Bail, O., Kourilsky, P. and Israel, A. (1991) Inhibition of transcription factors belonging to the rel/NK-kappaB family by a transdominant negative mutant. EMBO. J. 10:1827-1832.

Los, M., Van, D. C. M., Penning, L. C., Schenk, H., Westendorp, M., Baeuerle, P. A., Droge, W., Krammer, P. H., Fiers, W. and Schulze-Osthoff, K. (1995) Requirement of an ICE/CED-3 protease for Fas/APO-1-mediated apoptosis. Nature 375:81-83.

Macen, J. L., Graham, K. A., Lee, S. F., Schreiber, M., Boshkov, L. K. and McFadden, G. (1996) Expression of the myxoma virus tumor necrosis factor receptor homologue and M11L genes is required to prevent virus-induced apoptosis in infected rabbit T lymphocytes. Virology 218:232-237.

Marchini, A., Cohen, J. I., Wang, F. and Kieff, E. (1992a) A selectable marker allows investigation of a nontransforming Epstein-Barr virus mutant. J. Virol. 66:3214-3219.

Marchini, A., Longnecker, R. and Kieff, E. (1992b) Epstein-Barr virus (EBV)-negative B-lymphoma cell lines for clonal isolation and replication of EBV recombinants. J. Virol. 66:4972-4981.

Margulies, B. J. Browne, H. and Gibson, W. (1996) Identification of the human cytomegalovirus G protein-coupled receptor homologue encoded by UL33 in infected cells and envelope virus particles. Virology 225:111-125.

Martin, S., Moss, B., Berman, P. W., Laskey, L. A. and Rousse, B. T. (1987) Mechanisms of antiviral immunity induced by a vaccinia virus recombinant expressing herpes simplex virus type 1 glycoprotein D: cytotoxic T cells. J. Virol. 61:726-734.

McCarthy, N. J., Hazlewood, S. A., Huen, D. S., Rickinson, A. B. and Williams, G. T. (1996) The Epstein-Barr virus gene BHRF1, a homologue of the cellular oncogene Bcl-2, inhibits apoptosis induced by gamma radiation and chemotherapeutic drugs. Adv Exp. Med. Biol. 406:83-97.

McFadden, G. and Barry, M (1998) How pox viruses oppose apoptosis. Sem. Virol. 8:429-442.

McKenzie, R., Kotwal, G. J., Moss, B., Hammer, C. H. and Frank, M.M. (1992) Regulation of complement activity by vaccinia virus complement control protein. J. Infect. Dis. 166:1245-1256.

McNearney, T. A., Odell, C., Holers, V. M., Spear, P. G. and Atkinson, J. P. (1987) Herpes simplex virus glycoproteins gC-1 and gC-2 bind to the third component of complement and provide protection against complement-mediated neutralization of viral infectivity. J. Exp. Med. 166:1525-1535.

Meijer, I., Boot, A. J. M., Mahibin, G., Zantema, A. and van der Eb, A. J. (1992) Reduced binding activity of the transcription factor NF-κB accounts for the MHC class I repression in adenovirus 12 E1-transformed cells. Cell. Immunol. 145:56-65.

Meijer, I., Jochemsen, A. G., de Wit, C. M., Bos, J. L., Morello, D. and van der Eb, A. J. (1989) Adenovirus type 12 E1A down regulates expression of a transgene under control of a major histocompatibility complex class I promoter: evidence for transcriptional control. J. Virol. 63:4039-4042.

Meijer, I., van Dam, H., Boot, A. J. M., Bos, J. L., Zantema, A. and van der Eb, A. J. (1991) Co-regulated expression of *jun*B and MHC class I genes in adenovirus-transformed celss. Oncogene 6:911-916.

Miller, W. E., Earp, H. S. and Raab-Traub, N. (1995) The Epstein-Barr virus latent membrane protein 1 induces expression of the epidermal growth factor receptor. J. Virol. 69:4390-4398.

Miura, M., Zhu, H., Rotello, R., Hatweig, E. A. and Yuan, J. (1993) Induction of apoptosis in fibroplasts by IL-1β-converting enzyme, a mammalian homologue of the *C. elegans* cell death gene *ced*-3. Cell 75:653-660.

Muzio, M., Salvesen, G. S. and Dixit, V. M. (1997) FLICE induced apoptosis in a cell-free system: Cleavage of caspase zymogens. J. Biol. Chem. 400:15-18.

Nakagomi, H., Dolcetti, R., Bejarano, M. T., Pisa, P., Kiessling, R. and Masucci, M. G. (1994) The Epstein-Barr virus latent membrane protein-1 (LMP1) induces interleukin-10 production in Burkitt lymphoma lines. Int. J. Cancer 57:240-244.

Nash, A. A., Jayasuriya, A., Phelan, J., Cobbold, S. P., Waldmann, H. and Prospero, T. (1987) Different roles for L3T4+ and Lyt 2+ T cell subsets in the control of an acute herpes simplex virus infection of the skin and nervous system. J. Gen. Virol. 68:825-833.

Neote, K., DiGregorio, d., Mak, J. Y., Horuk, R. and Schall, T. J. (1993) Molecular cloning, functional expression, and signaling characteristics of a CC chemokine receptor. Cell 72:415-425.

Newmaster, R. S., Mylin, L. M., Fu, T.-M. and Tevethia, S. S. (1998) Role of a subdominant H-2K^b-restricted SV40 tumor antigen cytotoxic T lymphocyte epitope in tumor rejection. Virology 244:427-441.

Ng, S. C., Mertz, J. E., Sanden-Will, S. and Bina, M. (1985) Simian virus 40 maturation in cells harboring mutants deleted in the agnogene. J. Biol. Chem. 260:1127-1132.

Niedobitek, G., Young, L. S. and Herbst, H. (1997) Epstein-Barr virus infection and the pathogenesis of malignant lymphomas. Cancer Surveys 30:143-162.

Nong, Y., Kandil, O., Tobin, E. H., Rose, R. M. and Remold, H. G. (1991) The HIV core protein p24 inhibits interferon-gamma-induced increase of HLA-DR and cytochrome b heavy chain mRNA levels in the human monocyte-like cell line THP1. Cell. Immunol. 132:10-16.

Ortmann, B., Androlewicz, M. J. and Cresswell, P. (1994) MHC class I/β2-microglobulin complexes associate with transporters before peptide binding. Nature, 368:864-867.

Ozawa, K., Hagiwara, H., Tang, X., Saka, F., Kitabayashi, I., Shiroki, K., Fujinaga, K., Israel, A., Gachelin, G. and Yokoyama, K. (1993) Negative regulation of the gene for H-2K^b class I antigen by adenovirus 12-E1A is mediated by a CAA repeated element. J. Biol. Chem. 268:27258-27268.

Paabo, S., Nilsson, T. and Peterson, P. A. (1986) Adenoviruses of subgenera B, C, D, and E modulate cell-surface expression of major histocompatibility complex class I antigens. Proc. Natl. Acad. Sci. USA. 83:9665-9669.

Pan, S., Abramczuk, J. and Knowles, B. (1987) Immune control of SV40-induced tumors in mice. Int. J. Cancer 39:722-728.

Pereira, D. S., Rosenthal, K. L. and Graham, F. L. (1995) Identification of adenovirus E1A regions which affect MHC class I expression and susceptibility to cytotoxic T lymphocytes. Virology 211.268-277.

Perricaudet, M., Akusjarvi, G., Virtanen, A. and Pettersson, U. (1979) Structure of two spliced mRNAs from the transforming region of human subgroup C adenoviruses. Nature 281:694-696.

Phillips, J. H., Chang, C. W., Mattson, J., Gumperz, J. E., Parham, P. and Lanier, L. L. (1996) CD94 and a novel associated protein (94AP) from a NK cell receptor involved in the recognition of HLA-A, HLA-B and HLA-C allotypes. Immunity 5:163-172.

Phillips, R. E., Rowland-Jones, S., Nixon, D. F., Gotch, F. M., Edwards, J. P. Ogunlesi, A. O. Elvin, I. G., Rothbard, J. A., Bangham, C. R. M., Rizza, C. R. and McMichael, A. J. (1991) Human immunodeficiency virus genetic variation that can escape cytotoxic T cell recognition. Nature 354:453.

Proffitt, J. A. and Blair, G. E. (1997) The MHC-encoded TAP1/LMP2 bidirectional promoter is down-regulated in highly oncogenic adenovirus type 12 transformed cells. FEBS lett. 400:141-144.

Proffitt, J. L., Sharma, E. Blair, G. E. (1994) Adenovirus 12-mediated down-regulation of the major histocompatibility complex (MHC) class I promoter: identification of a negative regulatory element responsive to Ad12 E1A. Nucl. Acids Res. 22:4779-4788.

Puppo, F., Orlandini, A., Ruzzenenti, R., Comuzio, S., Salamito, A., Farrinelli, A., Stagnovo, R. and Indiveri, F. (1990) HLA class I soluble antigen serum levels in HIV-positive subjects - correlation with cellular and serological parameters. Cancer Detection and prevention 14:321-323.

Quan, L. T., Caputo, A., Bleakley, R. C., Pickup, D. J. and Salvesen, G. S. (1995) Granzyme B is inhibited by the cowpox virus serpin cytokine response modifier A. J. Biol. Chem. 270:10377-10379.

Radsak, K., Kern, H., Reis, B., Reschke, M., Mockenhaupt, T. and Eickmann, M. (1998) Human cytomegalovirus. Aspects of viral morphogenesis and of processing and transport of viral glycoproteins. In: DNA tumor viruses, Barbanti-Brodano, G., Bendinelli, M., Friedman, H. eds. Plenum Press.

Rapoport, T. A., Jungnickel, B. and Kutay, U. (1996) Protein transport across the eukaryotic endoplasmic reticulum and bacterial inner membranes. Annu. Rev. Biochem. 65:271-303.

Ray, C. A., Black, R. A., Kronheim, S. R., Greenstreet, T. A., Sleath. P. R., Salvesen, G. S. and Pickup, D. J. (1992) Viral inhibition of inflammation: cowpox virus encodes an inhibitor of the interleukin-1β converting enzyme. Cell 69:597-604.

Reyburn, H. O. M., Vales-Gomez, M., Sheu, E. G., Pazmany, L., Davis, D. M. and Strominger, J. L. (1997) Human NK cells: their ligands, receptors and functions. Immunol. Rev. 155:119-125.

Rooney, C. M., Edwards, C. F., Lenoir, G. M., Rupani, H. and Rickinson, A. B. (1986) Differential activation of cytotoxic responses by Burkitt's lymphoma (BL)-cell lines: relationship to the BL-cell surface phenotype. Cell. Immunol. 102:99-112.

Rooney, C. M., Rickinson, A. B., Moss, D. J., Lenoir, G. M. and Epstein, M. A. (1985a) Cell-mediated immunosurveillance mechanisms and the pathogenesis of Burkitt's lyphoma. In: Burkitt's lymphoma: A human cancer model, vol. 60. Lenoir, G. M., O'Connor, G. T., Olweny, C. L. M. ed. Lyon: International agency for research on cancer, p.249-264.

Rooney, C. M., Rowe, M., Wallace, L. E. and Rickinson, A. B. (1985b) Epstein-Barr virus-positive Burkitt's lymphoma cells not recognised by virus-specific T-cell surveillance. Nature 317:629-631.

Rotem-Yedudar, R., Winograd, S., Sela, S., Coligan, J. E. and Ehrlich, R. (1994) Down-regulation of peptide transporter genes in cell lines transformed with the highly oncogenic adenovirus 12. J. Exp. Med. 180:477-488.

Rotem-Yedudar, R., Groettrup, M., Soza, A., Kloetzel, P. M. and Ehrlich, R. (1996) LMP-associated proteolytic activities and TAP-dependent peptide transport for class I MHC molecules are suppressed in cell lines transformed by the highly oncogenic adenovirus 12. J. Exp. Med. 183:499-514.

Rowe, M. and Masucci, M. G. (1995) Cellular adhesion molecules and MHC antigens in cells infected with Epstein-Barr virus: implications for immune recognition. In: Modulation of MHC antigen expression and disease. Blair, G. E., Pringle, C. R. and Maudsley, D. J., eds. Cambridge University Press. p.261-277.

Rowe, W. P., Huebner, R. J., Gillmore, L. K., Parrott, R. H. and Ward, T. G. (1953) Isolation of a cytopathogenic agent from human adenoids undergoing spontaneous degeneration in tissue culture. Proc. Soc. Exp. Biol. Med. 84:570.

Sadasivan, B., Lehner, P. J., Ortmann, B., Spies, T. and Cresswell, P. (1996) Roles for calreticulin and a novel glycoprotein, tapasin, in the interaction of MHC class I molecules with TAP. Immunity 5:103-114.

Salazar-Onfray, F., Petersson, M. and Franksson, L., Matsuda, M., Blankenstein, T., Karre, K. and Kiessling, R. (1995) IL-10 converts mouse lymphoma cells to a CTL-resistant, NK-sensitive phenotype with low but peptide-inducible MHC class I expression. J. Immunol. 154:6291-6298.

Sample, J., Brooks, L., Sample, C., Young, L., Rowe, M., Gregory, C., Rickinson, A. and Kieff, E. (1991) Restricted Epstein-Barr virus protein expression in Burkitt lymphoma is due to a different Epstein-Barr nuclear antigen 1 transcriptional initiation site. Proc. Natl. Acad. Sci. USA. 88:6343-6347.

Sarnow, P., Ho, Y., Williams, J. and Levine, A. (1982) Adenovirus E1b-58kd tumor antigen and SV40 large tumor antigen are physically associated with the same 54 kd cellular protein in transformed cells. Cell 28:387-394.

Schall, T. J., Stein, B., Gorgone, G. and Bacon, K. B. (1994) Cytomegalovirus encodes a functional receptor for CC chemokines. In. Viroceptors, virokines and related immune modulators encoded by DNA viruses McFadden, G. ed. Landes, R. G. p.201-214.

Scheppler, J. A., Nicholson, K. A., Swan, D. C., Ahmed-Ansari, A. and McDougal, J. S. (1989) Downregulation of MHC-I in a CD4+ cell line, CEM-E5, after HIV-1 infection. J. Immunol. 143:2858.

Schmid, D. S. and Rousse, B. T. (1992) The role of T cell immunity in control of herpes simplex virus. Curr. Top. Microbiol. Immunol. 179:57-74.

Schmitz, M. L., Indorf, A., Limbourg, F. P., Stadtler, H., Traeckner, E B.-M. and Baeurle, P. A. (1996) The dual effect of adenovirus type 5 E1A 13S protein on NF-κB activation is antagonizedby E1B 19K. Mol. Cell. Biol. 15:4052-4063.

Schouten, G. J., van der Eb and Zantema, A. (1995) Down-regulation of MHC class I expression due to interference with p105-NF-κB1 processing by Ad12 E1A. EMBO. J. 14:1498-1507.

Schrier, P. I., Bernards, R., Vaessen, R. T. M. J., Houweling, A. and van der Eb, A. J. (1983) Expression of class I major histocompatibility antigens is switched off by highly oncogenic adenovirus 12 in transformed rat cells. Nature 305:771-775.

Schwartz, O., Marechal, V., Le Gall, S., Lemonnier, F. and Heard, J.-M. (1996) Endocytosis of major histocompatibility complex class I molecules is induced by the HIV Nef protein. Nature Med. 2:338.

Seidel-Dugan, C., Ponce de Leon, M., Friedman, H. M., Eisenberg, R. J. and Cohen, G. H. (1990) Identification of C3b-binding regions on herpes simplex virus type 2 glycoprotein C. J. Virol. 64:1897-1906.

Sester, M. and Burgert, H. G. (1994) Conserved cysteine residues within the E3/19K protein of adenovirus type 2 are essential for binding to major histocompatibility complex antigens. J. Virol. 68:5423-5432.

Sharipo, A., Imreh, M., Leonchiks, A., Imreh, S. and Massuci, M. G. (1998) A minimal glycine-alanine repeat prevents the interaction of ubiquitinated IκBα with the proteasome: a new mechanism for selective inhibition of proteolysis. Nature Medicine 4:939-944.

Shirayoshi, Y., Miyazaki, J., Burke, P., Hamada, K., Appella, E. and Ozato, K. (1987) Binding of multiple nuclear factors to the 5′upstream regulatory element of the murine major histocompatibility class I gene. Mol. Cell. Biol. 7:4542-4548.

Sivori, S., Vitale, M., Bottino, C., Marcenaro, E., Sanseverino, L., Parolini, S., Moretta, L. and Moretta, A. (1996) CD94 functions as a natural killer cell inhibitory receptor for different HLA class I alleles: Identification of the inhibitory form of CD94 by the use of novel monoclonal antibodies. Eur. J. Immunol. 26:2487-2492.

Smith, G. L., Chan, Y. S. and Howard, S. T. (1991) Nucleotide sequence of 42 kbp of vaccinia virus strain WR from near the right interted terminal repeat. J. Gen. Virol. 72:1349-1376.

Smith, G. L., Symons, J. A., Khanna, A., Vanderplasschen, A. and Alcami, A., (1997) Vaccinia virus immune evasion. Immunol. Revs. 159:137-154.

Smith, G. L., Symons, J. A. and Alcami, A. (1998) Poxviruses: interfering with interferon. Sem. Virol. 8:409-418.

Sparer, T. E. and Gooding, L. R. (1998) Suppression of MHC class I antigen presentation by human adenoviruses. Curr. Top. Microbiol. Immunol. 232:135-147.

Sprengel, J., Schmitz, B., Hens-Neitgel, D., Zock, C. and Doerfler, W. (1994) Nucleotide sequence of human adenovirus 12: comparative functional analysis. J. Virol. 68:379-389.

Spriggs, M. K., Hruby, D. E., Maliszewski, C. R., Pickup, D. J., Sims, J. E., Buller, R. M. and VanSlyke, J. (1992) Vaccinia and cowpox viruses encode a novel secreted interleukin-1 binding protein. Cell 71:145-152.

Stephens, C. and Harlow, E. (1987) Differential splicing yields novel adenovirus 5 E1A mRNAs that encode 30 kd and 35 kd proteins. EMBO. J. 6:2027-2035.

Suh, W. K., Cohen-Doyle, M. F., Fruh, K., Wang, K., Peterson, P. A. and Williams, D. B., (1994) Interaction of MHC class I molecules with the transporter associated with antigen processing. Scence 264: 1322-1326.

Symons, J. A., Alcami, A. and Smith, G. L. (1995) Vaccinia virus encodes a soluble type I interferon receptor of novel structure and broad species specificity. Cell 81:551-560.

Takeda, T., Nakajima, K., Kojima, H. and Hirano, T. (1994) E1A repression of IL-6 induced gene activation by blocking the assembly of IL 6 response element binding complexes. J. Immunol. 153:4573 4582.

Tanaka, K. and Tevethia, S. S. (1988) Differential effect of adenovirus 2 E3/19K glycoprotein on the expression of H-2K^b and H-2D^b restricted SV40-specific CTL-mediated lysis. Virology 165:357-366.

Tang, X., Li, H.-O., Sakatsuma, O., Ohta, T., Tsutsui, H., Smit, A. F. A., Horikoshi, M., Kourilsky, P., Israel, A., Gachelin, G. and Yokoyama, K. (1995) Cooperativity between an upstream TATA-like element mediates E1A-dependent negative repression of the H-2K^b class I gene. J. Biol. Chem. 270:2327-2336.

Telling, G. C. and Williams, J. (1994) Constructing chimeric type 12/type 5 adenovirus E1A genes and using them to identify an oncogenic determinant of adenovirus type 12. J. Virol. 68:877-887.

Tevethia, S. S. (1980) Immunology of simian virus 40. In: Viral oncology. Raven Press, New York. p. 581-601.

Tevethia, S. S. (1990) Recognition of simian virus 40 T antigen by cytotoxic T lymphocytes. Mol. Biol. Med. 7:83-96.

Tewari, M. and Dixit, V. M. (1995) Fas- and tumor necrosis factor-induced apoptosis is inhibited by the poxvirus crmA gene product. J. Biol. Chem. 270:3255-3260.

Thorley-Lawson, D. A. (1980) The suppression of Epstein-Barr virus *in vitro* occurs after infection but before transformation of the cell. J. Immunol. 124:745-751.

Thorley-Lawson, D. A., Chess, L. and Strominger, J. L. (1977) Suppression on *in vitro* Epstein-Barr virus infection. A new role for adult human lymphocytes. J. Exp. Med. 146:495-508.

Tigges, M. A., Koelle, D., Hartog, K., Sekulovich, R. E., Corey, L. and Burke, R. L. (1992) Human CD8+ herpes simplex virus-specific cytotoxic T-lymphocyte clones recognize diverse virion protein antigens. J. Virol. 66:1622-1634.

Tigges, M. A., Leng, S., Johnson, D. C. and Burke, R. L. (1996) Human herpes simplex virus (HSV)-specific CD8+ CTL clones recognize HSV-2-infected fibroblasts after treatment with IFN-gamma or when virion host shutoff functions are disabled. J. Immunol. 156:3901-3910.

Tomazin, R., Hill, A. B., Jugovic, P., York, I., van Endert, P., Ploegh, H. L., Andrews, D. W. and Johnson, D. C. (1996) Stable binding of the herpes simplex virus ICP47 protein to the peptide binding site of TAP. EMBO J. 15:3256-3266.

Tooze, J. ed. (1984) DNA Tumor Viruses. Cold Spring Harbour Laboratory, New York.

Torsteinsdottir, S., Brautbar, C., Ben Basset, H., Klein, E. and Klein, G. (1988) Differential expression of HLA antigens on human B-cell lines of normal and malignant origin: a consequence of immune surveillance or a phenotype vestige of the progenitor cells? Int. J. Cancer 41:913-919.

Torsteinsdottir, S., Masucci, M. G., Ehlin-Hendricksson, G., Brautbar, G., Basset, G. B., Klein, G. and Klein, E. (1986) Differential dependent sensitivity of human B-cel-derived major histocompatibility complex-restricted T-cell cytotoxicity. Proc. Natl. Acad. Sci. USA. 83:5620-5624.

Trentin, J. J., Yabe, Y. and Taylor, G. (1962) The quest for human cancer viruses. Science 137:835-841.

Tsomides, T. J., Aldovini, A., Johnson, R. P., Walker, B. D., Young, R. A. and Eisen, H. N. (1994) Naturally processed viral peptides recognised by cytotoxic T lymphocytes on cells chronically infected by human immunodeficiency virus type I. J. Exp. Med. 180:1283.

Ulfendahl, P. J., Linder, S. and Kreivi, J. P.,   (1987) A novel adenovirus-2 E1A mRNA encoding a protein with transcription activation properties. EMBO. J. 6:2037-2044.

van der Eb, A. J., van Kesteren, L. W. and van Bruggen, E. F. J. (1969) Structural properties of adenovirus DNAs. Biochem. Biophys. Acta 182:536-541.

Vanderplasschen, A., Hollinshead, M. and Smith, G. L., (1997) Antibodies against vaccinia virus do not neutralise extracellular enveloped virus but prevent virus release from infected cells and comet formation. J. Gen. Virol. 78:2041-2048.

Van Endert, P. M., Tampe, R., Meyer, T. H., Tisch, R., Bach, J-F. and McDevitt, H. O. (1994) A sequential model for peptide binding and transport by the transporters associated with antigen processing. Immunity 1:491-500.

Warren, A. P., Ducroq, D. H., Lehner, P. J. and Borysiewicz, L. K. (1994) Human cytomegalovirus-infected cells have unstable assembly of major histocompatibility complex class I complexes and are resistant to lysis by cytotoxic T lymphocytes. J. Virol. 68:2822-2829.

White, E. (1996) Life, death, and the pursuit of apoptosis. Genes and Dev. 10:1-15.

Wiertz, E. J. H. J., Tortorella, D., Bogyo, M., Yu, J., Mothes, W., Jones, T. R., Rapaport, T. A. and Ploegh, H. L. (1996a) Sec61-mediated transfer of a membrane protein from the endoplasmic reticulum to the proteasome for destruction. Nature 384:432-438.

Wiertz, E. J. H. J., Jones, T. R., Sun, L., Bogyo, M., Geuze, H. J. and Ploegh, H. L. (1996b) The human cytomegalovirus US11 gene product dislocates MHC class I heavy chains from the endoplasmic reticulum to the cytosol. Cell 84:769-779.

Wilcox, W. C., Ginsberg, H. S. and Anderson, T. F. (1963) Structure of type 5 adenovirus. J. Exp. Med. 118:307-313.

Williams, J., Williams, M., Liu, C. and Telling, G. (1995) Assessing the role of E1A in the differential oncogenicity of group A and group C human adenoviruses. Curr. Top. Microbiol. Immunol. 199:149-175.

Wolffe, E. J., Isaacs, S. N. and Moss, B. (1993) Deletion of the vaccinia virus B5R gene encoding a 42-kilodalton membrane glycoprotein inhibits extracellular virus envelope formation and dissemination. J. Virol. 67:4732-4741.

Wright, T. C. and Sun, X. W. (1996) Anogenital papillomavirus infection and neoplasia in immunodeficient women. Obstet. Gynecol. Clin. North Am. 23:861-893.

Yates, J., Warren, N., Reisman, D. and Sugden, B. (1984) A *cis*-acting element from the Epstein-Barr viral genome that permits stable replication of recombinant plasmids in latently infected cells. Proc. Natl. Acad. Sci. USA. 81:3806-3810.

Ye, X., McCarrick, J., Jewett, L. and Knowles, B. B. (1994) Timely immunization subverts the development of periperal nonresponsiveness and suppresses ttumor development in simian virus 40 tumor antigen-transgenic mice. Proc. Natl. Acad. Sci. USA. 91:3916-3920.

York, I. A. and Johnson, D. C. (1993) Direct contact with herpes simplex virus-infected cells results in inhibition of lymphokine-activated killer cells because of cell-to-cell spread of virus. J. Infect. Dis. 168:1127-1132.

York, I. A. and Johnson, D. C. (1994) Inhibition of humoral and cellular immune recognition by herpes simplex virus. In: McFadden, G. ed. Viroceptors, virokines and related immune modulators encoded by DNA viruses. Landes, Austin, p.89-110.

York, I. A., Roop, C., Andrews, D. W., Riddell, S. R., Graham, F. L. and Johnson, D. C. (1994) A cytosolic herpes simplex virus protein inhibits antigen presentation to CD8+ T lymphocytes. Cell 77:525-535.

Yoshida, M., Miyoshi, I. and Hinuma, Y. (1982) Isolation and characterisation of retrovirus from cell lines of human adult T-cell leukemia and its implication in disease. Proc. Natl. Acad. Sci. USA. 79:2031-2035.

Zaitseva, M. B., Mshnikov, S. A., Kozhich, A. T., Frolova, H. A., Makarova, O. D., Pavlikov, S. P., Sidorovich, I. G. and Brondz, B. B. (1992) Antibodies to MHC class II peptides are present in HIV-1-positive sera. Scandinavian J. Immunol. 35:267-273.

zur Hausen, H. (1991) Human papillomaviruses in the pathogenesis of anogenital cancer. Virology 184:9-13.

Zu, Y.-L., Takamatsu, Y. Zhoa, M.-J. Maekawa, T., Handa, H. and Ishii, S. (1992) Transcriptional regulation by a point mutation of adenovirus-2 E1A product lacking DNA binding activity. J. Biol. Chem. 267:20181-20187.

IMMUNITY TO HUMAN PAPILLOMAVIRUSES:

IMPLICATIONS FOR VACCINE DESIGN

Jane C. Steele

CRC Institute for Cancer Studies, University of Birmingham, UK

1. Introduction

Human papillomaviruses (HPVs) are small double-stranded DNA viruses which infect cutaneous and mucosal epithelia at a variety of locations. The HPV genome contains eight open reading frames (ORFs) and a non-coding region containing transcription regulatory sequences and the origin of replication. The early ORFs encode six proteins E1, E2, E4, E5, E6 and E7. Two ORFs in the late region encode the capsid proteins L1 and L2. The E1 and E2 genes are involved in viral DNA replication and transcriptional control (Lambert, 1991), E6 and E7 inhibit the actvity of negative regulators of the cell cycle (see Chapter 6 of this book) and the late proteins, L1 and L2 encode structural proteins. The function of the E4 protein is still unknown, although it has been shown to associate with cytokeratins (Doorbar, 1996; Doorbar et al., 1991; Roberts et al., 1993). Several properties of E5 have beeen observed; it activates both epidermal growth factor receptors and platelet-derived growth factor receptors; inhibits endosomal acidification; and possesses weak transforming activity (Banks and Matlashewski, 1996).

Approximately 130 types of HPV have been identified and classified on the basis of their DNA homology (deVilliers, 1997). A particularly well-studied group of these is associated with diseases of the genital tract and infection is sexually transmitted. These viruses are categorised according to their potential to cause malignancy, so that HPV types 6 and 11 are associated with low-risk disease such as genital warts, and high-risk HPVs such as types 16, 18, 31, 33 and 45 are associated with high-grade cervical intraepithelial lesions and invasive cancer of the cervix.

Other cutaneous types of HPV are also related in rare instances to skin cancer. Individuals with the skin disease epidermodysplasia verruciformis (EV) in particular, often develop skin carcinomas which harbour HPV type 5 or 8 (Orth, 1987). The same viruses are associated with the skin cancers common in immunosuppressed renal transplant recipients (Barr et al., 1989).

The wide acceptance that cell-mediated immunity is vitally involved in the control of HPV infection, and the fact that certain types of HPV are oncogenic, has led to intense research in this area worldwide with the ultimate aim of developing HPV-specific immunotherapies. This chapter reviews what is known about human immune responses against HPVs and goes on to discuss how such information is being used to develop immunotherapeutic strategies for both the prophylaxis and treatment of HPV-induced disease. Most of the work to date has understandably focussed on the genital types of HPV, as there is little doubt that the development of simple effective vaccines against

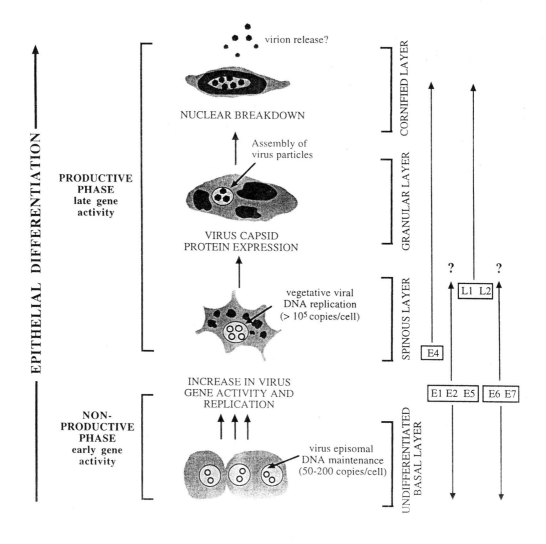

Figure 1. Schematic representation of the interrelationship between epithelial differentiation and the HPV life cycle indicating the stages at which different viral protein expression occurs.

HPV types 16/18 and 6/11 would have a considerable effect on the morbidity and mortality associated with these infections. By employing similar strategies, it should then be relatively straightforward in the future to treat the lesions induced by other types of HPV.

2. Natural History and Viral Life Cycle

In order to design effective immunotherapies against HPV it is important to have a knowledge of the life cycle of the virus and the natural history of infection. Understanding where and when different viral proteins are expressed will obviously help to determine the most appropriate target antigens and may also provide information about when to intervene.

Infection with one of the high risk HPVs on its own is not sufficient for full malignant transformation. This is illustrated by the fact that cancer development is actually rare compared to the incidence of infection with these HPVs. In addition, for cervical intraepithelial neoplasia (CIN) to develop into cancer generally takes a long time (up to 20 years), and the majority of lesions do not progress anyway. Clearly other genetic events and/or factors not yet fully characterized are necessary for progression to malignant disease.

HPV Life Cycle and Viral Gene Expression

HPVs are exclusively epitheliotropic and their infectious cycle is entirely dependent upon epithelial differentiation where cells migrate from the basal layer, differentiating as they progress, to be exfoliated from the surface and replaced by cells from below. Primary HPV infection is thought to occur in basal cells following penetration of the epithelium after wounding. The actual target cell of infection is believed to be some kind of primitive keratinocyte or stem cell which expresses the alpha (6) integrin identified as a candidate receptor for PVs (Roden et al., 1994; Evander et al., 1997). Following entry into the proliferating basal cell the viral genome is established extrachromosomally at a low copy number of between 50 and 200 copies per cell. In this 'non-productive' phase there is a steady-state level of virus DNA replication which is maintained until the infected basal cell enters the terminal differentiation pathway. The virus life cycle then switches to a 'productive' phase when the viral genome is amplified to a high copy number ($>10^5$ copies per cell). Infectious virus particles are only assembled in the most superficial terminally differentiated keratinocytes.

HPV protein expression follows a highly ordered sequence, with individual antigens first appearing in keratinocytes at specific points in the movement of cells from the basal layer to the epithelial surface (reviewed in Chow and Broker, 1997). This has been summarised in Figure 1 where it can be seen that the immediate early proteins (E1, E2 and E5), and the early transforming proteins (E6 and E7), first appear in basal/parabasal cells. The E4 protein is first detectable suprabasally in the spinous layer at the onset of vegetative viral DNA replication, whereas the L1 and L2 virion capsid proteins do not usually appear until the infected keratinocytes reach the upper spinous layers. E4, L1 and L2 persist in cells as they move up through the granular layer where progeny virus are assembled (Doorbar, 1998). Mature virions are released from exfoliating cells. This pattern of gene expression is characteristic of productive infections of both skin and mucosa although there are some differences. For example, the initiation of late events and the onset of vegetative viral DNA replication occurs earlier in plantar warts caused by HPV type 1 or 63. For other types of HPV studied these processes are retarded until the infected cell reaches the middle or upper spinous layers. The pathobiology of HPVs is covered in more detail in Chapter 5 of this book.

Viral Replication in Terminally Differentiating Epithelial Cells

The cellular environment of non-dividing terminally differentiating keratinocytes is not supportive of DNA replication since the cells have exited from the cell cycle. HPVs therefore have to reactivate the cellular DNA replication machinery in order to replicate themselves. In the case of the high risk genital types of HPV, this is believed to be mediated by the early transforming proteins E6 and E7 through their interactions with the tumor suppressor protein p53, and members of the retinoblastoma (Rb) protein family respectively (reviewed in Chapter 6).

The E6 and E7 proteins from oncogenic and non-oncogenic types of HPV show a number of biochemical and functional differences which probably relate to their differences in oncogenicity. It is not yet clear how the low-risk HPVs re-establish DNA replication, although this too is likely to involve a role for E6 and E7 in deregulation of the cell cycle. Interestingly, the oncogenic cutaneous HPVs associated with skin carcinomas appear to have different transformation strategies when compared to the high risk genital types. The HPV8 E6 protein does not appear to form complexes with p53, and HPV8 E7 does not bind Rb (Fuchs and Pfister, 1996).

Integration of HPV Genomes

In normal benign HPV-induced lesions the cells contain HPV DNA as circular episomes. Following infection of cervical tissue with the high risk HPV types, the HPV genome, although present initially as an episome, becomes integrated in more advanced lesions and invasive tumors (Cullen et al., 1991; Stoler et al., 1992). During integration, the E2 gene is disrupted and the E6 and E7 proteins are stably expressed. In fact, their continued expression is required for the maintenance of the transformed phenotype and they are the only two proteins constitutively expressed in cervical carcinomas. In contrast once again, the viral genomes of the oncogenic skin types of HPV are maintained as episomes in infected cells.

3. Natural Immunity to HPV

Most immunocompetent individuals clear HPV infections with no apparent consequences. Both cutaneous and genital lesions often regress spontaneously (Syrjanen, 1996) and the majority of women infected with genital HPV types do not develop cancer (Ho et al., 1998). Paradoxically, HPV infections can also be remarkably persistant. Precisely what role the immune system plays in this persistence, or in viral clearance, is not clear.

Evidence for Cell-Mediated Immunity to HPV

Deficiencies in humoral immunity do not result in an increase in HPV-associated lesions, which makes it unlikely that antibodies alone are responsible for controlling infection with HPV (Lutzner, 1985). There is however, considerable circumstantial evidence that cell-mediated immunity (CMI) is important. Firstly, HPV-associated lesions are more common in immunosuppressed individuals (reviewed by Benton et al., 1992) such as those receiving immunosuppressive therapy following kidney transplants (Halpert et al., 1986), or infected with human immunodeficiency virus (HIV) (Laga et al., 1992; Garzetti et al., 1994; Petry et al., 1994). Secondly, in humans, regressing cutaneous and genital warts are characterized by an infiltration of activated T-cells and macrophages (Tagami et al., 1985; Bender, 1986; Iwatsuki et al., 1986; Coleman et al., 1994). Similar observations have been made in animal models (Jarrett et al., 1991; Knowles et al., 1996; Selvakumar et al., 1997). A third piece of evidence suggesting that cellular immunity is important is that the presence of lymphocytes within HPV-associated lesions correlates with an improved prognosis in cervical carcinoma (Tosi et al., 1992).

HPV Persistence

In many healthy individuals, HPV infections can be remarkably persistent and although spontaneous regression nearly always occurs eventually, it can often take years. It is not really understood why HPV is so poorly immunogenic in these cases although a number of observations may be relevant.

ANTIGEN-PRESENTING CAPABILITIES OF INFECTED KERATINOCYTES
Under normal conditions epithelial keratinocytes do not usually express MHC class II molecules so that presentation of HPV antigens to CD4+ T-cells is unlikely. Neither do they express important co-stimulatory and adhesion molecules such as B7.1 (CD80), B7.2 (CD86) and intercellular adhesion molecule 1 (ICAM-1). This has been the explanation for the fact that, although keratinocytes are capable of delivering antigen-specific signals to T-cells, they cannot provide secondary co-stimulatory signals and therefore present antigen to the immune system in a manner which induces T-cell anergy rather than activation (Bal et al., 1990). Under certain conditions however, some of these important accessory molecules can be up-regulated and the potential for full T-cell

activation is greatly increased. This commonly occurs during inflammation in response to the release of soluble cytokines such as interferon-γ which increase the expression of both MHC class II (Barker et al., 1988) and ICAM-1 (Griffiths et al., 1989). Whether the B7 molecules are up-regulated under these conditions is still not clear although a related protein, B7/BB1, can be induced in response to IL-4 (Junghans et al., 1996). The importance of these proteins for effective antigen presentation has been demonstrated in epithelial cells by the transfection of keratinocytes with B7-like molecules and in B7.1 transgenic mice (Fleming et al., 1993; Gaspari et al., 1994; Williams et al., 1994; Kaufmann et al., 1997).

INFECTION WITH HPV DOES NOT CAUSE CELL LYSIS

The poor antigen presentation properties of epithelial keratinocytes, and the fact that HPV does not cause a systemic infection, may partly explain why HPV can apparently go unnoticed by the immune system for long periods of time. Another contributing factor is likely to be that when HPVs infect keratinocytes they do not lyse the infected cells. There is therefore little or no release of viral antigens into the surrounding tissue which could otherwise be taken up by professional antigen-presenting cells. There is also little or no local inflammation to up-regulate the expression of accessory molecules and MHC on the keratinocyte surface. How and why the spontaneous regression of HPV-induced lesions suddenly occurs against this background is not understood, but the possibility exists that it is initiated as a result of an inflammatory response following wounding or trauma (possibly in response to treatment).

DEPLETION OF LANGERHANS CELLS IN HPV-INFECTED TISSUE

Histological analysis of both HPV-induced cutaneous skin warts and cervical disease has shown that there are reduced numbers of Langerhans cells compared to normal tissue (Tay et al., 1987; Viac et al., 1990; Morelli et al., 1992; Lehtinen et al., 1993). Langerhans cells are specialised dendritic cells found suprabasally within epithelial surfaces. In common with the other types of professional antigen-presenting cells (APCs) such as macrophages and activated B-cells, they have high levels of MHC class II expression, are able to process antigens very efficiently, and are rich in the co-stimulatory molecules that are important for T-cell activation. Dendritic cells can stimulate both helper and cytotoxic T-cells (CTLs) and are particularly effective at initiating primary responses (reviewed by Cella et al., 1997; Bancherau and Steinman, 1998; Klagge and Schneider-Schaulies, 1999). It has recently been realised that dendritic cells also have the ability to process exogenous antigens for presentation on MHC class I molecules (Speidel et al., 1997; Albert et al., 1998). During infection with HPV this may be a particularly important mechanism for the induction of HPV-specific CTL responses if the keratinocytes themselves are poor antigen-presenters. Obviously if numbers of dendritic cells are low within HPV-infected lesions, this would contribute to poor local immunity.

IMMUNE EVASION

The oncogenic genital types of HPV, in common with other DNA tumor viruses (see Chapter 14), also appear to have developed other mechanisms for evading the immune response in immunocompetent hosts. These include the down-regulation of endogenous peptide processing machinery for MHC presentation (TAP-1 and TAP-2 proteins), the loss of expression of MHC class I alleles (Cromme et al., 1994; Keating et al., 1995; Bontkes et al., 1998) and point mutations in CTL epitopes (Ellis et al., 1995). These phenomena have not been observed in benign lesions associated with low risk HPVs.

HPV Serology

We know from the large number of serological studies carried out that a high proportion of infected individuals produce antibodies to various HPV antigens (reviewed by Galloway, 1996; Carter and Galloway, 1997). Infection with the genital types of HPV can also lead to the production of IgA antibodies in cervical secretions (Wang et al., 1996). Until fairly recently, it has been very difficult to correlate the results of the serological assays with disease progression or clearance. This has undoubtedly been due to difficulties in identifying and producing suitable antigens for measuring HPV antibodies, together with the fact that it is also very difficult to obtain accurate clinical histories. Many HPV infections are sub-clinical or are cleared before they become apparent.

In the earliest studies, before it became possible to express individual viral proteins, HPV virions purified from wart tissue were used as antigens. Nowadays, most serological assays take advantage of virus-like particles (VLPs) which are available for most of the common HPV types (Lowy and Schiller, 1998; Da Silva et al., 1999). It is beyond the scope of this chapter to review in detail the results of the many studies carried out over the years. However, recent assays using VLPs have used larger cohorts of people where the natural history of HPV infection and disease progression could be more closely monitored (Carter and Galloway, 1996; deGruijl et al., 1999). It has been noted that seroconversion does not generally occur until several months after detection of HPV DNA, that the antibody responses persist for years and are mostly type-specific. Antibody levels appear to correlate with disease severity and HPV persistence suggesting that the assays may be useful for identifying individuals infected with high risk viruses who are likely to develop invasive disease. Nevertheless, the fact remains that antibody responses do not predict HPV clearance, and we still do not know what role they play in eliminating virus.

T Helper Cell Responses

TYPE 1 AND TYPE 2 HELPER T-CELLS

T helper cells are usually CD4+ and stimulate different sorts of immunity depending on the pattern of cytokines they secrete (Mosman and Sad, 1996). Type 1 helper T-cells (Th1) secrete IFN-γ, TNF-α and IL-2. Their importance for both the induction and maintenance of cytotoxic T-cell (CTL) responses has only recently been fully recognised (Kalams and Walker, 1998), and they also play a role in the induction of delayed-type hypersensitivity (DTH) type reactions. It is now realised that antigen-stimulated Th1 cells can influence the direction of an immune response through their interaction with CD40 which is expressed on the surface of dendritic cells. The dendritic cell becomes activated and is then able to stimulate antigen-specific CTLs directly (Bennett et al., 1998; Ridge et al., 1998; Schoenberger et al., 1998).

Type 2 helper T-cells (Th2) principally support antibody responses through IL-4 and IL-5 production.

CLASS II PROCESSING OF HPV ANTIGENS

Helper T-cells recognise antigenic peptides which are presented in association with MHC class II molecules on the surface of professional APCs. These peptides are derived from 'exogenous' antigens which are taken up into the APC by endocytosis. Once inside, the protein encapsulates to form acidic endosomes and becomes degraded into peptide fragments 13-22 amino acids in length. The endosomes fuse with other vesicles which contain MHC class II molecules, the peptides bind to the appropriate class II, and the whole complex is transported to the cell surface for recognition by specific CD4+ T-cells. Unlike MHC class I which is expressed on all nucleated cells, class II expression is largely restricted to professional APCs.

During HPV infection, processing and presentation of viral antigens via MHC class II molecules to CD4+ T-cells could theoretically occur in a number of ways. Firstly there is the possibility that HPV proteins may be released into the extracellular space as a result of keratinocyte death or damage due to trauma or surgical treatment. These exogenous antigens could then be taken up and processed by local Langerhans cells and presented to CD4+ T-cells. This is particularly feasible for high grade CIN lesions and cervical carcinomas where inflammation is common, and both infiltrating lymphocytes and APCs have been observed (Ferguson et al., 1985; Tosi et al., 1992; Coleman and Stanley, 1994). However low grade CIN and benign HPV infections in general are characterized by the lack of markers for any ongoing local immune response and no inflammation or cell death (Tay et al., 1985).

There could also, in theory, be direct presentation of HPV antigens through MHC class II molecules, if and when they are expressed on the keratinocyte surface. Under normal circumstances this occurs following an inflammatory response, but it is interesting to note that in most cervical cancers there is up-regulation of MHC class II expression anyway (Glew et al., 1992). However, whether antigenic peptides presented in this way are able to fully activate the relevant T-cells is still unknown because of the lack of costimulation.

HPV-SPECIFIC HELPER T-CELLS

The most commonly used method to assess CD4+ T-cell responses *in vitro* is to test the ability of peripheral blood mononuclear cells (PBMCs) to proliferate in response to HPV antigens. Many of the early studies used antigen preparations prepared from skin warts or recombinant proteins to demonstrate proliferative responses *in vitro* (Ivanyi and Morison, 1976; Lee and Eisenger, 1976; Cubie et al., 1989; Charleson et al., 1992) and demonstrated low levels of lymphoproliferation in people with or without prior histories of HPV infection. More recently it has become possible to measure proliferative responses against individual HPV proteins and to map T-cell epitopes using synthetic peptides. Characterisation of proliferative T-cell responses to HPV type 1 E4 protein has been described (Steele et al., 1993), but most studies have again concentrated on the genital types of HPV, and several putative CD4+ epitopes have been mapped from the E6, E7 and L1 proteins of HPV 16 (Strang et al., 1990; Altmann et al., 1992). Some studies have found that proliferative T-cell responses are not significantly associated with the stage of the HPV-induced disease whereas others can show correlations with disease severity and viral persistence (Kadish et al., 1994; 1997; deGruijl et al., 1996; Luxton et al., 1996;1997; Shepherd et al., 1996; Gill et al., 1998). In an interesting study by Hong et al. (1997), wart-infiltrating lymphocytes (WILs) and PBMCs were isolated from patients with HPV6-induced genital warts and characterized according to phenotype and their proliferative responses to E7 and L1. Interesting differences in phenotype were observed between patients, and the L1 peptide epitopes recognized by the WILs differed from those recognized by peripheral T-cells.

Recent studies have also looked at the cytokine profiles of CD4+ T-cells during infection with HPV. The first by Clerici et al. (1997), using non-HPV antigens found that there was a trend towards production of the interleukins associated with immunosuppression (IL-10 and IL-4) in patients with extensive HPV-induced cervical disease. IL-2 production by CD4+ T-cells has been measured in response to stimulation by HPV16 E7 peptides (deGruijl et al., 1998b) or HPV16 L1 VLPs (deGruijl et al., 1999). Responses were observed in patients with both virus clearance and virus persistence, irrespective of CIN grade, but the highest responses were found in patients with the high grade cervical lesions and cervical cancer. An important HPV16 L1 Th epitope was identified which appeared to be closely associated with HPV exposure and CIN development.

A common finding amongst some of the helper T-cell studies has been the detection of high numbers of responders in the control groups. In some of the earlier work, the crude nature of the antigen preparations means that they may not have been measuring HPV-specific reactivities at all. The possibility also exists that the assay procedures are able to induce primary T-cell responses. It is more likely though that since many HPV infections go completely unnoticed it is very difficult to obtain accurate information about prior exposure to HPV and the asymptomatic control groups could therefore be making memory T-cell responses to the same, or a similar type of HPV. Since some of the viral proteins show a high degree of sequence homology, it is feasible that there may be some cross-reactive T-cell epitopes.

Cytotoxic T-Cell Responses

CLASS I PROCESSING OF HPV ANTIGENS

CTLs are generally CD8+, and are known to play a vital role in the clearance of most viral infections. They recognise short antigenic peptides (generally 8-10 amino acids in length) which are presented bound to MHC class I molecules on the surface of the virally-infected cell. The peptides are derived from viral proteins synthesised endogenously within the infected cell which undergo proteolytic breakdown by proteosomes within the cytoplasm. They are transported by specific transporter proteins (TAP-1 and TAP-2) from the cytosol into the endoplasmic reticulum where they associate with newly synthesised MHC class I molecules and β2-microglobulin. The antigenic complex then migrates to the cell surface where it can be recognised by CD8+ T-cells bearing T-cell receptors with the appropriate specificity. Since MHC class I molecules are present on the surface of all nucleated cells the potential is there for the appropriate CTL to kill virtually any virally-infected cell. The major effector mechanism responsible for killing by virus-specific CTLs is believed to be mediated by perforin, although both fas ligand interactions and tumor necrosis factor-mediated cell death play a secondary role (Griffiths, 1995).

Primary CTL responses are believed to be activated by the presentation of foreign antigens on the surface of professional APCs within local draining lymph nodes (Mehta-Damani et al., 1994; Stingl and Bergstresser, 1995; Tripp et al., 1995). Effector cells induced in the lymph nodes then recirculate via the blood to the site of infection to kill virally-infected cells 7-10 days after priming (Doherty, 1995). Effector T-cells usually die within 14-21 days and lifelong memory for the relevant virus is carried in T-cells resident in the spleen and elsewhere (Doherty et al., 1994).

Since HPVs do not infect the APCs themselves, there are presumably no endogenously synthesised viral antigens within the Langerhans cells available for the usual class I processing pathway. It is therefore not clear quite how HPV is able to prime specific CD8+ T-cell responses. If there were release of HPV antigens at some stage, or following cell trauma, then the dendritic cells may be able to process these exogenous proteins to produce class I-binding peptides and prime CTLs in this way.

The endogenous expression of viral proteins within the cytoplasm of the infected keratinocytes will presumably also generate class I-binding HPV peptides. In HPV-transformed cervical keratinocytes it is assumed that the constitutive expression of E6 and E7 will result in E6 or E7 derived peptides being presented by class I molecules at the cell surface. It is not known however, whether the infected keratinocytes themselves are able to directly activate CTLs due to their poor antigen-presenting function.

HUMAN CTL RESPONSES TO HPV

The search for naturally occurring HPV-specific CTLs in infected humans has been disappointing. Putative peptide epitopes derived from both HPV 16 E7 and HPV16 E2 proteins which bind the common haplotype HLA-A*0201 have been used to induce specific CTLs from normal donors (Ressing et al., 1995; Konya et al., 1997) but these are likely to represent primary responses. Other studies have used HPV16 E7 peptides to induce E7-specific CTLs from women with HPV-associated cervical disease (CIN3) and cervical cancer (Alexander et al., 1996; Ressing et al., 1996), and some of these CTLs have activity against HLA-matched tumor cells suggesting that they were able to recognise naturally processed HPV epitopes. The frequency of individuals where CTLs could be detected however, was low, which may reflect the fact that HPV-induced disease is highly localized and there may be fewer HPV-specific T-cells in peripheral blood. This has been demonstrated by the experiments of Evans et al. (1997). Again using HPV16 E7 peptides they compared lymphocytes isolated from blood, draining lymph nodes and infiltrating cervical tumors from cancer patients, and found that HPV-specific CTLs were more abundant at the site of exposure.

Some disadvantages of using peptides for the *in vitro* stimulation of HPV-specific CTLs are, firstly, that the peptides selected may not be representative of HPV epitopes expressed during the natural infection, and secondly, that experiments are restricted to only a few HLA alleles. In fact, studies using whole HPV proteins to restimulate CTL responses, either in a soluble form (Nakagawa et al., 1997) or expressed by recombinant viral vectors (Nimako et al., 1997), where the whole protein is naturally processed have been more successful with CTLs being found in the majority of patients with cervical disease.

Autologous dendritic cells loaded with A2-binding peptides from HPV11 E7 and HPV16 E7 have also been used to stimulate CTL responses from human donors *in vitro* (Tarpey et al., 1994; Jochmus et al., 1997) although it is not clear whether these represent primary or memory T-cell responses. The same approach has recently been extended to the use of autologous dendritic cells loaded with a recombinant HPV16 E6/E7 fusion protein to induce specific CTLs (Murakami et al., 1999). The use of intact protein in this way again overcomes the limitation of peptide epitopes for specific HLA haplotypes.

Overall, the results suggest that naturally occuring HPV-specific CTLs do exist in patients with HPV-associated disease, although their detection may depend on the methods used to reacitvate them *in vitro*. As with the proliferative T-cell work, the role of such responses in resolution, rather than as a consequence of disease, has not really been addressed, and the targets responsible for the immune regression of HPV-induced lesions have still not been clearly identified. For this it will be necessary to look at patients with regressing lesions, or who have resolved their disease, in order to determine which responses against which antigens are important. One other consideration is that most studies so far have looked at systemic responses to HPV, but in the case of the common genital types, we also need to examine mucosal immunity which has a bias towards T helper responses important for the induction of mucosal IgA responses.

4. HPV Vaccines

The involvement of certain mucosotropic HPVs (particularly HPV 16 and 18) with common carcinomas of the genital tract (Zur Hausen, 1991), and of some cutaneous HPVs (such as HPV 5 and 8) with squamous epithelial carcinomas (Pfister et al., 1985), emphasises the clinical importance of these agents. The evidence that HPV infection and their associated malignancies can induce humoral and cellular immunity to both capsid and non-structural viral proteins provides an opportunity for the design of therapeutic strategies based on immune intervention.

Although the skin cancers caused by cutaneous HPV types 5 and 8 are a problem in themselves, it is the development of vaccines to prevent and/or treat HPV-associated cervical disease which has been the major area of interest so far. Cervical neoplasia is classified histologically (CIN I - III) on the basis of progressive cellular atypia and disturbed epithelial architecture. Cancer of the cervix develops from pre-invasive CIN lesions and is the second most common cause of cancer-related death in women worldwide (Boyle, 1997). HPV DNA is found in over 94% of cervical cancers with types 16 and 18 being the most frequently detected (Bosch et al., 1995; Lehtinen et al., 1996). Current therapies are often of limited effectiveness and can be impractical in developing countries, so successful immunotherapies would be invaluable.

Immunological approaches to the treatment of benign cutaneous and mucosal warts would also be useful since these lesions cause significant problems in their own right and they affect many more people than cervical cancer. In particular, HPV types 6 and 11, which cause anogenital warts are difficult to treat and often reoccur. In young children these same viruses can cause recurrent laryngeal papillomas which need frequent laser treatment to keep the airways open (Derkay, 1995). Skin warts caused by the cutaneous types of HPV, apart from providing unique opportunities for immunological studies, also provide a safe system for the development of immunotherapies applicable to the high risk HPVs.

Considerations for the Design of HPV Vaccines

PROPHYLACTIC OR THERAPEUTIC?
A prophylactic vaccine would aim to prevent HPV infection by inducing neutralizing antibodies at the site and time of infection. This would benefit individuals at greatest exposure to HPV eg. for types 16 and 18, young men and women at the onset of sexual activity. Therapeutic vaccination is directed at the elimination of established infection and would aim to stimulate cell-mediated immunity so that virally-infected cells are killed by HPV-specific CTLs. This approach could be used in addition to conventional treatments in both benign and malignant disease.

Obviously both prophylactic and therapeutic vaccines could be of use in the treatment of HPV-associated disease, and their effectiveness may be influenced by several factors.

CHOICE OF TARGET ANTIGEN

In order to induce neutralizing antibodies, a prophylactic antigen would need to include the virus capsid proteins (L1 and L2) which contain the neutralizing epitopes. The design of therapeutic vaccines is not quite so simple and the target antigen(s) should be considered in light of what we know about the virus life cycle and the natural history of infection. For the treatment of invasive cervical carcinoma, the best candidates for therapeutic vaccines are obviously E6 and E7, since these are the only two viral proteins expressed. However, if the aim is to target individuals at earlier stages of disease, then it is just as valid to consider other early HPV proteins, such as E2 and E4, which are expressed at significant levels in premalignant lesions.

PRESENTATION OF ANTIGEN

It is now realised that the manner in which an antigen is presented to the immune system can have a profound effect on the magnitude and type of immune response that is generated. The most effective responses are likely to involve the activation of both CD4+ and CD8+ T-cells, and also the co-ordination of both Th1 and Th2 responses (Kelso, 1995; Allen and Maizels, 1997).

The choice of immunogen is important here once again, particularly with respect to the site of expression of the various viral proteins within differentiating epithelial tissue. The antigen-processing capabilities of the epithelial cells may influence whether or not virally-infected cells can be recognised and killed by the appropriate T-cells.

The mode of delivery of an immunogen, including the choice of adjuvant, is another important consideration. For example, the type of T helper response that is induced can depend upon how the vaccine is delivered and the route of administration (Pertmer et al., 1996; Feltquate et al., 1997). In the case of HPV, the highly localized nature of the infection means that the immunogen must be able to induce immunity at both mucosal and epidermal surfaces.

MULTIPLICITY OF INFECTION

HPV-associated lesions can be caused by more than one type of virus. For example, even though about half of cervical cancers contain HPV type 16, the remainder may contain HPV types 18, 31, 33 or 45. Since it is not clear whether related strains of viruses share at least some neutralizing epitopes (Roden et al., 1996 a;b; 1997; White et al., 1998), we might need to consider the design of polytope prophylactic vaccines capable of inducing responses to multiple virus types. For therapeutic purposes, it may be possible to screen individuals in order to determine which HPV type they are carrying before administering the appropriate vaccine. Generally speaking however, it is not feasible to tailor individual treatments in this way.

Candidate Vaccines

Based on research carried out on human immunity to HPVs, and in animal models, a number of HPV vaccines have been developed and are currently in Phase I/II clinical trials (see Table 1). For some of the earlier trials, results are now available and these are

Table 1. HPV vaccine trials

IMMUNOGEN	PROTOCOL	RESULTS
HPV11 VLPs (MEDI-501) University of Rochester Medical Centre MedImmune Inc USA Aluminium hydroxide adjuvant **HPV16 and HPV18 VLPs planned**	Phase I Healthy volunteers 60 individuals received 3 intramuscular injections over 16 weeks	Vaccine safe, well tolerated and immunogenic (Reichman et al., 1999) • All made IgG antibodies with titres increasing over time • Good neutralizing antibody responses • Some serological cross-reactivity with HPV6 VLPs
HPV16 L2E7 fusion protein (TA-GW) Alhydrogel adjuvant	Phase I Healthy male volunteers Phase IIa 27 indivuduals with recurrent genitalwarts received 3 intramuscular immunizations over 4 weeks	Vaccine safe and immunogenic (Thompson et al., 1999; Lacey et al., 1999) • All made IgG responses to L2E7 • 85% made antigen specificproliferative T-cell responses • Clinical results promising 1) 5 resolved warts completely 2) Further 8 resolved with treatment 3) No recurrence of warts in any individual vaccinated

HPV16 E7-GST fusion protein Algammulin adjuvant	Phase I/II 5 late stage cervical cancer patients	(Tindle, 1996) • All made E7 antibodies • 2 out of 3 evaluated made proliferative T-cell responses to E7 protein and peptides
Recombinant vaccinia virus expressing E6 and E7 from HPV 16 and HPV 18 (TA-HPV)	Phase I/II 8 late stage cervical cancer patients immunized once by dermal scarification Phase II CIN III, stage 1B and 2A cervical cancer patients in addition to conventional treatments	(Boursnell et al., 1996; Borysiewicz et al., 1996) • No significant side effects • All made antibody responses to vaccinia virus • 3 patients mounted HPV-specific antibody responses • HPV18 E6/E7 specific CTL response detected in 1 out of 3 evaluable patients • This patient experienced remission and was still tumor-free 15 months later Not complete
HPV16 E7 peptides 2 high affinity HLA-A*C201 binding peptides together with a synthetic T helper cell epitope Montanide ISA 51 adjuvant	Phase I/II 15 late stage cervical cancer patients unresponsive to conventional treatments received four subcutaneous injections over 3 months (Patients were HLA-A*0201 positive and had HPV16 positive tumors)	(Brandt et al., 1999) • 4 out of 12 evaluable patients showed proliferative T-cell responses to E7 peptides • No CTL responses to E7 peptides detected • Only 2 patients showing stable disease - remaining progressed

discussed below. HPV vaccines have also been reviewed elsewhere (Tindle, 1996; Duggan-Keene et al., 1998; Lowy and Schiller, 1998).

VIRUS-LIKE PARTICLES (VLPS)

VLP PRODUCTION AND IMMUNOGENICITY.

Most prophylactic viral vaccines have consisted of live attenuated, or formalin-inactivated virus. This is not possible for HPV because the dependence of the virus life cycle upon epithelial differentiation means that it is very difficult to produce enough virus particles *in vitro*. The discovery that the high-level expression of the major capsid protein L1 results in the self-assembly of VLPs was a considerable breakthrough and VLPs have now been produced for all major HPV types associated with human disease in a variety of expression systems including yeast, insect cells and bacteria (Zhou et al., 1991a; Kirnbauer et al., 1992;1993; Hagensee et al., 1993; Rose et al., 1993; Hofman et al., 1995; Sasagawa et al., 1995; Li et al., 1997). The coexpression of both the L1 and L2 structural proteins leads to VLPs containing both proteins with a ratio very similar to that found in native virions (Kirnbauer et al., 1993; Volpers et al., 1994). The L1 protein assumes the same conformation as the immunodominant epitopes on native virions so that VLPs are capable of inducing high levels of neutralizing antibodies (Kirnbauer et al, 1992). VLPs containing L2 as well self-asssemble more efficiently and retain similar antigenic characteristics to the L1 capsomeres (Roden et al., 1996a).

VACCINE STUDIES OF VLPS IN ANIMALS

The ability of HPV VLPs to mimic the conformation of natural HPV virions obviously makes them attractive candidates for prophylactic vaccines and there have been several successful vaccine trials of VLPs using animal models. Immunisation of rabbits with cottontail rabbit papillomavirus (CRPV) VLPs, dogs with canine oral papillomavirus (COPV) VLPs, and cattle with bovine papillomavirus type 4 (BPV4) VLPs, can all protect the animal against subsequent viral challenge (Breitburd et al., 1995; Jansen et al., 1995; Suzich et al., 1995; Christensen et al., 1996; Kirnbauer et al., 1996). This protection can be passively transferred and is type-specific, indicating that the success of VLP vaccination is due to the induction of neutralizing antibodies. In other animals it has been possible to induce mucosal immunity following vaccination with HPV VLPs. Both the systemic innoculation of monkeys with HPV11 VLPs, and the intranasal immunization of mice with HPV16 VLPs, can elicit neutralizing antibodies in cervico-vaginal secretions (Lowe et al., 1997; Balmelli et al., 1998). This suggests that, for VLPs at least, it may not be necessary to immunise at mucosal sites to elicit mucosal antibodies .

CHIMERIC VLPS

VLPs have proven to be good prophylactic vaccines in several animal models because they induce neutralizing antibodies, but in mice it has also been shown that HPV16 VLPs can induce cell-mediated immunity too (Dupuy et al., 1997). More recently, the efficacy of VLPs has been extended by the production of chimeric VLPs which incorporate relevant early region proteins as well as L1 and L2 (Muller et al., 1997).

The extra protein is usually fused onto L2, since L2 is not critical to the formation of the particle. For HPV16 VLPs, full length E2 or E7 have both been added to the C-terminus of L2 without interfering with particle assembly or its ability to induce neutralizing antibodies (Greenstone et al., 1997).

Chimeric particles again appear to be very promising as vaccines in animals. HPV16 VLPs containing E7 confer anti tumor immunity in mice (Greenstone et al., 1997) and strong CTL responses are elicited by hybrid BPV1 L1/HPV16 E7 VLPs (Peng et al., 1998). It is clear that VLPs can be taken up, processed and presented through both the HLA class I and II pathways to allow the induction of both CD4+ and CD8+ T-cells, as well as humoral immunity. Chimeric VLPs might therefore represent a one-agent vaccine suitable for combined prophylaxis and therapy.

CURRENT VLP TRIALS IN HUMANS

The advantages of VLPs are that they are safe, since they do not contain the viral genome, and that they are also highly immunogenic without adjuvant. A Phase I trial to evaluate HPV 11 L1 VLPs (MEDI-501) in healthy volunteers has recently been completed at the University of Rochester Medical Centre (USA) in association with MedImmune Inc. Sixty individuals received 3 intramuscular innoculations over a period of 16 weeks and their serum was evaluated for anti-HPV VLP IgG levels by ELISA and *in vitro* neutralization by an RT-PCR based assay. All subjects demonstrated rising antibody titres to HPV11 VLPs (some cross-reacting with HPV6 VLPs), and those receiving the higher doses showed high neutralization titres exceeding those observed in naturally infected individuals. Trials using HPV16 and 18 VLPs are planned.

WHOLE PROTEINS

Immunisation with whole HPV proteins has the advantage that antigenic peptides are produced by natural processing and so the HLA type of the individual is not a restriction. Immunity to soluble proteins is classically associated with the production of MHC class II binding peptides which stimulate CD4+ T helper cells, but exogenous proteins may also enter the class I processing pathway in professional APCs. It is possible therefore, that vaccination with whole HPV proteins may induce both CD4+ and CD8+ T-cell responses. With a few exceptions, natural viral proteins are not obtainable for HPVs and so much of the work in this area has focussed on the use of recombinant fusion proteins.

ANIMAL STUDIES

Once again vaccination studies in animals have been quite successful and demonstrate that both humoral and cellular immunity can be induced by the administration of recombinant HPV proteins. In cattle, cutaneous lesions induced by BPV2 were rejected after administration of an L2 vaccine (Jarrett et al., 1991). In the BPV4 model, immunization with E7 caused the regression of mucosal papillomas and the administration of L2 protected against subsequent viral challenge (Campo et al., 1993). E1 and E2 vaccines caused regression of CRPV-induced lesions in rabbits in which there was clear evidence of the involvement of CD8+ T-cells (Selvakumar et al., 1995;

1997; Jensen et al., 1997). In mice bearing experimental HPV16 tumors, both E6 and E7 vaccines caused tumor rejection believed to be mediated by CTLs (Meneguzzi et al., 1991; Chen et al., 1992; Zhu et al., 1995)

CLINICAL TRIALS IN HUMANS

Based on the observations made in the mucosotropic BPV4 model, an HPV6 L2/E7 fusion protein (TA-GW) was evaluated for safety and immunogenicity in Phase I trials using healthy male volunteers (Thompson et al., 1999). In Phase II, the TA-GW vaccine was administered intramuscularly to patients with recurrent genital warts. The results have recently been published and are very encouraging (Lacey et al., 1999). Twenty-seven patients received three injections over a period of four weeks. All made IgG antibodies against L2E7, and 85% made antigen-specific proliferative T-cell responses. The clinical responses were also promising in that 5 subjects cleared their warts completely within 8 weeks of receiving the vaccine. Remaining patients were offered conventional treatment and another 8 patients resolved their disease. Genital warts have not recurred in any of the individuals in either group who have received the vaccine.

In Australia another trial using a recombinant HPV protein as the immunogen has been completed. Five patients with end-stage cervical cancer received a GST-HPV16E7 fusion protein in adjuvant. All five women made antibodies to E7 and two out of the three patients evaluated also showed proliferative T-cell responses to E7 protein and peptides (Tindle, 1996).

PEPTIDES

Peptide vaccines for HPV have been aimed at inducing therapeutic CD8+ CTL responses but their success depends on the identification of peptide epitopes suitable for the HLA type of the individual. Most of the work has concentrated on identifying peptides restricted through the common HLA A*0201 haplotype. Using computer predictions and binding assays, several have been identified, but studies in mice suggest that epitopes predicted by these methods may not be naturally processed, and conversely, some immunogenic peptides would not be identified (Sadovnikova et al., 1994).

It is clear that peptide-based vaccines can be protective against HPV tumors in mice (Feltkamp et al., 1993; 1995; Lipford et al., 1995) and they are attractive candidates for human vaccines for a number of reasons. They are relatively cheap to produce and very easy to make in large amounts. It is also possible to produce cocktails of several peptides which could be used together as a single immunogen. In this way it would be possible to cover most of the common haplotypes and related HPV types in one vaccine.

Phase I/II clinical trials have been carried out in Holland using a mixture of two high affinity HLA A*0201-binding peptides from HPV16 E7 together with an HPV unrelated T helper cell epitope (Melief et al., 1996). The vaccine has been administered to 15 late stage cervical cancer patients who had not responded to conventional treatment. All received 4 subcutaneous injections over 3 months in a dose escalation scheme. No CTL responses against the E7 peptides were detectable, but peptide-specific proliferation was seen in 4 out of 12 evaluable patients. The clinical results have been mixed with the majority of subjects showing progressive disease - only 2 subjects, who had received the lowest dose of peptides, were stable more than a year later (Brandt et al., 1999). Several other peptide trials are currently underway in the USA (McNeil, 1997).

VIRAL VECTORS

The use of viral vectors to deliver the protein of choice again offers the advantage that the antigen will be naturally processed. The peptides produced will vary according to the HLA type of the host but all individuals will be eligible. A popular choice is the use of recombinant vaccinia viruses which we know from other systems can elicit CTL responses in humans (Cooney et al., 1991; Tsang et al., 1995). Any problems with toxicity could be addressed using the modified virus Ankara (MVA), a highly attenuated strain which replicates very inefficiently in human cells.

Work with papillomaviruses has shown that immunizing rabbits with recombinants expressing the L1 or L2 proteins of CRPV gives excellent protection mediated through the production of neutralizing antibodies (Lin et al., 1992). In mice too, vaccinia viruses expressing HPV16 L1, E6 or E7 proteins have been successful (Zhou et al., 1991b; Gao et al., 1994; Zhu et al., 1995; Lin et al., 1996).

An important Phase I/II trial using recombinant vaccinia viruses expressing E6 and E7 from HPV16 and 18 (TA-HPV) has been completed in Cardiff (Borysiewicz et al., 1996). The E7 portions of the proteins had been mutated to inactivate the Rb binding site and eight late stage cervical cancer patients received the vaccine by dermal scarification with no significant side effects. All developed IgG antibodies to the vaccinia virus, and out of the three that were evaluated, one patient showed an HPV18 E6/E7 specific CTL response nine weeks after immunisation which had disappeared by 14 weeks. This patient also went into remission and was still tumor free 15 months later. The TA-HPV vaccine has now been taken forward into Phase II trials and is currently being administered to patients with earlier stages of cervical cancer and CIN III as an adjunct to conventional treatments.

DNA

Another approach is to introduce DNA directly into the host cell so that the protein of interest can be synthesised by the cell. There is evidence in other systems that this can be quite successful and DNA vaccines are already in clinical trials for HIV, influenza, hepatitis B and malaria. In rabbits, the L1 gene of CRPV injected as naked DNA has been shown to confer protection against tumor challenge through the production of neutralizing antibodies (Donnelly et al., 1996).

DENDRITIC CELLS

Recent advances in our ability to expand dendritic cells *ex vivo* and use them for immunotherapies in other cancers such as B-cell lymphomas and melanoma, means that they could be considered for the treatment of HPV-associated disease. In mice, dendritic cells loaded with HPV16 E7-derived peptides conferred protection against tumor challenge, and were also able to eradicate existing tumors (Ossevoort et al., 1996; de Bruijn et al, 1998a). CTL responses from normal human donors *in vitro* using autologous dendritic cells pulsed with A2-binding peptides from HPV 11 E7 and HPV16 E7 have also been reported (Tarpey et al., 1994; Jochmus et al., 1997).

A big advantage to the use of dendritic cells is that they can be loaded with antigens in a variety of forms, but the treatment has to be carried out in autologous, or at least HLA-matched, systems which is obviously not always feasible.

5. Conclusions

Most of the vaccine trials so far reported have been carried out primarily to evaluate safety, and have involved fairly small numbers of patients often with very advanced disease. To take the trials forward we need larger cohorts, and also to think carefully about which groups of people to immunize. The immune response to the vaccine has to be monitored carefully and we have to decide how to assess the end-point with regards to the regression and reoccurrence of lesions. With this in mind, there is still a need for more basic research into the immunological events during natural regression, and the identification of the antigenic targets involved. In the case of the prophylactic vaccines for cervical cancer, it may be some time before the efficacy can be assessed because it usually takes many years for the cancer to develop.

Other problems likely to be encountered may be due to the poor antigen-presenting properties of the keratinocyte, so that even though a vaccine is capable of inducing the appropriate HPV-specific T-cells, they will be of limited use if they cannot recognise and kill their target cells. In order to address this, and related problems associated with immune evasion by the high risk viruses, we need to understand more about how differentiating epithelial tissue presents HPV antigens to the immune system.

Nevertheless, the results to the first clinical trials have been encouraging, and there is little doubt that HPV proteins and peptides can be immunogenic when administered to humans. Successful HPV vaccines remain a real possibilty for the future.

References

Albert, M.L., Sauter, B. and Bhardwaj, N. (1998) Dendritic cells acquire antigen from apoptotic cells and induce class I-restricted CTLs. Nature 392:86-89

Alexander, M., Salgaller, M.L., Sette, A., Barnes, W.A., Rosenberg, S.A. and Steller, M.A. (1996) Generation of tumor-specific cytolytic T lymphocytes from peripheral blood of cervical cancer patients by *in vitro* stimulation with a synthetic human papillomavirus type 16 E7 epitope. Am. J. Obstet. Gynecol. 175:1586-1593

Allen, J.E. and Maizels, R.M. (1997) Th1-Th2: reliable paradigm or dangerous dogma? Immunol. Today 18:387-392

Altmann, A., Jochmus-Kudielka, I., Rainer, F., Gausepohl, H., Moebius, U., Gissmann, L. and Meuer, S.C. (1992) Definition of immunogenic determinants of the human papillomavirus type 16 nucleoprotein E7. Eur. J. Cancer 28:326-333

Bal, V., McIndoe, A., Denton, G., Hudson, D., Lombardi, G. and Lamb, J. (1990) Antigen presentation by keratinocytes induces tolerance in human T-cells. Eur. J. Immunol. 20:1893-1897

Balmelli, C., Roden, R., Potts, A., Schiller, J., and De Grandi, P. and Nardelli-Haefliger, D. (1998) Nasal immunization of mice with human papillomavirus type 16 virus-like particles elicits neutralizing antibodies in mucosal secretions. J. Virol. 72:8220-82229

Banchereau, J. and Steinman, R.M. (1998) Dendritic cells and the control of immunity. Nature 392:245-252

Banks, L. and Matlashewski, G. (1996) Biochemical and biological activities of the HPV E5 proteins. In: Papillomavirus Reviews: Current research on Papillomaviruses. Eds: C. Lacey, Leeds University Press, Leeds. 39-46

Barker, J.N.W.N., Navsaria, H.A., Leigh, I.M., and MacDonald, D.M. (1988) Gamma-interferon induced human keratinocyte HLA-DR synthesis: the role of dermal activated T lymphocytes. Br. J. Dermatol. 119:567-572.

Barr, B.B.B., McClaren, K., Smith I.W., Benton, E.C., Bunney, M.H., Blessing, K. and Hunter, J.A.A. (1989) Papillomavirus infections and skin cancer in renal allograft recipients. Lancet (i):124-129

Bender, M.E. (1986) Concepts of wart regression. Arch. Dermatol. 122:644-647

Bennett, S.R.M., Carbone, F.R., Karamalis, F., Flavell, R.A., Miller, J.F.A.P. and Heath W.R. (1998) Help for cytotoxic T-cell responses is mediated by CD40 signalling. Nature 393:478-480

Benton, C., Shahdullah, H. and Hunter, J.A.A. (1992). Human papillomavirus in the immunocompromised. Papillomavirus Rep. 3:23-26

Bontkes, H.J., Walboomers, J.M.M., Meijer, C.J.L.M., Helmerhorst, T.J.M. and Stern, P.L. (1998). Specific HLA class I down-regulation is an early event in cervical dysplasia associated with clinical progression. The Lancet. 351:187-188

Borysiewicz, L.K., Fiander, A., Nimako, M., Man, S., Wilkinson, G.W.G., Westmorland. D., Evans, A.S., Adams, M., Stacey, S.M., Boursall, M.E.G., Rutherford, E., Hickling, J.K. and Inglis, S. (1996) A recombinant vaccinia virus encoding human papillomavirus types 16 and 18, E6 and E7 proteins as immunotherapy for cervical cancer. Lancet 347:1523-1527

Bosch, F.X., Manos, M.M., Munoz, M., Sherman, M., Jansen, A.M., Peto, J., Schiffman, M.H., Moreno, V., Kurman, R. and Shah, K.V. (1995) Prevalence of human papillomavirus in cervical cancer: a worldwide perspective. International Biological Study on Cervical Cancer (IBSCC) study group. J. Natl. Cancer Inst. 87:796-802

Boursnell, M.E., Rutherforf, E., Hickling, J.K., Rollinson, E.A., Munro, A.J., Rolley, N., McLean, C.S., Borysiewicz, L.K., Vousden, K. and Inglis, S. (1996) Construction and characterization of a recombinant vaccinia virus expressing human papillomavirus proteins for immunotherapy of cervical cancer. Vaccine 14:1485-1494

Boyle, P. (1997) Global burden of cancer. Lancet 349 (ii):23-26

Brandt, R.M.P., Ressing, M.E., de Jong, J.H., Kenter, G.G., van Driel, W.J., Kast, W.M. and Melief, C.J.M. (1999) The HPV16 E7 peptide based vaccine trial in end stage cervical carcinoma. J. Immunother. (In press)

Breitburd, F., Kirnbauer, R., Hubbert, N.L., Nonnenmacher, B., Trin-Dinh-Desmarquet, C., Orth, G., Schiller, J.T. and Lowy, D.R. (1995) Immunization with virus-like particles from cottontail rabbit papillomavirus (CRPV) can protect against experimental CRPV infection. J. Virol. 69:3959-3963

Campo, M.S., Grindlay, G.J., O'Neil, B.W., Chandrachud, L.M., McGarvie, G.M. and Jarrett, W.F.H. (1993) Prophylactic and therapeutic vaccination against a mucosal papillomavirus. J. Gen. Virol. 74:945-953

Carbone, F.R. and Bevan, M.J. (1990) Class I-restricted processing and presentation of exogenous cell-associated antigen *in vivo*. J. Exp. Med. 171:377-387

Carter, J.J., Koutsky, L.A., Wipf, G.C., Christensen, N.D., Lee, S.K., Kuypers, J., Kiviat, N. and Galloway, D.A. (1996) The natural history of human papillomavirus type 16 capsid antibodies among a cohort of university women. J. Infect. Dis. 145:927-936

Carter, J.J. and Galloway, D.A. (1997) Humoral immune response to human papillomavirus infection. Clin. Dermatol. 15(2):249-259

Cella, M., Sallusto, F. and Lanzavecchia, A. (1997) Origin, maturation and antigen presenting function of dendritic cells. Curr. Opin. Immunol. 9:10-16

Charleson, F.C., Norval, M., Benton, E.C. and Hunter, J.A.A. (1992) Lymphoproliferative responses to human papillomaviruses in patients with cutaneous warts. Br. J. Dermatol. 127:551-559

Chen, L.P., Kinney Thomas, E., Hu, S-L., Hellstrom, I. and Hellstrom, K.E. (1991) Human papillomavirus type 16 nucleoprotein E7 is a tumor rejection antigen. Proc. Natl. Acad. Sci. USA 88:110-114

Chen, L.P., Mizuno, M.T., Singhal, M.C., Hu, S-L., Galloway, D.A., Hellstrom, I. and Hellstrom, K.E. (1992) Induction of cytotoxic T lymphocytes specific for a syngeneic tumor expressing the E6 oncoprotein of human papillomavirus type 16. J. Immunol. 148:2617-2621

Chow, L.T. and Broker, T.R. (1997) Small DNA viruses. In: Viral Pathogenesis: Eds: N. Nathanson, R. Ahmed, F. Gonzalez-Scarano, D.E. Griffin, K.V. Holmes, F.A. Murphy and H.L. Robinson, Lippincott-Raven, Philadelphia. 267-301

Christensen, N.D., Reed, C.A., Cladel, N.M., Han, R. and Kreider, J.W. (1996) Immunisation with virus-like particles induces long-term protection of rabbits against challenge with cottontail rabbit papillomaviruses. J. Virol. 70:960-965

Clerici, M., Merola, M., Ferrario, E., Trabattoni, D., Villa, M.L., Stafanon, B., Venzon, D.J., Shearer, G.M., DePalo, G. and Clerici, E. (1997) Cytokine production patterns in cervical intraepithelial neoplasia: association with human papillomavirus infection. J. Natl. Cancer Inst. 89:245-250

Coleman, N. and Stanley, M.A. (1994) Analysis of HLA-DR expression on keratinocytes in cervical neoplasia. Int. J. Cancer 56:314-319

Coleman, N., Birley, H.D.L., Renton, A.M., Hanna, N.F., Ryait, B.K., Byrne, M., Taylor Robinson, D. and Stanley, M.A. (1994) Immunological events in regressing genital warts. Am. J. Clin. Pathol. 102:768-774

Cooney, E.L., Collier, A.C., Greenberg, P.D., Coombs, R.W., Zarling, J., Arditti, G.E., Hoffman, N.C., Hu, S. and Corey, L. (1991) Safety of and immunological response to a recombinant vaccinia virus vaccine expressing HIV envelope glycoprotein. Lancet 337:567-572

Cromme, F.V., Airey, J., Heemels, M.T., Ploegh, H.L., Keating, P.J., Stern, P.L., Meijer, C.J.L.M., and Walboomers, J.M.M. (1994) Loss of transporter protein, encoded by the Tap-1 gene, is highly correlated with loss of HLA expression in cervical carcinomas. J. Exp. Med. 179:335-340.

Cubie, H.A., Norval, M., Crawford, L., Banks, L. and Crook, T. (1989) Lymphoproliferative response to fusion proteins of human papillomaviruses in patients with cervical intraepithelial neoplasia. Epidemiol. Infect. 103:625-632

Cullen, A.P., Reid, R., Campion, M. and Lorincz, T. (1991) Analysis of the physical state of different human papillomavirus DNAs in intraepithelial neoplasia and invasive cervical carcinoma. J. Virol. 65:606-612

Da Silva, D.M., Velders, M.P., Rudolf, M.P., Schiller, J.T. and Kast, W.M. (1999) Papillomavirus virus-like particles as anti-cancer vaccines. Curr. Opin. Mol. Ther. 1(1):82-88

deGruijl, T.D., Bontkes, H.J., Stukart, M.J., Walboomers, J.M.M., Remmink, A.J., Verheijen, R.H.M., Helmerhorst, T.J.M., Meijer, C.J.L.M. and Scheper, R.J. (1996) T-cell proliferative responses against human papillomavirus type 16 E7 oncoprotein are most prominent in cervical intraepithelial neoplasia patients with a persistent viral infection. J. Gen. Virol. 77:2183-2191

deGruijl, T.D., Schuurhuis, D.H., Vierboom, M.P.M., Vermeulen, H., deCock, K.A.J., Ooms, M.E., Ressing, M.E., Toebes, M., Franken, K.L., Drijfhout, J.W., Ottenhoff, T.H.M., Offringa, R. and Melief, C.J.M. (1998a) Immunization with human papillomavirus type 16 (HPV16) oncoprotein-loaded dendritic cells as well as protein adjuvant induces MHC class I-restricted protection to HPV16-induced tumor cells. Cancer Res. 58:724-731

deGruijl, T.D. Bontkes, H.J., Wallboomers, J.M.M., Coursaget, P., Stukart, M.J., Dupuy, C., Kueter, E., Verheijen, R.H.M., Helmerhorst, T.J.M., Duggan-Keen, M., Stevens, F.R.A., Dyer, P.A., Stern, P.L., Meijer, C.J.L.M. and Scheper, R.J. (1998b) Differential T helper cell responses to human papillomavirus type 16 E7 related to viral clearance or persistence in patients with cervical neoplasia: a longitudinal study. Cancer Res. 58:1700-1706

deGruijl, T.D., Bontkes, H.J., Wallboomers, J.M.M., Coursaget, P., Stukart, M.J., Dupuy, C., Kueter, E., Verheijen, R.H.M., Helmerhorst, T.J.M., Duggan-Keen, M.F., Stern, P.L., Meijer, C.J.L.M. and Scheper, R.J. (1999) Immune responses against human papillomavirus (HPV) type 16 virus-like particles in a cohort study of women with cervical intraepithelial neoplasia: 1. Differential T helper and IgG responses in relation to HPV infection and disease outcome. J. Gen. Virol. 80(2):399-408

deVilliers, E.M. (1997) Papillomavirus and HPV typing. Clin. Dermatol. 15:199-206

Derkay, C.S. (1995) Task force on recurrent respiratory papillomas. Arch. Otolaryngol. Head Neck Surg. 121:1386-1391

Doherty, P. (1995) Anatomical environment as a determinant in viral immunity. J. Immunol. 155:1023-1027

Doherty, P.C., Hou, S. and Tripp, R.A. (1994) CD8+ T-cell memory to viruses. Curr. Opin. Immunol. 6:545-552

Donnelly, J.J., Martinez, D., Jansen, K.U., Ellis, R.W., Montgomery, M.A. and Liu, M.A. (1996) Protection against papillomavirus with a polynucleotide vaccine. J. Infect. Dis. 173:314-320

Doorbar, J. (1996) The E4 proteins and their role in the viral life cycle. In: Papillomavirus Reviews: Current research on Papillomaviruses. Eds: C. Lacey, Leeds University Press, Leeds. 31-38

Doorbar, J. (1998) Late stages in the papillomavirus life cycle. Papillomavirus Rep. 9:119-126

Doorbar, J., Ely, S., Coleman, N., Hibma, M., Davies, D.H. and Crawford, L. (1991) Specific interaction between HPV16 E1-E4 and cytokeratins results in collapse of the epithelial cell intermediate filament network. Nature 352:824-827

Duggan-Keene, M.F., Brown, M.D., Stacey, S.N. and Stern, P.L. (1998) Papillomavirus vaccines. Frontiers in Bioscience 3:d1192-1208

Dupuy, C., Buzoni Gatel, D., Touze, A., LeCann, P., Bout, D. and Coursaget, P. (1997) Cell-mediated immunity induced in mice by HPV16 L1 virus-like particles. Microb. Pathog. 22:219-225

Ellis, J.R.M., Keating, P.J., Baird, J., Hounsell, E.F., Renouf, D.V., Rowe, M., Hopkins, D., Duggan-Keen, M., Bartholomew, J.S., Young, L.S., and Stern, P.L. (1995). The association of an HPV16 oncogene variant with HLA-B7 has implications for vaccine design in cervical cancer. Nature Med. 1:464-470.

Evander, M., Frazer, I.H., Payne, E., Qi, Y.M., Hengst, K. and McMillan, N.A.J. (1997) Identification of the alpha (6) integrin as a candidate receptor for papillomaviruses. J. Virol. 71:2449-2456

Evans, E.M., Man, S., Evans, A.S. and Borysiewicz, L.K. (1997) Infiltration of cervical cancer tissue with human papillomavirus-specific cytotoxic T lymphocytes. Cancer Res. 57:2943-2950

Feltkamp, M.C.W., Smits, H.S., Vierboom, M.P.M., Minaar, R.P., de Jongh, B.M., Drijfhout, J.W., ter Schegget, J., Melief, C.J.M. and Kast, W.M. (1993) Vaccination with cytotoxic T lymphocyte epitope-containing peptide protects against a tumor induced by human papillomavirus type 16-transformed cells. Eur. J. Immunol. 23:2242-2249

Feltkamp, M.C.W., Vreugdenhil, G.R., Vierboom, M.P.M., Ras, E., van der Berg, S.H., ter Schegget, J., Melief, C.J.M. and Kast, W.M. (1995) Cytotoxic T lymphocytes raised against a sub-dominant epitope offered as a synthetic peptide eradicate human papillomavirus type 16-induced tumors. Eur. J. Immunol. 25:2638-2642

Feltquate, D.M., Heaney, S., Webster, R.G. and Robinson, H.L. (1997) Different Th-cell types and antibody isotypes generated by saline and gene gun DNA immunization. J. Immunol. 158:2278-2284

Ferguson A.. Moore, M. and Fox, H. (1985) Expression of MHC products and leucocyte differentiation antigens in gynaecological neoplasms: an immunohistological analysis of the tumor cells and infiltrating leucocytes. Br. J. Cancer 52:551-563

Fleming, T.E., Mirando, W.S., Trefzer, U., Tubesking, K.A., and Elmets, C.A. (1993) In situ expression of a B7-like adhesion molecule on keratinocytes from human epidermis. J. Invest. Dermatol. 101:754-75.

Fuchs, P.G. and Pfister. H. (1996) Papillomaviruses in epidermodysplasia verruciformis. In: Papillomavirus Reviews: Current research on Papillomaviruses. Eds: C. Lacey, Leeds University Press., Leeds. 253-262

Galloway, D.A. (1996) HPV serology: another update. In: Papillomavirus Reviews: Current research on Papillomaviruses. Eds: C. Laccy, Leeds University Press., Leeds. 113-119

Gao, L., Chain, B., Sinclair, C., Crawford, L., Zhou, J., Morris, J., Zhu, X. and Stauss, H. (1994) Immune response to human papillomavirus type 16 E6 gene in a live vaccinia vector. J. Gen. Virol. 75:157-164

Garzetti, G.G., Ciavattini, A., Buttini, L., Vecchi, A. and Montroni, M. (1994) Cervical dysplasia in HIV-seropositive women - role of human papillomavirus infection and immune status. Gynecol. Obstet. Invest. 40:52-56

Gaspari, A.A., Ferbel, B., Chen, Z., Razvi, F., and Polakowska, R. (1994). Accessory and alloantigen-presenting cell functions of A431 keratinocytes that stably express the B7 antigen. Cell. Immunol. 149:291-302

Gill, D.K., Bible, J.M., Biswas, C., Kell, B., Best, J.M., Punchard, N.A. and Cason, J. (1998) Proliferative T-cell responses to human papillomavirus type 16 E5 are decreased amongst women with high grade neoplasia. J. Gen. Virol. 79:1971-1976

Glew, S.S., Duggan-Keen, M., Cabrera, T. and Stern, P.L. (1992) HLA class II antigen expression in human papillomavirus-associated cervical cancer. Cancer Res. 52:4009-4016

Greenstone, H.L., Nieland, J.D., deVisser, K.E., DeBruijn, M.L.H., Kirnbauer, R., Roden, R.B.S., Lowy, D.R. and Schiller, J.T. (1998) Chimeric papillomavirus virus-like particles elicit anti-tumor immunity against the E7 oncoprotein in an HPV16 tumor model. Proc. Natl. Acad. Sci. USA. 95:1800-1805

Griffiths, G.M. (1995) The cell biology of CTL killing. Curr. Opin. Immunol. 7:343-348

Griffiths, C.E.M., Voorhees, J.J. and Nickoloff, B.J. (1989). Gamma interferon induces different keratinocyte cellular patterns of expression of HLA-DR, DQ and intercellular adhesion molecule-1 (ICAM-1) antigens. Br. J. Dermatol. 120:1-7.

Hagensee, M.E., Yaegashi, N. and Galloway, D.A. (1993) Self-assembly of human papillomavirus type 1 capsids by expression of the L1 protein alone or by the coexpression of the L1 and L2 capsid proteins. J. Virol. 67:315-322

Halpert, R., Fruchter, R.G., Sedlis, A., Butt, K., Boyce, J.G. and Sillman, F.H. (1986) Human papillomavirus and lower genital neoplasia in renal transplant patients. Obstet. Gynecol. 68:251-258

Ho, G.Y.F., Bierman, R., Beardsley, L., Chang, C.J. and Burk, R.D. (1998) Natural history of cervicovaginal papillomavirus infection in young women. N. Engl. J. Med. 338:423-428

Hofman, K., Cook, J., Joyce, J., Brown, D.R., Schulz, L.D., George, H.A., Rosolowsky, M., Fife, K.H. and Jansen, K.U. (1995) Sequence determination of human papillomavirus type 6a and assembly of virus-like particles in *Saccharomyces cerevisiae*. Virology 209:506-518

Hong, K., Greer. C.E., Ketter, N., Van Nest, G. and Paliard, X. (1997) Isolation and characterization of human papillomavirus type 6-specific T cells infiltrating genital warts. J. Virol. 71:6427-6432

Ivanyi, L. and Morison, W.L. (1976) *In vitro* lymphocyte stimulation by wart antigens in man. Br. J. Dermatol. 94:523-527

Iwatsuki, K., Tagami, M., Takigawa, M. and Yamanda, M. (1986) Plane warts under spontaneous regression. Immunopathologic study on cellular constituents leading to the inflammatory reaction Arch. Dermatol. 122:655-659

Jansen, K.U., Rosolowsky, M., Schultz, L.D., Markus, H.Z., Cook, J.C., Donnelly, J.J., Martinez, D., Ellis, R.W. and Shaw, A.R. (1995) Vaccination with yeast-expressed cottontail rabbit papillomavirus (CRPV) virus-like particles protects rabbits from CRPV-induced papillomavirus formation. Vaccine 13:1509-1514

Jarrett, W.F.H., Smith, K.T., O'Neill, B.W., Gaukroger, J.M., Chandrachaud, M., Grindlay, G.J., McGarvie, G.M. and Campo, M.S. (1991) Studies on vaccination against papillomaviruses: prophylactic and therapeutic vaccination with recombinant structural proteins. Virology 184:33-42

Jensen, E.R., Selvakumar, R., Shen, H., Ahmed, R., Wettstein, F.O. and Miller, J.F. (1997) Recombinant *Listeria monocytogenes* vaccination eliminates papillomavirus-induced tumors and prevents papilloma formation from viral DNA. J. Virol. 71:8467-8474

Jochmus, I., Osen, W., Altmann, A., Buck, G., Hofmann, B., Schneider, A., Gissmann, L. and Rammensee, H.G. (1997) Specificity of human cytotoxic T lymphocytes induced by a human papillomavirus type 16 E7-derived peptide. J. Gen. Virol. 78:1689-1695

Junghans, V., Jung, T., and Neumann, C. (1996). Human keratinocytes constitutively express IL-4 receptor molecules and respond to IL-4 with an increase in B7/BB1 expression. Exp. Dermatol. 5:316-324

Kadish, A.S., Romney, S.L., Ledwidge, R., Tindle, R., Fernando, J.P., Zee, S.Y., Vanrast, M.A. and Burk, R.D. (1994) Cell-mediated immune responses to E7 peptides of human papillomavirus (HPV) type 16 are dependent on the HPV type infecting the cervix whereas serological reactivity is not type-specific. J. Gen. Virol. 75:2277-2284

Kadish, A.S., Ho, G.F.Y., Burk, R.D., Wang, Y.X., Romney, S.L., Ledwidge, R. and Angeletti, R.H. (1997) Lymphoproliferative responses to human papillomavirus (HPV) type 16 proteins E6 and E7:outcome of HPV infection and associated neoplasia. J. Natl. Canc. Inst. 89:1285-1293

Kalams, S.A. and Walker, B.D. (1998) The critical need for CD4 help in maintaining effective cytotoxic T lymphocyte responses. J. Exp. Med. 188(12):2199-2204

Kaufmann, A.M., Gissmann, L., Schreckenberger, C., and Qiao, L. (1997) Cervical carcinoma cells transfected with the CD80 gene elicit a primary cytotoxic T lymphocyte responses specific for HPV16 E7 antigens. Cancer Gene Ther. 4:377-382

Keating, P.J., Cromme, F.V., Duggan-Keen, M., Snijders, P.J.F., Walboomers, J.M.M., Hunter, R.D., Dyer, P.A. and Stern, P.L. (1995). Frequency of down-regulation of individual HLA-A and -B alleles in cervical carcinomas in relation to TAP-1 expression. Br. J. Cancer. 72:405-411.

Kelso, A. (1995) Th1 and Th2 subsets: paradigms lost? Immunol. Today 16:374-379

Kirnbauer, R., Booy, F., Cheng, N., Lowy, D.R. and Schiller, J.T. (1992) Papillomavirus L1 major capsid protein self assembles into virus-like particles that are highly immunogenic. Proc. Natl. Acad. Sci. USA. 89:12180-12184

Kirnbauer, R., Taub, J., Greenstone, H., Roden, R.B.S., Durst, M., Gissman, L., Lowy, D.R. and Schiller, J.T. (1993) Efficient self-assembly of human papillomavirus type 16 L1 and L1-L2 into virus-like particles. J. Virol. 67:6929-6936

Kirnbauer, R., Chandrachud, L., O'Neil, B., Wagner, E., Grindlay, G., Armstrong, E., McGarvie, G., Schiller, J., Lowy, D. and Campo, M. (1996) Virus-like particles of bovine papillomavirus type 4 in prophylactic and therapeutic immunization. Virology 219:37-44

Klagge, I.M. and Schneider-Schaulies, S. (1999) Virus interactions with dendritic cells. J. Gen. Virol. 80:823-833

Knowles, G., O'Neil, B.W. and Campo, M.S. (1996) Phenotypical characterisation of lymphocytes infiltrating regressing papillomas. J. Virol. 70:8451-8458

Konya, J., Eklund, C., af Geijersstam, V., Yuan, F., Stuber, G. and Dillner, J. (1997) Identification of a cytotoxic T lymphocyte epitope in the human papillomavirus type 16 E2 protein. J. Gen. Virol. 78:2615-2620

Lacey, C.J.N., Thompson, H.S.G., Monteiro, E.F., O'Neill, T., Davies, M.L., Holding, F.P., Fallon, R.E. and Roberts, J.St.C. (1999) Phase IIa safety and immunogenicity of a therapeutic vaccine, TA-GW, in persons with genital warts. J. Infect. Dis. 179:612-618

Lambert, P.F. (1991) Papillomavirus DNA replication. J. Virol. 65:3417-3420

Laga, M., Icenogle, J.P., Marsella, R., Manoka, A.T., Nzila, N., Ryder, R.W., Vermund, S.H., Heyward, W.L., Nelson, A. and Reeves, W.C. (1992) Genital papillomavirus infection and cervical dysplasia - opportunistic complications of HIV infection. Int. J. Cancer 48:682-688

Lee, A.K. and Eisenger, M. (1976) Cell-mediated immunity to human wart virus and wart-associated tissue antigens. Clin. Exp. Immunol. 26:419-424

Lehtinen, M., Rantala, I., Tiovonen, A., Luoto, H., Aine, R., Lauslahti, K., Ylaoutinen, A., Romppanen, U. and Paavonen, J. (1993) Depletion of Langerhans cells in cervical HPV infection is associated with replication of the virus. APIMS 101:833-837

Lehtinen, M., Dillner, J., Knekt, P., Luostarinen, T., Aromaa, A., Kirnbauer, R., Koskela, P., Paavonen, J., Peto, R., Schiller, J.T. and Hakama, M. (1996) Serologically diagnosed infection with human papillomavirus type 16 and risk for subsequent development of cervical carcinoma: nested case-control study. Br. Med. J. 312:537-539

Li, M.L., Cripe, T.P., Estes, P.A., Lyon, M.K., Rose, R.C. and Garcea, R.L. (1997) Expression of the human papilllomavirus type 11 L1 capsid protein in *Escherichia coli*: characterization of protein domains involved in DNA binding and capsid assembly. J. Virol. 71:2988-2995

Lin, Y.L., Borenstein, L.A., Selvakumar, R., Ahmed, R. and Wettstein, F.O. (1992) Effective vaccination against papilloma development by immunization with L1 or L2 structural proteins of cottontail rabbit papillomavirus. Virology 187.612-619

Lin, K.Y., Guarnieri, F.G., Stavely-O'Carroll, K.F., Livitsky, H.I., August, J.T., Pardoll, D.M. and Wu, T.C. (1996) Treatment of established tumors with a novel vaccine that enhances major histocompatibility class II presentation of tumor antigen. Cancer Res. 56:21-26

Lipford, G.B., Bauer, S., Wagner, H. and Heeg, K. (1995) Peptide engineering allows cytotoxic T-cell vaccination against human papillomavirus tumor-antigen E6. Immunol. 84:298-303

Lowe, R.S., Brown, D.R., Bryan, J.T., Cook, J.C., George, H.A., Hofmann, K.J., Hurni, W.M., Joyce, J.G., Lehman, E.D., Markus, H.Z., Neeper, M.P., Schultz, L.D., Shaw, A.R. and Jansen, K.U. (1997) Human papillomavirus type 11 neutralizing antibodies in the serum and genital mucosal secretions of African green monkeys immunized with HPV11 virus-like particles expressed in yeast. J. Infect. Dis. 176:1141-1145

Lowy, D.R. and Schiller, J.T, (1998) Papillomaviruses: Prophylactic vaccine prospects. Biochim. Biophys. Acta 1423:M1-M8

Lutzner, M.A. (1985) Papillomavirus lesions in immunodepression and immunosuppression. Clin. Dermatol. 3:165-169

Luxton, J.C., Rowe, A.J., Cridland, J.C., Coletart, T., Wilson, P. and Shepherd, P.S. (1996) Proliferative T-cell responses to the human papillomavirus type 16 E7 protein in women with cervical dysplasia and cervical carcinoma and in healthy individuals. J. Gen. Virol. 77:1585-1593

Luxton, J.C., Rose, R.C., Coletart, T., Wilson, P. and Shepherd, P.S. (1997) Serological and T helper cell responses to human papillomavirus type 16 L1 in women with cervical dysplasia or cervical carcinoma and in healthy controls. J. Gen. Virol. 78:917-923

McNeil, C. (1997) HPV vaccine treatment trials proliferate, diversify. J. Natl. Cancer Inst. 89:280-281

Mehta-Damani, A., Markowicz, S. and Engleman, E.G. (1994) Generation of antigen-specific CD8+ CTLs from naive precursors. J. Immunol. 153:996-1003

Melief, C.J.M., Offringa, R., Toes, R.E.M. and Kast, W.M. (1996) Peptide-based cancer vaccines. Curr. Opin. Immunol. 8:651-657

Meneguzzi, G., Cerni, C., Kieny, M.P. and Lathe, R. (1991) Immunization against human papillomavirus 16 tumor cells with recombinant vaccinia viruses expressing E6 and E7. Virology 181:62-69

Murakami, M., Gurski, K.J., Marincola, F.M., Ackland, J. and Steller, M.A. (1999) Induction of specific CD8+ T-lymphocyte responses using a human papillomavirus 16 E6/E7 fusion protein and autologous dendritic cells. Cancer Res. 59:1184-1187

Morelli, A.E., Sananes, C., DiPaola, G., Paredes, A. and Fainboim, L. (1992) Relationship between types of human papillomavirus and Langerhans cells in cervical condyloma and intraepithelial neoplasia. Am. J. Clin. Pathol. 99:200-206

Mosman, T.R. and Sad, S. (1996) The expanding universe of T-cell subsets: Th1, Th2 and more. Immunol. Today 17:138-146

Muller, M., Zhou, J., Reed, T.D., Rittmuller, C., Burger, A., Gabelsberger, J., Braspenning, J. and Gissmann, L. (1997) Chimeric papillomavirus-like particles. Virology 234:93-111

Nakagawa, M., Stites, D.P., Farhat, S., Sisler, J.R., Kong, M.B.F., Moscicki, A.B. and Palefsky, J.M. (1997) Cytotoxic T lymphocyte responses to E6 and E7 proteins of human papillomavirus type 16: Relationship to cervical intraepithelial neoplasia. J. Infect. Dis. 175:927-931

Nimako, M., Fiander, A.N., Wilkinson, G.W.G., Borysiewicz, L.K. and Man, S. Human papillomavirus-specific cytotoxic T lymphocytes in patients with cervical intraepithelial neoplasia grade III. (1997) Cancer Res. 57:4855-4861

Orth, G. (1987) Epidermodysplasia verruciformis. In: The Papovaviridae. Eds: N.P. Salzman and P.M. Howley. Plenum Publishing Corporation. 2:199-243

Ossevoort, M.A., Feltkamp, M.C., van Veen, K.J.H., Melief, C.J.M. and Kast, W.M. (1995) Dendritic cells as carriers for a cytotoxic T-lympocyte epitope-based peptide vaccine in protection against a human papillomavirus type 16-induced tumor. J. Immunother. 18:86-94

Peng, S., Frazer, I.H., Fernando, G.J. and Zhou, J. (1998) Papillomavirus virus-like particles can deliver defined CTL epitopes to the MHC class I pathway. Virology 240:147-157

Pertmer, T.M., Roberts, T.R. and Haynes, J.R. (1996) Influenza virus nucleoprotein-specific immunoglobulin G subclass and cytokine responses elicited by DNA vaccination are dependent on the route of vector DNA delivery. J. Virol. 70:6119-6125

Petry, K.W., Scheffel, D., Bode, U., Gabrysiak, T., Kochel, H., Kupsch, E., Glaubitz, M., Niesert, S., Kuhnle, H. and Schedel, I. (1994) Cellular immunodeficiency enhances the progression of human papillomavirus-associated cervical lesions. Int. J. Cancer 57: 836-840

Pfister, H., Iftner, T. and Fuchs, P.G. (1985) Papillomaviruses from epidermodysplasia verruciformis patients and renal allograft recipients. In: Papillomaviruses: Molecular and clinical aspects. Eds: P.M. Howley and T.R. Broker, Liss, New York. 85-100

Ressing, M.E., Sette, A., Brandt, R.M.P., Ruppert, J., Wentworth, P.A., Hartman, M., Oseroff, C., Grey, H.M., Melief, C.J. and Kast, W.M. (1995) Human CTL epitopes encoded by human papillomavirus type 16 E6 and E7 identified through *in vivo* and *in vitro* immunogenicity studies of HLA-A*0201-binding peptides. J. Immunol. 154:5934-5943

Ressing, M.E., Van Driel, W.J., Celis, E., Sette, A., Brandt, R.M.P., Hartman, M., Anholts, J.D.H., Schreuder, G.M.T., Ter Harmsel, W.B. and Fleuren, G.R. (1996) Occasional memory cytotoxic T-cell responses of patients with human papillomavirus type 16-positive cervical lesions against a human leukocyte antigen-A*0201 restricted E7-encoded epitope. Cancer Res. 56:582-588

Reichman, R., Balsley, J., Carlin, D., Connor, E., White, W., Wilson, S., Suzich, J. and Koenig, S. (1999) Evaluation of the safety and immunogenicity of a recombinant HPV11 L1 virus-like particle vaccine in healthy adult volunteers. Abstract. 17th International Papillomavirus Conference, Charleston, SC, USA. p13.

Ridge, J.P., DiRosa, F. and Matzinger, P. (1998) A conditioned dendritic cell can be a temporal bridge between a CD4+ helper and a T-killer cell. Nature 393:474-478

Roberts, S., Ashmole, I., Johnson, G.D., Kreider, J.W. and Gallimore, P.H. (1993) Cutaneous and mucosal human papillomavirus E4 proteins form intermediate filament-like structures in epithelial cells. Virology 197:176-187

Roden, R.B., Kirnbauer, A., Jensen, A.B., Lowy, D.R. and Schiller, J.T. (1994) Interaction of papillomaviruses with the cell surface. J. Virol. 68:7260-7266

Roden, R.B.S., Hubbert, N.L., Kirnbauer, R., Christensen, N.D., Lowy, D.R. and Schiller, J.T. (1996a) Assessment of the serological relatedness of genital human papillomaviruses by haemagglutination inhibition. J. Virol. 70:3298-3301

Roden, R.B.S., Greenstone, H.L., Kirnbauer, R., Booy, F.P., Jessie, J., Lowy, D.R. and Schiller, J.T. (1996b) In vitro generation and type-specific neutralization of a human papillomavirus type 16 virion pseudotype. J. Virol. 70:5875-5883

Roden, R.B., Armstrong, A., Haderer, P., Christensen, N.D., Hubbert, N.L., Lowy, D.R., Schiller, J.T. and Kirnbauer, R. (1997) Characterization of a human papillomavirus type 16 variant-dependent neutralizing epitope. J. Virol. 71:6247-6252

Rose, R.C., Bonnez, W., Reichman, R.C. and Garcea, R.L. (1993) Expression of human papillomavirus type 11 L1 protein in insect cells: in vivo and in vitro assembly of virus-like particles. J. Virol. 67:1936-1944

Sadovnikova, E., Zhu, X.J., Collins, S.M., Zhou, J., Vousden, K., Crawford, L., Beverley, P. and Stauss, H.J. (1994) Limitations of predictive motifs revealed by cytotoxic T-lymphocyte epitope mapping of the human papillomavirus E7 protein. Int. Immunol. 6:289-296

Sasagawa, T., Pushko, P., Steers, G., Gschmeissner, S.E., Hajibagheri, M.A., Finch, J., Crawford, L. and Tomassino, M. (1995) Synthesis and assembly of virus-like particles of human papillomaviruses type 6 and type 16 in fission yeast Schizosaccharomyces pombe. Virology 206:126-135

Schoenberger, S.P., Toes, R.E.M., Van der Voort, E.I.H., Offringa, R. and Melief, C.J.M. (1998) T cell help for cytotoxic T lymphocytes is mediated by CD40-CD40L interactions. Nature 393:480-483

Selvakumar, R., Borenstein, L.A., Lin, Y.L., Ahmed, R., Wettstein, F.O. (1995) Immunization with nonstructural proteins E1 and E2 of cottontail rabbit papillomavirus stimulates regression of virus-induced papillomas. J. Virol. 69:602-605

Selvakumar, R., Scmitt, A., Iffner, T, Ahmed, R. and Wettstein, F.O. (1997) Regression of papillomas induced by cottontail rabbit papillomavirus is associated with infiltration of CD8+ cells and persistence of viral DNA after regression. J. Virol. 71:5540-5548

Shepherd, P.S., Rowe, A.J., Cridland, J.C., Coletart, T., Wilson, P. and Luxton, J.C. (1996) Proliferative T cell responses to human papillomavirus type 16 L1 peptides in patients with cervical dysplasia. J. Gen. Virol. 77:593-602

Speidel, K. et al (1997) Priming of cytotoxic T-lymphocytes by five heat-aggregated antigens in vivo: conditions, efficiency, and relation to antibody responses. Eur. J. Immunol. 27:2391-2399

Steele, J.C., Stankovic, T.J., and Gallimore, P.H. (1993) Production and characterization of human proliferative T-cell clones specific for human papillomavirus type 1 E4 protein. J. Virol. 67:2799-2806

Stingl, G. and Berstresser, P.R. (1995) Dendritic cells: a major story unfolds. Immunol. Today 16:330-333

Stoler, M.H., Rhodes, C.R., Whitbeck, A., Wolinsky, S.M., Chow, L.T. and Broker, T.R. (1992) Human papillomavirus type 16 and 18 gene expression in cervical neoplasias. Hum. Pathol. 23:117-128

Strang, G., Hickling, J.K., McIndoe, G.A.J., Howland, K., Wilkinson, D., Ikeda, H. and Rothbard, J.B. (1990) Human T-cell responses to human papillomavirus type 16 L1 and E6 synthetic peptides:

identification of T-cell determinants, HLA-DR restriction and virus type specificity. J. Gen. Virol. 71:423-431

Suzich, J.A., Ghim, S., Palmer-Hill, S.J., White, W.I., Tamura, J.K., Bell, J., Newsome, J.A., Jenson, A.B. and Schlegel, R. (1995) Systemic immunization with papillomavirus L1 protein completely prevents the development of viral mucosal papillomas. Proc. Natl. Acad. Sci. USA. 92:11553-11557

Syrjanen, K.J. (1996) Natural history of genital human papillomavirus infections. In: Papillomavirus Reviews: Current Research on Human Papillomaviruses. Eds. C. Lacey, Leeds University Press, Leeds. 189-206

Tagami, H., Oku, T. and Iwatsuki, K. (1985) Primary tissue culture of spontanously regressing flat warts. In vitro attack by mononuclear cells against wart-derived epidermal cells. Cancer 55:2437-2341

Tarpey, I., Stacey, S., Hickling, J., Birley, H.D.L., Renton, A., McIndoe, A. and Davies, D.H. (1994) Human cytotoxic T lymphocytes stimulated by endogenously processed human papillomavirus type 11 E7 recognize a peptide containing a HLA-A2 (0201) motif. Immunol. 81:222-227

Tay, S.K., Jenkins, D., Madox, P., Campion, M. and Singer, A. (1985) Sub-populations of Langerhans cells in cervical neoplasia. Br. J. Obstet. Gynaecol. 94:10-15

Thompson, H.S.G., Davies, M.L. and Holding, F.P. (1999) Phase I safety and antigenicity of TA-GW: a recombinant HPV6 L2E7 vaccine for the treatment of genital warts. Vaccine 16:1993-1999

Tindle, R. (1996) Human papillomavirus vaccines for cervical cancer. Curr. Opin. Immunol. 8:643-650

Tosi, P. Cintorino, M., Santopietro, R., Lio, R. Barbini, P., Ji, H.X. Chang, P., Kataja, V. and Syrjanan, K. (1992) Prognostic factors in invasive carcinoma associated with human papillomavirus. Path. Res. Pract. 188:866-873

Tripp, R.A., Hou, S., McMickle, A., Houston, J. and Doherty, P.C. (1995) Recruitment and proliferation of CD8+ T-cells in respiratory virus infections. J. Immunol. 154:6013-6021

Tsang, K.Y., Zaremba, S., Nieroda, C.A., Zhu, M.Z., Hamilton, M. and Schlom, J. (1995) Generation of human cytotoxic T cells for human carcinoembryonic antigen (CEA) epitopes from patients immunized with recombinant vaccinia-CEA vaccines. J. Natl. Canc. Inst. 87:982-990

Viac, J., Guerin, R.I., Chardonnet, Y. and Bremond, A. (1990) Langerhans cells and epithelial modifications in cervical intraepithelial neoplasia: correlation with human papillomavirus infections. Immunobiol. 180:328-338

Volpers, C., Schirmacher, P., Streeck, R.E. and Sapp, M. (1994) Assembly of the major and the minor capsid protein of human papillomavirus type 33 into virus-like particles and tubular structures in insect cells. Virology 200:504-512

Wang, Z.H., Hansson, B.G., Forslund, O., Dillner, L., Sapp, M., Schiller, J.T., Bjerre, B. and Dillner, J. (1996) Cervical-mucus antibodies against human papillomavirus type 16, type 18, and type 33 capsids in relation to presence of viral DNA. J. Clin. Microbiol. 34:3056-3062

White, W.I., Wilson, S.D., Bonnez, W., Rose, R.C., Koenig, S. and Suzie, J.A. (1998) In vitro infection and type-restricted antibody-mediated neutralization of authentic human papilllomavirus type 16. J. Virol. 72:959-964

Williams, I.R., Ort, R.J. and Kupper, T.S. (1994). Keratinocyte expression of B7.1 in transgenic mice amplifies the primary immune response to cutaneous antigens. Proc. Natl. Acad. Sci. USA. 91:12780-12784.

Zhou, J., Sun, X.Y., Stenzl, D.J. and Frazer, I.H. (1991a) Expression of vaccinia recombinant HPV 16 L1 and L2 ORF proteins in epithelial cells is sufficient for assembly of HPV virion-like particles. Virology. 185:251-257

Zhou, J., McIndoe, A., Davies, H., Sun, X.Y. and Crawford, L. (1991b) the induction of cytotoxic T lymphocyte precursor cells by recombinant vaccinia virus expressing human papillomavirus type 16 L1. Virology 181:203-210

Zhu, X., Tommasino, M., Vousden, K., Sadovnikava, E., Rappuoli, R., Crawford, L., Kast, M., Melief, C.J.M., Beverley, P.C.L. and Stauss, H.J. (1995) Both immunization with protein and recombinant vaccinia virus can stimulate CTL specific for the E7 protein of human papillomavirus 16 in H-2(D) mice. Scand. J. Immunol. 42:557-563

Zur Hausen, H. (1991) Human papillomaviruses in the pathogenesis of anogenital cancer. Virology 184:9-13

ADENOVIRUS CANCER GENE THERAPY

Martin B. Powell and Gavin W. G. Wilkinson

Department of Medicine, University of Wales
College of Medicine, Cardiff, UK

ABSTRACT

Recombinant adenoviruses are now used extensively in experimental protocols for the treatment of infectious, genetic and neoplastic disease. Adenovirus has emerged as of one the leading gene therapy vectors primarily because of its unrivalled capacity to deliver a transgene efficiently to a high proportion of target cells *in vitro*, *ex vivo* and *in vivo*. Most published studies use a standard first generation replication-deficient Ad vector with high level transgene expression being driven by a strong constitutive promoter. However, considerable research effort is now going into optimizing vectors for specific clinical applications. The virus particle is being manipulated so that it can be re-targeted to infect specific cell types. Tumor-specific promoters are also being exploited to restrict expression to malignant cells. Furthermore, the safety and performance of adenovirus vector systems are being enhanced by the deletion of additional essential genes from the vector backbone and the development of promoters that can be actively regulated *in vivo*.

A plethora of different therapies are being explored for cancer gene therapy using adenovirus vector systems and they are reviewed extensively within this chapter. The results of pre-clinical studies have been highly encouraging and already data from a series of human phase I clinical trials have been published. Most early studies naturally concentrated on assessing the effect of a single therapeutic agent including immunization with tumor specific antigens, cytokines, tumor suppressors, ribozymes/antisense technology, prodrug technology and suppressors of tumor angiogenesis. The complexity of the field is increasing rapidly with an increasing number of studies exploring the potential additive or synergistic benefits of combining multiple transgenes. Ad vectors will readily accommodate multiple gene delivery to a target cell population either using a single or multiple vectors.

1. Introduction

Gene therapy provides an exciting, novel approach that is applicable to the treatment of a wide range of diseases and yet our understanding of what can be achieved with this technology remains uncertain. Many of the early extravagant predictions for gene therapy were unrealistic because of the limitations of the available technology for gene transfer. Originally envisioned primarily as a mechanism for the correction of inherited somatic genetic defects (such as adenosine deaminase deficiency and cystic fibrosis), remarkably, the most common application in human gene transfer protocols submitted

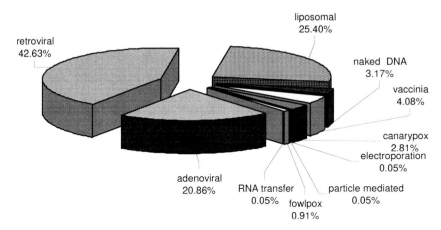

Figure 1. DNA delivery systems used in cancer gene therapy protocols registered for phase I/II clinical trials with the National Institute of Health (NIH) as of June 1998.

for approval by the NIH (USA) is currently for the treatment of cancers (Fig. 1). Cancer is now seen as an obvious and promising target disease for gene therapy. Although there has been remarkable progress in conventional cancer therapies, half of all patients still remain unresponsive to treatment. There is clearly an urgent need for innovative, effective regimes that can be used in combination with conventional procedures (surgery, radiotherapy, chemotherapy) to enhance further the prospects for these patients. The increased understanding of the molecular, genetic and immunological processes involved in the initiation and progression of tumors has led to the identification of numerous potential molecular targets that may be amenable to gene therapy strategies. Extensive experimentation *in vitro,* and *in vivo* using animal tumor models have tested, and continue to test, the validity of different intervention strategies and these studies have provided the basis for initial clinical trials.

The availability of an appropriate vehicle for the delivery and maintenance of a therapeutic genetic element is a key element in developing an effective gene therapy protocol, and frequently the rate-limiting step. While enhanced systems for direct DNA delivery are used extensively (e.g particle bombardment and cationic liposomes), virus-derived vectors provide the most efficient and robust systems for *in vivo* and *ex vivo* gene delivery and remain the preferred option in approved protocols for human gene therapy trials (Fig. 1). Classically, retrovirus-derived vectors have dominated gene therapy protocols, primarily because of their capacity to insert the transgene into the genome of the target cell, thus providing stable expression over prolonged periods of time. In contrast, adenovirus (Ad) vectors are associated with high efficiency gene delivery and 'transient' expression. The popularity of adenovirus vectors has, however, increased in recent years and their usage is beginning to rival that of retroviral systems (Fig. 1). The aim of this chapter is to review the biological properties of Ad vectors, both their merits and limitations, and to describe how they are currently being adapted and developed to be exploited in cancer gene therapy protocols.

2. Adenovirus vectors

2.1. *Adenovirus – a background to the vector*

Adenoviruses are primarily associated with mild upper respiratory tract infections but can cause acute respiratory disease (ARD), keratoconjunctivitis, gastroenteritis and occasionally severe disease in immunosuppressed individuals. There are some 47 human serotypes assigned to six subgenera with different serotypes being associated with distinct patterns of infection; e.g. Ad40 and Ad41 are associated with infantile diarrhea (Horwitz, 1996). Although certain Ad serotypes can induce transformation of cells in culture or tumor formation in animal models, there is no demonstrable association with any human cancer. The majority of recombinant adenoviral (RAd) vectors are based on Ad5, a common serotype associated with respiratory infections, although vectors based on other serotypes have been developed (Abrahamsen et al., 1997, Croyle et al., 1998).

Ads are well suited to manipulation in the laboratory. It is a robust non-enveloped virus, has a short replication cycle (~36h), grows to extremely high titer (>10^{11} pfu/ml) and can readily be purified by CsCl gradient centrifugation. This has facilitated extensive research into the molecular biology of the virus, which in turn has aided vector development. A range of simple, elegant systems have been developed for the generation of Ad recombinants, which we have reviewed recently (Scarpini, 1999). Some understanding of the molecular biology of Ad is useful in appreciating the rational behind vector design, development and ultimately their application in gene therapy protocols.

Ad5 has a ~35kb linear, double-stranded DNA genome and exhibits a complex pattern of gene expression. Both strands of the virus genome are transcribed with extensive use of both differential RNA splicing and alternate polyadenylation signals. As detailed in Fig. 2, four groups of early genes (E1, E2, E3 and E4) are transcribed prior to the onset of virus DNA replication, two genes (IX and IVa2) are expressed with intermediate kinetics while the vast majority of late transcription is driven by the major late promoter. Transcription from the major later promoter is complex but can be divided into 5 groups of transcripts designated L1-L5 (Fig. 2).

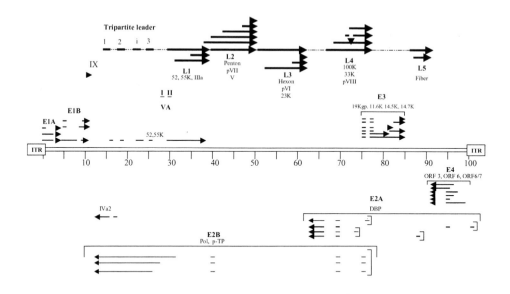

Figure 2. Transcriptional map of the Ad genome showing the location of Early phase (E1-E4) and Late phase (L1-L5) transcription). Genes encoding IX and IVa2 are expressed with intermediate kinetics while the small VA RNAs are transcribed by RNA polIII. The Ad genome is approximately 35kb (divided into 100 map units) and is transcribed in both directions. An inverted terminal repeat (ITR) is present at either end of the genome.

2.2. *Adenovirus vectors*

Virtually all Ad vectors currently in use are based on E1 gene deletion mutants which renders the virus replication-deficient by effectively disabling its capacity to activate early and late phase gene expression. The E1 gene products interact with a large number of cellular proteins in order to enhance the efficiency of viral replication (Shenk, 1996). E1A is the first gene to be expressed following infection and is required for activating virus early and late phase transcription. The E1A and E1B gene products are also required to induce the infected cell to progress to the S phase of the cell cycle. In this context, E1A has been shown to inhibit the phosphorylation of Rb and related proteins, while E1B-55Kd sequesters p53 and blocks transcriptional activation of WAF1. E1A also stabilizes p53, whilst the E1B proteins (55K and 19K) act to prevent the initiation of cell cycle arrest and apoptosis that would otherwise be induced by elevated levels of p53.

In contrast to E1, the E3 gene products are non-essential for replication *in vitro* (Kelly and Lewis, 1973) and thus E3 is often deleted from vectors to facilitate the cloning of larger inserts. Nevertheless, functions have been ascribed to E3 and the effect of their deletion from vectors should be considered. Five E3 gene products (E3-gp19K, 14.5K, 10.4K, 11.6K and 6.7K) are integral membrane proteins that act to modulate or evade the host immune response. E3-gp19K can impair antigen presentation to cytotoxic T-lymphocytes (CTL) by sequestering MHC class I molecules in the endoplasmic reticulum (Beier et al., 1994). Both E3-14.7K and an E3-10.4K/14.5K complex inhibit cell lysis and inflammation induced by tumor necrosis factor (TNF) by blocking the activation of cytosolic phospholipase A_2 ($cPLA_2$) and synthesis of leukotrienes and prostaglandins which are potent mediators of the inflammatory response (Zilli et al., 1992). E3-10.4K/14.5K downregulates the epidermal growth factor receptor (EGF-R) by inducing its internalization and degradation (Carlin et al., 1989, Tollefson et al., 1992), while E3-11.6, (the adenovirus death protein; ADP), promotes cell lysis and virus release late in infection by inducing apoptosis (Tollefson et al., 1996a, Tollefson et al., 1996b).

Although an E1 deletion results in an efficient blockade in early/late phase gene expression, *in vivo* gene delivery experiments revealed that first generation Ad E1⁻ vectors could be associated with the induction of an Ad-specific immune response as a consequence of breakthrough early/late phase expression (Englehardt et al., 1994). This induction of an immune response to Ad in the host is associated with a loss of *in vivo* transgene expression. Consequently, a series of second generation Ad vectors were constructed with deletions in additional essential early genes with the intention of minimising breakthrough expression. Three gene products encoded by the E2 gene cluster, the precursor terminal protein (pTP), DNA polymerase (pol) and DNA-binding protein (DBP), are essential for virus DNA replication and all have been deleted or mutated in 2nd generation vectors in an effort to prevent breakthrough Ad gene expression. The E4 gene region, through alternate splicing encodes numerous distinct transcripts and at least 6 polypeptides. The function of E4 is complex but is required (notably Orf3 or Orf6) for late phase gene expression (Leppard, 1997). Although deletion of E4 markedly reduces the potential for breakthrough gene expression, there is some doubt as to whether its deletion is beneficial because the presence of E4 in vectors has also been associated with sustained transgene expression (Brough et al., 1997). Vectors have also been constructed with deletions in the gene encoding pIX, required for efficient packaging of virus DNA into virus particles. Second generation vectors thus: (i) permit the insertion of larger transgenes, (ii) render the vector more disabled and thus safer and (iii) reduce the potential for breakthrough to early/late phase gene expression from the Ad vector.

Recently the emphasis in RAd vector development has shifted to 'gutless' or 'gutted' helper-dependent Ad vectors. In these vectors most, or all, Ad protein coding sequences are removed leaving the *cis*-acting sequences at either end of the genome required for DNA replication and packaging into the virus particle. With conventional replication-deficient Ad vectors the essential genes deleted from the vector are expressed in a complementing helper cell line. The provision of all Ad gene function in a helper cell line has proved to be problematical, so gutless vectors have to be propagated with the aid of a helper Ad. The production of substantial stocks of the gutless recombinant virus free from contamination with the helper Ad has been a major challenge, however, recent developments in vector systems have been encouraging. Once these vectors are more fully developed, the added containment associated with 'gutless' vectors and increased DNA packaging capacity will clearly be a benefit in many gene therapy applications.

2.3. *Vector Delivery*

A key property of Ad vectors is their currently unrivalled capacity to permit efficient *in vivo* gene delivery to a range of different tissues when directly administered. Gene delivery requires the virus to physically interact with the target cell. This interaction may be impaired by a range of factors, including: (i) virus neutralization by Ad-specific antibodies in the host, (ii) the extracellular matrix or mucus (e.g in respiratory tract) providing a physical barrier, or (iii) an absence of available receptors for the virus on the target cell. Receptor-mediated adenovirus cell entry is dependent on the knob domain of the adenoviral fiber protein (Louis et al., 1994) binding to the primary coxsackievirus/adenovirus receptor (CAR) (Bergelson et al., 1998). Following a subsequent secondary interaction between an RGD motif in the Ad penton base protein and α_v integrins on the cell surface (Bai et al., 1993) (Wickham et al., 1993) Ad enters the cell by receptor-mediated endocytosis. Cells that do not express the primary receptor (CAR), such as hematopoietic cells, are relatively resistant to infection with conventional Ad vectors. Additionally, cells with high levels of CAR on their surface can sequester virus, systemically delivered Ad preferentially targets the liver.

Ad vectors are being developed that will no longer recognize their natural receptors (CAR and α_v integrins) by mutation of receptor-defining sequences in the fiber and penton base proteins. Following deletion of their natural tropism Ad vector can be re-targeted to specific cell types including tumor cells. Small peptides containing specific receptor-binding motifs can be genetically inserted into specific sites within the Ad fibre or penton base proteins to alter the tropism of the vector (Krasnykh et al., 1996, Michael et al., 1995, Wickham et al., 1996). Alternatively, Ad have been redirected by conjugating a cell-specific ligand to a neutralizing anti-knob monoclonal antibody (Douglas et al., 1996) or a virus neutralizing scFv antibody fragment fused to a specific ligand (Watkins et al., 1997).

2.4. *Constitutive, tumor-specific and regulated promoters*

Ad vectors provide not only efficient gene delivery in terms of cell numbers but are also capable of producing extremely high levels of transgene expression. Surprisingly, using a replication-deficient vector the transgene product can constitute up 25% of total cell protein, rivaling levels achieved using baculovirus vector systems (Jacobs et al., 1992, Wilkinson and Akrigg, 1992). High levels of expression are associated with the use of strong constitutive viral promoters, notably in approximate order of strength: the murine cytomegalovirus (CMV) major IE promoter, the human CMV major immediate early (IE) promoter the, Rous sarcoma virus (RSV) LTR, and the SV40 early promoter (Addison et al., 1997). Expression levels can be controlled to some extent by the type of promoter used but will vary substantially in different cell types, different species and the local environment (e.g. inflammation) (Addison et al., 1997, Marr et al., 1998) (Tang et al., 1997).

As early as 1986, cell-specific promoters were used effectively in replication-deficient Ad vector to target and restrict transgene expression to specific cell types (Babiss et al., 1986). Restricting expression of a therapeutic gene to malignant cells can be beneficial in cancer gene therapy. The discrimination between tumor and normal cells is a major problem in both chemotherapy and radiotherapy as rapidly dividing healthy cells, notably in the bone marrow and gastrointestinal tract, are killed during treatment. In an effort to restrict cytocidal effects to cancer cells alone, tumor-specific control elements have been incorporated into Ad vectors. Such vectors currently developed for both *in vitro* or *in vivo* models of cancer gene therapy include;

(i) The tyrosinase promoter enhancer element for targeting melanocytes in malignant melanoma (Siders et al., 1998a).

(ii) The glial fibrillary acidic protein gene enhancer for targeting cells of glial origin including glioblastoma (Chen et al., 1998).

(iii) The osteocalcin promoter for targeting osteosarcomas (Cheon et al., 1997; Shirakawa et al., 1998).

(iv) The carcinoembryonic antigen (CEA) promoter for targeting CEA-producing pancreatic cancer cells (Ohashi et al., 1998).

(v) The α-fetoprotein promoter enhancer for targeting hepatocellular carcinoma (Kanai et al., 1997).

(vi) The E-selectin promoter is activated and provides 'transcriptional specificity' during tumor-mediated angiogenesis (Walton et al., 1998).

(vii) The DF3/MUC1 promoter for targeting DF3-positive breast carcinomas (Chen et al., 1996b)

(viii) The E2F-1 promoter has been used to target murine pRB-negative glioma (Parr et al., 1997).

There are situations in which the potential to be able to constantly regulate the level of an expressed therapeutic transgene *in vivo* may be beneficial either to optimize the production of the therapeutic product or to relieve toxicity due to excessive expression of the transgene. Substantial progress has been made in the development of tetracycline (Tet) controlled transcriptional activation systems. Tetracycline or its derivatives can be administered orally at sub-microcidal levels to control the level of transgene expression. Transgene expression can be tightly regulated by combining both transactivators and silencers of the Tet control element within one expression system (Blau and Rossi, 1999). Alternative promoter systems which efficiently regulate transgene expression *in vivo* are also being developed, most notably placing the transgene under the control of a hormonally regulated promoter (Burcin et al., 1999).

3. Replication-competent adenoviruses in tumor cells

As far back as 1956, patients with advanced cervical cancer were treated by direct intratumoral or intra-arterial injection of Ad. The treatment was inspired by the observation that Ad grows particularly well in HeLa cells (Smith, 1956). Patients were screened for antibodies to Ad and then treated with a serotype to which they were non-immune. Sixty-five percent of patients were shown to exhibit tumor necrosis and cavity formation within the pelvis, however, tumor regression was not observed. The application of fully replication competent Ads, however, raises obvious concerns in late stage cancer patients who are frequently immunosuppressed. Nevertheless, in specific therapeutic circumstances it could be envisaged that limited replication of a therapeutic adenovirus within a tumor could be a distinct advantage.

Loss of p53 function is the most common mutation in advanced tumors and is associated with resistance to chemotherapy and decreased survival. As described previously, E1B-55K binds p53 to prevent cell cycle arrest and apoptosis during adenovirus infections. Cells lacking functional p53 have been found to support productive infection by the AdE1B⁻ deletion *dl*1520 (Barker and Berk, 1987), now renamed ONYX-015 (Bischoff et al., 1996). The ONYX-015 virus was unable to establish a productive infection in human colon cancer RKO cells with normal p53 function although a cytopathic effect (cpe) was observed, but could replicate as efficiently as a wild-type virus in a subclone lacking functional p53. Tumor cells lacking p53, whether by mutation or degradation by HPV E6 have also been shown to support ONYX-015 replication (Bischoff et al., 1996). Some recent studies debate the basis of the growth defect in Ad E1B deletion mutants (Goodrum and Ornelles, 1997; Goodrum and Ornelles, 1998; Rothmann et al., 1998). Nevertheless, when tumor cell xenografts established in athymic nude mice were directly injected with ONYX-015 virus complete tumor regression observed in 7/13 cases. Furthermore, the anti-tumor activity of ONYX-015 was enhanced when used in combination with either cisplatin or 5-fluorouracil (5-FU) (Heise et al., 1997).

Preliminary results of Phase I and II clinical trials in patients with squamous cell carcinoma of the head and neck have been promising. Direct intratumoral injection of ONYX-015 virus resulted in no demonstrable toxicity and complete or partial tumor regression in several patients was associated with improved clinical signs, such as improved speech and pain reduction. Replication of virus could be demonstrated in tumor cells using electron microscopy and tumor necrosis correlated with clinical benefit. Clinical trials are now being extended to include ovarian carcinoma and colorectal hepatic metastases. Whilst this approach technically may not be 'gene therapy', the exploitation of conditionally replicating Ad mutants is both an innovative and extremely promising development.

4. Ad Vectors and Immunotherapy

It has long been postulated that immune surveillance plays a major role in controlling human malignancies. Cellular gene expression is perturbed in transformed cells and can result in their becoming potential targets for the humoral, cellular or innate immune responses. Indeed, tumor progression is frequently associated with immunsuppression. The aim of "immunomodulatory" cancer gene therapy is to induce, or stimulate, an immune response that will counteract tumor cell growth. Antigen-specific major histocompatibility complex (MHC)-restricted cytotoxic T-lymphocytes (CTLs) in particular have been proposed to play a major role in immune-mediated tumor regression both in animal models and human studies. Clearance of acute virus infection and the control of persistent viruses are also believed to be highly dependent on the induction of an appropriate MHC class I-restricted CTL response. MHC-molecules present peptides derived from both endogenous cellular proteins and foreign antigens present in the cell as a trimeric complex with β2-microglublin on the cell surface. CTLs recognize foreign peptides presented by specific MHC molecules but undergo selection *in vivo* to induce tolerance to self antigens.

4.1. *Induction of an immune response to an expressed transgene*

Viruses, including human papilloma virus (HPV), Epstein-Barr virus (EBV), human T cell leukemia virus (HTLV-1), human herpes virus 8 (HHV8) and hepatitis viruses B (HBV) and C (HCV), are estimated to be associated with approximately 20% of all human cancers worldwide. Considerable success has been achieved over the past 200 years in the application of vaccines and immunotherapies to combat viral diseases. Replication-competent and replication-deficient Ads have been used as immunization agents to protect against virus infection and this work has provided the basis for their application in cancer immunotherapy (Randrianarison-Jewtoukoff, 1995; Wilkinson and Borysiewicz, 1995).

Ads types 4 and 7 were identified as being associated with large outbreaks of a severe debilitating acute respiratory disease (ARD) in new recruits by the US military. To counteract this problem a vaccine was developed which involved oral administration of replication-competent Ad 4 and 7 virus encapsulated in 'enteric-coated' tablets. The vaccine viruses were not 'specifically' attenuated but elicited immunity and not disease when delivered by an enteric route. The vaccine has been used extensively in US military recruits since 1966 and has a good safety record (Rubin and Rocke, 1994). The success of the enteric Ad vaccine encouraged the development of replication-competent Ad vectors as immunization agents. Early studies focussed on replication-competent vectors expressing HBV surface antigen (HBsAg) which was able to induce a specific antibody response in various animal models (reviewed (Randrianarison-Jewtoukoff, 1995) and elicited protection following immunization of chimpanzees (Chengalvala et al., 1997, Lubeck et al., 1989). However, human enteric delivery of a replication-competent Ad7HBsAg recombinant did not elicit a detectable response (Tacket et al., 1992). A replication-competent Ad vector expressing HSV-1 gB was demonstrated to induce a comprehensive immune response (humoral, cellular and mucosal) to gB which protected against subsequent virus challenge in a murine model (Gallichan et al., 1993, Hanke et al., 1991). More recently a replication-competent Ad encoding SIV *env* in a combination vaccination regime with purified SIV gp120 induced a comprehensive immune response and elicited limited protection to virus challenge in rhesus macaques (Buge et al., 1997). Similarly, a replication-competent Ad encoding HIV *env* in a combination vaccination regime with HIV gp120 elicited limited protection in a chimpanzee model (Lubeck et al., 1997, Robert-Guroff et al., 1998). Replication-competent Ad vectors clearly are continuing to be developed and evaluated as potential vaccine delivery system.

Operationally replication-deficient Ad vectors (RDAd) are quite distinct from replication-competent vectors, being conceptually more like an ultra-efficient naked DNA delivery system. RDAd E1⁻ vectors can promote high level *in vivo* expression of a transgene for a period of a few days to many months depending on the route of administration, thus providing a sustained antigenic stimulus. Furthermore the transgene is expressed in the absence of any additional competing antigens from the vector so that the immune response is focussed on a single target antigen. Additionally, gene delivery is clearly independent of cell-to-cell spread by the vector, which may be inhibited by a specific or innate immune response. The replication-deficient nature of the vector makes it inherently safer, particularly in immunosuppressed individuals. However, RDAd-associated gene delivery permits long term survival of the infected cell and there are identifiable hazards associated with the potential integration of 'oncogenic' transgenes or prolonged overexpression of secreted bioactive proteins.

A single immunization with a RDAd vector induces a strong mucosal, humoral and MHC Class I restricted CTL response to the expressed transgene that is typically sustained at high levels over long periods of time (Juillard et al., 1995; Fooks et al., 1995; 1996). In gene therapy applications, when a RDAd is used to express a foreign protein characteristically the major immune response is to the expressed transgene, not the vector, and that immune response can limit the longevity of transgene expression (Juillard et al., 1995, Morral et al., 1997, Tripathy et al., 1996). The strength of the immune response will vary with the immunization regime, the level of transgene expression, antigenicity of the expressed protein and the host background. In a phase I clinical trial involving a single intratumoral (lung cancer) injection with 10^9 pfu of a RDAd encoding a β-gal reporter into four patients, strong humoral and cell-mediated immune responses were generated to β-gal (Gahery-Segard et al., 1997). In animal models RDAd recombinants have also been shown to be capable of inducing protection against virus infection in a range of viral systems including pseudorabies virus (Eloit et al., 1990), tick borne encephalitis virus (Jacobs et al., 1992; 1994), EBV (Ragot et al., 1993) and measles virus (Fooks et al., 1995). Direct comparisons demonstrated that RDAd vectors could obtain a similar level of protection to that achieved using vaccinia virus (Fooks et al., 1995, Gonin et al., 1996) and replication-competent Ad vectors (Mittal et al., 1996).

Human tumor-specific antigens of non-viral origin capable of inducing a CTL response were first identified in melanomas (van der Bruggen et al., 1991) and include

MAGE-1 (Romero et al., 1995) *MAGE*-3 (van der Bruggen et al., 1994) *BAGE* (Boel et al., 1995) and *GAGE* (Van den Eynde et al., 1995). These tumor-specific antigens are expressed in the majority of melanomas and provide potential targets for immunotherapeutic intervention in the treatment of malignant melanoma (Hirschowitz et al., 1998; Greenberg, 1991). Additional tumor-specific antigens have now been identified in other malignancies. Breast, ovarian and pancreatic carcinomas have all been demonstrated to express mucin (Jerome et al., 1993). When p53, (Nijman et al., 1994) ras (Van Elsas et al., 1995; Jung and Schluesener, 1991) HER-2/neu (Disis et al., 1994) and bcr/abl (Chen et al., 1992b) are either over-expressed or expressed in a mutated form, then they can also constitute potential targets recognized by CTLs. Differentiation antigens associated with cells of a specific lineage, such as melanocytes in malignant melanoma, can also constitute tumor-specific targets for CTLs; examples include tyrosinase (Brichard et al., 1993), Pmel17 (Kawakami et al., 1995), gp100 (Bakker et al., 1994), gp75[TRPI] (Wang et al., 1995) and MART-1 (Castelli et al., 1995, Kawakami et al., 1994).

Ad vectors can generate a comprehensive, long lasting immune response to an expressed transgene that can protect against virus challenge. The same approach can be used to induce a therapeutic immune response to a tumor-specific protein. Proof of this principle was elegantly demonstrated in an experiment by Chen et al (Chen et al., 1996c). Mice bearing tumor cells expressing the *E.coli* β-galactosidase (β-gal) were immunized with a RDAd encoding the same gene. Immunization resulted in tumor regression and, furthermore, passive transfer of splenocytes from an immunized mice could also protect syngeneic naïve mice from challenge with the tumor.

With a view to developing an immunotherapy to melanoma RDAd recombinants encoding MART-1 or gp100 were constructed (Zhai et al., 1996). Antigen-specific human CTL were able to induce lysis of MHC Class I-matched cells infected with either Ad/MART-1 or Ad/gp100. Furthermore, immunization of mice with Ad/gp100 could protect mice from a tumor challenge with murine melanoma B16 cells. Depletion of CD8$^+$, but not CD4$^+$ T cells *in vivo* eliminated the protective effect, thus demonstrating the importance of specific CD8$^+$ cells in tumor regression using this approach. Similar results have also been demonstrated for the murine gp75 melanoma (Hirschowitz et al., 1998). Such studies demonstrate that tumors antigens delivered by RDAd vectors are able to elicit a strong and specific CTL response *in vivo* and protect animals from tumor challenge, even against self-antigens to which there is normally tolerance. A phase I clinical trial has recently been initiated in which patient with metastatic melanoma were given escalating doses of Ad recombinant (10^4 to 10^{11} pfu). The patients coped well with even high doses of the virus and one (out of 16 patients) receiving the Ad MART1 construct 'experienced a complete response" (Rosenberg et al., 1998).

4.2. *Antigen Presentation in Dendritic Cells*

Immunization with Ad recombinants has proved effective *in vivo* when adminstered by a variety of routes including delivery to mucosal surfaces or by direct inoculation i.v., i.m. or i.p.. Theoretically the immune response to the expressed transgene should be further enhanced if it can be targeted to a 'professional' antigen presenting cell (APC). Dendritic cells (DC) are potent APC which are able to activate naïve T-cells (Gimmi et al., 1996) and prime antigen-specific CTL *in vivo* (Porgador and Gilboa, 1995). Peptide-pulsed DCs have proved to be highly effective at stimulating CTLs and this approach is being tested in melanoma patients with promising clinical results (Rosenberg et al., 1998). Since RDAds can infect DC relatively efficiently either *in vitro* or *ex vivo* (Arthur et al., 1997). RDAds can thus also be used to present antigen in DCs with the added advantages, over the peptide approach, that antigen presentation should be sustained longer and it is not restricted to defined peptides that will bind specifically to MHC Class I molecules of a single haplotype only.

Murine DC were infected with a RDAd encoding the DF3/MUC1 gene and injected into mice. The mice thus immunized were then observed to induce a DF3/MUC1-specific CTL response and be protected against with DF3/MUC1-positive tumors (Gong et al., 1997). In a similar study, the level of protection afforded by (i) fibrosarcoma (NFSA) cells stably transfected with MART-1 (ii) systemic administration of a RDAd encoding MART-1 and (iii) i.v. delivery of differentiated murine DCs infected with the AdMART-1 virus. Interestingly, superior levels of protection were achieved in this system with the recombinant Ad-infected DC. (Ribas et al., 1997). More recently, Butterfield and co-workers have established that human DC infected with RDAd MART-1 are also potent stimulators of MART-1-specific human CTL *in vitro,* even using 'naïve' PBL from normal donors. (Butterfield et al., 1998).

Preliminary results using RDAd-infected DCs to induce an efficient tumor-specific, cell-mediated immune response have been very encouraging. However, the expansion of the DC cultures *in vitro*, infection with the Ad recombinant and re-introduction of the autologous RDAd-transduced DCs is a relatively complex and expensive process. Consequently, the possibility of engineering Ad vectors to target professional APCs *in vivo* also needs to be explored.

4.3. *Co-stimulatory and Adhesion Molecule Therapy*

The interaction between MHC Class I or II complex and its associated receptors (TCR) is generally not sufficient to fully activate a T cell. The engagement of additional cell surface ligands on APC provide co-stimulatory signals that stimulate T cell function and promote cytokine production. The B7 family of co-stimulatory molecules expressed on APC interacts with CD28 on T cells to promote activation and IL-2 production. B7 family members also bind the CD28-related protein CTLA-4, which is expressed following activation on peripheral CD4+ and CD8+ T-cells. The adhesion molecules ICAM-1 and CD58 (LFA-3) on APC also interact with LFA-1 and CD2, respectively. The absence of appropriate co-stimulatory signals can induce tolerance or anergy, so that T cells are unable to carry out effector functions. Tumor cells that fail to express appropriate co-stimulatory molecules may constitute poor targets for host immune surveillance. Transfection of weakly immunogenic HPV16 E7[+] tumor cells with the co-stimulatory B7-1 gene enhanced immunogenicity sufficiently to elicit a curative and protective immune response in mice (Chen et al., 1992a, Townsend and Allison, 1993).

In a similar experiment using an *in vivo* murine model, transduction of a range of different tumor cell lines with a retroviral vector expressing B7-1 also generated a curative and protective immune response to 'immunogenic' tumor cells although 'non-immunogenic' cells did not respond to transduction with B7-1 (Chen et al., 1994a). The capacity of a co-stimulatory molecule to promote tumor rejection is thus dependent on the inherent immunogenicity of the tumor.

In order for this approach to be effective in a clinical context an effective method of delivering the co-stimulatory molecule to the tumor cell *in vivo* must be deployed. RDAd vectors can express high levels of B7-1, in both murine and human cells, and this expression will stimulate a T cell proliferation response to tumor cells *in vitro* and provide protection if the tumor cells are introduced in a mouse model (Lee et al., 1996a; Boxhorn et al., 1998). While murine melanoma K1735 cells expressing murine B7-1 following infection with a RDAd were rejected by syngeneic, immunocompetent mice, direct injection of the RDAd B7-1 was unable to eliminate an established K1735 tumor (Boxhorn et al., 1998). A recent study, using polyoma middle T-transformed breast adenocarcinoma tumor cells (PyMT) in a murine model, showed partial (38-42%) tumor elimination if RDAd expressing B7-1 or IL-2 were injected into the tumor. Complete regression was seen if a construct expressing both genes was used (Emtage et al., 1998). In a similar study, direct injection of an RDAd encoding both IL-12 and B7-1 into a mouse mammary tumor induced tumor regression in 70% of mice, while RDAd constructs encoding B7-1 or IL-12 alone only delayed tumor growth (Putzer et al., 1997). B7-1 expression is effective in stimulating an anti-tumor immune response, but may not always be sufficient to result in elimination of an established tumor. While more detailed studies are required, these investigations indicate that co-stimulatory molecules have significant therapeutic value if used in isolation but may act synergistically with other agents to provide a clear benefit.

5. Cytokine Gene Therapy

Cytokines (including interleukins, interferons, colony stimulating factors, chemokines and TNFs) are soluble intercellular signaling molecules that can be used very effectively to manipulate the immune response. The genetic modification of tumor cells to secrete various cytokines has been used in cancer immunization studies to stimulate the induction of an immune response to weakly immunogenic tumors or to counter an anergic response where lymphocytes can recognize an antigen but fail to respond to it. Systemic delivery of cytokines is frequently associated with an unacceptable level of toxicity and can be extremely expensive. Gene therapy provides for the local, sustained production of the therapeutic agent. Increased local production of cytokines, such as IL-2 or granulocyte/macrophage-colony stimulating factor (GM-CSF), also results in the recruitment of immune cells including CTLs and macrophages to the tumor site. RDAd vectors are clearly attractive candidates for this approach providing efficient *in vivo* delivery with low potential for lateral spread. Additionally, the fact that RDAd is a transient vector makes it particularly suited for gene therapy involving such potent bioactive therapeutic proteins.

The cytokine network is complex and there are numerous potential targets for therapeutic intervention. This area is the focus of an intensive research effort and holds great promise. However, this review is constrained to a limited number of cytokines actively investigated using Ad vector systems. Animal tumor models have demonstrated impressive levels of tumor regression in response to cytokine gene therapy with Ad vector systems and as a consequence a number of human gene therapy protocols have been submitted in this area.

5.1. *IL2*

Rosenberg and co-workers pioneered the use of IL-2 in cancer therapy. IL-2 plays a critical role in regulating the immune response being responsible for inducing proliferation of CTLs, helper T-cells and NK cells and activating the cytolytic properties of CTLs and NK cells (Rosenberg and Lotze, 1986). Systemic administration of IL-2 can induce regression of both murine and human tumors but often causes severe toxicity (Rosenberg et al., 1987, Rosenberg et al., 1985). The addition of high concentrations of IL-2 to peripheral blood mononuclear cells *in vitro* stimulates the growth of 'lymphokine-activated killer' (LAK) cells that exhibit a broad non-specific cytotoxic activity against NK cell-resistant tumor cells. LAK cells were also able to promote tumor regression in adoptive transfer experiments (Grimm et al., 1982; Vujanovic et al., 1988; Rosenberg, 1992). Similarly, tumor infiltrating lymphocytes (TILs) extracted from fresh tumor, when stimulated with IL-2, also show strong cytotoxic activity against tumor cells (Topalian et al., 1987; Rabinowich et al., 1987). LAKs cells are reported to be derived from the natural killer (NK) cell lineage, while TILs include MHC-restricted, tumor-specific T-cells (Itoh et al., 1986, Vose and Moore, 1985; Barth et al., 1990).

There have now been a substantial number of studies utilizing RDAd vectors encoding IL-2 in an impressive range of animal tumor models that have demonstrated tumor regression including: murine mammary adenocarcinoma (Addison et al., 1995; Addison et al., 1998, Emtage et al., 1998, Toloza et al., 1996), mastocytoma (Cordier et al., 1995, Haddada et al., 1993),renal cell carcinoma (Mulders et al., 1998), colorectal cancer (Diaz et al., 1998), metastatic colon carcinoma (Chen et al., 1996c), medullary thyroid carcinoma (Zhang et al., 1998a, Zhang et al., 1998b), lung adenocarcinoma (Heike et al., 1997), hepatocellular carcinoma (Bui et al., 1997, Huang et al., 1996), erythroleukemia (Ju et al., 1998), metastatic lung cancer (Kwong et al., 1997), fibrosarcoma, mammary carcinoma, melanoma (Toloza et al., 1996) and others. These studies demonstrated that *in vivo* introduction of RDAd IL2-infected tumor cells or direct injection of pre-established tumors infected with RDAdIL2 resulted in tumor regression. Histopathological examination in a number of instances demonstrated CD8+ T cell and macrophage infiltration associated with tumor regression (Huang et al., 1996; Cordier et al., 1995; O'Malley et al., 1997, Zhang et al., 1998a). The primary mechanism by which IL-2 functions in tumor eradication appears to by the induction of an antigen-specific CD8$^+$ MHC Class I CTL response which is then assisted by other immune mechanisms (Zatloukal et al., 1995).

While results obtained using RDAd IL-2 immunotherapy are clearly very impressive, there were a number of reports where administration of such a virus was unable to induce tumor regression (Donson and Foreman, 1998; O'Malley et al., 1996, 1997, Ram et al., 1994). Such failures could be due to an immunosuppressive property of the tumor, low immunogenicity of the tumor and/or a need to further optimize conditions (Toloza et al., 1996). In a murine squamous cell carcinoma model for head and neck cancer direct injection of a RDAd IL2 virus did not induce tumor regression. However, there was an increased rate of tumor regression, the induction of a CD8$^+$ CTL response and protection against subsequent challenge, when the RDAd IL2 virus was used in combination with a RDAd encoding thymine kinase (TK) and ganciclovir (see Section 8) (O'Malley et al., 1996; 1997). A combination of cytokine and prodrug therapy also proved successful in combating hepatic metastases of colon carcinoma in a mouse model. While direct injection of RDAd IL-2 into tumors was again ineffective, co-delivery with a therapeutic RDAd TK construct was required to elicit protection against subsequent challenge (Chen et al., 1995a; Kwong et al., 1997).

Following on from the generally encouraging results achieved *in vitro* and using animal models, there is a clear need to investigate the utility of this approach in the clinic. It has also been shown that delivery of a RDAd IL-2 construct to a metastatic renal cell carcinoma cell could stimulate the growth of human cytotoxic TILs *in vitro* (Mulders et al., 1998).Recently, the first report of a human phase I clinical trial using Ad-mediated delivery of IL-2 was reported (Stewart et al., 1999). Twenty-three metastatic breast cancer and melanoma patients were given intratumoral injections of escalating doses of RDAd encoding IL-2 (10^7-10^{10} pfu). Transgene expression could be detected at days 7 and 14 in biopsy samples, these also exhibited evidence of tumor necrosis and a lymphocyte infiltrate (predominantly CD8$^+$ T cells). Inflammation was often associated with delivery of the virus and a reduction in circulating CD4$^+$ and CD8$^+$ cells in blood by 24h was interpreted as resulting from a migration to the tumors. Encouragingly, 24% of tumors exhibited local, although incomplete, regression at the site of treatment.

5.2. *IL12*

Interleukin 12 (IL-12) acts to stimulate IFN-γ and TNF-α production by NK and T cells, and has a central role in stimulating proliferation and cytotoxicity of NK cells and CTLs. IL-12 has been shown to exhibit potent anti-tumor activity in a wide variety of murine tumor models including colon, kidney and lung carcinomas and melanomas (Brunda et al., 1993, Nastala et al., 1994, Tannenbaum et al., 1996). Both CD4$^+$ and CD8$^+$ T-cells are believed to play a critical role in tumor regression, with animals cured of established tumors by IL-12 therapy developing protection to further challenge (Brunda et al., 1993, Nastala et al., 1994). However, toxicity is associated with systemic delivery of IL-12 (Cohen, 1995). Since IL-12 (often acting synergistically with IL-2) is a key factor in driving a Th1 immune response, it represents an ideal candidate for cancer gene therapy and has been used with some success in RDAd vector systems.

The application of a RDAd encoding IL-12 has been systematically investigated in a murine breast cancer model (Bramson et al., 1996a, Bramson et al., 1996b, Bramson et al., 1997). Direct intratumoral injection of the Ad recombinant resulted in > 75% regression of treated tumors with a third of the animals remained tumor free. Animals exhibiting complete regression were shown to have a systemic immunity against challenge with the parental tumor. RDAd IL-12 inoculations also induced IFN-γ secretion within the tumor and within draining lymph nodes, suggesting activation of immune cells within the nodes. Similar levels of tumor regression were also demonstrated for hepatic metastases of colon carcinoma (Caruso et al., 1996) and murine bladder carcinoma (Chen et al., 1997a).

The liver is a primary site of RDAd localization after intravenous administration, making RDAd recombinant particularly suitable for the treatment of hepatic tumors, both primary and secondary. Systemic administration of RDAd IL-12 was found to dramatically reduce the formation of hepatic metastases in a murine model (Siders et al., 1998b). Although the inhibition of tumor formation was associated with perivascular infiltration by T-cells, macrophages and neutrophils, the therapeutic effect of the RDAd IL-12 virus was not affected by the depletion of CD4$^+$ T-cells, CD8$^+$ T-cells or NK cell, or indeed when the experiments were repeated in SCID mice. The authors suggest that in this system non-lymphocytic factors may also be important in IL-12 inhibition of tumor growth such as anti-angiogenic chemokines (Siders et al., 1998b)

A combination of RAD/IL-12 and the co-stimulatory molecule B7-1 has been demonstrated to act synergistically to inhibit tumor cell growth in a murine mammary adenocarcinoma model. A single intratumoral injection of a virus encoding both IL-12 and B7-1 resulted in complete regression in 70% of animals, whereas RDAd constructs encoding only one of the genes merely delayed tumor growth. Interestingly, administration of both genes using separate viruses only resulted in 30% total regression (Putzer et al., 1997). Using a similar approach, intratumoral injection with RDAd recombinants encoding both IL-2 or IL-12 resulted in more efficient tumor regression than the use of a single agent; in all cases tumor regression was associated with the induction of a tumor-specific CTL response (Addison et al., 1998). The expression of multiple transgenes aimed at enhancing the Th1 immune response to the tumor clearly has the potential to provide for more efficient cancer gene therapy.

5.3. *Ad and GM-CSF immunotherapy*

Granulocyte/macrophage-colony stimulating factor (GM-CSF) was originally identified by its ability to stimulate neutrophil, monocyte, macrophage and eosinophil colony formation, but it is now known to possess a range of functions also affecting hematopoietic cells. The value of GM-CSF in tumor therapy may be in promoting differentiation of hematopoietic precursors to DCs and their recruitment to the tumor. Dranoff and co-workers compared a wide range of cytokines using a retrovirus vector in an *in vivo* system and identified GM-CSF as having the most potent anti tumor activity

(Dranoff et al., 1993). High level constitutive *in vivo* GM-CSF expression associated with conventional RDAd vectors, however, may not be ideal. Routine administration of a RDAd CM-CSF construct was reported to induce eosinophilia, granuloma and fibrosis (Gauldie et al., 1996). Tumor cells expressing GM-CSF following transduction with a retrovirus vector also elicited better protection in an animal model than following infection with an Ad GM-CSF recombinant, even though the level of GM-CSF expression was lower (Abe et al., 1995). Since high level expression is associated with may toxicity and an inferior response, Ad vectors or gene delivery protocols may need to be modified to provide reduced levels of GM-CSF expression, possibly under the control of a promoter that can be regulated *in vivo*.

A small number of studies have been performed using RDAd GM-CSF recombinants and the results have been very encouraging. Tumor regression was observed in mice (with pre-established tumors) immunized with syngeneic irradiated Lewis lung carcinoma cells infected with a RDAd GM-CSF recombinant. CTL were demonstrated, DCs were observed to accumulate at the tumor site and a tumor-specific CTL was detected. (Lee et al., 1997). Using a similar approach, Nagai and co-workers found that vaccination with irradiated mouse colon carcinoma cells infected with a RDAd GM-CSF construct protected 90% of mice from challenge with the parental tumor cell. Protection was both long-lived and dependent on CD8+ cells (Nagai et al., 1998). Furthermore, a comparative study in a murine melanoma model demonstrated that u.v.-irradiated syngeneic cells infected with an RDAd encoding GM-CSF elicited a higher degree of protection (88% reduction) than RDAd viruses encoding IL-2 (72%) or TNFα (no effect) alone (Bonnekoh et al., 1998). When the experiment was repeated, although this time combined with a prodrug therapy, by direct intratumoral inoculation, the RDAd GM-CSF construct again provided greatest benefit (Bonnekoh et al., 1998)

5.4. *Ad and interferons*

Interferons (IFNs) (α,β and γ) have exhibited efficacy in a range of experimental models by inhibiting tumor proliferation. Systemic administration of interferons has proved beneficial in a range of clinical conditions. Hematological malignancies have proved particularly responsive to IFN-α or β, solid tumors have proved refractory. Patients with hairy cell leukemia (up to 80% experience partial or complete remission) (Thompson and Fefer, 1987) and chronic myelogenous leukemia (CML; up to 70% experience complete remission) are particularly responsive to IFN treatment.

Ad recombinants have been used to deliver the IFN-α gene to CD34[+] hematopoietic stem cells and CML mononuclear cell *ex vivo* and promote high level transgene expressions without any overt toxicity (Ahmed et al., 1998, Feldman et al., 1997). However, infection of hematopoietic cells with standard Ad vectors is relatively inefficient and expression tends to be of short duration. A limited number of attempts have been made to use Ad IFN constructs in experimental solid tumors. Direct-intratumoral inoculation with a replication-competent Ad vector encoding the IFN-con1 gene inserted at the E3 locus was able to induce tumor regression when introduced in tumors produced with human breast cancinoma cells (MDA-MB-435), myelogenous leukemic (K562) cells or Syrian hamster melanoma (RPMI1846) cells in athymic nude mice. In this case high levels of IFN may inhibit tumor growth but some, although not all, of the anti-tumor effect could be explained by virus-induced 'oncolysis' or cytoxicity of infected tumor cells (Zhang et al., 1996). More recently, a RDAd IFN-α recombinant was demonstrated to induce complete tumor regression when injected into tumors induced by human prostatic cancer (PC-3) and hepatocellular cancer (Hep3B) cells an athymic nude mice (Ahmed et al., 1999). Additionally, direct intratumoral administration of an RDAd-IFNβ construct into a human breast carcinoma induced in immune-deficient mice resulted in sufficiently high levels of IFN-β locally to induce tumor regression (Qin et al., 1998). Indeed, infection of as few as 1% of the tumor cells prior to implant was sufficient to prevent tumor formation (Qin et al., 1998). Ad vectors are capable of providing local high level expression of IFNs by direct intratumoral inoculation. Studies in the animal models indicate that therapeutic levels are achievable even following relatively inefficient *in vivo* gene delivery to solid tumors.

The adoptive transfer of *in vitro* stimulated and expanded CTL has been utilized clinically as an immunotherapy. Abe and co-workers reported that adoptive transfer of TILs in a murine B16 melanoma was only effective in reducing tumor formation when the cells were infected with a RDAd IFN-γ recombinant (Abe et al., 1996). This study demonstrates the potential to optimize or modify an adoptive immunotherapy protocol by *ex vivo* gene delivery to CTL using RDAd vectors.

5.5. *Other cytokines*

There is a need to examine more extensively the potential therapeutic value of a wide range of cytokines in cancer gene therapy. A RDAd expressing an IL-4 construct has been shown to inhibit the growth of rat C6 glioma cells in an *in vivo* subcutaneous tumor models (Wei et al., 1998). Limited studies with RDAd encoding IL-1, IL-3 and IL6 have not been encouraging (Felzmann et al., 1997) (Esandi et al., 1998). The major obstacle in using TNFα as an anticancer agent is its acknowledged toxicity even in the context of localized delivery with an Ad vector. A RDAd recombinant encoding TNFα under the control of the strong MCMV major IE promoter induced tumor necrosis but was associated with systemic toxicity killing 8/20 mice tested (Marr et al., 1998). A number of approaches have been taken to overcome this problem. The toxicity of RDAd TNFα constructs has been reduced successfully by: (i) using a less efficient promoter in the murine system (Marr et al., 1998, Staba et al., 1998), (ii) placing the gene under the control of a tetracycline-inducible promoter (Hu et al., 1997) or (iii) using an artificial membrane bound form of TNF (Marr et al., 1997). While the capacity of TNFα alone to induce tumor regression in animal models was disappointing, the efficiency was much enhanced when combined with radiotherapy, this was attributed to the combined affect of both treatments on the tumor microvasculature (Staba et al., 1998).

6. Tumor Suppressor Gene Therapy and Anti-oncogenes

Tumor suppressor genes act primarily, although not exclusively, by the negative modulation of cellular proteins which regulate transcription and cell division. A number of tumor suppressors are involved in the cell cycle control such that their loss of function leads to unrestrained cell division. Inherited or somatic mutations of both alleles can abrogate their functions leading to tumor development.

6.1. *p53*

It has been demonstrated by many investigators that the introduction of functional p53 into tumor cells can often either suppress tumor growth or induce apoptosis (Cai et al., 1993, Chen et al., 1991, Cheng et al., 1992, Takahashi et al., 1992). Consequently, a gene therapy approach resulting in transduction of cancer cells *in vivo* with p53 has the potential to correct the neoplastic phenotype in tumors lacking functional p53. RDAds encoding p53 can induce dose-dependent inhibition of cell growth *in vitro* in a wide variety of tumor cells, including those derived from tumors of the head and neck (Liu et al., 1995, Mobley et al., 1998, Overholt et al., 1997), the cervix (Hamada et al., 1996), breast (Seth et al., 1997), lung (Nguyen et al., 1997, Zhang and Roth, 1994), ovaries (Mujoo et al., 1996); Santoso, (Santoso et al., 1995), osteosarcoma (Marcellus et al., 1996), colorectal (Spitz et al., 1996a) prostate [(Ko et al., 1996)] and others known to lack wt-p53 expression (Wills et al., 1994). Tumor cells infected with RDAd p53 constructs *ex vivo* and then injected into nude mice have demonstrated extensive and in most instances complete tumor growth suppression (Ko et al., 1996, Kock et al., 1996, Wills et al., 1994) (Mujoo et al., 1996). These observations have been extended in pre-clinical experiments using *in vivo* tumor model systems. Injection of the RAd-p53 directly into established tumors in animal models has been shown to decrease the tumorigenic phenotype and increase survival times in a range of experimental tumor systems including glioma (Badie et al., 1995, Kock et al., 1996), head and neck (Clayman et al., 1996), prostatic (Gotoh et al., 1997, Ko et al., 1996) ovarian (Mujoo et al., 1996), small cell lung (Wills et al., 1994) and cervical (Hamada et al., 1996) carcinomas.

Cellular p53 levels increase in response to DNA damaging agents used in cancer therapy, including radiation and certain chemotherapeutic agents. Normal p53 function is associated with increased sensitivity to the cell damage induced by these agents. DNA damage induced by either chemotherapy or radiotherapy causes cells expressing wt-p53 to arrest in G_1 phase, whilst cells lacking functional p53 proceed to S-phase despite DNA damage. Thus the effect of DNA damage by agents used in cancer therapy is related to the expression of functional p53. If DNA damage can not be repaired, wt-p53 will induce apoptosis following G_1 arrest.

Restoration of normal p53 function to the tumor cell thus not only suppresses tumor growth but also makes the cell sensitive to radiotherapy. Enhanced sensitivity to radiotherapy following RDAd-mediated transfer of p53 has been demonstrated for the following tumor cell types: glioblastoma (Badie et al., 1995) (Geng et al., 1998) (Lang et al., 1998), colorectal (Spitz et al., 1996b) and ovarian cancer (Gallardo et al., 1996). The rate of apoptosis also increased in cells infected with the RDAd p53 construct. Restoration of p53 function by using a RDAd recombinant was predicted to increase sensitivity to chemotherapeutic agents and this has indeed been demonstrated for mitomycin C and adriamycin (Blagosklonny et al., 1998), cisplatin (Fujiwara et al., 1994), etoposide (Meng et al., 1999) and topotecan (Yang et al., 1996). A problem for p53 gene therapy, even using an Ad vector system, is that it is not feasible to expect all cells in a solid tumor mass to be infected/transduced. Gene therapy using p53 will be expected to affect primarily cells receiving the gene, although a limited bystander effect has been reported following RDAd p53 infection (Frank et al., 1998). However, the additional tumor damage induced by combining gene therapy with a RDAd-p53 virus with radiotherapy and/or chemotherapy is highly effective in inducing tumor regression, at least in animal models.

A phase 1 clinical trial has been conducted in which 33 patients with advanced head and neck squamous cell carcinoma were treated by multiple direct intratumoral inoculation with up to 10^{11} pfu of a RDAd p53 construct (Clayman et al., 1998). Even with high virus dosage, no serious adverse affects were attributed to the treatment although the virus could be recovered in blood, urine and sputum. Most encouragingly, a significant therapeutic effect was observed, in particular two patients exhibited 'objective tumor regression' (Clayman et al., 1998).

6.2. $p21^{Waf}$

Following DNA damage p53 activates transcription of the gene encoding $p21^{Waf}$. $p21^{Waf}$ binds and inhibits multiple cyclins and cyclin-dependent kinases (CDKs) by forming a quaternary complexes with CDKs, cyclins and proliferating cellular nuclear antigen (PCNA), thereby arresting cell growth. In many tumors CDK activity is not repressed due to a loss of $p21^{Waf}$ function, thus contributing to unregulated cell growth.

Infection with a RDAd $p21^{Waf}$ recombinant virus induced over-expression of $p21^{Waf}$ in both p53-deficient and p53 wt-type human astrocytoma lines and resulted in a suppression of cell growth both *in vitro* and *in vivo*, using peripheral and intracerebral murine xenograft models (Chen et al., 1996a). The anti-proliferative and tumor suppressive properties of $p21^{Waf}$ thus appear not to be affected by the p53 status of the cell. Several other groups have also reported on the effect of RDAd $p21^{Waf}$ infection of cancer cells with similar results (Chen et al., 1995b, Eastham et al., 1995, Joshi et al., 1998a, Joshi et al., 1998b, Mobley et al., 1998, Yang et al., 1995) although variation was observed between different tumors types. In most, but not all (Eastham et al., 1995), cases, RDAd recombinants encoding $p21^{Waf}$ were reported to be inferior to RDAd p53 constructs in inhibiting cell growth *in vitro* (Clayman et al., 1996) and tumorogenesis in animal models (Gotoh et al., 1997). Interestingly, however, the efficacy of a p21-based RDAd therapy was found to be significantly enhanced by using a $p21^{Waf}$ C-terminal deletion mutant (unable to interact with PCNA). An RDAd encoding the $p21^{Waf}$ deletion inhibited the growth of a tumor cell line more effectively that either RDAd p53 and an Ad p21wt constructs (Prabhu et al., 1996).

6.3. $p16^{INK4}$

The major transitions in the cell cycle are triggered by cyclin-dependent kinases (CDK's). CDK4 promotes progression through G_1 phase, however, its activity is repressed by displacement of the activating subunit with the inhibitory subunit, $p16^{INK4}$. $p16^{INK4}$ can act as a tumor suppressor, indeed homozygous deletions and mutations of the $p16^{INK4}$ gene are frequent in human tumors. This ability of $p16^{INK4}$ to suppress cell cycle progression has made it a popular candidate to target for cancer gene therapy. RDAd-mediated transfer of $p16^{INK4}$ has been demonstrated to suppress the growth of a range of different tumor cell types; including lung (Jin et al., 1995, Lee et al., 1998), glioma (Chintala et al., 1997, Fueyo et al., 1996), mesothelioma (Frizelle et al., 1998), head and neck (Mobley et al., 1998, Rocco et al., 1998), bladder (Grim et al., 1997) and esophageal (Schrump et al., 1996) tumors. Consistent with an acknowledged function of $p16^{INK4}$ as an inhibitor of Rb phosporylation, tumor cells with functional Rb are significantly more sensitive to growth suppression following RDAd $p16^{INK4}$ infection (Craig et al., 1998). Expression of exogenous $p16^{INK4}$ correlates with G1 cell cycle arrest blocking entry to S-phase and inhibition of tumor growth both *in vivo* and *in vitro* (Frizelle et al., 1998, Jin et al., 1995, Rocco et al., 1998). Interestingly, simultaneous infection with RDAd recombinants encoding both p53 and p16 results in enhanced apoptotic tumor cell death *in vitro* and a substantial enhancement of tumor regression in an *in vivo* model (Sandig et al., 1997). This is another example of where the combination of two therapeutic genes can have an additive or synergistic effect.

6.4. Rb

The loss of the retinoblastoma (Rb) gene function is associated with the initiation and progression of many common cancers. Furthermore, the restoration of Rb function in Rb-deficient tumor cells is often sufficient to suppress tumorigenic activity in many distinct tumor cell types (Goodrich and Lee, 1993, Zhou et al., 1994). Infection with RDAd recombinants encoding Rb has also been shown to inhibit tumor cell growth *in vitro* (Demers et al., 1998, Simeone et al., 1997). Infection of human glioma cells *in vitro* with an RDAd Rb construct was also sufficient to prevent them forming tumors in nude mice (Demers et al., 1998). Spontaneous pituitary melanotroph tumors arising in immunocompetent *Rb*-heterozygous mice could also be effectively treated by direct intratumoral injection with a RDAd Rb construct. Treatment produced long term tumor growth suppression and a significantly enhanced survival rate which correlated well with the stage of tumor progression when treatment was started (Riley et al., 1996).

In gene therapy the potential always exists to manipulate a transgene to enhance its function. A truncated form of the Rb protein (lacking 112 amino acids at the N-terminus) has a slower turnover rate and tends to remain in an unphosphorylated form in tumor cells. This mutant form of Rb exerts a growth inhibitory effect in normal cells and Rb-deficient tumors cells (Xu et al., 1994). Using RDAd to infect tumor cells with truncated and full length Rb constructs, growth was suppressed. This resulted in partial or complete regression of small newly established tumor xenografts in nude mice although the response in larger tumours was less effective. Rather than use a normal functional Rb gene, Simeone and coworkers have also demonstrated the efficacy of an RDAd recombinant encoding a constitutively active (non-phosphorylatable) form of Rb in inhibiting the proliferation human pancreatic tumor cell in vitro without stimulating of apoptosis (Simeone et al., 1997).

6.5. *PML*

The 15:17 chromosomal translocation associated with acute promyelocytic leukemia (APL) results from a recombination event between the genes encoding PML and RARα (retinoic acid receptor-α) and the subsequent expression of a PML/ RARα fusion protein. PML is normally associated with discrete nuclear domains (known commonly as PML-bodies, PODs or ND10), but the PML/ RARα fusion protein acts dominantly to disrupt this domain. PML is a tumor/growth suppressor protein that forms multiple interactions. The association of PML with PML-bodies has a role in caspase-dependent and caspase-independent induction of apoptosis, the transformed APL cells being resistant to apoptosis. Infection with a RDAd encoding PML has been demonstrated to suppress the growth rate of prostate cancer cells *in vitro* and suppress tumor growth following direct intratumoral inoculation in a murine model (He et al., 1997). A similar study demonstrated that infection of human breast cancer cells with a RDAd PML recombinant induced cell cycle arrest in G1 phase, apoptosis. Following intratumoral injection *in vivo* RDAd PML induced apoptosis resulted in 80% tumor regression (Le et al., 1998). Although the function of PML has only been partially elucidated, gene therapy with a RDAd PML recombinant has attracted interest because of its capacity to both inhibit cell cycle progression and induce the apoptotic pathway in tumor cells.

7. Ribozyme Gene Therapy

The majority of gene therapy protocols aim to complement a defect in a cellular gene or to induce the expression of a novel therapeutic function, such as a cytokine or a 'suicide' gene. An alternative approach to cancer gene therapy is to inhibit the expression of a gene responsible, or required, for a malignant phenotype. Whereas mutations in tumor suppressor genes lead to malignancies by their loss of function, the active expression of an oncogene leads directly to neoplasia. Proto-oncogenes (the normal cellular homologues of oncogenes) have essential roles in normal cell functions, including signal transduction and transcription. Since a mutant oncogene characteristically exhibits a dominant phenotype, it cannot readily be repaired by expression of the normal function. It is, however, possible to attempt to ablate the expression of an oncogene by a number of approaches including antisense or ribozyme technology. Ribozymes are catalytic RNA molecules that are designed to cleave specific phosphodiester bonds in target RNA molecules. The potential exists therefore to use RDAd to deliver genes directly to the tumor cells to inactivate the expression of a malignant gene.

RDAd recombinants have been constructed that encode hammerhead ribozymes directed against transcripts encoded by Her-2/neu and the growth factor pleiotrophin (Czubayko et al., 1997). Her-2/neu is a member of the epidermal growth factor tyrosine kinase receptor family that has been implicated in modulation of hormone responsiveness in breast cancer cells (Pietras et al., 1995), while pleiotrophin is a critical factor in angiogenesis and metastasis associated with melanoma (Czubayko et al., 1996). Both Ad recombinants directed high level ribozyme expression resulting in a substantial decrease in the level of expression of their respective target genes and, most importantly, infection with the recombinant viruses can virtually eliminate proliferation of ovarian and breast cancer cells *in vitro* (Czubayko et al., 1997).

The insulin-like growth factor I receptor can play an important role in the maintenance of a transformed cell phenotype (Sell et al., 1993). Antisense to IGF-I transcripts has been shown to suppress the tumorigenicity of a rat glioblastoma and elicit regression of pre-established tumors (Trojan et al., 1993). In certain lung cancer cell lines, IGF-I and its receptor can mediate autocrine proliferation (Ankrapp and Bevan, 1993, Nakanishi et al., 1988). A RDAd recombinant was constructed encoding an antisense transcript to the IGF-1 receptor that, following infection of lung cancer cells *in vitro,* reduced IGF-R expression and cell proliferation. *In vivo* administration of the RDAd recombinant also prolonged the survival times in nude mice bearing pre-established tumors (Lee et al., 1996b). A well-characterized ribozyme has been also described that directs sequence specific cleavage of H-*ras* transcripts in a variety of tumor cell lines (Kashani-Sabet et al., 1994). Consequently, a RDAd construct encoding the H-*ras* ribozyme was generated that was capable of promoting high-level ribozyme expression in neoplastic cells *in vitro*. Expression of the H-*ras* resulted in decreased H-*ras* mRNA, growth suppression *in vitro* and complete growth suppression of xenografts in athymic mice (Feng et al., 1995). Such reports clearly demonstrate the feasibility of using Ad vectors to deliver high level expression of ribozymes or antisense construct therapeutically to nullify the expression of a malignant gene.

8. Genetic Prodrug Therapy

Prodrug gene therapy has proved one of the most effective strategies for cancer gene therapy using a range of different gene delivery systems. The principle involves the expression of a 'suicide' gene that can convert a non-toxic prodrug substrate to a cytotoxic product. Such systems have been used to incorporate a 'suicide gene' into recombinant vectors and CTLs used for adoptive transfer to patients. The therapeutic agent can then be inactivated *in vivo* by administering the prodrug. Gene therapy can also be used to deliver 'suicide' genes to tumor cells either *in vivo* or *ex vivo*, which are then sensitive and can be killed by pro-drug treatment.

A wide range of enzyme systems have been adapted for prodrug therapy but perhaps the most intensely investigated combines a herpes virus-encoded thymidine kinase (TK) with the antiviral ganciclovir (GC) or an appropriate analogue (Moolten, 1986). TK converts the prodrug ganciclovir to ganciclovir monophosphate, which cellular enzymes modify to ganciclovir triphosphate. Ganciclovir triphosphate inhibits DNA polymerase thus becoming toxic to cells in S-phase (Mar et al., 1985). Transfection of the TK gene specifically into tumor cells and subsequent GC treatment results in tumor cell death and regression of the tumor mass (Culver et al., 1992).

When prodrug gene therapy was first proposed, it was envisaged that only target cells receiving and expressing the therapeutic gene would be affected. Studies *in vitro*, however, show that tumor cells that do not express the suicide gene can also be killed by prodrug therapy, however, this effect is not observed when cells are grown at low density (Moolten, 1986). A similar effect – known as the bystander effect - was also observed *in vivo* (Freeman et al., 1993). Several mechanisms have been suggested to explain the bystander effect. One proposes apoptotic vesicles containing the toxic triphosphate form of ganciclovir are phagocytized by surrounding cells (Freeman et al., 1993). Cells capable of converting the prodrug are able to transfer the low molecular weight active drug metabolites to neighboring cells via gap junctions (Bi et al., 1993). Finally, certain active drug metabolites (e.g. 5-fluorouracil) are able to pass freely between cells by non-facilitated diffusion (Domin et al., 1993).

RDAd vectors encoding the HSV TK gene have been highly effective at inducing tumor regression in a number of cancer models including glioma (Chen et al., 1994b, Perez-Cruet et al., 1994), mesothelioma (Smythe et al., 1994a; 1994b; 1995), hepatocellular carcinoma (Wills et al., 1995), and squamous cell carcinoma of head and neck (O'Malley et al., 1995). RDAd TK- infected human malignant mesothelioma cells were used to establish subcutaneous tumors in Fischer rats. Although the induction of an anti-tumor immune response is considered to be highly desirable; somewhat surprisingly tumor suppression induced by RDAd TK recombinant was more efficient in immunodeficient than immunocompetent mice. In this system, the elimination of RDAd TK-infected cells by the immune systems appear to reduce the efficiency of prodrug therapy (Elshami et al., 1995).

Tumor cell contamination of hematopoietic stem cells constitutes a potential hazard for patients receiving autografts following high dose chemotherapy in breast cancer. Ad vectors, however, infect breast carncinoma cells much more efficiently than hematopoietic stem cells. The potential exists therefore to utilize Ad vectors to preferentially kill the contaminating tumor cells in hematopoietic stem cell autografts. *Ex vivo* infection with a RDAd recombinant encoding TK under the control of the DF3/MUC1 carcinoma-specific promoter provided for selective infection, expression and effective purging of contaminating breast carcinoma cells from a population of hematopoietic stems (Chen et al., 1996b; Wroblewski et al., 1996).

The *E. coli* cytosine deaminase gene converts the non-toxic prodrug 5-fluorocytosine (5-FC) to the toxic product 5-fluorouracil (5-FU)(Danielsen et al., 1992). This suicide gene/prodrug combination has been used effectively with a RDAd vector in a number of different experimental tumor models, including a rat gliosarcoma (Dong et al., 1996), murine pancreatic carcinoma (Evoy et al., 1997), human colon carcinoma (Hirschowitz et al., 1995) and human breast cancer (Li et al., 1997). A potent dose-dependent growth inhibition was demonstrated after administration of 5-FC *in vitro,* and *in vivo* following tumor cell transplant to nude mice. The bystander effect observed using cytosine deaminase has been shown to be even more effective than that observed with TK. In a comparative system, when less than 10% of tumor cells expressed TK there was no significant antitumor effect following treatment with ganciclovir; however, when fewer than 4% of cells expressed cytosine deaminase, treatment with 5-FC still provided significant growth inhibition (Freeman et al., 1993, Huber et al., 1994). Tumor cell-specific promoters have also been used effectively to limit cytosine deaminase expression, in the context of a RDAd vectors, to malignant cells; for example expression from the alpha fetoprotein promoter provided selective expression of the 'suicide' gene in an experimental in vivo hepatocellular carcinoma (Kanai et al., 1997).

Cyclophosphamide is an alkylating prodrug activated by liver cytochrome P450 enzymes but its clinical application was limited by renal, hematological and cardiac toxicity. Cyclophosphamide is of value, however, in prodrug therapies. A RDAd vector encoding liver cytochrome P450 was used to infect human breast MCF-7 cancer cells, which consequently became sensitive to cyclophosphamide (Chen et al., 1997b). As is the case with cytosine deaminase there is a strong bystander effect that does not require direct cell-to-cell contact. When MCF-7 tumor cells were transplanted into nude mice there was an extremely significant growth inhibition when compared to MCF-7 cells which had not been infected (15-20 fold greater effect).

The combination of efficient *in vivo* gene delivery associated with the Ad vector system and a need only to deliver the therapeutic gene to a small proportion of cells makes Ad prodrug gene therapy a potent combination.

9. Suppression of Tumor Angiogenesis

The growth of a tumor is critically dependent upon the development of new blood vessels (neovascularisation), without which cells in prevascular tumors or metastases reach equilibrium with their rate of death and cease to expand. A balance between negative and positive regulators of endothelial cell proliferation, invasion, migration and capillary tube formation within the tumors local environment is important for the development of vessels (Hanahan and Folkman, 1996). Under normal physiological conditions, angiogenesis is quiescent except under specific conditions such as wound healing and the menstrual cycle.

Although a number of growth factors expressed by tumor cells have been implicated in angiogenesis, vascular endothelial growth factor (VEGF) clearly plays a central role. VEGF is expressed in most human tumors and tumor cell lines (Senger et al., 1986, Shibuya, 1995) and induced by tumor cell hypoxia and necrosis. VEGF stimulates endothelial cells to proliferate, migrate and form capillaries via interaction with the *flt-1* and/or *flk-1/* KDR receptors found almost exclusively on endothelial cells. One method of blocking angiogenesis is to infuse a tumor with a truncated, soluble form of a VEGF receptor which is then able to sequester any VEGF produced by the tumor and interact with native receptors to block their function (Kendall and Thomas, 1993, Kendall et al., 1996). The challenge, when using a truncated VEGF receptor, is to provide high enough concentrations of the therapeutic protein within the tumor, without impeding wound repair or provoking systemic anti-angiogenesis in organs such as the ovaries and uterus. Anti-VEGF therapy has been evaluated for the inhibition of tumor angiogenesis using RDAd-mediated transfer of a secreted form of the extracellular domain of human *flt-1* VEGF receptor (RAd-s*flt*) (Kong et al., 1998). Using subcutaneous, liver metastatic and lung metastatic murine tumor models, it has been demonstrated that regional delivery of RAd-s*flt* inhibited the growth of pre-established tumors only in those organs receiving the recombinant virus.

The amino-terminal fragment of murine urokinase (ATF/uPA) is a broad-spectrum cell invasion inhibitor that antagonizes uPA binding to its cell surface receptor (uPAR). ATF has been shown to exert a direct effect on tumor cells and inhibits metastasis in experimental models (Crowley et al., 1993, Kobayashi et al., 1994, Lu et al., 1994). Infection with an adenovirus recombinant (AdmATF) encoding secreted murine ATF/uPA can inhibit tumor angiogenesis in murine tumor models. A single intratumoral injection of AdmATF into a pre-established human breast cancer xenograft grown in athymic mice or into pre-established Lewis lung carcinoma led to tumor growth inhibition and inhibition of neovascularisation both within the tumor and in the immediately adjacent normal tissue. AdmATF was also demonstrated to affect tumor growth at remote sites, dissemination of Lewis lung carcinoma after intratumoral injection at the primary site was inhibited and systemic administration inhibited hepatic metastases in colon carcinoma xenograft models (Li, 1998).

Platelet factor 4 (PF4) inhibits angiogenesis and tumor growth both *in vitro* and *in vivo* (Maione et al., 1990). A RDAd encoding soluble PF4 (sPF4) has been demonstrated to significantly inhibit growth of endothelial cells but not glioma cells *in vitro* (Tanaka et al., 1997). Solid tumors directly infected with RDAd-sPF4 were shown to become hypovascular and both glioma cells within the tumor and the vasculature cells demonstrated high apoptotic indices. The mechanism involved in inducing apoptosis in both the endothelial and glioma cells is not known, however, hypoxia can induce tumor cell apoptosis in a p53-dependent fashion (Graeber et al., 1996).

Tie2 is an endothelium-specific receptor tyrosine kinase known to play a role in tumor angiogenesis (Lin et al., 1997). Infection with a RDAd recombinant (AdExTek) engineered to express a soluble Tie2 receptor is capable of blocking Tie2 activation (Lin et al., 1998). Adminstration of AdExTek to mice with either a well-established murine mammary carcinoma (4T1) or a murine melanoma (B16F10.9) was shown to significantly inhibit significantly growth of both tumors. In order to study the effect on metastases, both cell lines were co-injected intravenously with either AdExTek or a control virus. Mice co-injected with the control virus developed numerous large, well-vascularised lung metastases. Mice co-injected with AdExTEK developed few metastases and histological examination demonstrated only small avascular clusters of tumor cells. AdExTek was also shown to inhibit tumor metastases when delivered at the time of surgical excision of the primary tumor.

An internal peptide fragment of plasminogen, angiostatin, found in the serum and urine of mice with Lewis lung carcinoma, has been shown to have potent anti-angiogenic properties (O'Reilly et al., 1994). Metastatic tumor growth was shown to be suppressed in animals after removal of the primary tumor if animals were systemically treated with angiostatin, however, once treatment was discontinued, tumor growth restarted. Long term delivery of angiostatin and other anti-angiogenic proteins, poses a number of pharmacological problems and may not be required for treating locally, aggressive tumors such as gliomas. Infection with a RDAd recombinant encoding angiostatin (RAd/Agst) has been shown to successfully promote transgene expression in human vein endothelial cells (HUVECs) and to inhibit cell proliferation *in vitro*. Similar results were shown by intratumoral injection of RAd/Agst into human glioblastoma cell xenografts in the subrenal capsule of nude mice. Intracerebral xenografts in nude mice infected with RAd/Agst were shown to have significantly lower vascularisation and higher apoptotic indices than tumors infected with a control virus, resulting in greater survival in treated animals (Tanaka et al., 1998).

Apart from the induction of p53-mediated apoptosis, RDAd expression of p53 has also been demonstrated to inhibit tumor angiogenesis, by affecting endothelial cell differentiation *in vitro* and angiogenesis *in vivo* (Riccioni et al., 1998). The mechanism of action has been proposed to be due to the down-regulation of thrombospondin-1, an angiogenesis inhibitor, (Dameron et al., 1994; Volpert et al., 1995).

The varied mechanisms available for inhibiting tumor angiogenesis, especially in metastases, is an area of intense research with encouraging preliminary results currently generating intense interest in the field of gene therapy. By switching therapeutic emphasis from the tumor cell itself to the blood supply directing oxygen and nutrients to the whole tumor, an Achilles' heal common to many diverse tumor types may be attacked.

10. Combination Therapies

Modern RDAd vectors can accommodate large inserts (up to 35Kb) and multiple genes can be expressed from the same construct using different promoters, internal ribosomal entry initiation sites and alternate splicing. An individual cell can also be infected and support expression using multiple Ad vectors. In devising a cancer gene therapy strategy the possible combinations of RDAd vectors, promoters and therapeutic genes are endless. The effect of combining therapeutic genes may be antagonistic, neutral, additive or synergistic and furthermore may have an impact on the efficacy of conventional therapeutic regimes that may be performed in parallel. A primary concern therefore is that a gene therapy treatment should first do no harm. The underlying toxicity of therapeutic genes may be enhanced when they are used in combination. The stimulation of an immune response to a tumor also has the potential to ablate the expression of a second therapeutic transgene (Elshami et al., 1995). One should consider that expression of a cytostatic gene may make a tumor resistant to a more potent second gene, for example one that induces apoptosis in the tumor, and could also make the tumor less sensitive to conventional radiotherapy or chemotherapy regimes (Gorospe et al., 1997).

Although research is at an early stage, the majority of studies have demonstrated an extraordinary benefit in combining multiple therapeutic genes. While the use of genes that provide no obvious advantage is to be avoided, certain genes can also be ineffective when delivered independently but may be extremely beneficial when used in combination therapies. A single intratumoral injection of a virus encoding both IL-12 and B7-1 resulted in complete regression in 70% of animals, whereas RDAd constructs encoding only one of the genes merely delayed tumor growth (Putzer et al., 1997). This is also an example of a situation in which two genes with related purposes, stimulating a cellular immune response, can lead to enhanced tumor rejection. The combined use of genes targeting different intervention strategies may have the capacity to provide not only a more effective response to a single tumor but may be better able to cope with genetic variability within and between tumors. A combination of cytokine and prodrug therapy proved successful in combating hepatic metastases of colon carcinoma in a mouse model. While direct injection of RDAd IL-2 into tumors was ineffective, co-delivery with a therapeutic RDAd TK construct was required to elicit protection against subsequent challenge (Chen et al., 1995a, Kwong et al., 1997).

This review describes many examples of multiple genes working together to protect against tumors in animal models. Recent developments in cancer gene therapy aimed at preventing tumor angiogenesis have been highly encouraging and this is an approach that is well suited to incorporation into combination therapies. Well-designed gene therapy protocols may also have the capacity to enhance conventional treatments. Restoration of normal p53 function to a tumor cell thus not only suppresses tumor growth but also makes the cell sensitive to radiotherapy. (Badie et al., 1995; Geng et al., 1998) and chemotheraputic agents (Blagosklonny et al., 1998; Fujiwara et al., 1994; Meng et al., 1999; Yang et al., 1996).

Acknowledgments

The authors wish to thank Prof LK Borysiewicz and Dr Steve Man for their encouragement and helpful discussions. We are also grateful to the Wellcome Trust and the Welsh Scheme for the Development of Health and Social Research for their support.

References

Abe, J., Wakimoto, H., Tsunoda, R., Okabe, S., Yoshida, Y., Aoyagi, M., Hirakawa, K. and Hamada, H. (1996). In vivo antitumor effect of cytotoxic T lymphocytes engineered to produce interferon-gamma by adenovirus-mediated genetic transduction. Biochem Biophys Res Commun 218, 164-70.

Abe, J., Wakimoto, H., Yoshida, Y., Aoyagi, M., Hirakawa, K. and Hamada, H. (1995). Antitumor effect induced by granulocyte/macrophage-colony-stimulating factor gene-modified tumor vaccination: comparison of adenovirus- and retrovirus-mediated genetic transduction. J Cancer Res Clin Oncol 121, 587-92.

Abrahamsen, K., Kong, H. L., Mastrangeli, A., Brough, D., Lizonova, A., Crystal, R. G. and Falck-Pedersen, E. (1997). Construction of an adenovirus type 7a E1A- vector. J Virol 71, 8946-51.

Addison, C. L., Braciak, T., Ralston, R., Muller, W. J., Gauldie, J. and Graham, F. L. (1995). Intratumoral injection of an adenovirus expressing interleukin 2 induces regression and immunity in a murine breast cancer model. Proc Natl Acad Sci U S A 92, 8522-6.

Addison, C. L., Bramson, J. L., Hitt, M. M., Muller, W. J., Gauldie, J. and Graham, F. L. (1998). Intratumoral coinjection of adenoviral vectors expressing IL-2 and IL- 12 results in enhanced frequency of regression of injected and untreated distal tumors. Gene Ther 5, 1400-9.

Addison, C. L., Hitt, M., Kunsken, D. and Graham, F. L. (1997). Comparison of the human versus murine cytomegalovirus immediate early gene promoters for transgene expression by adenoviral vectors. J Gen Virol 78, 1653-61.

Ahmed, C. M., Sugarman, B. J., Johnson, D. E., Bookstein, R. E., Saha, D. P., Nagabhushan, T. L. and Wills, K. N. (1999). In vivo tumor suppression by adenovirus-mediated interferon alpha2β gene delivery [In Process Citation]. Hum Gene Ther 10, 77-84.

Ahmed, T., Lutton, J. D., Feldman, E., Tani, K., Asano, S. and Abraham, N. G. (1998). Gene transfer of alpha interferon into hematopoietic stem cells. Leuk Res 22, 119-24.

Ankrapp, D. P. and Bevan, D. R. (1993). Insulin-like growth factor-I and human lung fibroblast-derived insulin- like growth factor-I stimulate the proliferation of human lung carcinoma cells in vitro. Cancer Res 53, 3399-404.

Arthur, J. F., Butterfield, L. H., Roth, M. D., Bui, L. A., Kiertscher, S. M., Lau, R., Dubinett, S., Glaspy, J., McBride, W. H. and Economou, J. S. (1997). A comparison of gene transfer methods in human dendritic cells. Cancer Gene Ther 4, 17-25.

Babiss, L. E., Friedman, J. M. and Darnell, J. E., Jr. (1986). Cellular promoters incorporated into the adenovirus genome: effects of viral regulatory elements on transcription rates and cell specificity of albumin and beta-globin promoters. Mol Cell Biol 6, 3798-806.

Badie, B., Drazan, K. E., Kramar, M. H., Shaked, A. and Black, K. L. (1995). Adenovirus-mediated p53 gene delivery inhibits 9L glioma growth in rats. Neurol Res 17, 209-16.

Bai, M., Harfe, B. and Freimuth, P. (1993). Mutations that alter an Arg-Gly-Asp (RGD) sequence in the adenovirus type 2 penton base protein abolish its cell-rounding activity and delay virus reproduction in flat cells. J Virol 67, 5198-205.

Bakker, A. B., Schreurs, M. W., de Boer, A. J., Kawakami, Y., Rosenberg, S. A., Adema, G. J. and Figdor, C. G. (1994). Melanocyte lineage-specific antigen gp100 is recognized by melanoma- derived tumor-infiltrating lymphocytes. J Exp Med 179, 1005-9.

Barker, D. D. and Berk, A. J. (1987). Adenovirus proteins from both E1B reading frames are required for transformation of rodent cells by viral infection and DNA transfection. Virology 156, 107-121.

Barth, R. J., Jr., Bock, S. N., Mule, J. J. and Rosenberg, S. A. (1990). Unique murine tumor-associated antigens identified by tumor infiltrating lymphocytes. J Immunol 144, 1531-7.

Beier, D. C., Cox, J. H., Vining, D. R., Cresswell, P. and Engelhard, V. H. (1994). Association of human class I MHC alleles with the adenovirus E3/19K protein. J Immunol 152, 3862-72.

Bergelson, J. M., Krithivas, A., Celi, L., Droguett, G., Horwitz, M. S., Wickham, T., Crowell, R. L. and Finberg, R. W. (1998). The murine CAR homolog is a receptor for coxsackie B viruses and adenoviruses. J Virol 72, 415-9.

Bi, W. L., Parysek, L. M., Warnick, R. and Stambrook, P. J. (1993). In vitro evidence that metabolic cooperation is responsible for the bystander effect observed with HSV tk retroviral gene therapy. Hum Gene Ther 4, 725-31.

Bischoff, J. R., Kirn, D. H., Williams, A., Heise, C., Horn, S., Muna, M., Ng, L., Nye, J. A., Sampson-Johannes, A., Fattaey, A. and McCormick, F. (1996). An adenovirus mutant that replicates selectively in p53-deficient human tumor cells [see comments]. Science 274, 373-6.

Blagosklonny, M. V., Giannakakou, P., Wojtowicz, M., Romanova, L. Y., Ain, K. B., Bates, S. E. and Fojo, T. (1998). Effects of p53-expressing adenovirus on the chemosensitivity and differentiation of anaplastic thyroid cancer cells. J Clin Endocrinol Metab 83, 2516-22.

Blau, H. M. and Rossi, F. M. V. (1999). Tet B or not tet B: Advances in tetracycline-inducible gene expression. Proc. Natl. Acad. Sci. USA 96, 797-799.

Boel, P., Wildmann, C., Sensi, M. L., Brasseur, R., Renauld, J. C., Coulie, P., Boon, T. and van der Bruggen, P. (1995). BAGE: a new gene encoding an antigen recognized on human melanomas by cytolytic T lymphocytes. Immunity 2, 167-75.

Bonnekoh, B., Greenhalgh, D. A., Chen, S. H., Block, A., Rich, S. S., Krieg, T., Woo, S. L. and Roop, D. R. (1998). Ex vivo and in vivo adenovirus-mediated gene therapy strategies induce a systemic anti-tumor immune defence in the B16 melanoma model. J Invest Dermatol 110, 867-71.

Boxhorn, H. K., Smith, J. G., Chang, Y. J., Guerry, D., Lee, W. M., Rodeck, U., Turka, L. A. and Eck, S. L. (1998). Adenoviral transduction of melanoma cells with B7-1: antitumor immunity and immunosuppressive factors. Cancer Immunol Immunother 46, 283-92.

Bramson, J., Hitt, M., Gallichan, W. S., Rosenthal, K. L., Gauldie, J. and Graham, F. L. (1996a). Construction of a double recombinant adenovirus vector expressing a heterodimeric cytokine: in vitro and in vivo production of biologically active interleukin-12. Hum Gene Ther 7, 333-42.

Bramson, J. L., Hitt, M., Addison, C. L., Muller, W. J., Gauldie, J. and Graham, F. L. (1996b). Direct intratumoral injection of an adenovirus expressing interleukin- 12 induces regression and long-lasting immunity that is associated with highly localized expression of interleukin-12. Hum Gene Ther 7, 1995-2002.

Bramson, J. L., Hitt, M., Gauldie, J. and Graham, F. L. (1997). Pre-existing immunity to adenovirus does not prevent tumor regression following intratumoral administration of a vector expressing IL-12 but inhibits virus dissemination. Gene Ther 4, 1069-76.

Brichard, V., Van Pel, A., Wolfel, T., Wolfel, C., De Plaen, E., Lethe, B., Coulie, P. and Boon, T. (1993). The tyrosinase gene codes for an antigen recognized by autologous cytolytic T lymphocytes on HLA-A2 melanomas. J Exp Med 178, 489-95.

Brough, D. E., Hsu, C., Kulesa, V. A., Lee, G. M., Cantolupo, L. J., Lizonova, A. and Kovesdi, I. (1997). Activation of transgene expression by early 4 region 4 is responsible for a high level of persistent transgene expression from adenovirus vectors. J. Virol. 1997, 9206-9213.

Brunda, M. J., Luistro, L., Warrier, R. R., Wright, R. B., Hubbard, B. R., Murphy, M., Wolf, S. F. and Gately, M. K. (1993). Antitumor and antimetastatic activity of interleukin 12 against murine tumors. J Exp Med 178, 1223-30.

Buge, S. L., Richardson, E., Alipanah, S., Markham, P., Cheng, S., Kalyan, N., Miller, C. J., Lubeck, M., Udem, S., Eldridge, J. and Robert-Guroff, M. (1997). An adenovirus-simian immunodeficiency virus env vaccine elicits humoral, cellular, and mucosal immune responses in rhesus macaques and decreases viral burden following vaginal challenge. J Virol 71, 8531-41.

Bui, L. A., Butterfield, L. H., Kim, J. Y., Ribas, A., Seu, P., Lau, R., Glaspy, J. A., McBride, W. H. and Economou, J. S. (1997). In vivo therapy of hepatocellular carcinoma with a tumor-specific adenoviral vector expressing interleukin-2 [see comments]. Hum Gene Ther 8, 2173-82.

Burcin, M. M., Schiedner, G., Kochanek, S., Tsai, S. Y. and O'Malley, B. W. (1999). Adenovirus-mediated regulable target gene expression in vivo [In Process Citation]. Proc Natl Acad Sci U S A 96, 355-60.

Butterfield, L. H., Jilani, S. M., Chakraborty, N. G., Bui, L. A., Ribas, A., Dissette, V. B., Lau, R., Gamradt, S. C., Glaspy, J. A., McBride, W. H., Mukherji, B. and Economou, J. S. (1998). Generation of melanoma-specific cytotoxic T lymphocytes by dendritic cells transduced with a MART-1 adenovirus [In Process Citation]. J Immunol 161, 5607-13.

Cai, D. W., Mukhopadhyay, T., Liu, Y., Fujiwara, T. and Roth, J. A. (1993). Stable expression of the wild-type p53 gene in human lung cancer cells after retrovirus-mediated gene transfer. Hum Gene Ther 4, 617-24.

Carlin, C. R., Tollefson, A. E., Brady, H. A., Hoffman, B. L. and Wold, W. S. (1989). Epidermal growth factor receptor is down-regulated by a 10,400 MW protein encoded by the E3 region of adenovirus. Cell 57, 135-44.

Caruso, M., Pham-Nguyen, K., Kwong, Y. L., Xu, B., Kosai, K. I., Finegold, M., Woo, S. L. and Chen, S. H. (1996). Adenovirus-mediated interleukin-12 gene therapy for metastatic colon carcinoma. Proc Natl Acad Sci U S A 93, 11302-6.

Castelli, C., Storkus, W. J., Maeurer, M. J., Martin, D. M., Huang, E. C., Pramanik, B. N., Nagabhushan, T. L., Parmiani, G. and Lotze, M. T. (1995). Mass spectrometric identification of a naturally processed melanoma peptide recognized by CD8+ cytotoxic T lymphocytes. J Exp Med 181, 363-8.

Chen, J., Bezdek, T., Chang, J., Kherzai, A. W., Willingham, T., Azzara, M. and Nisen, P. D. (1998). A glial-specific, repressible, adenovirus vector for brain tumor gene therapy. Cancer Res 58, 3504-7.

Chen, J., Willingham, T., Shuford, M., Bruce, D., Rushing, E., Smith, Y. and Nisen, P. D. (1996a). Effects of ectopic overexpression of p21(WAF1/CIP1) on aneuploidy and the malignant phenotype of human brain tumor cells. Oncogene 13, 1395-403.

Chen, L., Ashe, S., Brady, W. A., Hellstrom, I., Hellstrom, K. E., Ledbetter, J. A., McGowan, P. and Linsley, P. S. (1992a). Costimulation of antitumor immunity by the B7 counterreceptor for the T lymphocyte molecules CD28 and CTLA-4. Cell 71, 1093-102.

Chen, L., Chen, D., Block, E., O'Donnell, M., Kufe, D. W. and Clinton, S. K. (1997a). Eradication of murine bladder carcinoma by intratumor injection of a bicistronic adenoviral vector carrying cDNAs for the IL-12 heterodimer and its inhibition by the IL-12 p40 subunit homodimer. J Immunol 159, 351-9.

Chen, L., McGowan, P., Ashe, S., Johnston, J., Li, Y., Hellstrom, I. and Hellstrom, K. E. (1994a). Tumor immunogenicity determines the effect of B7 costimulation on T cell-mediated tumor immunity. J Exp Med 179, 523-32.

Chen, L., Pulsipher, M., Chen, D., Sieff, C., Elias, A., Fine, H. A. and Kufe, D. W. (1996b). Selective transgene expression for detection and elimination of contaminating carcinoma cells in hematopoietic stem cell sources [see comments]. J Clin Invest 98, 2539-48.

Chen, L., Yu, L. J. and Waxman, D. J. (1997b). Potentiation of cytochrome P450/cyclophosphamide-based cancer gene therapy by coexpression of the P450 reductase gene. Cancer Res 57, 4830-7.

Chen, P. W., Wang, M., Bronte, V., Zhai, Y., Rosenberg, S. A. and Restifo, N. P. (1996c). Therapeutic antitumor response after immunization with a recombinant adenovirus encoding a model tumor-associated antigen. J Immunol 156, 224-31.

Chen, S. H., Chen, X. H., Wang, Y., Kosai, K., Finegold, M. J., Rich, S. S. and Woo, S. L. (1995a). Combination gene therapy for liver metastasis of colon carcinoma in vivo. Proc Natl Acad Sci U S A 92, 2577-81.

Chen, S. H., Shine, H. D., Goodman, J. C., Grossman, R. G. and Woo, S. L. (1994b). Gene therapy for brain tumors: regression of experimental gliomas by adenovirus-mediated gene transfer in vivo. Proc Natl Acad Sci U S A 91, 3054-7.

Chen, W., Peace, D. J., Rovira, D. K., You, S. G. and Cheever, M. A. (1992b). T-cell immunity to the joining region of p210BCR-ABL protein. Proc Natl Acad Sci U S A 89, 1468-72.

Chen, Y. M., Chen, P. L., Arnaiz, N., Goodrich, D. and Lee, W. H. (1991). Expression of wild-type p53 in human A673 cells suppresses tumorigenicity but not growth rate. Oncogene 6, 1799-805.

Chen, Y. Q., Cipriano, S. C., Arenkiel, J. M. and Miller, F. R. (1995b). Tumor suppression by p21WAF1. Cancer Res 55, 4536-9.

Cheng, J., Yee, J. K., Yeargin, J., Friedmann, T. and Haas, M. (1992). Suppression of acute lymphoblastic leukemia by the human wild-type p53 gene. Cancer Res 52, 222-6.

Chengalvala, M. V., Bhat, B. M., Bhat, R. A., Dheer, S. K., Lubeck, M. D., Purcell, R. H. and Murthy, K. K. (1997). Replication and immunogenicity of Ad7-, Ad4-, and Ad5-hepatitis B virus surface antigen recombinants, with or without a portion of E3 region, in chimpanzees. Vaccine 15, 335-9.

Cheon, J., Ko, S. C., Gardner, T. A., Shirakawa, T., Gotoh, A., Kao, C. and Chung, L. W. (1997). Chemogene therapy: osteocalcin promoter-based suicide gene therapy in combination with methotrexate in a murine osteosarcoma model. Cancer Gene Ther 4, 359 65.

Chintala, S. K., Fueyo, J., Gomez-Manzano, C., Venkaiah, B., Bjerkvig, R., Yung, W. K., Sawaya, R., Kyritsis, A. P. and Rao, J. S. (1997). Adenovirus-mediated p16/CDKN2 gene transfer suppresses glioma invasion in vitro. Oncogene 15, 2049-57.

Clayman, G. L., el-Naggar, A. K., Lippman, S. M., Henderson, Y. C., Frederick, M., Merritt, J. A., Zumstein, L. A., Timmons, T. M., Liu, T. J., Ginsberg, L., Roth, J. A., Hong, W. K., Bruso, P. and Goepfert, H. (1998). Adenovirus-mediated p53 gene transfer in patients with advanced recurrent head and neck squamous cell carcinoma. J Clin Oncol 16, 2221 32.

Clayman, G. L., Liu, T. J., Overholt, S. M., Mobley, S. R., Wang, M., Janot, F. and Goepfert, H. (1996). Gene therapy for head and neck cancer. Comparing the tumor suppressor gene p53 and a cell cycle regulator WAF1/CIP1 (p21). Arch Otolaryngol Head Neck Surg 122, 489-93.

Cohen, J. (1995). IL-12 deaths: explanation and a puzzle [news]. Science 270, 908.

Cordier, L., Duffour, M. T., Sabourin, J. C., Lee, M. G., Cabannes, J., Ragot, T., Perricaudet, M. and Haddada, H. (1995). Complete recovery of mice from a pre-established tumor by direct intratumoral delivery of an adenovirus vector harboring the murine IL-2 gene. Gene Ther 2, 16-21.

Craig, C., Kim, M., Ohri, E., Wersto, R., Katayose, D., Li, Z., Choi, Y. H., Mudahar, B., Srivastava, S., Seth, P. and Cowan, K. (1998). Effects of adenovirus-mediated p16INK4A expression on cell cycle arrest are determined by endogenous p16 and Rb status in human cancer cells. Oncogene 16, 265-72.

Crowley, C. W., Cohen, R. L., Lucas, B. K., Liu, G., Shuman, M. A. and Levinson, A. D. (1993). Prevention of metastasis by inhibition of the urokinase receptor. Proc Natl Acad Sci U S A 90, 5021-5.

Croyle, M. A., Stone, M., Amidon, G. L. and Roessler, B. J. (1998). In vitro and in vivo asessment of adenovirus 41 as a vector for gene delivery to the intestine [In Process Citation]. Gene Ther 5, 645-54.

Culver, K. W., Ram, Z., Wallbridge, S., Ishii, H., Oldfield, E. H. and Blaese, R. M. (1992). In vivo gene transfer with retroviral vector-producer cells for treatment of experimental brain tumors [see comments]. Science 256, 1550-2.

Czubayko, F., Downing, S. G., Hsieh, S. S., Goldstein, D. J., Lu, P. Y., Trapnell, B. C. and Wellstein, A. (1997). Adenovirus-mediated transduction of ribozymes abrogates HER-2/neu and pleiotrophin expression and inhibits tumor cell proliferation. Gene Ther 4, 943-9.

Czubayko, F., Schulte, A. M., Berchem, G. J. and Wellstein, A. (1996). Melanoma angiogenesis and metastasis modulated by ribozyme targeting of the secreted growth factor pleiotrophin. Proc Natl Acad Sci U S A 93, 14753-8.

Dameron, K. M., Volpert, O. V., Tainsky, M. A. and Bouck, N. (1994). Control of angiogenesis in fibroblasts by p53 regulation of thrombospondin-1. Science 265, 1582-4.

Danielsen, S., Kilstrup, M., Barilla, K., Jochimsen, B. and Neuhard, J. (1992). Characterization of the Escherichia coli codBA operon encoding cytosine permease and cytosine deaminase. Mol Microbiol 6, 1335-44.

Demers, G. W., Harris, M. P., Wen, S. F., Engler, H., Nielsen, L. L. and Maneval, D. C. (1998). A recombinant adenoviral vector expressing full-length human retinoblastoma susceptibility gene inhibits human tumor cell growth. Cancer Gene Ther 5, 207-14.

Diaz, R. M., Todryk, S., Chong, H., Hart, I. R., Sikora, K., Dorudi, S. and Vile, R. G. (1998). Rapid adenoviral transduction of freshly resected tumour explants with therapeutically useful genes provides a rationale for genetic immunotherapy for colorectal cancer. Gene Ther 5, 869-79.

Disis, M. L., Smith, J. W., Murphy, A. E., Chen, W. and Cheever, M. A. (1994). In vitro generation of human cytolytic T-cells specific for peptides derived from the HER-2/neu protooncogene protein. Cancer Res 54, 1071-6.

Domin, B. A., Mahony, W. B. and Zimmerman, T. P. (1993). Transport of 5-fluorouracil and uracil into human erythrocytes. Biochem Pharmacol 46, 503-10.

Dong, Y., Wen, P., Manome, Y., Parr, M., Hirshowitz, A., Chen, L., Hirschowitz, E. A., Crystal, R., Weichselbaum, R., Kufe, D. W. and Fine, H. A. (1996). In vivo replication-deficient adenovirus vector-mediated transduction of the cytosine deaminase gene sensitizes glioma cells to 5- fluorocytosine. Hum Gene Ther 7, 713-20.

Donson, A. M. and Foreman, N. K. (1998). Adenovirus mediated gene therapy in a glioblastoma vaccine model; specific antitumor immunity and abrogation of immunosuppression [In Process Citation]. J Neurooncol 40, 205-14.

Douglas, J. T., Rogers, B. E., Rosenfeld, M. E., Michael, S. I., Feng, M. and Curiel, D. T. (1996). Targeted gene delivery by tropism-modified adenoviral vectors. Nat Biotechnol 14, 1574-8.

Dranoff, G., Jaffee, E., Lazenby, A., Golumbek, P., Levitsky, H., Brose, K., Jackson, V., Hamada, H., Pardoll, D. and Mulligan, R. C. (1993). Vaccination with irradiated tumor cells engineered to secrete murine granulocyte-macrophage colony-stimulating factor stimulates potent, specific, and long-lasting anti-tumor immunity. Proc Natl Acad Sci U S A 90, 3539-43.

Eastham, J. A., Hall, S. J., Sehgal, I., Wang, J., Timme, T. L., Yang, G., Connell-Crowley, L., Elledge, S. J., Zhang, W. W., Harper, J. W. and et al. (1995). In vivo gene therapy with p53 or p21 adenovirus for prostate cancer. Cancer Res 55, 5151-5.

Eloit, M., Gilardi-Hebenstreit, P., Toma, B. and Perricaudet, M. (1990). Construction of a defective adenovirus vector expressing the pseudorabies virus glycoprotein gp50 and its use as a live vaccine. J Gen Virol 71, 2425-31.

Elshami, A. A., Kucharczuk, J. C., Sterman, D. H., Smythe, W. R., Hwang, H. C., Amin, K. M., Litzky, L. A., Albelda, S. M. and Kaiser, L. R. (1995). The role of immunosuppression in the efficacy of cancer gene therapy using adenovirus transfer of the herpes simplex thymidine kinase gene. Ann Surg 222, 298-307; 307-10.

Emtage, P. C., Wan, Y., Bramson, J. L., Graham, F. L. and Gauldie, J. (1998). A double recombinant adenovirus expressing the costimulatory molecule B7-1 (murine) and human IL-2 induces complete tumor regression in a murine breast adenocarcinoma model. J Immunol 160, 2531-8.

Englehardt, J. F., Ye, X., Doranz, B. and Wilson, J. M. (1994). Ablation of E2a in recombinant adenoviruses improves transgene persistence and and decreases inflamatory response in mouse liver. Proc. Natl. Acad. Sci. USA 91, 6196-6200.

Esandi, M. C., van Someren, G. D., Bout, A., Mulder, A. H., van Bekkum, D. W., Valerio, D. and Noteboom, J. L. (1998). IL-1/IL-3 gene therapy of non-small cell lung cancer (NSCLC) in rats using 'cracked' adenoproducer cells. Gene Ther 5, 778-88.

Evoy, D., Hirschowitz, E. A., Naama, H. A., Li, X. K., Crystal, R. G., Daly, J. M. and Lieberman, M. D. (1997). In vivo adenoviral-mediated gene transfer in the treatment of pancreatic cancer. J Surg Res 69, 226-31.

Feldman, E., Ahmed, T., Lutton, J. D., Farley, T., Tani, K., Freund, M., Asano, S. and Abraham, N. G. (1997). Adenovirus mediated alpha interferon (IFN-alpha) gene transfer into CD34+ cells and CML mononuclear cells. Stem Cells 15, 386-95.

Felzmann, T., Ramsey, W. J. and Blaese, R. M. (1997). Characterization of the antitumor immune response generated by treatment of murine tumors with recombinant adenoviruses expressing HSVtk, IL-2, IL-6 or B7-1. Gene Ther 4, 1322-9.

Feng, M., Cabrera, G., Deshane, J., Scanlon, K. J. and Curiel, D. T. (1995). Neoplastic reversion accomplished by high efficiency adenoviral- mediated delivery of an anti-ras ribozyme. Cancer Res 55, 2024-8.

Fooks, A. R., Jeevarajah, D., Warnes, A., Wilkinson, G. W. and Clegg, J. C. (1996). Immunization of mice with plasmid DNA expressing the measles virus nucleoprotein gene. Viral Immunol 9, 65-71.

Fooks, A. R., Schadeck, E., Liebert, U. G., Dowsett, A. B., Rima, B. K., Steward, M., Stephenson, J. R. and Wilkinson, G. W. (1995). High-level expression of the measles virus nucleocapsid protein by using a replication-deficient adenovirus vector: induction of an MHC-1- restricted CTL response and protection in a murine model. Virology 210, 456-65.

Frank, D. K., Frederick, M. J., Liu, T. J. and Clayman, G. L. (1998). Bystander effect in the adenovirus-mediated wild-type p53 gene therapy model of human squamous cell carcinoma of the head and neck. Clin Cancer Res 4, 2521-8.

Freeman, S. M., Abboud, C. N., Whartenby, K. A., Packman, C. H., Koeplin, D. S., Moolten, F. L. and Abraham, G. N. (1993). The "bystander effect": tumor regression when a fraction of the tumor mass is genetically modified. Cancer Res 53, 5274-83.

Frizelle, S. P., Grim, J., Zhou, J., Gupta, P., Curiel, D. T., Geradts, J. and Kratzke, R. A. (1998). Re-expression of p16INK4a in mesothelioma cells results in cell cycle arrest, cell death, tumor suppression and tumor regression. Oncogene 16, 3087-95.

Fueyo, J., Gomez-Manzano, C., Yung, W. K., Clayman, G. L., Liu, T. J., Bruner, J., Levin, V. A. and Kyritsis, A. P. (1996). Adenovirus-mediated p16/CDKN2 gene transfer induces growth arrest and modifies the transformed phenotype of glioma cells. Oncogene 12, 103-10.

Fujiwara, T., Grimm, E. A., Mukhopadhyay, T., Zhang, W. W., Owen Schaub, L. B. and Roth, J. A. (1994). Induction of chemosensitivity in human lung cancer cells in vivo by adenovirus-mediated transfer of the wild-type p53 gene. Cancer Res 54, 2287-91.

Gahery-Segard, H., Molinier-Frenkel, V., Le Boulaire, C., Saulnier, P., Opolon, P., Lengagne, R., Gautier, E., Le Cesne, A., Zitvogel, L., Venet, A., Schatz, C., Courtney, M., Le Chevalier, T., Tursz, T., Guillet, J. G. and Farace, F. (1997). Phase I trial of recombinant adenovirus gene transfer in lung cancer. Longitudinal study of the immune responses to transgene and viral products. J Clin Invest 100, 2218-26.

Gallardo, D., Drazan, K. E. and McBride, W. H. (1996). Adenovirus-based transfer of wild-type p53 gene increases ovarian tumor radiosensitivity. Cancer Res 56, 4891-3.

Gallichan, W. S., Johnson, D. C., Graham, F. L. and Rosenthal, K. L. (1993). Mucosal immunity and protection after intranasal immunization with recombinant adenovirus expressing herpes simplex virus glycoprotein B. J Infect Dis 168, 622-9.

Gauldie, J., Graham, F., Xing, Z., Braciak, T., Foley, R. and Sime, P. J. (1996). Adenovirus-vector-mediated cytokine gene transfer to lung tissue. Ann N Y Acad Sci 796, 235-44.

Geng, L., Walter, S., Melian, E. and Vaughan, A. T. (1998). Transfection of a vector expressing wild-type p53 into cells of two human glioma cell lines enhances radiation toxicity. Radiat Res 150, 31-7.

Gimmi, C. D., Morrison, B. W., Mainprice, B. A., Gribben, J. G., Boussiotis, V. A., Freeman, G. J., Park, S. Y., Watanabe, M., Gong, J., Hayes, D. F., Kufe, D. W. and Nadler, L. M. (1996). Breast cancer-associated antigen, DF3/MUC1, induces apoptosis of activated human T cells. Nat Med 2, 1367-70.

Gong, J., Chen, L., Chen, D., Kashiwaba, M., Manome, Y., Tanaka, T. and Kufe, D. (1997). Induction of antigen-specific antitumor immunity with adenovirus- transduced dendritic cells. Gene Ther 4, 1023-8.

Gonin, P., Oualikene, W., Fournier, A. and Eloit, M. (1996). Comparison of the efficacy of replication-defective adenovirus and Nyvac poxvirus as vaccine vectors in mice. Vaccine 14, 1083-7.

Goodrich, D. W. and Lee, W. H. (1993). Molecular characterization of the retinoblastoma susceptibility gene. Biochim Biophys Acta 1155, 43-61.

Goodrum, F. D. and Ornelles, D. A. (1997). The early region 1B 55-kilodalton oncoprotein of adenovirus relieves growth restrictions imposed on viral replication by the cell cycle. J Virol 71, 548-61.

Goodrum, F. D. and Ornelles, D. A. (1998). p53 status does not determine outcome of E1B 55-kilodalton mutant adenovirus lytic infection [In Process Citation]. J Virol 72, 9479-90.

Gorospe, M., Cirielli, C., Wang, X., Seth, P., Capogrossi, M. C. and Holbrook, N. J. (1997). p21(Waf1/Cip1) protects against p53-mediated apoptosis of human melanoma cells. Oncogene 14, 929-35.

Gotoh, A., Kao, C., Ko, S. C., Hamada, K., Liu, T. J. and Chung, L. W. (1997). Cytotoxic effects of recombinant adenovirus p53 and cell cycle regulator genes (p21 WAF1/CIP1 and p16CDKN4) in human prostate cancers. J Urol 158, 636-41.

Graeber, T. G., Osmanian, C., Jacks, T., Housman, D. E., Koch, C. J., Lowe, S. W. and Giaccia, A. J. (1996). Hypoxia-mediated selection of cells with diminished apoptotic potential in solid tumours [see comments]. Nature 379, 88-91.

Greenberg, P. D. (1991). Adoptive T cell therapy of tumors: mechanisms operative in the recognition and elimination of tumor cells. Adv Immunol 49, 281-355.

Grim, J., D'Amico, A., Frizelle, S., Zhou, J., Kratzke, R. A. and Curiel, D. T. (1997). Adenovirus-mediated delivery of p16 to p16-deficient human bladder cancer cells confers chemoresistance to cisplatin and paclitaxel. Clin Cancer Res 3, 2415-23.

Grimm, E. A., Mazumder, A., Zhang, H. Z. and Rosenberg, S. A. (1982). Lymphokine-activated killer cell phenomenon. Lysis of natural killer- resistant fresh solid tumor cells by interleukin 2-activated autologous human peripheral blood lymphocytes. J Exp Med 155, 1823-41.

Haddada, H., Ragot, T., Cordier, L., Duffour, M. T. and Perricaudet, M. (1993). Adenoviral interleukin-2 gene transfer into P815 tumor cells abrogates tumorigenicity and induces antitumoral immunity in mice. Hum Gene Ther 4, 703-11.

Hamada, K., Alemany, R., Zhang, W. W., Hittelman, W. N., Lotan, R., Roth, J. A. and Mitchell, M. F. (1996). Adenovirus-mediated transfer of a wild-type p53 gene and induction of apoptosis in cervical cancer. Cancer Res 56, 3047-54.

Hanahan, D. and Folkman, J. (1996). Patterns and emerging mechanisms of the angiogenic switch during tumorigenesis. Cell 86, 353-64.

Hanke, T., Graham, F. L., Rosenthal, K. L. and Johnson, D. C. (1991). Identification of an immunodominant cytotoxic T-lymphocyte recognition site in glycoprotein B of herpes simplex virus by using recombinant adenovirus vectors and synthetic peptides. J Virol 65, 1177-86.

He, D., Mu, Z. M., Le, X., Hsieh, J. T., Pong, R. C., Chung, L. W. and Chang, K. S. (1997). Adenovirus-mediated expression of PML suppresses growth and tumorigenicity of prostate cancer cells. Cancer Res 57, 1868-72.

Heike, Y., Takahashi, M., Kanegae, Y., Sato, Y., Saito, I. and Saijo, N. (1997). Interleukin-2 gene transduction into freshly isolated lung adenocarcinoma cells with adenoviral vectors. Hum Gene Ther 8, 1-14.

Heise, C., Sampson-Johannes, A., Williams, A., McCormick, F., Von Hoff, D. D. and Kirn, D. H. (1997). ONYX-015, an E1B gene-attenuated adenovirus, causes tumor-specific cytolysis and antitumoral efficacy that can be augmented by standard chemotherapeutic agents [see comments]. Nat Med 3, 639-45.

Hirschowitz, E. A., Leonard, S., Song, W., Ferris, B., Leopold, P. L., Lewis, J. J., Bowne, W. B., Wang, S., Houghton, A. N. and Crystal, R. G. (1998). Adenovirus-mediated expression of melanoma antigen gp75 as immunotherapy for metastatic melanoma [In Process Citation]. Gene Ther 5, 975-83.

Hirschowitz, E. A., Ohwada, A., Pascal, W. R., Russi, T. J. and Crystal, R. G. (1995). In vivo adenovirus-mediated gene transfer of the Escherichia coli cytosine deaminase gene to human colon carcinoma-derived tumors induces chemosensitivity to 5-fluorocytosine. Hum Gene Ther 6, 1055-63.

Horwitz, M. S. (1996). Adenoviruses. In Fields Virology., pp. 2149-2171. Edited by B. N. Fields, Knipe, D.M. and Howley, P.M. Philidelphia: Lippincott-Raven.

Hu, S. X., Ji, W., Zhou, Y., Logothetis, C. and Xu, H. J. (1997). Development of an adenovirus vector with tetracycline-regulatable human tumor necrosis factor alpha gene expression. Cancer Res 57, 3339-43.

Huang, H., Chen, S. H., Kosai, K., Finegold, M. J. and Woo, S. L. (1996). Gene therapy for hepatocellular carcinoma: long-term remission of primary and metastatic tumors in mice by interleukin-2 gene therapy in vivo. Gene Ther 3, 980-7.

Huber, B. E., Austin, E. A., Richards, C. A., Davis, S. T. and Good, S. S. (1994). Metabolism of 5-fluorocytosine to 5-fluorouracil in human colorectal tumor cells transduced with the cytosine deaminase gene: significant antitumor effects when only a small percentage of tumor cells express cytosine deaminase. Proc Natl Acad Sci U S A 91, 8302-6.

Itoh, K., Tilden, A. B. and Balch, C. M. (1986). Interleukin 2 activation of cytotoxic T-lymphocytes infiltrating into human metastatic melanomas. Cancer Res 46, 3011-7.

Jacobs, S. C., Stephenson, J. R. and Wilkinson, G. W. (1992). High-level expression of the tick-borne encephalitis virus NS1 protein by using an adenovirus-based vector: protection elicited in a murine model. J Virol 66, 2086-95.

Jacobs, S. C., Stephenson, J. R. and Wilkinson, G. W. (1994). Protection elicited by a replication-defective adenovirus vector expressing the tick-borne encephalitis virus non-structural glycoprotein NS1. J Gen Virol 75, 2399-402.

Jerome, K. R., Domenech, N. and Finn, O. J. (1993). Tumor-specific cytotoxic T cell clones from patients with breast and pancreatic adenocarcinoma recognize EBV-immortalized B cells transfected with polymorphic epithelial mucin complementary DNA. J Immunol 151, 1654-62.

Jin, X., Nguyen, D., Zhang, W. W., Kyritsis, A. P. and Roth, J. A. (1995). Cell cycle arrest and inhibition of tumor cell proliferation by the p16INK4 gene mediated by an adenovirus vector. Cancer Res 55, 3250-3.

Joshi, U. S., Chen, Y. Q., Kalemkerian, G. P., Adil, M. R., Kraut, M. and Sarkar, F. H. (1998a). Inhibition of tumor cell growth by p21WAF1 adenoviral gene transfer in lung cancer. Cancer Gene Ther 5, 183-91.

Joshi, U. S., Dergham, S. T., Chen, Y. Q., Dugan, M. C., Crissman, J. D., Vaitkevicius, V. K. and Sarkar, F. H. (1998b). Inhibition of pancreatic tumor cell growth in culture by p21WAF1 recombinant adenovirus. Pancreas 16, 107-13.

Ju, D. W., Wang, B. M. and Cao, X. (1998). Adenovirus-mediated combined suicide gene and interleukin-2 gene therapy for the treatment of established tumor and induction of antitumor immunity. J Cancer Res Clin Oncol 124, 683-9.

Juillard, V., Villefroy, P., Godfrin, D., Pavirani, A., Venet, A. and Guillet, J. G. (1995). Long-term humoral and cellular immunity induced by a single immunization with replication-defective adenovirus recombinant vector. Eur J Immunol 25, 3467-73.

Jung, S. and Schluesener, H. J. (1991). Human T lymphocytes recognize a peptide of single point-mutated, oncogenic ras proteins. J Exp Med 173, 273-6.

Kanai, F., Lan, K. H., Shiratori, Y., Tanaka, T., Ohashi, M., Okudaira, T., Yoshida, Y., Wakimoto, H., Hamada, H., Nakabayashi, H., Tamaoki, T. and Omata, M. (1997). In vivo gene therapy for alpha-fetoprotein-producing hepatocellular carcinoma by adenovirus-mediated transfer of cytosine deaminase gene. Cancer Res 57, 461-5.

Kashani-Sabet, M., Funato, T., Florenes, V. A., Fodstad, O. and Scanlon, K. J. (1994). Suppression of the neoplastic phenotype in vivo by an anti-ras ribozyme. Cancer Res 54, 900-2.

Kawakami, Y., Eliyahu, S., Jennings, C., Sakaguchi, K., Kang, X., Southwood, S., Robbins, P. F., Sette, A., Appella, E. and Rosenberg, S. A. (1995). Recognition of multiple epitopes in the human melanoma antigen gp100 by tumor-infiltrating T lymphocytes associated with in vivo tumor regression. J Immunol 154, 3961-8.

Kawakami, Y., Eliyahu, S., Sakaguchi, K., Robbins, P. F., Rivoltini, L., Yannelli, J. R., Appella, E. and Rosenberg, S. A. (1994). Identification of the immunodominant peptides of the MART-1 human melanoma antigen recognized by the majority of HLA-A2-restricted tumor infiltrating lymphocytes. J Exp Med 180, 347-52.

Kelly, T. J., Jr. and Lewis, A. M., Jr. (1973). Use of nondefective adenovirus-simian virus 40 hybrids for mapping the simian virus 40 genome. J Virol 12, 643-52.

Kendall, R. L. and Thomas, K. A. (1993). Inhibition of vascular endothelial cell growth factor activity by an endogenously encoded soluble receptor. Proc Natl Acad Sci U S A 90, 10705-9.

Kendall, R. L., Wang, G. and Thomas, K. A. (1996). Identification of a natural soluble form of the vascular endothelial growth factor receptor, FLT-1, and its heterodimerization with KDR. Biochem Biophys Res Commun 226, 324-8.

Ko, S. C., Gotoh, A., Thalmann, G. N., Zhau, H. E., Johnston, D. A., Zhang, W. W., Kao, C. and Chung, L. W. (1996). Molecular therapy with recombinant p53 adenovirus in an androgen- independent, metastatic human prostate cancer model. Hum Gene Ther 7, 1683-91.

Kobayashi, H., Gotoh, J., Fujie, M., Shinohara, H., Moniwa, N. and Terao, T. (1994). Inhibition of metastasis of Lewis lung carcinoma by a synthetic peptide within growth factor-like domain of urokinase in the experimental and spontaneous metastasis model. Int J Cancer 57, 727-33.

Kock, H., Harris, M. P., Anderson, S. C., Machemer, T., Hancock, W., Sutjipto, S., Wills, K. N., Gregory, R. J., Shepard, H. M., Westphal, M. and Maneval, D. C. (1996). Adenovirus-mediated p53 gene transfer suppresses growth of human glioblastoma cells in vitro and in vivo. Int J Cancer 67, 808-15.

Kong, H. L., Hecht, D., Song, W., Kovesdi, I., Hackett, N. R., Yayon, A. and Crystal, R. G. (1998). Regional suppression of tumor growth by in vivo transfer of a cDNA encoding a secreted form of the extracellular domain of the flt-1 vascular endothelial growth factor receptor. Hum Gene Ther 9, 823-33.

Krasnykh, V. N., Mikheeva, G. V., Douglas, J. T. and Curiel, D. T. (1996). Generation of recombinant adenovirus vectors with modified fibers for altering viral tropism. J Virol 70, 6839-46.

Kwong, Y. L., Chen, S. H., Kosai, K., Finegold, M. and Woo, S. L. (1997). Combination therapy with suicide and cytokine genes for hepatic metastases of lung cancer. Chest 112, 1332-7.

Lang, F. F., Yung, W. K., Raju, U., Libunao, F., Terry, N. H. and Tofilon, P. J. (1998). Enhancement of radiosensitivity of wild-type p53 human glioma cells by adenovirus-mediated delivery of the p53 gene. J Neurosurg 89, 125-32.

Le, X. F., Vallian, S., Mu, Z. M., Hung, M. C. and Chang, K. S. (1998). Recombinant PML adenovirus suppresses growth and tumorigenicity of human breast cancer cells by inducing G1 cell cycle arrest and apoptosis. Oncogene 16, 1839-49.

Lee, C. T., Ciernik, I. F., Wu, S., Tang, D. C., Chen, H. L., Truelson, J. M. and Carbone, D. P. (1996a). Increased immunogenicity of tumors bearing mutant p53 and P1A epitopes after transduction of B7-1 via recombinant adenovirus. Cancer Gene Ther 3, 238-44.

Lee, C. T., Wu, S., Ciernik, I. F., Chen, H., Nadaf-Rahrov, S., Gabrilovich, D. and Carbone, D. P. (1997). Genetic immunotherapy of established tumors with adenovirus-murine granulocyte-macrophage colony-stimulating factor. Hum Gene Ther 8, 187-93.

Lee, C. T., Wu, S., Gabrilovich, D., Chen, H., Nadaf-Rahrov, S., Ciernik, I. F. and Carbone, D. P. (1996b). Antitumor effects of an adenovirus expressing antisense insulin-like growth factor I receptor on human lung cancer cell lines. Cancer Res 56, 3038-41.

Lee, J. H., Lee, C. T., Yoo, C. G., Hong, Y. K., Kim, C. M., Han, S. K., Shim, Y. S., Carbone, D. P. and Kim, Y. W. (1998). The inhibitory effect of adenovirus-mediated p16INK4a gene transfer on the proliferation of lung cancer cell line. Anticancer Res 18, 3257-61.

Leppard, K. (1997). E4 function in adenovirus, adenovirus vector and adeno-associated virus infections. J. Gen Virol 78, 2131-2138.

Li, H., H. Lu, F. Griscelli, P. Opolon, L-Q. Sun, T. Ragot, Y. Legrand, D. Belin, J. Soria, C. Soria, M. Perricaudet and P. Yeh. (1998). Adenovirus-mediated delivery of a uPA/uPAR antagonist suppresses angiogenesis-dependent tumor growth and dissemination in mice. Gene Therapy 5, 1105-1113.

Li, Z., Shanmugam, N., Katayose, D., Huber, B., Srivastava, S., Cowan, K. and Seth, P. (1997). Enzyme/prodrug gene therapy approach for breast cancer using a recombinant adenovirus expressing Escherichia coli cytosine deaminase. Cancer Gene Ther 4, 113-7.

Lin, P., Buxton, J. A., Acheson, A., Radziejewski, C., Maisonpierre, P. C., Yancopoulos, G. D., Channon, K. M., Hale, L. P., Dewhirst, M. W., George, S. E. and Peters, K. G. (1998). Antiangiogenic gene therapy targeting the endothelium-specific receptor tyrosine kinase Tie2. Proc Natl Acad Sci U S A 95, 8829-34.

Lin, P., Polverini, P., Dewhirst, M., Shan, S., Rao, P. S. and Peters, K. (1997). Inhibition of tumor angiogenesis using a soluble receptor establishes a role for Tie2 in pathologic vascular growth. J Clin Invest 100, 2072-8.

Liu, T. J., el-Naggar, A. K., McDonnell, T. J., Steck, K. D., Wang, M., Taylor, D. L. and Clayman, G. L. (1995). Apoptosis induction mediated by wild-type p53 adenoviral gene transfer in squamous cell carcinoma of the head and neck. Cancer Res 55, 3117-22.

Louis, N., Fender, P., Barge, A., Kitts, P. and Chroboczek, J. (1994). Cell-binding domain of adenovirus serotype 2 fiber. J Virol 68, 4104-6.

Lu, H., Yeh, P., Guitton, J. D., Mabilat, C., Desanlis, F., Maury, I., Legrand, Y., Soria, J. and Soria, C. (1994). Blockage of the urokinase receptor on the cell surface: construction and characterization of a hybrid protein consisting of the N-terminal fragment of human urokinase and human albumin. FEBS Lett 356, 56-9.

Lubeck, M. D., Davis, A. R., Chengalvala, M., Natuk, R. J., Morin, J. E., Molnar-Kimber, K., Mason, B. B., Bhat, B. M., Mizutani, S., Hung, P. P. and et al. (1989). Immunogenicity and efficacy testing in chimpanzees of an oral hepatitis B vaccine based on live recombinant adenovirus. Proc Natl Acad Sci U S A 86, 6763-7.

Lubeck, M. D., Natuk, R., Myagkikh, M., Kalyan, N., Aldrich, K., Sinangil, F., Alipanah, S., Murthy, S. C., Chanda, P. K., Nigida, S. M., Jr., Markham, P. D., Zolla-Pazner, S., Steimer, K., Wade, M., Reitz, M. S., Jr., Arthur, L. O., Mizutani, S., Davis, A., Hung, P. P., Gallo, R. C., Eichberg, J. and Robert-Guroff, M. (1997). Long-term protection of chimpanzees against high-dose HIV-1 challenge induced by immunization. Nat Med 3, 651-8.

Maione, T. E., Gray, G. S., Petro, J., Hunt, A. J., Donner, A. L., Bauer, S. I., Carson, H. F. and Sharpe, R. J. (1990). Inhibition of angiogenesis by recombinant human platelet factor-4 and related peptides. Science 247, 77-9.

Mar, E. C., Chiou, J. F., Cheng, Y. C. and Huang, E. S. (1985). Inhibition of cellular DNA polymerase alpha and human cytomegalovirus- induced DNA polymerase by the triphosphates of 9-(2-hydroxyethoxymethyl)guanine and 9-(1,3-dihydroxy-2- propoxymethyl)guanine. J Virol 53, 776-80.

Marcellus, R. C., Teodoro, J. G., Charbonneau, R., Shore, G. C. and Branton, P. E. (1996). Expression of p53 in Saos-2 osteosarcoma cells induces apoptosis which can be inhibited by Bcl-2 or the adenovirus E1B-55 kDa protein. Cell Growth Differ 7, 1643-50.

Marr, R. A., Addison, C. L., Snider, D., Muller, W. J., Gauldie, J. and Graham, F. L. (1997). Tumour immunotherapy using an adenoviral vector expressing a membrane- bound mutant of murine TNF alpha. Gene Ther 4, 1181-8.

Marr, R. A., Hitt, M., Muller, W. J., Gauldie, J. and Graham, F. L. (1998). Tumour therapy in mice using adenovirus vectors expressing human TNFa. Int J Oncol 12, 509-15.

Meng, R. D., Phillips, P. and El-Deiry, W. S. (1999). p53-independent increase in E2F-1 expression enhances the cytotoxic effects of etoposide and of adriamycin. Int J Oncol 14, 5-14.

Michael, S. I., Hong, I. S., Curiel, D. T. and Engler, I. A. (1995). Addition of a short peptide ligand to the adenovirus fiber protein. Gene Ther 2, 660-8.

Mittal, S. K., Papp, Z., Tikoo, S. K., Baca-Estrada, M. E., Yoo, D., Benko, M. and Babiuk, L. A. (1996). Induction of systemic and mucosal immune responses in cotton rats immunized with human adenovirus type 5 recombinants expressing the full and truncated forms of bovine herpesvirus type 1 glycoprotein gD. Virology 222, 299-309.

Mobley, S. R., Liu, T. J., Hudson, J. M. and Clayman, G. L. (1998). In vitro growth suppression by adenoviral transduction of p21 and p16 in squamous cell carcinoma of the head and neck: a research model for combination gene therapy. Arch Otolaryngol Head Neck Surg 124, 88-92.

Moolten, F. L. (1986). Tumor chemosensitivity conferred by inserted herpes thymidine kinase genes: paradigm for a prospective cancer control strategy. Cancer Res 46, 5276-81.

Morral, N., O'Neal, W., Zhou, H., Langston, C. and Beaudet, A. (1997). Immune responses to reporter proteins and high viral dose limit duration of expression with adenoviral vectors: comparison of E2a wild type and E2a deleted vectors. Hum Gene Ther 8, 1275-86.

Mujoo, K., Maneval, D. C., Anderson, S. C. and Gutterman, J. U. (1996). Adenoviral-mediated p53 tumor suppressor gene therapy of human ovarian carcinoma. Oncogene 12, 1617-23.

Mulders, P., Tso, C. L., Pang, S., Kaboo, R., McBride, W. H., Hinkel, A., Gitlitz, B., Dannull, J., Figlin, R. and Belldegrun, A. (1998). Adenovirus-mediated interleukin-2 production by tumors induces growth of cytotoxic tumor-infiltrating lymphocytes against human renal cell carcinoma. J Immunother 21, 170-80.

Nagai, E., Ogawa, T., Kielian, T., Ikubo, A. and Suzuki, T. (1998). Irradiated tumor cells adenovirally engineered to secrete granulocyte/macrophage-colony-stimulating factor establish antitumor immunity and eliminate pre-existing tumors in syngeneic mice. Cancer Immunol Immunother 47, 72-80.

Nakanishi, Y., Mulshine, J. L., Kasprzyk, P. G., Natale, R. B., Maneckjee, R., Avis, I., Treston, A. M., Gazdar, A. F., Minna, J. D. and Cuttitta, F. (1988). Insulin-like growth factor-I can mediate autocrine proliferation of human small cell lung cancer cell lines in vitro. J Clin Invest 82, 354-9.

Nastala, C. L., Edington, H. D., McKinney, T. G., Tahara, H., Nalesnik, M. A., Brunda, M. J., Gately, M. K., Wolf, S. F., Schreiber, R. D., Storkus, W. J. and et al. (1994). Recombinant IL-12 administration induces tumor regression in association with IFN-gamma production. J Immunol 153, 1697-706.

Nguyen, D. M., Wiehle, S. A., Koch, P. E., Branch, C., Yen, N., Roth, J. A. and Cristiano, R. J. (1997). Delivery of the p53 tumor suppressor gene into lung cancer cells by an adenovirus/DNA complex. Cancer Gene Ther 4, 191-8.

Nijman, H. W., Van der Burg, S. H., Vierboom, M. P., Houbiers, J. G., Kast, W. M. and Melief, C. J. (1994). p53, a potential target for tumor-directed T cells. Immunol Lett 40, 171-8.

O'Malley, B. W., Jr., Chen, S. H., Schwartz, M. R. and Woo, S. L. (1995). Adenovirus-mediated gene therapy for human head and neck squamous cell cancer in a nude mouse model. Cancer Res 55, 1080-5.

O'Malley, B. W., Cope, K. A., Chen, S. H., Li, D., Schwarta, M. R. and Woo, S. L. (1996). Combination gene therapy for oral cancer in a murine model. Cancer Res 56, 1737-41.

O'Malley, B. W., Jr., Sewell, D. A., Li, D., Kosai, K., Chen, S. H., Woo, S. L. and Duan, L. (1997). The role of interleukin-2 in combination adenovirus gene therapy for head and neck cancer. Mol Endocrinol 11, 667-73.

O'Reilly, M. S., Holmgren, L., Shing, Y., Chen, C., Rosenthal, R. A., Moses, M., Lane, W. S., Cao, Y., Sage, E. H. and Folkman, J. (1994). Angiostatin: a novel angiogenesis inhibitor that mediates the suppression of metastases by a Lewis lung carcinoma [see comments]. Cell 79, 315-28.

Ohashi, M., Kanai, F., Tanaka, T., Lan, K. H., Shiratori, Y., Komatsu, Y., Kawabe, T., Yoshida, H., Hamada, H. and Omata, M. (1998). In vivo adenovirus-mediated prodrug gene therapy for carcinoembryonic antigen-producing pancreatic cancer. Jpn J Cancer Res 89, 457-62.

Overholt, S. M., Liu, T. J., Taylor, D. L., Wang, M., El-Naggar, A. K., Shillitoe, E., Adler-Storthz, K., John, L. S., Zhang, W. W., Roth, J. A. and Clayman, G. L. (1997). Head and neck squamous cell growth suppression using adenovirus-p53- FLAG: a potential marker for gene therapy trials. Clin Cancer Res 3, 185-91.

Parr, M. J., Manome, Y., Tanaka, T., Wen, P., Kufe, D. W., Kaelin, W. G., Jr. and Fine, H. A. (1997). Tumor-selective transgene expression in vivo mediated by an E2F- responsive adenoviral vector. Nat Med 3, 1145-9.

Perez-Cruet, M. J., Trask, T. W., Chen, S. H., Goodman, J. C., Woo, S. L., Grossman, R. G. and Shine, H. D. (1994). Adenovirus-mediated gene therapy of experimental gliomas. J Neurosci Res 39, 506-11.

Pietras, R. J., Arboleda, J., Reese, D. M., Wongvipat, N., Pegram, M. D., Ramos, L., Gorman, C. M., Parker, M. G., Sliwkowski, M. X. and Slamon, D. J. (1995). HER-2 tyrosine kinase pathway targets estrogen receptor and promotes hormone-independent growth in human breast cancer cells. Oncogene 10, 2435-46.

Porgador, A. and Gilboa, E. (1995). Bone marrow-generated dendritic cells pulsed with a class I-restricted peptide are potent inducers of cytotoxic T lymphocytes. J Exp Med 182, 255-60.

Prabhu, N. S., Blagosklonny, M. V., Zeng, Y. X., Wu, G. S., Waldman, T. and El-Deiry, W. S. (1996). Suppression of cancer cell growth by adenovirus expressing p21(WAF1/CIP1) deficient in PCNA interaction. Clin Cancer Res 2, 1221-9.

Putzer, B. M., Hitt, M., Muller, W. J., Emtage, P., Gauldie, J. and Graham, F. L. (1997). Interleukin 12 and B7-1 costimulatory molecule expressed by an adenovirus vector act synergistically to facilitate tumor regression. Proc Natl Acad Sci U S A 94, 10889-94.

Qin, X. Q., Tao, N., Dergay, A., Moy, P., Fawell, S., Davis, A., Wilson, J. M. and Barsoum, J. (1998). Interferon-beta gene therapy inhibits tumor formation and causes regression of established tumors in immune-deficient mice. Proc Natl Acad Sci U S A 95, 14411-6.

Rabinowich, H., Cohen, R., Bruderman, I., Steiner, Z. and Klajman, A. (1987). Functional analysis of mononuclear cells infiltrating into tumors: lysis of autologous human tumor cells by cultured infiltrating lymphocytes. Cancer Res 47, 173-7.

Ragot, T., Finerty, S., Watkins, P. E., Perricaudet, M. and Morgan, A. J. (1993). Replication-defective recombinant adenovirus expressing the Epstein- Barr virus (EBV) envelope glycoprotein gp340/220 induces protective immunity against EBV-induced lymphomas in the cottontop tamarin. J Gen Virol 74, 501-7.

Ram, Z., Walbridge, S., Heiss, J. D., Culver, K. W., Blaese, R. M. and Oldfield, E. H. (1994). In vivo transfer of the human interleukin-2 gene: negative tumoricidal results in experimental brain tumors. J Neurosurg 80, 535-40.

Randrianarison-Jewtoukoff, V. a. P., M. (1995). Recombinant adenoviruses as vaccines. Biologicals 23, 145-157.

Ribas, A., Butterfield, L. H., McBride, W. H., Jilani, S. M., Bui, L. A., Vollmer, C. M., Lau, R., Dissette, V. B., Hu, B., Chen, A. Y., Glaspy, J. A. and Economou, J. S. (1997). Genetic immunization for the melanoma antigen MART-1/Melan-A using recombinant adenovirus-transduced murine dendritic cells. Cancer Res 57, 2865-9.

Riccioni, T., Cirielli, C., Wang, X., Passaniti, A. and Capogrossi, M. C. (1998). Adenovirus-mediated wild-type p53 overexpression inhibits endothelial cell differentiation in vitro and angiogenesis in vivo. Gene Ther 5, 747-54.

Riley, D. J., Nikitin, A. Y. and Lee, W. H. (1996). Adenovirus-mediated retinoblastoma gene therapy suppresses spontaneous pituitary melanotroph tumors in Rb+/- mice. Nat Med 2, 1316-21.

Robert-Guroff, M., Kaur, H., Patterson, L. J., Leno, M., Conley, A. J., McKenna, P. M., Markham, P. D., Richardson, E., Aldrich, K., Arora, K., Murty, L., Carter, L., Zolla-Pazner, S. and Sinangil, F. (1998). Vaccine protection against a heterologous, non-syncytium-inducing, primary human immunodeficiency virus. J Virol 72, 10275-80.

Rocco, J. W., Li, D., Liggett, W. H., Jr., Duan, L., Saunders, J. K., Jr., Sidransky, D. and O'Malley, B. W., Jr. (1998). p16INK4A adenovirus-mediated gene therapy for human head and neck squamous cell cancer. Clin Cancer Res 4, 1697-704.

Romero, P., Pannetier, C., Herman, J., Jongeneel, C. V., Cerottini, J. C. and Coulie, P. G. (1995). Multiple specificities in the repertoire of a melanoma patient's cytolytic T lymphocytes directed against tumor antigen MAGE-1.A1. J Exp Med 182, 1019-28.

Rosenberg, S. A. (1992). Karnofsky Memorial Lecture. The immunotherapy and gene therapy of cancer. J Clin Oncol 10, 180-99.

Rosenberg, S. A. and Lotze, M. T. (1986). Cancer immunotherapy using interleukin-2 and interleukin-2-activated lymphocytes. Annu Rev Immunol 4, 681-709.

Rosenberg, S. A., Lotze, M. T., Muul, L. M., Chang, A. E., Avis, F. P., Leitman, S., Linehan, W. M., Robertson, C. N., Lee, R. E., Rubin, J. T. and et al. (1987). A progress report on the treatment of 157 patients with advanced cancer using lymphokine-activated killer cells and interleukin-2 or high-dose interleukin-2 alone. N Engl J Med 316, 889-97.

Rosenberg, S. A., Mule, J. J., Spiess, P. J., Reichert, C. M. and Schwarz, S. L. (1985). Regression of established pulmonary metastases and subcutaneous tumor mediated by the systemic administration of high-dose recombinant interleukin 2. J Exp Med 161, 1169-88.

Rosenberg, S. A., Zhai, Y., Yang, J. C., Schwartzentruber, D. J., Hwu, P., Marincola, F. M., Topalian, S. L., Restifo, N. P., Seipp, C. A., Einhorn, J. H., Roberts, B. and White, D. E. (1998). Immunizing patients with metastatic melanoma using recombinant adenoviruses encoding MART-1 or gp100 melanoma antigens. J Natl Cancer Inst 90, 1894-900.

Rothmann, T., Hengstermann, A., Whitaker, N. J., Scheffner, M. and zur Hausen, H. (1998). Replication of ONYX-015, a potential anticancer adenovirus, is independent of p53 status in tumor cells [In Process Citation]. J Virol 72, 9470-8.

Rubin, B. A. and Rocke, L. B. (1994). Adenovirus vaccines. In Vaccines, 2nd edn. Edited by S. A. Plotkin and E. A. Mortimer. Philadelphia: W.B. Saunders.

Sandig, V., Brand, K., Herwig, S., Lukas, J., Bartek, J. and Strauss, M. (1997). Adenovirally transferred p16INK4/CDKN2 and p53 genes cooperate to induce apoptotic tumor cell death. Nat Med 3, 313-9.

Santoso, J. T., Tang, D. C., Lane, S. B., Hung, J., Reed, D. J., Muller, C. Y., Carbone, D. P., Lucci, J. A., 3rd, Miller, D. S. and Mathis, J. M. (1995). Adenovirus-based p53 gene therapy in ovarian cancer [see comments]. Gynecol Oncol 59, 171-8.

Scarpini, C., Arthur, J., Efstathiou, S., McGrath, Y. and Wilkinson, G. (1999). Herpes simplex and adenovirus vectors. In DNA viruses, pp. In Press. Edited by A. J. Cann: Oxford University Press.

Schrump, D. S., Chen, G. A., Consuli, U., Jin, X. and Roth, J. A. (1996). Inhibition of esophageal cancer proliferation by adenovirally mediated delivery of p16INK4. Cancer Gene Ther 3, 357-64.

Sell, C., Rubini, M., Rubin, R., Liu, J. P., Efstratiadis, A. and Baserga, R. (1993). Simian virus 40 large tumor antigen is unable to transform mouse embryonic fibroblasts lacking type 1 insulin-like growth factor receptor. Proc Natl Acad Sci U S A 90, 11217-21.

Senger, D. R., Perruzzi, C. A., Feder, J. and Dvorak, H. F. (1986). A highly conserved vascular permeability factor secreted by a variety of human and rodent tumor cell lines. Cancer Res 46, 5629-32.

Seth, P., Katayose, D., Li, Z., Kim, M., Wersto, R., Craig, C., Shanmugam, N., Ohri, E., Mudahar, B., Rakkar, A. N., Kodali, P. and Cowan, K. (1997). A recombinant adenovirus expressing wild type p53 induces apoptosis in drug-resistant human breast cancer cells: a gene therapy approach for drug-resistant cancers. Cancer Gene Ther 4, 383-90.

Shenk, T. (1996). Adenoviridae: The viruses and their replication. In Fields Virology., pp. 2111-2148. Edited by B. N. Fields, Knipe, D.M . and Howley, P.M. Philidelphia: Lippincott-Raven.

Shibuya, M. (1995). Role of VEGF-flt receptor system in normal and tumor angiogenesis. Adv Cancer Res 67, 281-316.

Shirakawa, T., Ko, S. C., Gardner, T. A., Cheon, J., Miyamoto, T., Gotoh, A., Chung, L. W. and Kao, C. (1998). In vivo suppression of osteosarcoma pulmonary metastasis with intravenous osteocalcin promoter-based toxic gene therapy [In Process Citation]. Cancer Gene Ther 5, 274-80.

Siders, W. M., Halloran, P. J. and Fenton, R. G. (1998a). Melanoma-specific cytotoxicity induced by a tyrosinase promoter- enhancer/herpes simplex virus thymidine kinase adenovirus [In Process Citation]. Cancer Gene Ther 5, 281-91.

Siders, W. M., Wright, P. W., Hixon, J. A., Alvord, W. G., Back, T. C., Wiltrout, R. H. and Fenton, R. G. (1998b). T cell- and NK cell-independent inhibition of hepatic metastases by systemic administration of an IL-12-expressing recombinant adenovirus. J Immunol 160, 5465-74.

Simeone, D. M., Cascarelli, A. and Logsdon, C. D. (1997). Adenoviral-mediated gene transfer of a constitutively active retinoblastoma gene inhibits human pancreatic tumor cell proliferation. Surgery 122, 428-33; discussion 433-4.

Smith, R., R., et al. (1956). Cancer. 9, 1211.

Smythe, W. R., Hwang, H. C., Amin, K. M., Eck, S. L., Davidson, B. L., Wilson, J. M., Kaiser, L. R. and Albelda, S. M. (1994a). Use of recombinant adenovirus to transfer the herpes simplex virus thymidine kinase (HSVtk) gene to thoracic neoplasms: an effective in vitro drug sensitization system. Cancer Res 54, 2055-9.

Smythe, W. R., Hwang, H. C., Elshami, A. A., Amin, K. M., Eck, S. L., Davidson, B. L., Wilson, J. M., Kaiser, L. R. and Albelda, S. M. (1995). Treatment of experimental human mesothelioma using adenovirus transfer of the herpes simplex thymidine kinase gene. Ann Surg 222, 78-86.

Smythe, W. R., Kaiser, L. R., Hwang, H. C., Amin, K. M., Pilewski, J. M., Eck, S. J., Wilson, J. M. and Albelda, S. M. (1994b). Successful adenovirus-mediated gene transfer in an in vivo model of human malignant mesothelioma [see comments]. Ann Thorac Surg 57, 1395-401.

Spitz, F. R., Nguyen, D., Skibber, J. M., Cusack, J., Roth, J. A. and Cristiano, R. J. (1996a). In vivo adenovirus-mediated p53 tumor suppressor gene therapy for colorectal cancer. Anticancer Res 16, 3415-22.

Spitz, F. R., Nguyen, D., Skibber, J. M., Meyn, R. E., Cristiano, R. J. and Roth, J. A. (1996b). Adenoviral-mediated Wild-Type p53 Gene Expression Sensitizes Colorectal Cancer Cells to Ionizing Radiation. Clin Cancer Res 2, 1665-1671.

Staba, M. J., Mauceri, H. J., Kufe, D. W., Hallahan, D. E. and Weichselbaum, R. R. (1998). Adenoviral TNF-alpha gene therapy and radiation damage tumor vasculature in a human malignant glioma xenograft. Gene Ther 5, 293-300.

Stewart, A. K., Lassam, N. J., Quirt, I. C., Bailey, D. J., Rotstein, L. E., Krajden, M., Dessureault, S., S., G., Cappe, D., Wan, Y., Addison, C. L., Moen, R. C., Gauldie, J. and Graham, F. (1999). Adenovector-mediated gene delivery of interleukin-2 in metastatic breast cancer and melanoma: results of a phase I clinical trial. Gene Therapy 6, 350-363.

Tacket, C. O., Losonsky, G., Lubeck, M. D., Davis, A. R., Mizutani, S., Horwith, G., Hung, P., Edelman, R. and Levine, M. M. (1992). Initial safety and immunogenicity studies of an oral recombinant adenohepatitis B vaccine. Vaccine 10, 673-6.

Takahashi, T., Carbone, D., Nau, M. M., Hida, T., Linnoila, I., Ueda, R. and Minna, J. D. (1992). Wild-type but not mutant p53 suppresses the growth of human lung cancer cells bearing multiple genetic lesions. Cancer Res 52, 2340-3.

Tanaka, T., Cao, Y., Folkman, J. and Fine, H. A. (1998). Viral vector-targeted antiangiogenic gene therapy utilizing an angiostatin complementary DNA. Cancer Res 58, 3362-9.

Tanaka, T., Manome, Y., Wen, P., Kufe, D. W. and Fine, H. A. (1997). Viral vector-mediated transduction of a modified platelet factor 4 cDNA inhibits angiogenesis and tumor growth. Nat Med 3, 437-42.

Tang, D. C., Jennelle, R. S., Shi, Z., Garver, R. I., Jr., Carbone, D. P., Loya, F., Chang, C. H. and Curiel, D. T. (1997). Overexpression of adenovirus-encoded transgenes from the cytomegalovirus immediate early promoter in irradiated tumor cells. Hum Gene Ther 8, 2117-24.

Tannenbaum, C. S., Wicker, N., Armstrong, D., Tubbs, R., Finke, J., Bukowski, R. M. and Hamilton, T. A. (1996). Cytokine and chemokine expression in tumors of mice receiving systemic therapy with IL-12. J Immunol 156, 693-9.

Thompson, J. A. and Fefer, A. (1987). Interferon in the treatment of hairy cell leukemia. Cancer 59, 605-9.

Tollefson, A. E., Ryerse, J. S., Scaria, A., Hermiston, T. W. and Wold, W. S. (1996a). The E3-11.6-kDa adenovirus death protein (ADP) is required for efficient cell death: characterization of cells infected with adp mutants. Virology 220, 152-62.

Tollefson, A. E., Scaria, A., Hermiston, T. W., Ryerse, J. S., Wold, L. J. and Wold, W. S. (1996b). The adenovirus death protein (E3-11.6K) is required at very late stages of infection for efficient cell lysis and release of adenovirus from infected cells. J Virol 70, 2296-306.

Tollefson, A. E., Scaria, A., Saha, S. K. and Wold, W. S. (1992). The 11,600-MW protein encoded by region E3 of adenovirus is expressed early but is greatly amplified at late stages of infection. J Virol 66, 3633-42.

Toloza, E. M., Hunt, K., Swisher, S., McBride, W., Lau, R., Pang, S., Rhoades, K., Drake, T., Belldegrun, A., Glaspy, J. and Economou, J. S. (1996). In vivo cancer gene therapy with a recombinant interleukin-2 adenovirus vector. Cancer Gene Ther 3, 11-7.

Topalian, S. L., Muul, L. M., Solomon, D. and Rosenberg, S. A. (1987). Expansion of human tumor infiltrating lymphocytes for use in immunotherapy trials. J Immunol Methods 102, 127-41.

Townsend, S. E. and Allison, J. P. (1993). Tumor rejection after direct costimulation of CD8+ T cells by B7 transfected melanoma cells [see comments]. Science 259, 368-70.

Tripathy, S. K., Black, H. B., Goldwasser, E. and Leiden, J. M. (1996). Immune responses to transgene-encoded proteins limit the stability of gene expression after injection of replication-defective adenovirus vectors. Nat Med 2, 545-50.

Trojan, J., Johnson, T. R., Rudin, S. D., Ilan, J. and Tykocinski, M. L. (1993). Treatment and prevention of rat glioblastoma by immunogenic C6 cells expressing antisense insulin-like growth factor I RNA [see comments]. Science 259, 94-7.

Van den Eynde, B., Peeters, O., De Backer, O., Gaugler, B., Lucas, S. and Boon, T. (1995). A new family of genes coding for an antigen recognized by autologous cytolytic T lymphocytes on a human melanoma. J Exp Med 182, 689-98.

van der Bruggen, P., Szikora, J. P., Boel, P., Wildmann, C., Somville, M., Sensi, M. and Boon, T. (1994). Autologous cytolytic T lymphocytes recognize a MAGE-1 nonapeptide on melanomas expressing HLA-Cw*1601. Eur J Immunol 24, 2134-40.

van der Bruggen, P., Traversari, C., Chomez, P., Lurquin, C., De Plaen, E., Van den Eynde, B., Knuth, A. and Boon, T. (1991). A gene encoding an antigen recognized by cytolytic T lymphocytes on a human melanoma. Science 254, 1643-7.

Van Elsas, A., Nijman, H. W., Van der Minne, C. E., Mourer, J. S., Kast, W. M., Melief, C. J. and Schrier, P. I. (1995). Induction and characterization of cytotoxic T-lymphocytes recognizing a mutated p21ras peptide presented by HLA-A*0201. Int J Cancer 61, 389-96.

Volpert, O. V., Stellmach, V. and Bouck, N. (1995). The modulation of thrombospondin and other naturally occurring inhibitors of angiogenesis during tumor progression. Breast Cancer Res Treat 36, 119-26.

Vose, B. M. and Moore, M. (1985). Human tumor-infiltrating lymphocytes: a marker of host response. Semin Hematol 22, 27-40.

Vujanovic, N. L., Herberman, R. B. and Hiserodt, J. C. (1988). Lymphokine-activated killer cells in rats: analysis of tissue and strain distribution, ontogeny, and target specificity. Cancer Res 48, 878-83.

Walton, T., Wang, J. L., Ribas, A., Barsky, S. H., Economou, J. and Nguyen, M. (1998). Endothelium-specific expression of an E-selectin promoter recombinant adenoviral vector. Anticancer Res 18, 1357-60.

Wang, R. F., Robbins, P. F., Kawakami, Y., Kang, X. Q. and Rosenberg, S. A. (1995). Identification of a gene encoding a melanoma tumor antigen recognized by HLA-A31-restricted tumor-infiltrating lymphocytes [published erratum appears in J Exp Med 1995 Mar 1;181(3):1261]. J Exp Med 181, 799-804.

Watkins, S. J., Mesyanzhinov, V. V., Kurochkina, L. P. and Hawkins, R. E. (1997). The 'adenobody' approach to viral targeting: specific and enhanced adenoviral gene delivery. Gene Ther 4, 1004-12.

Wei, M. X., Li, F., Ono, Y., Gauldie, J. and Chiocca, E. A. (1998). Effects on brain tumor cell proliferation by an adenovirus vector that bears the interleukin-4 gene. J Neurovirol 4, 237-41.

Wickham, T. J., Mathias, P., Cheresh, D. A. and Nemerow, G. R. (1993). Integrins alpha v beta 3 and alpha v beta 5 promote adenovirus internalization but not virus attachment. Cell 73, 309-19.

Wickham, T. J., Roelvink, P. W., Brough, D. E. and Kovesdi, I. (1996). Adenovirus targeted to heparan-containing receptors increases its gene delivery efficiency to multiple cell types. Nat Biotechnol 14, 1570-3.

Wilkinson, G. W. and Akrigg, A. (1992). Constitutive and enhanced expression from the CMV major IE promoter in a defective adenovirus vector. Nucleic Acids Res 20, 2233-9.

Wilkinson, G. W. and Borysiewicz, L. K. (1995). Gene therapy and viral vaccination: the interface. Br Med Bull 51, 205-16.

Wills, K. N., Huang, W. M., Harris, M. P., Machemer, T., Maneval, D. C. and Gregory, R. J. (1995). Gene therapy for hepatocellular carcinoma: chemosensitivity conferred by adenovirus-mediated transfer of the HSV-1 thymidine kinase gene. Cancer Gene Ther 2, 191-7.

Wills, K. N., Maneval, D. C., Menzel, P., Harris, M. P., Sutjipto, S., Vaillancourt, M. T., Huang, W. M., Johnson, D. E., Anderson, S. C., Wen, S. F. and et al. (1994). Development and characterization of recombinant adenoviruses encoding human p53 for gene therapy of cancer. Hum Gene Ther 5, 1079-88.

Wroblewski, J. M., Lay, L. T., Van Zant, G., Phillips, G., Seth, P., Curiel, D. and Meeker, T. C. (1996). Selective elimination (purging) of contaminating malignant cells from hematopoietic stem cell autografts using recombinant adenovirus. Cancer Gene Ther 3, 257-64.

Xu, H. J., Xu, K., Zhou, Y., Li, J., Benedict, W. F. and Hu, S. X. (1994). Enhanced tumor cell growth suppression by an N-terminal truncated retinoblastoma protein. Proc Natl Acad Sci U S A 91, 9837-41.

Yang, B., Eshleman, J. R., Berger, N. A. and Markowitz, S. D. (1996). Wild-Type p53 Protein Potentiates Cytotoxicity of Therapeutic Agents in Human Colon Cancer Cells. Clin Cancer Res 2, 1649-1657.

Yang, Z. Y., Perkins, N. D., Ohno, T., Nabel, E. G. and Nabel, G. J. (1995). The p21 cyclin-dependent kinase inhibitor suppresses tumorigenicity in vivo [see comments]. Nat Med 1, 1052-6.

Zatloukal, K., Schneeberger, A., Berger, M., Schmidt, W., Koszik, F., Kutil, R., Cotten, M., Wagner, E., Buschle, M., Maass, G. and et al. (1995). Elicitation of a systemic and protective anti-melanoma immune response by an IL-2-based vaccine. Assessment of critical cellular and molecular parameters. J Immunol 154, 3406-19.

Zhai, Y., Yang, J. C., Kawakami, Y., Spiess, P., Wadsworth, S. C., Cardoza, L. M., Couture, L. A., Smith, A. E. and Rosenberg, S. A. (1996). Antigen-specific tumor vaccines. Development and characterization of recombinant adenoviruses encoding MART1 or gp100 for cancer therapy. J Immunol 156, 700-10.

Zhang, J. F., Hu, C., Geng, Y., Selm, J., Klein, S. B., Orazi, A. and Taylor, M. W. (1996). Treatment of a human breast cancer xenograft with an adenovirus vector containing an interferon gene results in rapid regression due to viral oncolysis and gene therapy. Proc Natl Acad Sci U S A 93, 4513-8.

Zhang, R., Baunoch, D. and DeGroot, L. J. (1998a). Genetic immunotherapy for medullary thyroid carcinoma: destruction of tumors in mice by in vivo delivery of adenoviral vector transducing the murine interleukin-2 gene [In Process Citation]. Thyroid 8, 1137-46.

Zhang, R., Minemura, K. and De Groot, L. J. (1998b). Immunotherapy for medullary thyroid carcinoma by a replication- defective adenovirus transducing murine interleukin-2. Endocrinology 139, 601-8.

Zhang, W. W. and Roth, J. A. (1994). Anti-oncogene and tumor suppressor gene therapy—examples from a lung cancer animal model. In Vivo 8, 755-69.

Zhou, Y., Li, J., Xu, K., Hu, S. X., Benedict, W. F. and Xu, H. J. (1994). Further characterization of retinoblastoma gene-mediated cell growth and tumor suppression in human cancer cells. Proc Natl Acad Sci U S A 91, 4165-9.

Zilli, D., Voelkel-Johnson, C., Skinner, T. and Laster, S. M. (1992). The adenovirus E3 region 14.7 kDa protein, heat and sodium arsenite inhibit the TNF-induced release of arachidonic acid. Biochem Biophys Res Commun 188, 177-83.

Lawrence Banks
International Centre for Genetic Engineering and
  Biotechnology
Padriciano 99
I-34012 Trieste
Italy

Eric Blair
School of Biochemistry and Molecular Biology
University of Leeds
Leeds
LS2 9JT
Tel: 0113-233 3112; Fax: 0113-233 3167
Email: BMB@leeds.ac.uk

Stephen M. Dilworth
Department of Metabolic Medicine
Imperial College School of Medicine
Hammersmith Hospital
Du Cane Road
London. W12 0NN
U.K.
Phone: 0181-383-2155; Fax: 0181-746-1159
Email: sdilwort@rpms.ac.uk

R.J.A. Grand
CRC Institute for Cancer Studies
University of Birmingham
Edgbaston
Birmingham B15 2TT
UK
Tel: 0121-414 4471; Fax: 0121-414 4486
Email: R.J.A.Grand@bham.ac.uk

Ester M. Hammond
Dept. of Radiation Oncology
School of Medicine
Stanford University
Stanford, CA
USA
E.mail: emh24@cam.ac.uk

Ruth F. Jarrett
LRF Virus Centre
Department of Veterinary Pathology
University of Glasgow
GLASGOW G61 1QH
Tel: 44 141 330 5775; Fax: 44 141 330 5733
e-mail: r.f.jarreyy@vet.gla.ac.uk

Parmjit Jat
Ludwig Institute for Cancer Research

University College London
  Middlesex School of Medicine Branch
Courtauld Building
91 Riding House Street
London, W1P 8BT
UK
Tel: +44 171 878 4099; Fax: +44 171 878 4040
E-mail: parmjit@ludwig.ucl.ac.uk

Kuan-Teh Jeang
Laboratory of Molecular Microbiology
National Institutes of Allergy and Infectious
  Diseases
9000 Rockville Pike
Bethesda, MD 20892
USA

Kenneth G. Low
Lead Discovery Screening
Dept 114, F447A
Bristol-Myers Squibb
5 Research Parkway
Wallingford, CT 06492
USA

Edgar Meinl
Max-Planck Institute of Neurobiology
Am Klopferspitz 18 a
D-82152 Martinsried
Germany
Tel. +49 89 8578 3519; Fax +49 89 8995 0163

Tarik Möröy
Institut für Zellbiologie (Tumorforschung)
IFZ, Universitätsklinikum Essen
Virchowstrasse 173
D-45122 Essen
Germany
Tel.: +49 201 723 3380 ; Fax: +49 201 723 5904
Email: moeroey@uni-essen.de

Philippa R. Nicholson
Department of Metabolic Medicine
Imperial College School of Medicine
Hammersmith Hospital
Du Cane Road
London. W12 0NN
U.K.
Phone: 0181-383-2155; Fax: 0181-746-1159
Frank Neipel
Institut für Klinische und Molekulare Virologie
Friedrich-Alexander-Universität Erlangen-Nürnberg
Schlossgarten 4

D-91054 Erlangen
Germany
Tel. +49 9131 8526483; Fax +49 9131 8526493
E-mail: neipel@viro.med.uni-erlangen.de

Nicola Philpott
School of Biochemistry and Molecular Biology
University of Leeds
Leeds
LS2 9JT
Tel: 0113-233 3112; Fax: 0113-233 3167
E.mail: BMB@leeds.ac.uk

David Pim
International Centre for Genetic Engineering
   and Biotechnology
Padriciano 99
I-34012 Trieste
Italy

Martin B. Powell
Department of Medicine
Tenovus Building
University of Wales College of Medicine
Cardiff CF4 4XX,
Wales, UK.
Tel: 01222 745215; Fax: 01222 745003

Stephan Schaefer
Institut für Medizinische Virologie
Justus-Liebig-Universität
Frankfurter Str. 107
D-35392 Giessen, Germany
Tel.: xx49-641-99-41220; Fax: xx49-641-99-41209
email: stephan.schaefer@viro.med.uni-giessen.de

Thorsten Schmidt
Institut für Zellbiologie (Tumorforschung)
IFZ, Universitätsklinikum Essen
Virchowstrasse 173
D-45122 Essen
Germany

Dr Margaret A Stanley
Department of Pathology
Tennis Court Road
Cambridge CB2 1QP
UK
Tel: +44 1 223 333736; Fax: +44 1 223 333730
E-mail: mas@mole.bio.cam.ac.uk

Jane C. Steele
CRC Institute for Cancer Studies
Edgbaston
University of Birmingham
Birmingham B15 2TT
UK
Tel: 0121 414 4471; Fax: 0121 414 4486
E-mail: j.c.steele@bham.ac.uk

Miranda Thomas
International Centre for Genetic Engineering
   and Biotechnology
Padriciano 99
I-34012 Trieste
Italy

Gavin W. G. Wilkinson
Department of Medicine
Tenovus Building
University of Wales College of Medicine,
Cardiff CF4 4XX,
Wales, UK.
Tel: 01222 745215; Fax: 01222 745003
E.mail: wmdgww@cardiff.ac.uk

Lawrence S.Young
CRC Institute for Cancer Studies
University of Birmingham Medical School
Birmingham B15 2TA
Phone: 0121 414 7144; Fax: 0121 414 5376
E-mail: L.S.Young@bham.ac.uk

Martin Zörnig
Biochemistry of the Cell Nucleus Laboratory
Imperial Cancer Research Fund
44, Lincoln's Inn Fields
London WC2A 3PX
UK